Pharmaceutical Preformulation and Formulation

DRUGS AND THE PHARMACEUTICAL SCIENCES

A Series of Textbooks and Monographs

For information on volumes 1–149 in the *Drugs and Pharmaceutical Science* Series, please visit www.informahealthcare.com

150. Laboratory Auditing for Quality and Regulatory Compliance, *Donald Singer, Raluca-Ioana Stefan, and Jacobus van Staden*

151. Active Pharmaceutical Ingredients: Development, Manufacturing, and Regulation, *edited by Stanley Nusim*

152. Preclinical Drug Development, *edited by Mark C. Rogge and David R. Taft*

153. Pharmaceutical Stress Testing: Predicting Drug Degradation, *edited by Steven W. Baertschi*

154. Handbook of Pharmaceutical Granulation Technology: Second Edition, *edited by Dilip M. Parikh*

155. Percutaneous Absorption: Drugs–Cosmetics–Mechanisms–Methodology, Fourth Edition, *edited by Robert L. Bronaugh and Howard I. Maibach*

156. Pharmacogenomics: Second Edition, *edited by Werner Kalow, Urs A. Meyer and Rachel F. Tyndale*

157. Pharmaceutical Process Scale-Up, Second Edition, *edited by Michael Levin*

158. Microencapsulation: Methods and Industrial Applications, Second Edition, *edited by Simon Benita*

159. Nanoparticle Technology for Drug Delivery, *edited by Ram B. Gupta and Uday B. Kompella*

160. Spectroscopy of Pharmaceutical Solids, *edited by Harry G. Brittain*

161. Dose Optimization in Drug Development, *edited by Rajesh Krishna*

162. Herbal Supplements-Drug Interactions: Scientific and Regulatory Perspectives, *edited by Y. W. Francis Lam, Shiew-Mei Huang, and Stephen D. Hall*

163. Pharmaceutical Photostability and Stabilization Technology, *edited by Joseph T. Piechocki and Karl Thoma*

164. Environmental Monitoring for Cleanrooms and Controlled Environments, *edited by Anne Marie Dixon*

165. Pharmaceutical Product Development: In Vitro-In Vivo Correlation, *edited by Dakshina Murthy Chilukuri, Gangadhar Sunkara, and David Young*

166. Nanoparticulate Drug Delivery Systems, *edited by Deepak Thassu, Michel Deleers, and Yashwant Pathak*

167. Endotoxins: Pyrogens, LAL Testing and Depyrogenation, Third Edition, *edited by Kevin L. Williams*

168. Good Laboratory Practice Regulations, Fourth Edition, *edited by Anne Sandy Weinberg*

169. Good Manufacturing Practices for Pharmaceuticals, Sixth Edition, *edited by Joseph D. Nally*

170. Oral-Lipid Based Formulations: Enhancing the Bioavailability of Poorly Water-soluble Drugs, *edited by David J. Hauss*

171. Handbook of Bioequivalence Testing, *edited by Sarfaraz K. Niazi*

172. Advanced Drug Formulation Design to Optimize Therapeutic Outcomes, *edited by Robert O. Williams III, David R. Taft, and Jason T. McConville*

173. Clean-in-Place for Biopharmaceutical Processes, *edited by Dale A. Seiberling*

174. Filtration and Purification in the Biopharmaceutical Industry, Second Edition, *edited by Maik W. Jornitz and Theodore H. Meltzer*

175. Protein Formulation and Delivery, Second Edition, *edited by Eugene J. McNally and Jayne E. Hastedt*

176. Aqueous Polymeric Coatings for Pharmaceutical Dosage Forms, Third Edition, *edited by James McGinity and Linda A. Felton*

177. Dermal Absorption and Toxicity Assessment, Second Edition, *edited by Michael S. Roberts and Kenneth A. Walters*

178. Preformulation Solid Dosage Form Development, *edited by Moji C. Adeyeye and Harry G. Brittain*

179. Drug-Drug Interactions, Second Edition, *edited by A. David Rodrigues*

180. Generic Drug Product Development: Bioequivalence Issues, *edited by Isadore Kanfer and Leon Shargel*

181. Pharmaceutical Pre-Approval Inspections: A Guide to Regulatory Success, Second Edition, *edited by Martin D. Hynes III*

182. Pharmaceutical Project Management, Second Edition, *edited by Anthony Kennedy*

183. Modified Release Drug Delivery Technology, Second Edition, Volume 1, *edited by Michael J. Rathbone, Jonathan Hadgraft, Michael S. Roberts, and Majella E. Lane*

184. Modified-Release Drug Delivery Technology, Second Edition, Volume 2, *edited by Michael J. Rathbone, Jonathan Hadgraft, Michael S. Roberts, and Majella E. Lane*

185. The Pharmaceutical Regulatory Process, Second Edition, *edited by Ira R. Berry and Robert P. Martin*

186. Handbook of Drug Metabolism, Second Edition, *edited by Paul G. Pearson and Larry C. Wienkers*

187. Preclinical Drug Development, Second Edition, *edited by Mark Rogge and David R. Taft*

188. Modern Pharmaceutics, Fifth Edition, Volume 1: Basic Principles and Systems, *edited by Alexander T. Florence and Juergen Siepmann*

189. Modern Pharmaceutics, Fifth Edition, Volume 2: Applications and Advances, *edited by Alexander T. Florence and Juergen Siepmann*

190. New Drug Approval Process, Fifth Edition, *edited by Richard A.Guarino*

191. Drug Delivery Nanoparticulate Formulation and Characterization, *edited by Yashwant Pathak and Deepak Thassu*

192. Polymorphism of Pharmaceutical Solids, Second Edition, *edited by Harry G. Brittain*

193. Oral Drug Absorption: Prediction and Assessment, Second Edition, *edited by Jennifer J. Dressman, hans Lennernas, and Christos Reppas*

194. Biodrug Delivery Systems: Fundamentals, Applications, and Clinical Development, *edited by Mariko Morista and Kinam Park*

195. Pharmaceutical Process Engineering, Second Edition, *edited by Anthony J. Hickey and David Ganderton*

196. Handbook of Drug Screening, Second Edition, *edited by Ramakrishna Seethala and Litao Zhang*

197. Pharmaceutical Powder Compaction Technology, Second Edition, *edited by Metin Celik*

198. Handbook of Pharmaceutical Granulation Technology, *Dilip M. Parikh*

199. Pharmaceutical Preformulation and Formulation: A Practical Guide from Candidate Drug Selection to Commercial Dosage Form, Second Edition, *edited by Mark Gibson*

Pharmaceutical Preformulation and Formulation

Second Edition

A Practical Guide from Candidate Drug Selection to Commercial Dosage Form

edited by
Mark Gibson
AstraZeneca R&D Charnwood
Loughborough, Leicestershire, UK

informa
healthcare

New York   London

Informa Healthcare USA, Inc.
52 Vanderbilt Avenue
New York, NY 10017

© 2009 by Informa Healthcare USA, Inc.
Informa Healthcare is an Informa business

International Standard Book Number-10: 1-4200-7317-6 (Hardcover)
International Standard Book Number-13: 978-1-4200-7317-1 (Hardcover)

Library of Congress Cataloging-in-Publication Data

Pharmaceutical preformulation and formulation: A practical guide from candidate drug selection to commercial dosage form / edited by Mark Gibson.
—2nd ed.
     p. ; cm. — (Drugs and the pharmaceutical sciences ; 199)
  Includes bibliographical references and index.
  ISBN-13: 978-1-4200-7317-1 (hb : alk. paper)
  ISBN-10: 1-4200-7317-6 (hb : alk. paper) 1. Drugs—Dosage forms.
I. Gibson, Mark, 1957- II. Series: Drugs and the pharmaceutical
sciences ; v. 199.
  [DNLM: 1. Drug Compounding. 2. Biopharmaceutics—methods. 3.
Dosage Forms. 4. Drug Discovery. 5. Drug Evaluation. W1 DR893B v.199
2009 / QV 778 P53535 2009]
  RS200.P425 2009
  615′.1—dc22

                       2009012458

For Corporate Sales and Reprint Permissions call 212-520-2700 or write to: Sales Department, 52 Vanderbilt Avenue, 16th floor, New York, NY 10017.

**Visit the Informa Web site at
www.informa.com**

**and the Informa Healthcare Web site at
www.informahealthcare.com**

Preface

The first edition of this book published in 2001 has been more successful than I ever imagined, as indicated by the excellent reviews it has received, the continued demand, and impressive sales! I believe that the main reasons for its popularity are that there was a significant gap in the literature and also that the information presented was based on the extensive experiences of the various contributors who were all actively working in the industry and were willing to share "best practice" from their knowledge and experiences. The book is intended to be a practical guide to pharmaceutical preformulation and formulation to be used as a reference source or a guidance tool to those working in the pharmaceutical industry or related industries, such as biopharmaceuticals or medical devices, or anyone wanting an insight into the subject area. Indeed, this book has also proved to be a valuable text for undergraduate and postgraduate courses in industrial pharmacy and pharmaceutical technology. A second edition is required because preformulation and formulation technology continues to develop and also because there are bound to be some gaps and improvements to be filled.

The second edition still meets the main objectives of the first edition, that is, to

- provide a logical and structured approach to product development, with key stages identified and the preformulation, biopharmaceutics, and formulation activities and typical issues at each stage discussed, wherever possible with real or worked examples,
- emphasize what practical studies need to be undertaken for what reasons and during what key stages of the drug development process, and
- provide separate chapters on the formulation development of each route and type of dosage forms.

The pressure to accelerate the drug development process, shorten the development timelines, and launch new pharmaceutical products is even more intense than before, with fewer registrations year on year. Having a structured approach and doing the right things first time are essential elements for achieving this. The chapters on product design and product optimization are still very relevant but have been updated to include the quality by design (QbD) and International Conference on Harmonisation (ICH) Q8 (product development), ICH Q9 (quality risk management), process analytical technology (PAT), and lean manufacturing principles that aim to link regulatory expectations to good science.

Another significant change since the first edition is the growth of biopharmaceuticals, compared with small molecules, that deserves more attention. Pharmaceutical companies are shifting from developing small molecules to developing biopharmaceuticals to treat a wide range of diseases, and today approximately one in four drugs introduced to the market is a biopharmaceutical. Since the majority of biopharmaceuticals will be delivered by injection or infusion, the chapter on parenteral dosage forms has been updated to reflect this. Focus has been given to the steps after purification, formulation, and subsequent fill-finish. Consideration has also been given in the other chapters for handling and developing biopharmaceutical dosage forms where there is some potential for drug delivery, for example, intranasal dosage forms.

Elsewhere in the second edition, there are updates throughout the book to reflect on some omissions and developments since the first edition and make it up-to-date; for example, to reflect emerging "cutting-edge" technologies such as polymorph and salt selection and prediction, molecular modeling and automation in preformulation studies, and more consideration for packaging technology during development of the various dosage forms.

Once again I am indebted to all the contributors for giving up their time and energy in producing this updated version. I am also indebted to my wife, Alison, and my family for their support and understanding during the time I have been busy working on this book.

Mark Gibson

Contents

Preface   *vii*

Contributors   *xi*

1. **Introduction and Perspective**   1
   Mark Gibson

2. **Aiding Candidate Drug Selection: Introduction and Objectives**   11
   Mark Gibson

3. **Preformulation Investigations using Small Amounts of Compound as an Aid to Candidate Drug Selection and Early Development**   17
   Gerry Steele and Talbir Austin

4. **Biopharmaceutical Support in Candidate Drug Selection**   129
   Anna-Lena Ungell and Bertil Abrahamsson

5. **Early Drug Development: Product Design**   172
   Mark Gibson

6. **Preformulation as an Aid to Product Design in Early Drug Development**   188
   Gerry Steele

7. **Biopharmaceutical Support in Formulation Development**   247
   Bertil Abrahamsson and Anna-Lena Ungell

8. **Product Optimization**   289
   Mark Gibson

9. **Parenteral Dosage Forms**   325
   Joanne Broadhead and Mark Gibson

10. **Inhalation Dosage Forms**   348
    Paul Wright

11. **Oral Solid Dosage Forms**   367
    Peter Davies

12. **Ophthalmic Dosage Forms**   431
    Mark Gibson

13. **Aqueous Nasal Dosage Forms**   456
     Nigel Day

14. **Topical and Transdermal Delivery**   475
     Kenneth A. Walters and Keith R. Brain

Index   527

Contributors

Bertil Abrahamsson   AstraZeneca, Mölndal, Sweden

Talbir Austin   AstraZeneca R&D Charnwood, Loughborough, Leicestershire, U.K.

Keith R. Brain   Cardiff University, Cardiff, U.K.

Joanne Broadhead   AstraZeneca R&D Charnwood, Loughborough, Leicestershire, U.K.

Peter Davies   Shire Pharmaceutical Development Ltd., Basingstoke, U.K.

Nigel Day   AstraZeneca R&D Charnwood, Loughborough, Leicestershire, U.K.

Mark Gibson   AstraZeneca R&D Charnwood, Loughborough, Leicestershire, U.K.

Gerry Steele   AstraZeneca R&D Charnwood, Loughborough, Leicestershire, U.K.

Anna-Lena Ungell   AstraZeneca, Mölndal, Sweden

Kenneth A. Walters   An-eX Analytical Services Ltd., Cardiff, U.K.

Paul Wright   AstraZeneca R&D Charnwood, Loughborough, Leicestershire, U.K.

1 | Introduction and Perspective

Mark Gibson

AstraZeneca R&D Charnwood, Loughborough, Leicestershire, U.K.

INTRODUCTION

This book is intended to be a practical guide to pharmaceutical preformulation and formulation. It can be used as a reference source and a guidance tool for those working in the pharmaceutical industry or related industries, for example, medical devices and biopharmaceuticals, or anyone wanting an insight into this subject area. The information presented is essentially based on the extensive experiences of the editor and various other contributors who are all actively working in the industry and have learned "best practice" from their experiences.

There are various excellent books already available that cover the theoretical aspects of different types of pharmaceutical dosage forms and processes. A variety of books are also available that focus on the drug development process, business, and regulatory and project management aspects. The popularity of the first edition of this book, *Pharmaceutical Preformulation and Formulation: A Practical Guide from Candidate Drug Selection to Commercial Formulation*, confirms my opinion that there is a need for a pragmatic guide to pharmaceutical preformulation and formulation with an emphasis on what practical studies need to be undertaken, for what reasons, and during what key stages of the drug development process. Preformulation, biopharmaceutics, and formulation are all important for candidate drug selection and through the various stages of product development as shown in Figure 3. This book has been written to try and address this need.

A logical approach to product development is described in the book, with the key stages identified and the preformulation, biopharmaceuticals, and formulation activities and typical issues at each stage discussed. Wherever possible, the book is illustrated with real or worked examples from contributors who have considerable relevant experience of preformulation, biopharmaceuticals, and formulation development.

Jim Wells' book on preformulation (Wells, 1988) made a strong impact on trainees and pharmaceutical scientists (including myself) working in this field of the pharmaceutical industry when it was introduced two years ago. It describes the important concepts and methods used in preformulation with the underlying theory. To his credit, Wells' book is still useful today, but sadly, the book is now out of print, and existing copies are hard to obtain. It also requires updating to include the abundance of modern preformulation instrumental techniques that have emerged, such as thermogravimetric analysis (TGA), hot-stage microscopy (HSM), X-ray powder diffraction (XRPD), Raman and infrared spectroscopy, and solid-state nuclear magnetic resonance (NMR). These techniques can be used to provide valuable information to characterize the drug substance and aid formulation development using the minimal amounts of compound.

Pharmaceutical Preformulation and Formulation: A Practical Guide from Candidate Drug Selection to Commercial Formulation covers a wider subject area than just preformulation. Topics include biopharmaceutics, drug delivery, formulation, and process development aspects of product development. The book also describes a logical and structured approach to the product development process, recommending at what stages appropriate preformulation, biopharmaceutics, and formulation work are best undertaken.

DRUG DEVELOPMENT DRIVERS, CHALLENGES, RISKS, AND REWARDS

It is important that the reader is aware of the nature of pharmaceutical research and development (R&D) to appreciate the importance of preformulation and formulation in the overall process.

Table 1   Major Hurdles to Successful Product Registration and Sale

Activity	Requirements
Research	Novel compound (Is it patentable?)
	Novel biological mechanism (Is it patentable?)
	Unmet medical needs
	Potent and selective
Safety	High margin of safety
	Nontoxic (not carcinogenic, tetratogenic, mutagenic, etc.)
Clinical	Tolerable side effects profile
	Efficacious
	Acceptable duration of action
Drug process	Bulk drug can be synthesized/scaled up
Pharmaceutical	Acceptable formulation/pack (meets customer needs)
	Drug delivery/product performance acceptable
	Stable/acceptable shelf life
	Robust clinical trial process, which can be scaled up and transferred into operations
Regulatory	Quality of data/documentation
Manufacturing	Manufacturable
	Acceptable cost of goods
	Able to pass preapproval inspection
Marketing/commercial	Competitive
	Meets customer needs
	Value for money
	Commercial return

In simple terms, the objective *of pharmaceutical R&D* can be defined as "converting ideas into candidate drugs for development" and the objective of *product development* as "converting candidate drugs into products for registration and sale." In reality, these goals are extremely challenging and difficult to achieve because of the many significant hurdles a pharmaceutical company has to overcome during the course of drug development. Some of the major hurdles are listed in Table 1.

The high risk of failure in drug discovery and development throughout the pharmaceutical industry statistically shows that, on average, only 1 in 5000 compounds screened in research will reach the market. For those that are nominated for development, the failure rate will vary from one in five to one in ten compounds that will achieve registration and reach the marketplace. Most failures in early development are due to drug toxicity or safety issues, whereas a lack of efficacy is the primary reason for late-stage attrition (Lowe, 2008). The relatively high attrition rates of new medicines is a major challenge, particularly when they are expensive phase III clinical failures that have occurred in recent years. Regulators are being more selective in what they approve, and they are demanding more data on efficacy and side effects. Only about 20 new drugs are now approved every year, down from 40 or 50 a decade ago and despite an approximate 70% increase in R&D investment over the last 10 years. On top of this, there is a significant commercial risk from those that are marketed; only 3 out of 10 are likely to achieve a fair return on investment. The products that give poor return on investment are often the result of poor candidate drug selection (the compound does not have the desired properties of safety, selectivity, efficacy, potency, or duration) and/or poor product development (the development program does not establish the value of the product). The latter scenario should, and can be, avoided by careful assessment at the "product design" stage of development. Product design is discussed further in chapter 5.

There has been a recent worrying trend of marketed products being withdrawn a few years after launch. This may be because once it is used by many thousands, or even millions, of people, rare but significant side effects can emerge. For example, Merck's blockbuster arthritis drug, Vioxx, was approved in 1999 but withdrawn five years later when linked to increased cardiovascular risks. Another example is the surprise announcement by Pfizer when it withdrew the world's first inhalable insulin product, Exubera, from the market in 2007 following disappointing sales. It would seem that the company had failed to appreciate the customer requirements well enough during the product design phase of development.

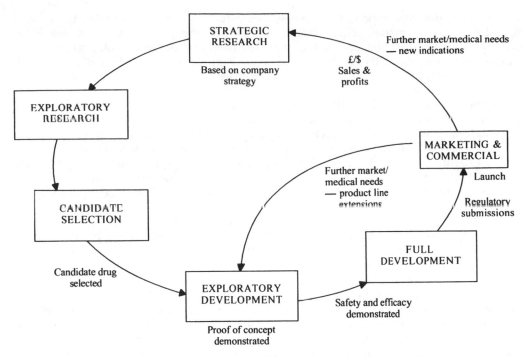

Figure 1 Product life cycle.

To be successful and competitive, research-based pharmaceutical companies must ensure that new discoveries are frequently brought to the market to generate cash flow. This is required to fund the next generation of compounds to meet the therapeutic needs of patients, and of course, to benefit the shareholders. This cycle of events is sometimes referred to as the "product life cycle" and is further illustrated in Figure 1.

The overall costs of drug discovery and development to bring a new medicine to the market are increasing at an alarming rate. It is currently estimated that US$1 billion is required to recoup the costs of research, development, manufacturing, distribution, marketing, and sales for a new chemical entity (NCE). Cost estimates are even higher for a new biopharmaceutical product at US$1.2 billion and take longer to develop than a NCE, but tend to enjoy much greater success rates (DiMari and Grabowski, 2007). A significant proportion of this total is for the cost of failures, or in other words, the elimination of unsuccessful compounds. R&D expenditure tends to increase substantially as the compound progresses from drug discovery research through the various clinical trial phases of development. The pivotal phase III patient trials are usually the largest, involving thousands of patients, and hence the most expensive. To reduce development costs, some companies selectively screen and eliminate compounds earlier in the drug development process on the basis of results from small-scale, less expensive studies in human and progress fewer, more certain compounds to later clinical phases.

In spite of the high risks and high costs involved, there is still a huge incentive for pharmaceutical companies to seek the financial rewards from successful marketed products, especially from the phenomenal success of the rare "blockbuster" (reaching sales of >US$1 billion per year). This can earn the company significant profits to reinvest in research and fund the product development pipeline.

Another factor, the risk of delay to registration and launch, can also have a significant impact on the financial success of a marketed product. McKinsey & Company, a management consultancy, assessed that a product that is six months late to market will miss out on one-third of the potential profit over the product's lifetime. In comparison, they found that a development cost overspend of 50% would reduce profits by just 3.5%, and a 9% overspend in production costs would reduce profits by 22% (McKinsey & Co., 1991). The loss of product revenue is often due to competitor companies being first to market, capturing the market share, and dictating the market price, in addition to the loss of effective patent life. Hence, the importance of accelerating and optimizing drug discovery and development, and getting to the market first with a new therapeutic class of medicinal product, cannot be underestimated. The second product to market in the same class will usually be compared with the market leader, often unfavorably.

The average time from drug discovery to product launch is currently estimated to be 10 to 12 years. Several factors may have contributed to lengthening development times over the years, including an increase in the preclinical phase to select the candidate drug and also an increase in the duration of the clinical and regulatory period required for marketing approval because regulatory agencies are requesting comparator efficacy studies and extensive safety profiling. Benchmarking studies show wide gaps between industry average or worst performance compared with what is achievable as best practice performance (Spence, 1997). On average, the preclinical phase currently takes four to six years to complete, whereas the time from candidate drug nomination to regulatory submission takes on average six to eight years, and longer for treatments of chronic conditions. Most forward-looking pharmaceutical companies are aiming to reduce these times by reevaluation and subsequently streamlining the development process, for example, by introducing more effective clinical programs and more efficient data reporting systems, forward planning, and conducting multiple activities in parallel. However, this in turn may put formulation development and clinical supplies on the critical path, with pressures to complete these activities in condensed time scales. Suggestions are offered throughout this book on how preformulation, biopharmaceuticals, and formulation can be conducted in the most efficient way to avoid delays in development times.

Any reduction in the total time frame of drug discovery to market should improve the company's profitability. In a highly competitive market, product lifetimes are being eroded because of the pace of introduction of competitor products, the rapid introduction of generic products when patents expire and move to "over-the-counter" (OTC) status. Successful pharmaceutical companies are focusing on strategies for optimum "product life cycle management" to maximize the early growth of the product on the market, sustain peak sales for as long as the product is in patent, and delay the post-patent expiry decline for as long as possible. This should maximize the return on investment during a product life cycle to enable the company to recover development costs and make further investments in R&D. Figure 2 shows a classic cash flow profile for a new drug product developed and marketed.

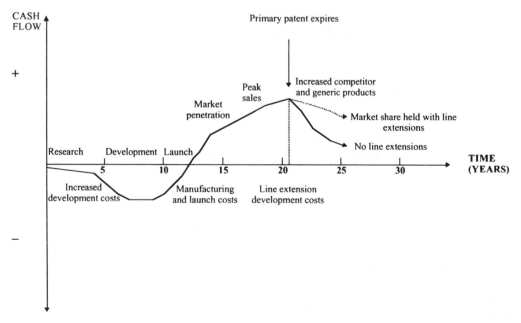

Figure 2   Product life cycle management.

During development there is a negative cash flow, and it may be some time after launch before sales revenue crosses from loss to profit because of manufacturing, distribution, and advertising costs. Profits continue to increase as the market is established to reach peak sales, after which sales decrease, especially after the primary patent expires and generic competition is introduced.

Throughout the life span of a product, it is in a company's interest to ensure the best patent protection to achieve the longest possible market exclusivity. Prior to the primary patent expiring (normally for the chemical drug substance), it is imperative to introduce new indications, formulations, manufacturing processes, devices, and general technology, which are patent protected, to extend the life of the product and maintain revenue. A patent generally has a term of about 20 years, but as development times are getting longer, there will be a limited duration of protection remaining once the product is marketed (the effective patent life). A comparison of effective patent life for pharmaceutical NCEs in various countries around the world shows the same downward trend between the 1960s and the 1980s (Karia et al., 1992; Lis and Walker, 1988). In the EU, products typically enjoy 10 years of patent exclusivity, whereas in the United States, it is typically only 5 years.

Getting to the market quickly is a major business-driving force, but this has to be balanced with the development of a product of the appropriate quality. There is a need to generate sufficient information to enable sound decisions on the selection of a candidate drug for development, as well as to develop dosage forms that are "fit for purpose" at the various stages of development. Anything more is wasting precious resources (people and drug substance), adding unnecessary cost to the program, and, more importantly, extending the development time. Perfect quality should not be the target if good quality is sufficient for the intended purpose. This can only be achieved if there is a clear understanding of the customer requirements.

For example, if a simple, non-optimized formulation with a relatively short shelf life is acceptable for phase I clinical studies, any further optimization or stability testing might be considered wasteful, unless the data generated can be used later in the development program.

There can be a significant risk associated with doing a minimum development program and cutting corners to fast track to market. Post launch, the cost of a retrospective fix due to poor product/process design and/or development can be extremely high. The additional financial cost from work in product/process redevelopment, manufacturing and validation, technical support, regulatory submission, and sales and marketing (due to a product recall) can easily wipe out the profit from an early launch. This can have several unpleasant knock-on effects; it may affect the market share and the company's relationship with the regulatory authorities, and its credibility with customers (both externally and internally within the company) may be threatened. These factors need to be taken into account when planning preformulation/formulation studies, which can directly influence the progress of a product to market and final product quality.

CURRENT TRENDS IN THE PHARMACEUTICAL INDUSTRY

Increasing competition and threats to the pharmaceutical industry with respect to maintaining continued sales growth and income mean that successful companies going forward will be those that have a portfolio of products capable of showing volume growth. However, to show volume growth, innovative new products are required. The cost of drug discovery and development is escalating because there are no easy targets left and the cost of development and the cost of goods (CoG) sold are increasing. There have been several mergers and acquisitions of research-based pharmaceutical companies since the 1980s, and increased collaborations and inward licensing of products and technologies, in attempts to acquire new leads, to share costs, to reduce the time to license, and to maintain growth. Unfortunately, mergers and acquisitions also result in streamlining and job losses, which improve efficiency and decrease overhead costs at the same time.

There is a changing trend in the nature of the candidate drug emerging from pharmaceutical R&D, from a low molecular weight chemical to a more complex macromolecule (biopharmaceuticals). Biopharmaceuticals comprise "biologics" such as vaccines and blood and plasma products, and products derived using biotechnology such as monoclonal antibodies or recombinant proteins that are engineered or derived from mammalian or other cells. Some of these compounds have been derived from biotechnological processes to produce biotechnological medicinal products that fight infection and disease. A typical biotechnology process consists of three major phases to produce the purified bulk active pharmaceutical ingredient (API): (*i*) fermentation of cells (generally mammalian cell lines for antibody manufacture), (*ii*) downstream processing to clear up any contamination, and (*iii*) characterization and testing of impurities. The bulk API is then either processed further or just filled in vials or ampoules to produce the drug product.

It is estimated that today there are more than one hundred biotechnological medicinal products on the market, and many more in clinical trials are being developed to treat a wide variety of diseases. Those currently on the market account for 60% of absolute annual sales growth in major pharmaceutical companies, with the remaining 40% being from small molecules (Mudhar, 2006). Biopharmaceuticals possess some advantages over small molecules, for example, some can affect human drug targets, which is not possible with small molecules. They are also difficult to copy when the patent expires, thus keeping the generics at bay. However, there are also some significant disadvantages of using biopharmaceuticals, such as the almost unavoidable loss of any oral dosing route because they tend to be denatured in the gastrointestinal tract or are too large to be absorbed. It can be a major challenge for the formulator to develop self-administered formulations to deliver macromolecules such as proteins and polypeptides into the body. Even if administered by injection, the pharmacokinetics of biopharmaceuticals can be complicated because of built-in clearance mechanisms.

For both small molecules and biopharmaceuticals, more sophisticated drug delivery systems are being developed to overcome the limitations of conventional forms of drug delivery systems [e.g., tablets and intravenous (IV) solutions], problems of poor drug absorption, noncompliance of patients, and inaccurate targeting of therapeutic agents. One example of emerging drug delivery technology is the use of low-level electrical energy to assist the transport of drugs across the skin in a process known as electrophoresis. This method could be particularly useful for the delivery of peptides and proteins, which are not adequately transported by passive transdermal therapy. The drug absorption rate is very rapid and more controlled compared with passive diffusion across the skin. Another example is the pulmonary delivery of proteins and peptides. The recent successful delivery of insulin using a dry-powder inhaler is impressive since it had to pass so many hurdles including the narrow therapeutic index of insulin and the need for tight particle size control to reach the alveolar surface. This provides encouragement for the delivery of other protein and peptide products delivered by this route. A third example is the use of bioerodable polymers that can be implanted or injected within the body to administer drugs from a matrix, which can be formulated to degrade over a long duration from one day to six months and do not require retrieval. Some of these specific delivery systems are explained in more detail in later chapters on the various dosage forms.

Futuristic drug delivery systems are being developed, which are hoped to facilitate the transport of a drug with a carrier to its intended destination in the body and then release it there. Liposomes, monoclonal antibodies, and modified viruses are being considered to deliver "repair genes" by IV injection to target the respiratory epithelium in the treatment of cystic fibrosis. These novel drug delivery systems not only offer clear medical benefits to the patient, but can also create opportunities for commercial exploitation, especially useful if a drug is approaching the end of its patent life.

There are pressures on the pharmaceutical industry, which affect the way products are being developed. For example, there is a trend for more comprehensive documentation to demonstrate compliance with current good manufacturing practice (cGMP) and good laboratory practice (GLP) and to demonstrate that systems and procedures have been validated. The latest trend is for more information required on the "design space" for the manufacturing process prior to regulatory submission, as discussed later in chapter 8 on product optimization. A benefit of doing this is to provide more flexibility for changes to the process within the design space limits once submitted. However, the pressure is for a company to submit early and develop the product "right first time" with a thorough understanding of the product and manufacturing process.

In spite of efforts to harmonize tests, standards, and pharmacopoeias, there is still diversity between the major global markets—Europe, the United States, and Japan—which have to be taken into account in the design of preformulation and formulation programs (Anonymous, 1993). This is discussed further in chapter 5 on product design.

Other pressures facing the pharmaceutical industry are of a political/economical or environmental nature. Some governments are trying to contain healthcare costs by introducing healthcare reforms, which may lead to reduced prices and profit margins for companies, or restricted markets where only certain drugs can be prescribed. Although the beneficial effect of drugs is not questioned in general, the pressure to contain the healthcare costs is acute. Healthcare costs are increasing partly because people are living longer and more treatments are available. This may influence the commercial price that can be obtained for a new product entering the market and, in turn, the "CoG target." The industry average for the CoG target is 5% to 10% of the commercial price, with pressure to keep it as low as possible. This may impact on the choice and cost of raw materials, components and packaging for the product, and the design and cost of manufacturing the drug and product.

Environmental pressures are to use environmentally friendly materials in products and processes and to accomplish the reduction of waste emissions from manufacturing processes. A good example is the replacement of chlorofluorocarbon (CFC) propellants in pressurized metered-dose inhalers (pMDIs) with hydrofluorocarbons (HFAs). The production of CFCs in developed countries was banned by the Montreal Protocol (an international treaty) apart from "essential uses," such as propellants in pMDIs, to reduce the damage to the earth's ozone layer. However, there is increasing pressure to phase out CFCs altogether. The transition from CFC to HFA products involves a massive reformulation exercise with significant technical challenges and costs for pharmaceutical companies involved in developing pMDIs, as described in chapter 10 "Inhalation Dosage Forms." However, this can be turned into a commercial opportunity for some companies, which have developed patent-protected delivery systems to extend the life cycle of their CFC pMDI products.

LESSONS LEARNT AND THE WAY FORWARD

To achieve the best chance of a fast and efficient development program to bring a candidate drug to market, several important messages can be gleaned from projects that have gone well and from companies with consistently good track records.

There are benefits for pharmaceutical development to get involved early with preclinical research during the candidate drug selection phase. This is to move away from an "over-the-wall" handover approach of the candidate drug to be developed from "research" to "development." The drug selection criteria will be primarily based on pharmacological properties such as potency, selectivity, duration of action, and safety/toxicology assessments. However, if all these factors are satisfactory and similar, there may be an important difference between the pharmaceutical properties of candidate drugs. A candidate drug with preferred pharmaceutical properties, for example, good aqueous solubility, crystalline, nonhygroscopic, and good stability, should be selected to minimize the challenges involved in developing a suitable formulation. This is discussed further in chapter 2.

Another important factor is good long-term planning, ideally from candidate drug nomination to launch, with consideration for the safety, clinical and pharmaceutical development, manufacturing operations, and regulatory strategies involved to develop the product. There is a need for one central, integrated company project plan that has been agreed on by all parties with a vested interest in the project. Needless to say, the plan should contain details of activities, timings, responsibilities, milestones, reviews, and decision points. Reviews and decision points are required at the end of a distinct activity to ensure that the project is still meeting its objectives and should progress to the next stage of development. However, these reviews should not cause any delays to the program, rather, they should ratify what is already progressing. The traditional sequential phases of product development (chapter 2) must be

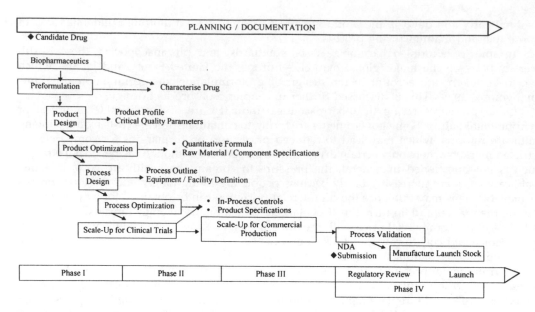

Figure 3 Framework for product development.

overlapped to accelerate the product to market. In reality, plans will inevitably change with time; they should be "living" documents, which are reviewed and updated at regular intervals and then communicated to all parties. There may be several more detailed, lower-level plans focusing on departmental activities, for example, pharmaceutical development, but these plans must be linked to the top-level central project plan.

Forward planning should provide the opportunity for a well thought out and efficient approach to product development, identifying requirements up front so as to avoid too much deliberation and backtracking along the way. It should also provide a visible communication tool.

Good planning is supported by adopting a systematic and structured approach to product development. The development process can be broken down into several key defined stages—product design, process design, product optimization, process optimization, scale-up, and so on. Each stage will have inputs and outputs as shown in Figure 3, a simplified framework for product development. The appropriate definition and requirements at each stage are described in chapters 5 and 8.

As product development can take several years to complete, it is important to have an effective document management system in place to record the work. The primary reference source for recording experimental work will usually be a laboratory notebook (paper or electronic). The work should be checked, dated, and countersigned to satisfy GLP and intellectual property requirements. Experimental protocols are sometimes useful for defining programs of work, explaining the rationale for the studies, and defining the acceptance criteria. When the studies are completed, the results can be reported with reference to the protocol and acceptance criteria. Laboratory notebooks are referenced in the protocols and reports so that the raw data can be retrieved in the event of an audit.

At the completion of key stages of the work, summary reports can be written, referencing all other protocols and reports relevant to that stage and highlighting the major recommendations and conclusions. In this way, a product development document file can be built up for transfer of information and technology, including the development history and rationale for progression. The file will also be vital for data retrieval in the event of a regulatory inspection.

Finally, successful product development is often associated with good teamwork. The process is multidisciplinary, relying on people with different specialist skills working together to make it happen. This is particularly important at the key interfaces such as preclinical research with pharmaceutical development and pharmaceutical development with manufacturing operations at the final production site. It is therefore useful to have representation on the project teams from all the key specialist functions to ensure buy-in to the plans, strategies, and decisions, and to have a good project management system in place.

SCOPE OF THE BOOK

This book is structured in a logical order to cover the various stages of drug development from candidate drug selection to development of the intended commercial dosage form.

In chapter 2, the key stages of the R&D process are explained in some detail, with the outputs expected from each stage, to afford an appreciation of the entire process. The remainder of the book concentrates on candidate drug selection for development and development of the commercial dosage form where preformulation, biopharmaceutics, and formulation play a vital role. Initial emphasis is on candidate drug selection and the importance of preformulation, formulation, and biopharmaceutics input at this stage. Traditionally, not all pharmaceutical companies operate in this way, and the result from experience is often that pharmaceutical development has to accept whatever candidate drug comes out of research and address any unforeseen difficulties during development. The disadvantages of this approach, and the opportunities and benefits of pharmaceutical input to the candidate selection process, are clearly explained in the early chapters.

Available drug substance for preformulation and biopharmaceutics studies at the candidate drug selection stage can be a major challenge. Chapter 3 describes the preformulation studies that can be undertaken to maximize the information gained from small amounts of drug substance to select the preferred candidate drug for development. Various modern preformulation techniques that use minimal amounts of drug are described to evaluate the physicochemical properties of compounds, salts and polymorphs.

Chapter 4 describes the importance of drug delivery and biopharmaceutical factors in the candidate drug selection phase. Consideration is given to the intended route of administration, what predictions can be made, and useful information gained from biopharmaceutical assessment of the candidate drug.

Following candidate selection, usually, one candidate drug is nominated for development. The importance of establishing the product design attributes is discussed in chapter 5. The value of this exercise is often underestimated in the rush to develop products quickly. However, the quality of the product design can often influence the success of developing a commercially viable product with a desired product profile in a timely manner to market.

Chapters 6 and 7 focus on preformulation and biopharmaceutics, respectively, as an aid to product design. The emphasis is on generating the appropriate data to characterize the candidate drug and aid product design and development. The objective at this stage is to determine the physicochemical properties of the candidate drug, which are considered important in the development of a stable, effective, and safe formulation. Use of a limited amount of available drug substance and the speed and program of work depending on the intended dosage form and route, are all carefully considered here and illustrated with the aid of worked examples. Modern instrumental techniques and personal computer (PC)-based "expert systems" are discussed as useful tools.

To develop a product from inception to market, the product and process have to be optimized and the process scaled up and transferred to commercial production. Definitions and descriptions of the requirements for all these stages of development are discussed in chapter 8, although the major discussion is on the preformulation/formulation input to product optimization. The many factors that a formulator should consider in the selection of pharmaceutical excipients and packaging are discussed. Useful sources of information and techniques for selection such as expert systems and experimental design tools are included.

Drugs are generally administered via the mouth, eyes, nose, or skin or by inhalation or injection, and so these routes are covered in more detail in separate chapters. Special considerations and issues for the formulation development of each route and type of dosage form are discussed on the basis of considerable relevant experience of the various contributors.

REFERENCES

Anonymous. Global differences in registration requirements. Pharm J 1993; 251:610–611.

DiMari JA, Grabowski HG. The cost of biopharmaceutical R&D: is biotech different? Manage Decis Econ 2007; 28:469–479.

Karia R, Lis Y, Walker SR. The erosion of effective patent life—an international comparison. In: Griffin JP, ed. Medicines, Regulation, Research and Risk. 2nd ed. Belfast: Queen's University Press, 1992:287–301.

Lis Y, Walker SR. Pharmaceutical patent term erosion—a comparison of the UK, USA and Federal Republic of Germany (FRG). Pharm J 1988; 240:176–180.

Lowe D. Opininion – in the pipeline. It's been a rough year, but the future looks bright. Chem World 2008; January: 23.

McKinsey & Co. In: Burall P, ed. Managing Product Creation, a Management Overview. London: The Design Council for the UK Department of Trade and Industry, 1991.

Mudhar P. Biopharmaceuticals: insight into today's market and a look to the future. Pharm Technol Eur 2006; 9:20–25.

Spence C, ed. The Pharmaceutical R&D Compendium: CMR International/SCRIP's Guide to Trends in R&D. Surrey, UK: CMR International/SCRIP Publication, 1997.

Wells JI. Pharmaceutical Preformulation. The Physicochemical Properties of Drug Substances. Chichester: Ellis Horwood; and New York: Wiley, 1988.

2 | Aiding Candidate Drug Selection: Introduction and Objectives

Mark Gibson
AstraZeneca R&D Charnwood, Loughborough, Leicestershire, U.K.

STAGES OF THE DRUG DISCOVERY AND DEVELOPMENT PROCESS

The development of a new medicinal product from a novel synthesized chemical compound, a chemical extracted from a natural source or a compound produced by biotechnological processes, is a long and complex procedure and involves many different disciplines working together. The drug discovery and development process for a typical research-based pharmaceutical company can be broken down into five distinct stages as described briefly below. At each stage, there will be several activities running in parallel, with the overall objective of discovering a candidate drug and developing it to market as efficiently as possible. It should be noted that different companies may use slightly different terminology and perform some activities sooner or later, but the overall process is essentially the same.

Strategic Research

Feasibility studies are conducted to demonstrate whether interfering in a particular biological mechanism has an effect that might be of therapeutic value.

The strategic research of a particular company is usually guided by factors such as its inherent research competence and expertise, therapeutic areas of unmet medical need, and market potential/commercial viability. Companies often wish to develop a portfolio of products within a specific therapeutic area to capture a segment of the market. By focusing on a particular therapeutic area, a company can build on its existing expertise and competence in all of its functions with the aim of becoming a leading company in that field. Product life cycle management is important in achieving this aim.

Exploratory Research

Exploratory research is an investigation of the biological mechanism and identification of a "chemical or biological lead" that interferes with it.

During the exploratory research stage, diverse compounds are screened for the desired biological activity. The aim is to find a chemical or molecular entity that interferes with the process and to provide a valuable probe of the underlying therapeutic problem. Traditionally, this has been achieved by the organic chemist synthesizing compounds one at a time for the biologist to test in a linear fashion. Over the last two decades, there has been a rapid development in the technologies for creating very large and diverse quantities of synthetic and biosynthetic molecules and for testing large numbers of activity in less time. These technologies have been labeled "combinatorial chemistry" and automated "high-throughput screening" (HTS), respectively. The key impact has been to accelerate the synthesis of new compounds from, say, 50 compounds per chemist year to many tens of thousands and to be able to test these against many biological targets (e.g., biological receptors or biochemical pathways) very quickly (Doyle et al., 1998).

The rate of technology development specifically associated with HTS for pharmaceutical drug discovery has increased markedly over recent years, with automated techniques involving miniaturization, to allow assays on very small samples (e.g., 1 µL volume), and the ability to analyze thousands of samples a day using well microplates (Burbaum, 1998). In addition to the use of HTS for pharmacological activity, HTS tests have been developed for assessing metabolism and pharmacokinetic and toxicity factors to speed up the drug discovery process.

In simple terms, a biologically active compound can be considered to consist of a supportive framework with biofunctional groups attached that bind to a target to induce a biological response. Each compound is, in effect, a unique combination of numerous possible groups. Combinatorial techniques have replaced traditional synthetic approaches to generate many possible combinations rapidly for biological testing.

Approaches to lead generation during exploratory research often depend on how much is already known about the therapeutic target under consideration. For example, if the three-dimensional structure of the target (such as an enzyme-inhibitor complex) is known, chemical leads could be found and optimized through combinatorial chemistry and HTS. Alternatively, in some cases, the only available biochemical knowledge might be the structure of a ligand for the enzyme. If there were no information at all, then the only approach might be limited to HTS of batches of compounds from combinatorial libraries.

Even with combinatorial chemistry and HTS, lead generation can be extremely laborious because of the vast number of different molecules possible (framework and biofunctional group combinations). To ease this burden, some rational drug design and quantitative structure activity relationships (QSARs) are often introduced to direct the program and utilize a company's finite screening resource as efficiently as possible.

"Representative" libraries of compounds, where each member is selected to give information about a larger cluster of compounds, are designed and used to reduce the amount of compounds that have to be made and tested.

There have been recent advances to create diverse biopharmaceutical molecules for evaluation, for example, through antibody engineering to produce anticancer treatments (Morrow, 2007). Protein and glycosylation engineering can be employed to generate antibodies with enhanced effector functions. The presence or absence of one sugar residue can result in a two-orders-of-magnitude difference in the ability to kill cancer cells by antibody-dependent cell cytotoxicity, which could result in reduced dose and cost.

Together with combinatorial chemistry and rational drug design, genomics is rapidly emerging as a useful technique to enable companies to significantly increase the number of drug targets and improve on candidate selection success. A number of companies have seen the potential in defining patient groups based on their genotypes and are now investing lots of money to gain a clearer understanding of the genes that are important to drug action. Personal medicine has been in development since the 1980s: "Personalized treatment" is where the doctor prescribes the best treatment for a patient based on his or her genetic profile, whereas personalized products involve drugs that are actually made for an individual patient. A patient's DNA can be rapidly sequenced and recombinant protein can be produced. For example, it is possible to look at the DNA sequences (biomarkers) of cancer patients, which tell the doctor what the best treatment would be for that patient. If personalized products are not available yet, the doctor can identify which general therapy, such as chemotherapy, antibodies, or radiation, would be the most statistically effective for a particular cancer type based on the genetic screening.

Candidate Drug Selection

The chemical or biological lead is used to generate specific chemical compounds with the optimal desired characteristics, for example, potency, specificity, duration, safety, and pharmaceutical aspects. One or more candidate drugs are nominated for development.

During the candidate drug selection stage, the molecular lead is optimized by testing a range of selected compounds in in vitro and in vivo (animal) studies. The objective is to select one or more candidate drugs for development with the most desired characteristics. Pharmacological characteristics might include acceptable absorption, potency, duration of action, and selectivity for the receptor or enzyme. Safety characteristics will normally include noncarcinogenicity, nonteratogenicity, nonmutagenicity, and general nontoxicity. The potential for these characteristics can be predicted from relatively short-term preclinical toxi-pharmacological animal studies and in vitro tests.

The U.S. Food and Drug Administration (FDA) has recently recommended that drug developers conduct phase 0 studies, a designation for exploratory, first-in-human microdosing studies. These are conducted prior to phase I studies and intended to speed up the

Table 1 Preferred Drug Synthesis and Dosage Form Pharmaceutical Properties for Chemical Compounds Intended for Oral Solid Development

Drug synthesis factors	Formulation/drug delivery factors
Least complex structure (none/few chiral centers)	Exists as a stable polymorphic form
Few synthesis steps as possible	Nonhygroscopic
High yields as possible	Crystalline
Nonexplosive route or safety issues	Acceptable solid-state stability of candidate drug
Commercial availability of building blocks and contract manufacturers	Acceptable oral bioavailability
Low cost of goods compared with overall cost of product on market	Not highly colored or strong odor (to ensure batch reproducibility and reduce problems with blinding in clinical studies)
	No predicted problems in scale-up of manufacturing process
No predicted problems in scale-up of batch size	Compatible with key excipients

development of promising drugs or imaging agents by establishing very early on whether the drug or agent behaves in human subjects as was anticipated from preclinical studies (FDA, 2006). Phase 0 studies involve the administration of single, subtherapeutic dose of the new drug candidate to a small number of human subjects (10–15) to gather preliminary data on the pharmacokinetics (how the body processes the drug) and pharmacodynamics (how the drug works in the body). A phase 0 study gives no data on safety or efficacy, but drug developers can carry out these studies to rank drug candidates to decide which to take forward. They enable decisions to be made based on human data instead of relying on animal data, which can be unpredictive and vary between species. The potential advantages of phase 0 studies are to aid candidate drug selection by getting an insight into the human pharmacokinetics, but also to help to establish the likely pharmacological dose and also the first dose for the subsequent phase I study. They may also identify early failures and save the company costs of further development.

In the interests of rapid drug development, it is also important to select a chemical lead with preferred pharmaceutical and chemical synthesis properties at this stage. A list of preferred characteristics for a compound intended for oral solid dosage form development is given in Table 1.

Higher priority in the selection process will, in most cases, be given to a compound's optimal pharmacological and safety characteristics. However, in the event of having a choice from a range of compounds all possessing similar pharmacological and safety properties, there may be a significant advantage for formulation development in selecting a compound with the most preferred pharmaceutical development properties. It is useful to conduct preformulation studies and biopharmaceutics studies at the candidate drug selection stage to determine the most relevant physicochemical and biopharmaceutical properties of potential candidate drugs to aid candidate selection.

Biopharmaceutics is the study of how the physicochemical properties of the candidate drugs, the formulation/delivery system, and the route of administration affect the rate and extent of drug absorption. Appropriate biopharmaceutical information generated at this stage can also be very important in directing the candidate selection process and for future dosage form design during development.

The benefits of providing preformulation and biopharmaceutics input during the candidate drug selection stage, to characterize the candidate drug and provide useful information to support the selection of the optimal compound for pharmaceutical development, are emphasized in chapters 3 and 4. Generally, any pharmaceutical issues can be discovered earlier, before the candidate drug reaches development, and any implications for product design and development considered in advance. The involvement of pharmaceutical development in the selection process and "buy-in" to the nomination decision can often enhance the team's working relationship with their research colleagues. The objective is to achieve a seamless transition from research to development, as opposed to the traditional "over-the-wall" approach that many pharmaceutical companies experience to their costs.

Earlier involvement by the pharmaceutical development group at the preclinical stage should also result in better planning for full development.

In spite of all these potential advantages of early pharmaceutical involvement to candidate drug selection, there may be several barriers within a company, which can hinder this way of working. Distance between the research group and the development group should not really be considered a barrier, although this can be the case for groups on different continents with different cultures and languages. The important factor for success seems to be the development of a formal mechanism for interaction, supported by senior management in the company. This often takes the form of a joint project team with regular meetings to review progress. However, there may still be a lack of appreciation of what input or expertise pharmaceutical development can offer at the candidate drug selection stage. Opportunities to demonstrate what can be done and to educate research colleagues should be sought to try and overcome this attitude.

Another potential barrier is any overlapping expertise there may be in research and development groups. For example, overlap may occur between preformulation in pharmaceutical development and physical chemistry in research, or between biopharmaceutics in development and drug metabolism in research. In these cases, it is important to clarify and agree which group does what activity.

A common perceived barrier to providing early preformulation and biopharmaceutics input can be the quantity of compound required for evaluation at this stage. The research group may believe that significantly more compound is required; with modern instrumental techniques; however, this is often not the case.

Other potential barriers that can influence the success of the relationship with research at the candidate drug selection stage are the pharmaceutical development response time not being fast enough to support research and the lack of resources that pharmaceutical development can give to support the candidate drug selection program. Several compounds may have to be evaluated simultaneously to generate comparative data to aid the selection process. Preformulation and biopharmaceutics have to keep pace with the pharmacological and safety testing; otherwise there is no point in generating the data. One way of achieving this is to allocate dedicated resources to these projects using people trained to rapidly respond to the preformulation and biopharmaceutics requirements. Fit-for-purpose, simple formulations can be used at this stage, and rank order information is often acceptable, rather than definitive quantitative information. Analytical methods should not require rigorous validation at this stage to provide these data. Excessive documentation and rigid standard operating procedures that can slow down the work are not usually necessary and should be avoided.

Exploratory Development

The aim of exploratory development is to gauge how the candidate drug is absorbed and metabolized in healthy human volunteers before studying its effect on those actually suffering from the disease for which it is intended. Occasionally, it is necessary to conduct further small-scale studies in patients to make a decision whether to progress the candidate drug into full development. This stage is often referred to as phase I clinical studies or concept testing (proof of concept). Usually a small number of healthy volunteers (20–80 who do not have the condition under investigation or any other illness) receive the drug candidate provided as a simple formulation, which can be different from the intended commercial formulation. For example, a simple aqueous oral solution or suspension may be used, rather than a capsule or tablet, to minimize the formulation development work at this early stage. Phase I studies are the first stage of testing in human subjects to assess the safety (pharmacovigilance), tolerability, pharmacokinetics, and pharmacodynamics of a new drug. The trials are usually conducted in an inpatient clinic where the subjects can be observed by full-time medical staff. These studies often include dose ranging or dose escalation so that the appropriate dose for therapeutic use can be found. There are different kinds of phase I trials.

SAD: Single ascending dose studies where human subjects are given a single dose of the drug. If there are no adverse side effects, the dose is escalated until intolerable side effects start to be observed. This is where the drug reaches its maximum tolerated dose (MTD).

MAD: Multiple ascending dose studies are conducted to better understand the pharmacokinetics and pharmacodynamics of multiple doses of the drug. Patients receive multiple low doses of the drug, and then the dose is subsequently escalated to a predetermined level.

Food effect: A short trial designed to investigate any differences in absorption of the drug by the body caused by eating before the drug is given. These are usually designed as crossover studies, with volunteers being given two identical doses of the drug on different occasions, one while fasted and one after being fed.

If the candidate drug does not produce the expected effects in human studies, or produces unexpected and unwanted effects, the development program is likely to be stopped at this stage. Since the introduction of the EU Clinical Trial Directive 2001/20/EC in 2001, there is now a requirement for all EU countries, including the United Kingdom when it came into force in May 2004, to make a submission to the local regulatory authorities for permission to conduct the trials in human volunteers.

Full Development

Completion of longer-term safety and clinical studies (phases II and III) in patients suffering from the disease are accomplished at this stage. Phase II studies are dose-ranging studies in a reasonable patient population (several hundred) to evaluate the effectiveness of the drug and common side effects. During phase II, the intended commercial formulation should be developed, and the product/process optimized and eventually scaled up to commercial production scale. The candidate drug should ideally be in the intended commercial formulation for the phase III trials. After the satisfactory completion of phase II trials, large patient populations (several hundred to thousands) are involved to statistically confirm efficacy and safety. Some patients will be given the drug, some a placebo product (required to be identical in appearance), and some may be given a known market leader (with all products appearing identical). The doctors and patients in the study will not know whether the patients are getting the test drug, placebo, or market leader; by switching the medication in a controlled way (double -blind trials), objectivity and statistical assessment of the treatment under investigation are assured. Most regulatory authorities, including the FDA, the Medicines and Healthcare products Regulatory Agency (MHRA) in the United Kingdom, and the European Agency for the Evaluation of Medicinal Products (EMEA), require three phases of clinical trials and sufficient data to demonstrate that the new product can be licensed as safe, effective, and of acceptable quality. Once these clinical studies are complete, the company can decide whether it wishes to submit a marketing authorization application to a regulatory authority for a medicinal drug product. Approval is usually followed by product launch to market.

There are also phase IV trials, also known as post-marketing surveillance trials, conducted to evaluate the safety surveillance (pharmacovigilance) of a drug after it receives permission to be sold. This may be a requirement of the regulatory authorities or maybe undertaken by a drug-developing company to find a new market for the drug or for other reasons. For example, the drug may not have been tested for interactions with other drugs or on certain population groups such as pregnant women or pediatrics. The objective of phase IV studies is to detect any long-term or rare adverse effects over a much larger patient population and longer time period than phases I to III trials. If harmful effects are discovered, it may result in a drug no longer being sold or a restriction to certain uses.

SUMMARY

Pharmaceutical companies with the best track records for drug discovery and rapid development to market tend to have a seamless transfer from research to development. There are many opportunities and benefits to be gained by the involvement of pharmaceutical development groups, such as preformulation and biopharmaceutics, during the candidate drug selection stage. It may be surprising what valuable information can be obtained using modern preformulation instrumental techniques and biopharmaceutical techniques from relatively small quantities of compound. These topics are discussed further in chapters 3 and 4 of this text.

REFERENCES

Burbaum J. Engines of discovery. Chem Br 1998; 6:38–41.

Doyle PM, Barker E, Harris CJ, et al. Combinatorial technologies—a revolution in pharmaceutical R&D. Pharm Technol Eur 1998; 4:26–32.

Food and Drug Administration (FDA). Guidance for Industry, Investigators, and Reviewers—Exploratory IND Studies. Available at: http://www.fda.gov/cder/guidance/7086fnl.htm. Accessed January 2006.

Morrow JM Jr. Glycosylation and the demands of antibody engineering. BioPharm Int 2007; 10:126–129.

3 | Preformulation Investigations using Small Amounts of Compound as an Aid to Candidate Drug Selection and Early Development

Gerry Steele and Talbir Austin

AstraZeneca R&D Charnwood, Loughborough, Leicestershire, U.K.

INTRODUCTION

In recent years, there has been a significant increase in pressure on pharmaceutical companies to discover and develop new medicines ever faster to replace those coming off patent and to counter generic manufacturer competition (Frantz, 2007). Despite the expenditure of many billons of dollars, Joshi (2007) reports that since 1990 an average of only 28 drugs have been approved each year, with the Food and Drug Administration (FDA) approving only 17 new chemical entities (NCEs) in 2002, the lowest number of new drug approvals for the decade leading up to that year (Kola and Landis, 2004). Indeed, the success rate achieved by the industry of bringing a candidate drug (CD) to market is no more than 10% (Schmid and Smith, 2006), and it is estimated that of 30,000 compounds synthesized only 0.003% of discovery compounds will show a satisfactory return on investment (Federsel, 2003). The majority of the attrition occurs in phase II and phase III of development, with approximately 62% of compounds entering phase II undergoing attrition (Kola and Landis, 2004). So, not only does the number of compounds being brought through from discovery phase need to increase, but the amount of effort expended on them needs to reflect the attrition that will occur as they are progressed through early development. One idea being mooted to increase the productivity of the drug discovery process is the concept of lean thinking, which has been used in pharmaceutical manufacturing for process improvement (Petrillo, 2007). Simply put, lean concepts aim to eliminate those steps in the process that do not add value to the process chain. It has been estimated that utilizing lean concepts in the discovery phase, combined with other methods of increasing productivity, would lead to an increase (from 1 in 5 to 1 to 3) in compounds entering clinical trials.

Drug discovery and development is characterized by a number of distinct stages, and typically, the drug discovery process falls into two phases, lead generation (LG) followed by lead optimization (LO) (Davis et al., 2005). The LG period is further subdivided into the active-to-hit (AtH) and the hit-to-lead (HtL) phases (Baxter et al., 2006). The HtL phase utilizes high-throughput screening (HTS) and generates actives, hits, and leads: leads are those compounds that meet predefined chemical and biological criteria to allow selection of the chemistry that provides molecules with drug-like properties (Leeson et al., 2004). Drug-like compounds can be defined as those with pharmacokinetic and pharmacodynamic properties that are independent of the pharmacological target (Vieth et al., 2004). Leeson and Springthorpe (2007) have discussed how drug-like concepts can influence decision making in the medicinal chemistry arena. In this paper, they argue that the wave of molecules presently being synthesized possess significantly different physicochemical properties to those already in clinical development.

One important aspect of the HTS and HtL approach is that it provides multiple chemical series to de-risk future LO work. Thus, the aim of this phase is to increase the drug-like properties (e.g., improve potency, selectivity, pharmacokinetic properties, and decrease toxicity) of lead compounds against a CD target profile (CDTP). During the LO phase, structure-activity relationships (SARs), which correlate molecular properties with biological effects, are derived. When SARs can be measured quantitatively, they become quantitative SARs (QSARs) (Andricopula and Montanari, 2005). Two specific examples of LO programs for the systematic optimization of compound series are given by Guile et al. (2006) and Baxter et al. (2006).

The iterative assessment of optimized leads against selection criteria allows identification of the most promising lead candidates. Once the lead candidates have been identified, then assessment of the material characteristics by the development scientists can be initiated (Venkatesh and Lipper, 2000). This phase has traditionally been termed "prenomination" and typically lasts around three to six months. It encompasses investigations into the physicochemical characterization of the solid and solution properties of CD compounds and has been the subject of the books by, for example, Wells (1988) and Carstensen (2002). Essentially the aim of this phase is to provide an initial evaluation of compounds from a development perspective and support the tolerability studies of compounds.

The scope of prenomination and early development studies to be carried out largely depends on the expertise, equipment, and drug substance available, and also on any organizational preferences or restrictions. In some organizations, detailed characterization studies are performed, while other companies prefer to do the minimum amount of work required to progress compounds as quickly as possible into development. There are advantages and disadvantages to both approaches, but an important consideration is to balance the studies that allow an appropriate understanding of the CD with the significant possibility of attrition. However, for the smooth progression of compounds through the preformulation phase, a close interaction between Medicinal Chemistry, Safety Assessment, Pharmaceutical Sciences, Analytical Chemistry, and Process Research and Development departments is essential to assess the physicochemical properties and toxicology of compounds and their progression to the first human dose as quickly as possible (Li, 2004). If the compound passes these assessments, it can then pass into the late-phase development, which will be dealt with in subsequent chapters.

In the case of development studies that can be undertaken to support the nomination of a compound for development, Balbach and Korn (2004) have proposed "the 100 mg approach" for the evaluation of early development CDs. However, as pointed out by Ticehurst and Docherty (2006), if a complete package of work is carried out too early, it may lead to much wasted effort. On the other hand, if insufficient work is performed, then it may lead to increased pressure to characterize the compound to meet accelerated project demands. Thus, they recommend a "fit for purpose" solid form in the early studies, followed by selection of solid form for a commercial development. For convenience, these phases can be termed early and late development, respectively. The goal of early development can be defined as that to secure a quick, risk-managed processes for testing the CD in animals and human volunteers for phase I studies.

During prenomination, compounds need to be evaluated in animals for exposure/toxicity purposes [7-day tox and 28-day single and multiple ascending doses (SADs and MADs)] (Kramer et al., 2007). The compound, in a suitable form to ensure systemic exposure (Gardner et al., 2004), needs to be formulated into an appropriate formulation for delivery in the first good laboratory practice (GLP) dose typically as either a suspension or solution. Reference is made to Chaubal (2004) for a review of this area and Mansky et al. (2007) for a method for rapidly screening preclinical vehicles that enhance the solubility of low solubility compounds. Hitchingham and Thomas (2007) have developed a semiautomated system to determine the stability of the dosing formulations.

During this stage, there may be a number of compounds with sufficient activity to merit consideration, and so studies must be designed appropriately to allow efficient assessment and selection of suitable compounds for development. Clear differences in in vivo activity may be sufficient to determine which of the candidates are selected. However, other factors that may be important from a pharmaceutical and drug synthesis point of view should also be considered if there is a choice. For example, physicochemical and biopharmaceutical characteristics of the compound(s), ease of scale-up for compound supply, cost of goods, and the nature of the anticipated dosage form should also be part of the decision process.

Ideally, for an oral solid dosage form, a water-soluble, nonhygroscopic, stable, and easily processed crystalline compound is preferred for development purposes; however, other formulation types will have their own specific requirements. For example, inhalation compounds need to be micronized for formulation into a pressurized metered dose or dry

Table 1 Suggested Physicochemical Tests Carried Out During Prenomination

Test/activity	Tier 1 Guidance to amount	Timing/comments
Elemental analysis	4 mg	LO
Initial HPLC methodology	2 mg	LO
NMR spectroscopy	5 mg	LO
Mass spectroscopy	5 mg	LO
General, e.g., MW, structural and empirical formulae	–	LO
IR/UV-visible spectroscopy	5 mg	LO
Karl Fischer	20 mg	LO
PK_a	10 mg	LO
Log P/log D	10 mg	LO
Initial solubility	10 mg	LO/prenomination
Initial solution stability	Done on above samples	LO//prenomination
Crystallinity investigations	20–30 mg	LO/prenomination
Hygroscopicity	5–10 mg	LO/prenomination
Initial solid stability	10 mg	Prenomination
Salt selection		
Decide/manufacture salts		Prenomination
Characterize salts—use DVS, X ray, DSC, solubility/stability tests	10–50 mg each salt	Prenomination
Initial polymorphism studies, etc. Investigations of selected salt or neutral compound. Production—use different solvents, cooling rates, precipitation, evaporation techniques, etc	100 mg	Prenomination Also included is the propensity of the CD to form hydrates, solvates, and amorphs
Polymorphism, etc. Investigations of selected salt or neutral compound. Characterization		Prenomination
DSC/TGA/HSM	2 mg per technique/sample	Prenomination
X-ray powder diffraction, including temperature and RH	10 mg/sample, 0 background holder	Prenomination
FTIR/Raman	2 mg/sample	Prenomination
Crystal habit–microscopy, light, and SEM	10 mg	Prenomination
Stability-stress wrt temperature/humidity	100 mg	Prenomination
Choose polymorph, amorph, or hydrate		Prenomination

Abbreviations: LO, lead optmization; CD, candidate drug; HPLC, high-performance liquid chromatography; NMR, nuclear magnetic resonance; MW, molecular weight; IR/UV, infrared/ultraviolet; DVS, dynamic vapor sorption; DSC, differential scanning calorimetry; TGA, thermogravimetric analysis; HSM, hot-stage microscopy; RH, relative humidity; FTIR, Fourier transform infrared; SEM, scanning electron microscopy; wrt, with respect to.

powder inhaler. This is an energy-intensive process and can change the crystallinity of compounds, and thus their subsequent interaction with moisture may be important. For a solution formulation, however, the stability of the compound will be paramount, and if instability is a major issue, then alternative measures such as freeze-drying may be required. Table 1 summarizes the prenomination studies that could be carried out on a CD. These are considered to be the minimum tests that should be undertaken, recognizing that during the prenomination phase only a limited quantity of compound, for example, 50 to 100 mg is typically available to the pharmaceutical scientist for characterization. However, it should be emphasized that this is a critical decision period that can profoundly affect the subsequent development of a CD. Thus, the tests shown are considered to be those important for making a rational decision as to which compound, salt, or polymorph to proceed with into development. A poor decision at this point may mean some revisionary work, such as, a change of salt or polymorph being necessary later and a possible delay to the development of the drug for the market.

After first-time-in-human (FTIH) studies in early development, if the compound progresses into full development, a more complete physicochemical characterization of the chosen compound(s), with particular emphasis on the dosage form, should be carried out, thus allowing a rational, stable, and bioavailable formulation to be progressed through to launch. This is discussed in more detail in chapter 6.

From a development point of view, perhaps the biggest change in the last decade has been the introduction and utilization of HTS technologies, whereby large number of compounds can be assessed in parallel to allow efficient physicochemical profiling as well as salt and polymorph screening (Desrosiers, 2004; Storey et al., 2004; Seadeek et al., 2007; Wyttenbach et al., 2007).

MOLECULAR PROPERTIES

Initial Physicochemical Characterization

Initial physicohemical characterization explores the two-dimensional structural properties. Many of the tests carried out, such as proof of structure, are normally performed by the Discovery department, for example, nuclear magnetic resonance (NMR), mass spectra, and elemental analysis. Although important from a physicochemical point of view, these measurements will not be discussed in this chapter. Rather, the text will focus on those tests carried out during prenomination that will have an important bearing on the selection of a potential CD in relation to the proposed formulation/dosage form.

pK_a Determinations

Potential CDs that possess ionizable groups, as either weak acids or bases, can be exploited to vary biological and physical properties such as binding to target enzyme or receptor, binding to plasma proteins, gastrointestinal (GI) absorption, central nervous system (CNS) penetration, solubility, and rate of dissolution (as will be discussed later in the chapter). Therefore, one of the most important initial determinations carried out prior to their development is the pK_a or ionization constant(s). Avdeef (2001) and Kerns (2001) have comprehensively reviewed this aspect of discovery work, and the reader is referred to these papers for a detailed account.

Strong acids such as HCl are ionized at all relevant pH values, whereas the ionization of weak acids is pH dependent. It is essential to know the extent to which the molecule is ionized at a certain pH, because it affects the properties noted above. The basic theory of the ionization constant is covered by most physical chemistry textbooks, and a most useful text is that by Albert and Sargeant (1984). Fundamental to our appreciation of the determination of this parameter, however, is the Brønstead and Lowry theory of acids and bases. This states that an acid is a substance that can donate a hydrogen ion, and a base is one that can accept a proton.

For a weak acid, the following equilibrium holds:

$$HA \rightleftharpoons H^+ + A^-$$

For the sake of brevity, a detailed discussion and derivation of equations will be avoided; however, it is important that the well-known Henderson–Hasselbach equation is understood (equation 1). This equation relates the pK_a to the pH of the solution and the relative concentrations of the dissociated and undissociated parts of a weak acid (equation 1).

$$pH = pK_a + \log \frac{[A^-]}{[HA]} \tag{1}$$

where [A$^-$] is the concentration of the dissociated species and [HA] the concentration of the undissociated species. This equation can be manipulated into the form given by equation (2) to yield the percentage of a compound that will be ionized at any particular pH.

$$\%\text{Ionization} = \frac{100}{1 + (pH - pK_a)} \tag{2}$$

Table 2 Some Reported Methods for the Determination of pK_as

Method	Reference
Potentiometric titration	Rosenberg and Waggenknecht, 1986
UV spectroscopy	Asuero et al., 1986
Solubility measurements	Zimmermann, 1982, 1986
HPLC techniques	Gustavo González, 1993
Capillary zone electrophoresis	Lin et al., 2004
Foaming activity	Alverez Núñez and Yalkowsky, 1997

Abbreviations: UV, ultraviolet; HPLC, high-performance liquid chromatography.

One simple point to note about equation (1) is that at 50% dissociation (or ionization) the pK_a = pH. It should also be noted that usually pK_a values are preferred for bases instead of pK_b values (pK_w = pK_a + pK_b).

Measurement of pK_a

Table 2 summarizes some methods used in the determination of ionization constants.

If a compound is poorly soluble in water, the aqueous pK_a may be difficult to measure. One way to circumvent this problem is to measure the apparent pK_a of the compound in solvent-water mixtures, and then extrapolate the data back to a purely aqueous medium using a Yasuda–Shedlovsky plot. The organic solvents most frequently used are methanol, ethanol, propanol, dimethylsulfoxide (DMSO), dimethyl formamide (DMF), acetone, and tetrahydrofuran (THF). However, methanol is by far the most popular, since its properties bear the closest resemblance to water. Takács-Novák et al. (1997) have reported a validation study in water-methanol mixtures, and the determination of the pK_as of ibuprofen and quinine in a range of organic solvent-water mixtures has been described by Avdeef et al. (1999).

If the compound contains an ultraviolet (UV) chromophore that changes with the extent of ionization, then a method involving UV spectroscopy can be used. This method involves measuring the UV spectrum of the compound as a function of pH. Mathematical analysis of the spectral shifts can then be used to determine the pK_a(s) of the compound. This method is most suitable for compounds where the ionizing group is close to or actually within an aromatic ring, which usually results in large UV shifts upon ionization. The UV method requires only 1 mg of compound, and the potentiometric method around 3 mg of compound.

Another method of determining pK_a is the pH indicator titration described by Kong et al. (2007). This appears to be quite a novel approach insofar that it utilizes a universal indicator solution with spectrophotometric detection for the determination of the pK_a instead of a pH electrode. The method works by calculating the pH from the indicator spectra in the visible region and then obtaining the spectra in the UV. Favorable results were obtained from a test set of five compounds.

The screening of pK_as can be carried out by using an instrumentation known as good laboratory practice pK_a (GLpK_a), so called because it conforms to the criteria laid down for instruments performing analyzes to the code of GLP. However, one of the limitations of this technique is that a solution concentration of at least 5×10^{-4} M is needed for the pK_a to be calculated from the amount of titrant versus pH data. Alternatively, the UV method appears to work at lower concentrations ($<10^{-5}$ M) using diode array detection. It should be noted, however, that some ionizable groups do not show great changes in their UV-absorption spectra when the pH changes.

High-throughput pK_a measurements were the subject of a paper by Box et al. (2003). They described a system whereby the pK_a of a compound could be determined in four minutes. Like many high-throughput systems, the determinations were conducted in 96-well plates using 10-mM DMSO solutions, which were diluted with water. These solutions were then injected into a gradient that contains a mixture of weak acids and bases, formulated to give a linear pH gradient. Determination of the pK_a is via the change in UV absorbance at multiple wavelengths as a function of pH.

Recent developments for the determination water-insoluble compounds include GLpK_a + D-PAS, and to deal with the ever-increasing numbers of compounds, the Sirius ProfilerSGA (spectral gradient analysis) instrument for high-throughput applications has been introduced. As noted earlier, to overcome the low solubility exhibited by modern CDs, pK_a measurements are carried out in, for example, methanol-water mixtures. However, to overcome extreme solubility limitations of some compounds, a ternary solvent system has been developed (Volgyi et al., 2007). This medium consists of methanol, dioxane, and acetonitrile in equal proportions, which appears to have a good balance of properties and was able to solubilize a wide range (50) of compounds (Box et al. 2006, 2007).

Wan et al. (2003) have reported a HTS method for pK_a values based on pressure-assisted capillary electrophoresis and mass spectrometry.

Prediction of pK_a

The pK_a of a compound may be estimated using a number of software packages, for example, PALLAS, MARVIN, ACDpK_a, and SPARC (Meloun and Bordovská, 2007). These authors looked at the accuracy of the pK_a data generated by these packages and concluded that ACDpK_a provided the most accurate prediction of this value. In addition, ACDpK_a also contains a large database of measured pK_a data.

The Partition and Distribution Coefficients

It has been shown that many biological phenomena can be correlated with the partition coefficient (log P), such that QSARs can be deduced. These include solubility, absorption potential, membrane permeability, plasma protein binding, volume of distribution, and renal and hepatic clearance. The lipophilicity of an organic compound is usually described in terms of a partition coefficient, log P, which can be defined as the ratio of the concentration of the unionized compound, at equilibrium, between organic and aqueous phases (equation 3).

$$\log P = \frac{[\text{unionized compound}]_{\text{org}}}{[\text{unionized compound}]_{\text{aq}}} \tag{3}$$

It is worth noting that this is a logarithmic scale, therefore, a log $P = 0$ means that the compound is equally soluble in water and the partitioning solvent. If the compound has a log $P = 5$, then the compound is 100,000 times more soluble in the partitioning solvent. A log $P = -2$ means that the compound is 100 times more soluble in water, that is, it is quite hydrophilic.

Log P values have been studied in approximately 100 organic liquid–water systems However, since it is virtually impossible to determine log P in a realistic biological medium, the octanol-water system has been widely adopted as a model of the lipid phase (Leo et al., 1971). While there has been much debate about the suitability of this system (Dearden et al., 1988), it is still the most widely used measure of compound lipophilicity in pharmaceutical studies. Octanol and water are immiscible when mixed, but some water does dissolve in octanol in a hydrated state. This hydrated state contains 16 octanol aggregates, with the hydroxyl head groups surrounded by trapped aqueous solution. Lipophilic (unionized) species dissolve in the aliphatic regions of the octanol, while ionized species (see later in the chapter) are drawn to the polar regions (Franks et al., 1993). The partitioning of solutes in different solvent systems has been reported by El-Tayar et al. (1991).

According to Lipinski (1997), log P values of less than 5 are best from a drug-like perspective. Generally compounds with log P values between 1 and 3 show good absorption, whereas those with log P values greater than 6 or less than 3 often have poor transport characteristics. Highly lipophilic molecules have a preference to reside in the lipophilic regions of membranes, and very polar compounds show poor bioavailability because of their inability to penetrate membrane barriers. Thus, there is a parabolic relationship between log P and drug transport such that CDs that exhibit a balance between these two properties will probably show the best oral bioavailability. However, it has been noted that lipophilicity (and molecular weight) increases with time from LG and through LO and accounts for the generic value of log $P = 3$ stipulated for candidates at the LG stage (Davis et al., 2005). Overall, however, Leeson and Davis (2004) have shown that the log P of compounds has not changed significantly when they reviewed the data for oral compounds gathered over a number of years.

By using data gleaned from the literature, Leeson and Springthorpe (2007) have designated lipophilicity as the most important drug-like physical property, and any increase in this parameter will lead to a lack of selectivity and an increase in attrition. Indeed, they cautioned that although larger lipophilic compounds may exhibit greater binding affinity, they may also show greater binding to, for example, the human ether-a-go-go related gene (HERG) ion channel or cause tissue toxicity by the promotion of cellular phospholipidosis. Thus, by lowering the lipophilicity of compounds, they argue that the attrition rate would be reduced and that even a 5% improvement in attrition would result in a doubling of the number of new medicines.

The partition coefficient refers to the intrinsic lipophilicity of the drug in the context of the equilibrium of unionized drug between the aqueous and organic phases. However, if the drug has more than one ionization center, the distribution of species present will depend on the pH. The concentration of the ionized drug in the aqueous phase will therefore have an effect on the overall observed partition coefficient. This leads to the definition of the distribution coefficient (log D) of a compound, which takes into account the dissociation of weak acids and bases. For a weak acid this is defined by equation (4).

$$D = \frac{[\text{HA}]_{\text{org}}}{[\text{HA}]_{\text{aq}} + [\text{A}^-]_{\text{aq}}} \qquad (4)$$

It can be seen that combining this equation with equation (1) gives an expression relating the distribution to the intrinsic lipophilicity (log P), the pK_a of the molecule, and the pH of the aqueous phase (equation 5).

$$\log\left(\frac{P}{D-1}\right) = \text{pH} - \text{p}K_a \qquad \text{for acids}$$

$$\log\left(\frac{P}{D-1}\right) = \text{p}K_a - \text{pH} \qquad \text{for bases}$$

$$(5)$$

Figure 1 shows the effect of ionization on the partitioning of a proton pump inhibitor compound. This compound has a log P of 3.82 and three pK_a values, that is, ≤ 1, 5.26, and 8.63. At low pH, both the benzimidazole and diethylamine nitrogens are protonated, and hence the tendency of the compound is to reside in the aqueous phase. As the pH increases,

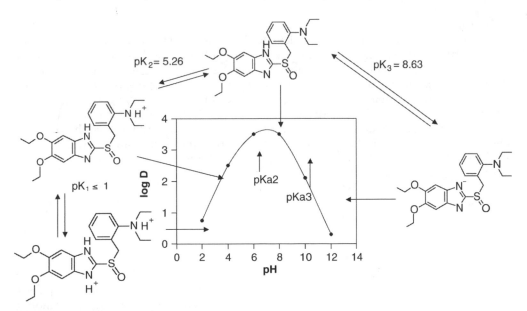

Figure 1 Ionization and partitioning scheme for a proton pump inhibitor.

deprotonation of the protonated nitrogen of the benzimidazole takes place, and as the compound is less ionized, the compound resides more in the octanol phase. At neutral pH, deprotonation of the diethylamine nitrogen renders the molecule neutral and hence its lipophilicity is a maximum. A further increase in the pH results in deprotonation of the second nitrogen to form an anion, which, being ionized, is more hydrophilic and hence causes a decrease in log D. As a consequence of the pH effect on the log P value of a compound, Bhal et al. (2008) have argued that log D is a better descriptor in the context of Lipinski's rule, since it more physiologically relevant, that is, it takes into account the ionizable nature of many pharmaceutical molecules.

Methods for Determining Log P and Log D
The most common technique for determining partition and distribution coefficients is the shake-flask method. In this method, the compound is equilibrated with an octanol-aqueous buffer mixture for 30 minutes, and the resulting emulsion is centrifuged to separate the two constituent phases. Once separated, the concentration of each layer is determined by high-performance liquid chromatography (HPLC) and log D/log P is calculated. In experimental conditions, the value of the partition coefficient obtained from this type of experiment is affected by such factors as temperature, insufficient mutual phase saturation, pH, buffer ions and their concentration, as well as the nature of the solvents used and solute examined (Dearden and Bresnen, 1988). Bearing in mind the drive to determine the maximum amount of information from the minimum quantity of compound, high-throughput techniques are now employed to determine these parameters. For example, Wilson et al. (2001) have reported a high-throughput log D determination methodology using liquid chromatography-mass spectrometry (LC-MS) of DMSO solutions (5 µL) on a microtiter plate. Other high-throughput procedures for lipophilicity measurements include immobilized artificial membranes (Barbeto et al., 2004; Faller et al., 2005) and the PAMPA (parallel artificial membrane permeability assays) techniques (Ottaviani et al., 2008).

Valkó (2007) reviewed HPLC techniques that have been used to determine log P values and concluded that retention data obtained from a C_{18} column gave reasonable results for neutral molecules, but was less good for ionizable compounds. Log D_{mem} is another way of measuring the lipophilicity of a compound (Austin et al., 1995). In this technique the compound is partitioned into liposomes and the log D is calculated; however, it is fair to say that it is much less frequently used than the octanol-water partitioning systems already described.

Prediction of Log P and Log D
Computer methods have been devised to calculate these values. The first approach is where the molecule is broken down into fragments of known lipophilicity, and the log P is calculated using various computer routines. Alternatively, there are atom-based methods, and the lipophilicity is calculated by summing the atom-type values. Although discrepancies do occur between measured and calculated log Ps (clog Ps), agreement is reasonably good and has the advantage that it does not physically require any compound and can be a useful starting place for these types of measurements. Machatha and Yalkowsky (2005) have compared the partition coefficients, calculated using the ClogP®, ACDlogP, and KowWin® programs, and concluded that the ClogP program gave the most accurate predicted value for log P. With regard to the calculation of log D, Tetko and Bruneau (2004) have described the application of ALOGPS to predict the 1-octanol/water distribution coefficients, log P, and log D, using the AstraZeneca in-house database. A notable feature of this program was the use of an associative neural network (ANN) in the prediction process.

INITIAL SOLUBILITY INVESTIGATIONS

The solubility of a CD may be the critical factor determining its usefulness, since aqueous solubility dictates the amount of compound that will dissolve and, therefore, the amount available for absorption (Bhattachar et al., 2006). If a compound has a low aqueous solubility, it may be subject to dissolution rate-limited absorption within the GI residence time. The importance of solubility, in biopharmaceutical terms, has been highlighted by its use in the biopharmaceutics classification system (BCS) described by Amidon et al. (1995). In this system, compounds are defined in terms of combinations of their solubility and permeability, for example, high solubility and high permeability or low solubility and high permeability. High solubility is defined as the highest dose strength that is soluble in 250 mL or less of aqueous media across the physiological pH range. Poorly soluble drugs can be defined as those with an aqueous solubility of less than 100 μg/mL. If a drug is poorly soluble, then it will only slowly dissolve, perhaps leading to incomplete absorption (Hörter and Dressman, 1997). For further details, the reader may refer to a study by Stegmann et al. (2007) that discusses the importance of solubility in the drug discovery and development arenas.

From a physicochemical perspective, James (1986) has provided some general rules regarding solubility:

1. Electrolytes dissolve in conducting solvents.
2. Solutes containing hydrogen capable of forming hydrogen bonds (H-bonds) dissolve in solvents capable of accepting H-bonds and vice versa.
3. Solutes having significant dipole moments dissolve in solvents having significant dipole moments.
4. Solutes with low or zero dipole moments dissolve in solvents with low or zero dipole moments.

The United States Pharmacopeia (USP) (Table 3) gives the following definitions of solubility (extended by Stegmann et al., 2007).

Solvents can be classed into various classes, and Table 4 gives some examples (Chasette, 1985).

For a Lewis acid, the molecule must be electron deficient and, in particular, contain an atom bearing only a sextet of electrons. A Lewis base is where the molecule must have an electron pair for sharing.

Table 3 Solubility Definitions

Descriptive term	Parts of solvent required for 1 part of solute	Solubility range (mg/mL)	Solubility assigned (mg/mL)
Very soluble	<1	>1000	1000
Freely soluble	1–10	100–1000	100
Soluble	10–30	33–100	33
Sparingly soluble	30–100	10–33	10
Slightly soluble	100–1000	1–10	1
Very slightly soluble	1000–10,000	0.1–1	0.1
Practically insoluble or insoluble	≥10,000	<0.1	0.01

Source: From Stegmann et al., 2007 with permission from Elsevier.

Table 4 Classification of Solvents

Dipolar aprotic	Protic	Lewis basic	Lewis acidic	Aromatic	Nonpolar
DMF	Water	Acetone	Chloroform	Toluene	Heptane
DMSO	Ethanol	THF	Dichloromethane-methane	*p*-Xylene	Hexanes
N-Methyl-2-pyrolidinone	Methanol	Ethyl acetate		Pyridine	Cyclohexane
Acetonitrile	*n*-Butanol	2-Pentanone		Anisole	
	Acetic acid	Methyl-*t*-butyl ether		Ethylbenzene	
	n-Propanol	Butyl acetate			
	2-Propanol				

Abbreviations: DMF, dimethyl formamide; DMSO, dimethylsulfoxide; THF, tetrahydrofuran.

The properties of solvents can be classified further. For example, Gu et al. (2004) have classified 96 solvents using a number of physicochemical parameters, that is, H-bond acceptor and donor propensity, polarity, dipole moment, dielectric constant, viscosity, surface tension, and cohesive energy density. By using a cluster statistical analysis method, they classified the solvents into 15 groups. Similarly, Xu and Redman-Furey (2007) used a clustering principal components analysis (PCA) technique (on 17 different solvent descriptors) of 57 class 2 and class 3 International Council of Harmonization (ICH) solvents. These were reduced to a set of 20 clusters, with the goal of producing an efficient solid-state screening solvent system.

Solubility Prediction

As is the case with log P, the prediction of solubility is of obvious interest, and various approaches to this problem have been reported by, for example, Chen and Song (2004), Faller and Ertl (2007), and Duchowicz et al. (2007). Faller and Ertl (2007) classified the various solubility prediction methods available as:

1. Fragment-based models
2. Models based on log P
3. Models based on solvation properties
4. Hybrid models

In their paper they posed a very pertinent question, "When can one trust the computed value?" They argued with a variety of physicochemical reasons that since the accuracy of a high-quality solubility assay is within 0.6 log units, it was unrealistic for any computed value to be more accurate than 0.5 log units or a factor of 3 to 5. More recently, Palmer et al. (2008) have adopted an ab initio thermodynamic approach to solubility prediction, and Tsung et al. (2008) have described the prediction of solubility using the nonrandom segment activity coefficient model (NRTL-SAC) and COSMO-SAC methods. Kokitkar et al. (2008) used the NTRL-SAC model for exploring solvent systems for crystallization from which a solvent or mixture of solvents are chosen to carry out the process. While the predicted data are not an exact match to experimental values, they are sufficiently accurate to allow the investigating scientist to move in a particular direction.

Solubility of a compound in various solvents is also important from a crystallization process point of view and polymorphism screening. By using data extracted from the Cambridge Structural Database (CSD), Hosokawa et al. (2005) attempted to predict the solvents that would be suitable for the crystallization of small molecules. Data collected from 6397 compounds and 15 single solvents that were used to obtain single crystals, were assessed by chemometric analysis to show that ethanol was the best solvent for crystallization (1328 compounds) followed by methanol (1030 compounds).

Phase Solubility Analysis

Methods used for the estimation of the aqueous solubility of organic compounds have been presented in a book by Yalkowsky and Banerjee (1992). Solubilities can also be estimated by visual observation as follows. The solubility of a compound is initially determined by weighing out 10 mg (or other suitable amount) of the compound. To this is added 10 µL of the solvent of interest. If the compound does not dissolve, a further 40 µL of solvent is added and its effect noted. Successive amounts of the solvent are then added until the compound is observed to dissolve. This procedure should give an approximate value of the solubility.

It should be noted that this is a crude method of solubility determination and takes no account of the kinetic aspects of the dissolution processes involved in solubility measurements. To more accurately determine the concentration of a saturated solution of a compound, the following procedure can be used. A known volume of the solvent, water or buffer, is pipetted into a vial and the compound of interest is added until saturation is observed to occur. The solution is then stirred or shaken for approximately one hour at the desired temperature. If the compound dissolves, then more compound is added and the experiment restarted. It is recommended that the experiment is conducted at least overnight, but longer time periods may be required if the compound has a very low solubility, for example, saturation of morphine in water at 35°C was obtained only after approximately 48 hours (Roy and Flynn, 1989).

Depending on the amount of compound available, replicate experiments should be carried out. After stirring or shaking, the solvent should be separated from the suspension by centrifugation or filtration using polytetrafluoroethylene (PTFE) filters. The filtrate is then assayed preferably by HPLC, although UV-visible spectroscopy can also be used to determine the solubility, if compound stability or impurities are not an issue. This is termed the thermodynamic solubility. It may also be useful to measure the pH of the filtrate if the experiment is conducted in water, and to analyze any undissolved material by differential scanning calorimetry (DSC) or X-ray powder diffraction (XRPD) to detect any phase changes that may have occurred during the course of the experiment.

For HTS of solubilities, where the amount of compound may be severely restricted, reporting kinetic solubilities may be adequate. In this respect Quarterman et al. (1998) have described a technique based on a 96-well microtiter technique with an integral nephelometer. The process of determining kinetic solubilities by this method was summarized as follows. Aliquots of the aqueous solution are placed in the microtiter wells, to which are added 1 µL of the compounds in DMSO and the plate is shaken. The turbidity of the solutions is then measured using the nephelometer; this process is repeated up to 10 times. If turbity is detected in a cell, the experiment is terminated, that is, solution additions are stopped and the solutions ranked in terms of number of additions that caused turbidity. The authors emphasized, however, that the purpose of this experiment is to rank the compounds in terms of their solubility and not to give a precise measure of a compound's solubility. A high-throughput solubility measurement in the drug discovery and development arena was the subject of a review by Alsenz and Kansy (2007).

Because of the differences in melting point and other characteristics of polymorphs, solubility differences are often observed. Usually the most stable form of the compound has the lowest solubility in any solvent. It has already been noted that solids can undergo phase changes by way of the solution phase (Davey et al., 1986). When the solvent is in contact with the metastable phase, it dissolves and the stable phase nucleates and grows from solution. So it is always worth slurrying a compound and assessing the solid phase to determine whether a solution-mediated phase transformation to the stable phase has taken place.

If solubility of a compound is accompanied by degradation, the quotation of a solubility figure is problematic. In this case, it is preferable to quote a solubility figure, but with the caveat that a specified amount of degradation was found. Obviously, large amounts of degradation will render the solubility value meaningless. A technique to estimate the water solubility of a number of water-unstable prodrugs of 5-fluorouracil has been reported by Beall et al. (1993).

Many CDs are ionizable organic compounds, and thus there are a number of parameters that will determine the solubility of a compound, for example, molecular size and substituent groups on the molecule, degree of ionization, ionic strength, salt form, temperature, crystal properties, and complexation.

Effect of Molecular Size on Solubility

Because of interactions between the nonpolar groups and water, large organic molecules have a smaller aqueous solubility than smaller molecules, that is, it is dependent on the number of solvent molecules that can pack around the solute molecule (James, 1986). Figure 2 shows the effect of molecular weight on the solubility of some amino acids in water (data taken from James, 1986).

Effect of Ionization on Solubility

The solubility of a compound, at a given pH, is a function of the solubility of the ionized form and the limiting solubility of the neutral molecule. This gives rise to equations (6) and (7), which describe the relationship between the intrinsic solubility of the free acid or base S_0, pK_a, and pH.

$$S = [HA] + [A^-] \qquad \text{for acids} \tag{6}$$

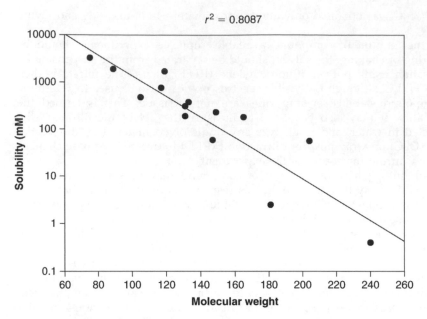

$r^2 = 0.8087$

Figure 2 Solubility of amino acids in water as a function of molecular weight. *Source*: From Ref. James, 1986.

$$S = [B] + [BH^+] \qquad \text{for bases} \tag{7}$$

By setting $S_0 = [HA]$ for acids or $[B]$ for bases and recalling our definition of the ionization constant, it follows that for weak acids with only one ionization center, the change in solubility with respect to pH is given by the Henderson–Hasselbach equation (equation 8).

$$S = S_0\left(1 + 10^{pH-pK_a}\right) \tag{8}$$

Thus, it is possible to calculate the solubility of a compound at any pH if the intrinsic solubility of the free acid or base is known along with its pK_a.

A weak acid with two ionizable acid groups show a more dramatic increase in solubility with respect to pH as described by equation (9) (Zimmerman, 1986a,b).

$$S = S_0\left\{1 + \frac{K_{a1}}{[H^+]} + \frac{K_{a1}K_{a2}}{[H^+]^2}\right\}$$

or

$$S = S_0(1 + 10^{pH-pK_{a1}} + 10^{2pH-pK_{a1}+pK_{a2}}) \tag{9}$$

Figure 3 shows the pH-solubility profile of the nedocromil sodium, demonstrating that the solubility reaches a plateau at approximately pH 5. This is the limiting solubility (S^*) of the dianion under these experimental conditions.

The experimentally determined pH-solubility curve for remacemide hydrochloride is shown in Figure 4. The observed behavior can be attributed to a number of physical-chemical phenomena (Serajuddin and Mufson, 1985). For example, at low pH the solubility is suppressed because of the common ion effect. However, the rise in solubility at pH values greater than 5 is more difficult to explain. In this case, supersaturation due to self-association appears to be the most likely explanation (Ledwidge and Corrigan, 1998).

Using conventional techniques, it is unlikely that a complete solubility profile can be generated in the prenomination phase because of a lack of compound. However, if the intrinsic solubility of the free base or acid is known, then the solubility can be calculated at any pH.

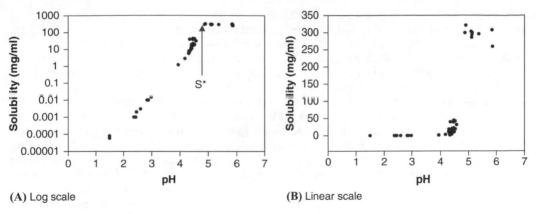

(A) Log scale   (B) Linear scale

Figure 3   The pH-solubility curve of nedocromil sodium.

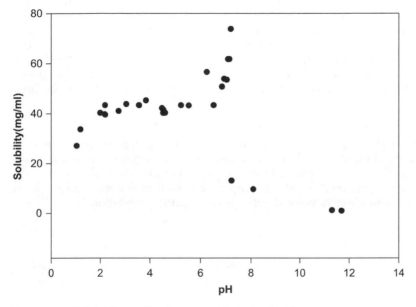

Figure 4   pH-Solubility profile of remacemide hydrochloride.

      In the case of amphoteric compounds, equation (10) is relevant at pHs below the isoelectric point and equation (11) above the isoelectric point.

$$pH - pK_a = \log\left(\frac{S - S_0}{S_0}\right) \text{ for weak acids} \tag{10}$$

$$pH - pK_a = \log\left(\frac{S_0}{S_0 - S}\right) \text{ for weak bases} \tag{11}$$

      An instrument for determining intrinsic solubility and solubility pH profiles has been introduced. Known as pSOL^{TM}, it claims that with as little as 0.1 mg a complete solubility profile can be derived (Avdeef et al., 2000). Stuart and Box (2005) have introduced a new technique for determining the intrinsic solubility of weak acids and bases, which they have termed "chasing equilibrium." Utilizing the GLpK_a titrator with a D-PAS spectrometer (marketed by Sirius Analytical Instruments Ltd., Forest Row, East Sussex, U.K.), the compound under investigation is taken into solution at a pH where it is dissolved. The pH is then adjusted to precipitate the neutral form of the compound. The pH is then readjusted to dissolve and precipitate the compound over and over again until equilibrium is attained. The authors claim that this methodology can operate down to 2 to 5 mg in 10 mL. By using diclofenac as a typical example of a monoprotic acid (pK_a 3.99), they performed 10 alternating pH titrations, changing the pH gradient eight times, and found good agreement with the published equilibrium solubility figure (0.87 cf. 0.82 mg/mL). Another potential advantage is the speed of the determination, whereby this technique actively seeks the equilibrium solubility compared to a conventional experiment, which can take many hours for equilibrium to be established.

Glomme et al. (2005) have described a miniaturized shake-flask methodology for solubility measurement, which they compared to those obtained from acid/base titrations and computationally derived values. They found that it gave comparable results to those obtained from potentiometric titrations; however, one significant advantage of this way of determining solubility was that it was applicable to all types of compounds (not just weak acids and bases) in a range solvent systems. Another type of miniaturized instrument, based on a multichannel cartridge pump, filter, and HPLC analysis, for solubility measurement has been reported by Chen and Venkatesh (2004). They claimed that with as little as 1 mg of compound they could determine the entire pH-solubility profile.

Bergström et al. (2005) have studied the applicability of the Henderson–Hasselbach (equation 8) solubility-pH relationship of a range of amines in divalent buffer solutions. From this investigation, they showed that the Henderson–Hasselbach equation was only useful as a first estimate in these calculations. They concluded that significant error arose because of the neglect of the solubility product of the charged molecule and the phosphate ion used to buffer the solution. The net result of this inaccuracy would then be the error propagation in programs for the calculation of other physicochemical properties, for example, log P and permeability.

Impact of Additives

Additives may increase or decrease the solubility of a solute in a given solvent. Salts that increase the solubility are said to "salt in" the solute, and those that decrease the solubility are said to "salt out" the solute. The effect of the additive depends very much on the influence it has on the structure of the water or on its ability to compete with solvent water molecules. Both effects are described by the empirically derived Setschenow equation (equation 12).

$$\log \frac{S_0}{S} = kM \tag{12}$$

where S_0 is the solubility of the nonelectrolyte in pure water, S the solubility of the nonelectrolyte in the salt solution, M the concentration of the salt, and k the salting out constant, which is equal to $0.217/S_0$ at low concentrations of added salt.

Another aspect of the effect of electrolytes on the solubility of a salt is the concept of the solubility product for poorly soluble substances. The experimental consequences of this phenomenon is that if the concentration of a common ion is high, then the other ion must become low in a saturated solution of the substance, that is, precipitation will occur. Conversely, the effect of foreign ions on the solubility of sparingly soluble salts is just the opposite, and the solubility increases. This is the so-called salt effect.

Setchenow (salting out) constants have been determined for eight hydrochloride salts of some α-adrenergic agonists and β-adregenic agonist/blocker drugs (Thomas and Rubino, 1996). The constant was calculated by determining the solubility of the salts in sodium chloride water, and the results showed that they were greatest for those with the lowest aqueous solubility and highest melting point. In addition, the number of aromatic rings and aromatic ring substituents appeared to contribute to the values of the salting out constants. Larsen et al. (2007) have investigated the use of the common ion effect as a means to extend the release of bupivacaine from mixed salt suspensions.

Impact of Temperature

Since dissolution is usually an endothermic process, increasing solubility of solids with a rise in temperature is the general rule. Therefore, many investigations of solubility plotted as a function of temperature show a rise. For example, Gracin and Rasmuson (2002) investigated the solubilities of phenylacetic acid, *p*-hydroxyphenylacetic acid, *p*-aminophenylacetic acid, *p*-hydroxybenzoic acid, and ibuprofen in a range of solvents as a function of temperature. In this study, ibuprofen reported a general increase in solubility with increasing temperature, with high solubilities being recorded in the polar solvents, methanol, and ethanol. However, there are exceptions, for example, the solubility of hexamethylenetetramine in water decreases with increasing temperature (Blanco et al., 2006). Of course, binary mixtures of solvents can be employed; however, it is worth pointing out that many compounds show a parabolic relationship with respect to solvent composition. For example, Granberg and Rasmuson (2000) have reported the solubility behavior of paracetamol in mixtures of water and acetone as well as in data for paracetamol in water, ethanol, and toluene. Since cooling crystallization is a common method regarding the production of compounds, knowledge of the solubility with respect to temperature is essential.

The theoretical solubility of a compound may be calculated by the ideal solubility equation (Qing-Zhu et al., 2006), using the enthalpy of melting, ΔH_{fus}, and melting temperature, T_m, using equation (13).

$$\ln(x_a) = \frac{\Delta H_{fus}}{R}\left(\frac{1}{T_m} - \frac{1}{T}\right) \tag{13}$$

Williams-Seton et al. (1999) have discussed solvent-solute interactions with regard to crystallization. By comparing the theoretical solubility-temperature curve calculated from equation (13) with data obtained for saccharin in ethanol and acetone, they hypothesized that in acetone solutions the saccharin molecules were monomers; however, in ethanol they were associated, like in the crystal structure, as dimers via an amide H-bond. Furthermore, they correlated the surface chemistry of crystals grown from ethanol and acetone, which appeared to support their theory of the self-association of the molecules in ethanol and not in acetone. In this situation, ethanol would not be recommended as a suitable solvent for a cooling crystallization because of its poor solubility-temperature relationship. On the other hand, ethanol may be a potential antisolvent and may be considered for a "drown out" crystallization.

As another example, the solubility of cefotaxime sodium with respect to temperature in a range of organic solvents of varying polarity has been studied by Pardillo-Fontdevila et al. (1998). As might be expected for a salt, cefotaxime was not found in hexane, ethyl acetate, dichloromethane, and diethyl ether in the 5°C to 40°C temperature range. The solubility in the other solvents, that is, methanol, acetone, and ethanol was described by the van't Hoff equation shown below (equation 14):

$$\ln C_s(g/100\,g\,\text{solvent}) = \alpha + \frac{\beta}{T(K)} \tag{14}$$

where C_s is the solubility of cefotaxime and T the temperature. The slope β yields the heat of solution. Zhu (2001) has reported the solubilities of the disodium salt hemiheptahydrate of ceftriaxone in water and ethanol at 10°C, 20°C, and 30°C. As expected, the solubility of this compound increased with the increase in temperature and decreased as the proportion of ethanol increased.

INITIAL STABILITY INVESTIGATIONS

Knowledge about the chemical and physical stability of a CD in the solid and liquid state is extremely important in drug development for a number of reasons. In the longer term, the stability of the formulation will dictate the shelf life of the marketed product; however, to achieve this formulation, careful preformulation work will have characterized the compound such that a rational choice of conditions and excipients are available to the formulation team. The ICH specifies the amount of impurities allowed from product storage, and for most drugs the allowable levels of a single impurity permissible without toxicological cover is much less than 1%. In early development, accelerated stability therefore needs to be undertaken to assess how the CDs will stand up to a longer term (Waterman et al., 2005).

CDs being evaluated for development are often one of a series of related compounds that may have similar chemical properties, that is, similar paths of degradation may be deduced. However, this rarely tells us the rate at which they will decompose, which is of more importance in pharmaceutical development terms. To elucidate their stability with respect to, for example, temperature, pH, light, and oxygen, a number of experiments need to be performed. The major objectives of preformulation team are therefore to (1) identify conditions to which the compound is sensitive and (2) identify degradation profiles under these conditions.

The main routes of drug degradation in solution are via hydrolysis, oxidation, or photochemical means. In their book, Connors et al. (1986) have dealt with the physical chemistry involved in the kinetic analysis of degradation of pharmaceuticals very well, and the reader is referred there for a detailed discussion.

Although hydrolysis and oxidation constitute the main mechanisms by which drugs can decompose, racemization is another way in which the compound can change in solution. For example, Yuchun et al. (2000) reported the kinetics of the base-catalyzed racemization of ibuprofen enantiomers. Although ibuprofen is highly resistant to racemization in acids, it will racemize in basic solutions through a keto-enol mechanism.

Solution Stability

Hydrolysis

Mechanistically, hydrolysis takes place in two stages. In the first instance, a nucleophile, such as water or the OH^- ion adds to, for example, an acyl carbon to form an intermediate from which the leaving group then breaks away. The structure of the compound will affect the rate at which this reaction takes place, and the stronger the leaving conjugate acid, the faster the degradation reaction will take place.

Degradation by hydrolysis is affected by a number of factors, of which solution pH, buffer salts, and ionic strength are the most important. In addition, the presence of cosolvents, complexing agents, and surfactants can also affect this type of degradation.

As noted, solution pH is one of major determinants of the stability of a compound. Hydroxyl ions are stronger nucleophiles than water, thus degradation reactions are usually faster in alkaline solutions than in water, that is, OH^- ions catalyze the reaction. In solutions of low pH, H^+ can also catalyze hydrolysis reactions. In this case, catalysis by H^+ and OH^- is termed specific acid base catalysis. Of course, H^+ and OH^- ions are not the only ions that may be present during an experiment or in a formulation. It is well known that buffer ions such as acetate or citrate can catalyze degradation, and in this case the effect is known as general acid-base degradation. Therefore, although it is prudent to adjust the pH to the desired value to optimize stability, this should always be done with the minimum concentration necessary.

Stewart and Tucker (1985) provide a useful, simple guide to hydrolysis where the mechanism of hydrolysis is discussed. Table 5 shows some examples of the functional groups that undergo hydrolysis.

Oxidation

The second most common way a compound can decompose in solution is via oxidation. Reduction/oxidation (redox) reactions involve one of the following processes: (1) transfer of

Table 5 Examples of Classes of Drugs That are Subject to Hydrolysis

Class	Example
Ester	Aspirin
Thiol ester	Spirolactone
Amide	Chloramphenicol
Sulfonamide	Sulfapyrazine
Imide	Phenobarbitone
Lactam	Methicillin
Lactone	Spirolactone
HalogenatedAliphatic	Chlorambucil

Source: From Stewart and Tucker (1985), reproduced with permission.

oxygen or hydrogen atoms or (2) transfer of electrons. Oxidation is promoted by the presence of oxygen, and the reaction can be initiated by the action of heat, light, or trace metal ions that produce organic free radicals. These radicals propagate the oxidation reaction that proceeds until inhibitors destroy them or by side reactions that eventually break the chain. A typical oxidation sequence is that shown by dopamine Mayers and Jeneke (1993). To test whether a compound is sensitive to oxygen, simply bubble air through the solution, or add hydrogen peroxide, and assess the amount of degradation that takes place.

Kinetics of Degradation

Essentially we must determine the amount of the compound remaining with respect to time under the conditions of interest. Alternatively, the appearance of degradation product could also be used to monitor the reaction kinetics.

Thus, the rate of a reaction can be defined as the rate of change of concentration of one of the reactants or products.

For a simple drug decomposition, therefore, the following situation holds

Drug → product(s)

The concentration of the compound will decrease with time; equation (15) relating to these quantities is as follows:

$$-\frac{d[D]}{dt} = k[D]^n \tag{15}$$

where k is the rate constant for the reaction at that particular temperature and n is the reaction order, which is the dependence of the rate on the reactant concentrations.

Zero-Order Reactions

In this case, the rate of reaction is independent of concentration and does not change (with time) until the reactant has been consumed (equation 16).

$$\text{Rate} = -\frac{d[D]}{dt} = k_0 \tag{16}$$

The final form of the zero-order equation is given by equation (17).

$$[D]_t = [D]_0 - k_0 t \tag{17}$$

Therefore, if we plot the concentration $[D]_0$ = initial and $[D]_t$ = at time t, directly as a function of time, the slope is equal to the rate constant, k_0, for this reaction. Moreover, the time required for any specific amount of reactant to disappear is proportional to the initial amount present. Many reactions in the solid state or in suspensions undergo decomposition by zero-order kinetics.

First-Order Reactions

In first-order reactions, the rate of reaction decreases with time as the concentration of the reactant decreases, according to equation (18),

$$\text{Rate} = -\frac{d[D]}{dt} = k_1[D] \tag{18}$$

The final form of the first-order equation is give by equation (19),

$$\log_{10}[D] = \log_{10}[D_0] - \frac{k_1}{2.303} \tag{19}$$

Therefore, if the logarithm of the concentration of the compound (for convenience, % log remaining is often used) is plotted against time, a line with slope equal to $-k_1/2.303$ is obtained, where k is known as the rate constant. Further manipulation of the rate equation yields the expression for the half-life [time taken for the concentration to fall to half its initial value and half in concentration thereafter (equation 20)]. The unit of the rate constant is time^{-1}.

$$t_{1/2} = \frac{0.693}{k_1} \tag{20}$$

It should be noted that the half-life of the reaction is independent of the initial concentration.

Many hydrolysis reactions technically follow second-order kinetics, but since water is present in a large excess, there is only a negligible change in its concentration with time. Thus, the rate is dependent only on the rate of decomposition of the drug in solution; this type of reaction is termed a pseudo–first order. Most compounds that degrade in solution follow this order. Second-order kinetics are observed when a reactant reacts with itself or when the reaction rate depends on the concentration of more than one reactant.

Temperature can affect reactions and, in general, an increase in temperature will increase the rate of reaction. The effect of temperature on reaction is described by the Arrhenius relationship (equation 21).

$$\log k = \log A - \frac{E_a}{2.303RT} \tag{21}$$

where k is the observed pseudo–first-order rate constant for the reaction, A is a constant, and E_a is the observed energy of activation of the reaction. R is the gas constant (8.314 J/mol K).

Because of insufficient drug, a complete degradation profile will probably not be possible during prenomination studies, but it should be possible to assess the stability of the CD at a few pHs (acid, alkali, and neutral) to establish the approximate stability of the compound with respect to hydrolysis. To accelerate the reaction, temperature elevation will probably be necessary to generate the data. Although it is difficult assign a definite temperature for these studies, 50°C to 90°C in the first instance is a reasonable compromise; exposure to light may also be undertaken. This should be followed by extrapolation via the Arrhenius equation to 25°C. Hydrolytic stability of greater than 100 days at 25°C should be taken as a goal of these studies. In CD selection, if all other factors are equal, the compound that is most stable should be the one taken forward into development.

THE ORGANIC SOLID STATE

Solid phases or molecular solids are defined in thermodynamic terms as states of matter that are uniform throughout in chemical composition and also in physical state (Wunderlich, 1999). Molecular solids can exist as crystalline or noncrystalline (amorphous) phases depending on the extent of three-dimensional order and the relative thermodynamic stability hierarchy. Crystalline states can be described as a periodic array of molecules within a three-dimensional framework. Whereas noncrystalline materials (as will be described later in the chapter) lack significant three-dimensional order, but may exhibit lower-dimensional short-range order. Gavazotti (2007) has set a range of criteria by which he judges the solid state of organic compounds. In this paper, a "crystal proper" is defined as one in which the molecule is repeated to 10,000 to 100,000 times its size through a set of translationally periodic symmetry operations.

The crystalline state, as molecular crystals, is a class of solids that are composed of discrete molecules arranged in a structural framework. The structures of molecular crystals are influenced by both intramolecular and intermolecular interactions. Intramolecular forces determine molecular shape, which in turn contributes to the way the molecules pack in the crystal (Wright, 1995). Intermolecular forces are relatively weak, and thus their effect is largely short range. As a consequence of this short-range effect, diversity in the arrangement of molecules within the molecular crystals is brought about, which also gives rise to differences in properties and performance of the molecular crystals. Furthermore, a variation in spatial arrangement can give rise to the enhanced possibility of structural dynamics within molecular crystals, leading to a variation in performance and behavior of the resultant material. Thus, an understanding of molecular crystals, and in particular the intermolecular interactions driving the molecular packing within the structure, allows an understanding of the material properties.

Any change in the physical or spatial arrangement of the molecules or inclusion of other molecule types (to give a heterogeneous material) results in the formation of different phases termed polymorphs and hydrates/co-crystals, respectively. A significant interest in molecular crystals originates from the ability to use molecular level "crystal engineering" strategies to rationally design crystal packing to control specific physical properties (Ward et al., 1997). The crystal engineering approach utilizes additives and other molecules to direct the self-assembly of the parent molecules to give a desired solid-state motif. Thus, control or understanding of arrangements in molecular crystals leads to control or understanding of various physical properties. In addition to pharmaceuticals, molecular crystals cover a diverse range of materials used in dyes and speciality chemicals, conductors, nonlinear optical materials, and agrochemicals.

Crystalline States and Structural Assessment

Polymorphism and Related Phenomena

In 2002, Bernstein pointed out that structural diversity is present in almost every facet of nature, and crystal polymorphism is one manifestation of this diversity. Polymorphism, in a chemical sense, is a solid-state phenomenon where the crystal structures of a chemical entity are different, but correspond to identical liquid and vapor states (McCrone, 1965). A variation in crystal structure is brought about by differences in molecular packing and intermolecular interactions within the three-dimensional framework of the crystalline state. The way the molecules pack is defined in part by the molecular structure itself, and there is also the possibility of forming stable intermolecular interactions such as H-bonds, giving rise to structures with differences in density. Consequently, polymorphs will have different lattice energies, which in turn govern the physical properties and behaviors of the material (Pudipeddi and Serajuddin, 2005).

An understanding and control of this phenomenon is of paramount importance in the fields of crystal engineering or material selection, crucial to the pharmaceutical, chemical, food, and agrochemical industries. Figure 5 shows the various polymorphs of estrone (Busetta et al., 1973).

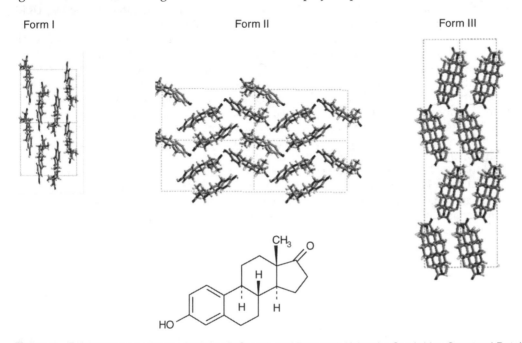

Figure 5 Polymorphs of estrone. *Source*: 3D Search and Research Using the Cambridge Structural Database, Allen, F. H. and Kennard O. Chemical Design Automation News, 8 (1) pp 1 & 31–37, 1993.

Polymorphism is a common phenomenon in small organic molecules, and the occurrence of polymorphs has been documented extensively (Borka and Haleblain, 1990; Byrn et al., 1999; Bernstein, 2002). Specifically, in the area of pharmaceutical material selection, polymorphs are selected on the basis of physical and chemical stability, behavior to processing and formulation, and biopharmaceutical properties as an assessment of in vivo performance. Knowledge of the relative behavior of the polymorphs with respect to the properties outlined above allows a rationalized selection. For instance, differences in solubility and dissolution rate between polymorphs can have a pronounced impact on the oral bioavailability (i.e., dissolution and absorption from the GI tract) of pharmaceuticals as exemplified by investigations of formulations of tolbutamide (Kimura et al., 1999). Other differences in properties also include thermodynamic and kinetic variations between polymorphs. Such differences encompass distinctions in reactivity involving both physical (e.g., involving interconversion of a metastable to a stable form) and chemical changes. Physical changes can occur in either the solid state or via a solution-mediated process, but are driven in accordance to Ostwald's law of stages (Threlfall; 2003), which states that a highly metastable form should transform to the most stable form via a series of thermodynamically driven phase transitions. Differences in chemical reactivity, such as those exemplified by the three physical forms of trans-2-ethoxy cinnamic acid (Cohen and Green, 1973), for which the α and β forms dimerize under UV irradiation, whereas the γ form gives no reaction, illustrate the importance of selecting a stable and robust polymorph.

McCrone stated, in 1965, that the number of polymorphs identified is directly proportional to the time and effort spent looking for them. Many approaches can be taken to induce polymorphic changes to explore its occurrence. These include solution-mediated transitions such as recrystallization and solution maturation studies (Cardew and Davey, 1985) and thermally induced (Giron, 1995) and mechanical/pressure-induced changes such as those exhibited by chlorpropamide (Wildfong et al., 2005). Other solvent-free methods of isolating polymorphs involve quenching from the molten liquid or gaseous state (sublimation experiments), as are used to isolate polymorphs of venlafaxine hydrochloride (Roy et al., 2005). The occurrence of polymorphism can also be explored using computational methodology (Beyer et al., 2001; Neumann 2008). The basis of these approaches involves in silico generation of all plausible crystal structures, which are subsequently ranked in order of calculated lattice energies. While the applicability has been demonstrated for small rigid structures, there are many limitations in the wider use of this approach—in particular for structures with significant conformational flexibility. Furthermore, the veracity of such approaches depends on the quality of the force fields used to model thermodynamic and kinetic properties satisfactorily (Gavezzotti, 2002), which renders the current approaches applicable only to a small subset of organic structures.

In addition to simple variations in hydrogen bonding, polymorphism can also be induced by conformational differences, that is, the existence of different conformers of the same molecule in different polymorphic modifications. When a molecule is conformationally flexible with a number of energetically accessible conformations (typically differing by <2 kcal/mol), then there is a potential that different crystallization conditions can lead to conformational polymorphism (Nangia, 2008). An example of conformational polymorphism is spiperone (Azibi et al., 1983), and the two conformers are shown in Figure 6.

Conformational polymorphism has also been reported for ritonavir (Bauer et al., 2001). Two polymorphs have been identified, where the conformers in each form sterically drive the three-dimensional packing and subsequent hydrogen-bonding motif. This in turn resulted in

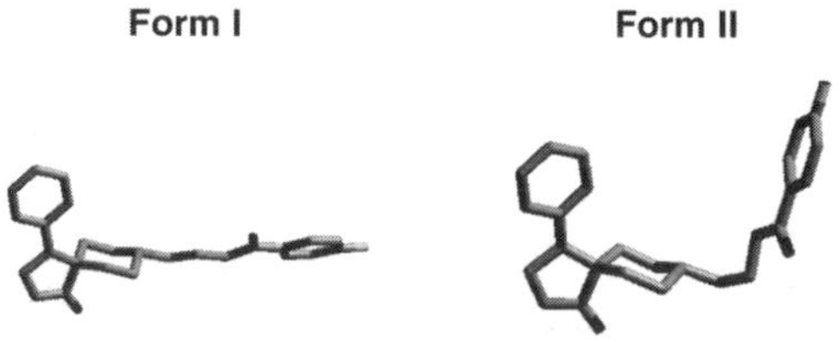

Form I   **Form II**

Figure 6 Conformers in spiperone forms I and II. *Source*: From Azibi et al., 1983.

stabilization of the lattice of each polymorph to a differing extent and hence significantly different solubility properties. Furthermore, conformational polymorphism can also result in diversity in bulk properties such as polychromism, as exemplified by the three main polymorphs of 5-XII (an aromatic carbonitrile), each of which exhibits a different color, red, yellow, and orange (Yu et al., 2000). The polymorphism in this case, and hence the different coloration, was directly due to a variation in the molecular conformation, giving rise to different three-dimensional packing (Yu, 2002).

Bhatt and Desiraju (2007) describe the case of polymorphism of omeprazole, which is due to tautomerism, whereby the crystalline phases of this molecule are solid solutions of the two tautomers existing in a continuous composition range. From a series of experiments where the compositions of the solid solutions were changed, the authors were able to identify the stable form. Furthermore, these investigations identified a number of questions regarding the classification of tautomers as polymorphism or different compounds. It was proposed that distinctions should be made in terms of a structural landscape, which includes a number of solvated and nonsolvated variations of the same molecular species, rather than absolute structural assignments. An interesting extension of tautomerism-induced polymorphism is where two valence tautomers, that is, different electronic structures where nonpolar N-atom (sp^3 hybridization) and polar structures (sp^2 hybridization) were observed in the crystal structure of 7-amino-4-methylcoumarin (Niedzialek and Urbanczyk-Lipowska, 2007).

Polymorph Screening
In the prenomination phase, any polymorphism screen will be somewhat restricted due to the amount of compound that is available at this stage. As such, an appropriate strategy to optimize the scope for assessing the polymorph hypersurface must therefore be employed to reflect this situation. An initial assessment into the propensity for polymorphism is achieved by assessing physical reproducibility of the early batches prepared by medicinal chemists. Furthermore, the process research and development chemists will also be working on the synthesis and crystallization of the compound (Kim et al., 2005), and physical integrity assessment of these laboratory scale test batches further supplements any polymorphism screens that have or will be conducted. In both these situations, a range of solvents and crystallization conditions may be explored, thus allowing (potentially) a wide area of the polymorphism hypersurface to be evaluated. Moreover, this strategy allows (to a certain degree) an evaluation into the role that impurities play in either templating or prohibiting growth of specific physical forms. Additionally, initial screens, usually using a single large-scale batch, are also conducted in parallel on a micro- or semi-microscale. There are a number of literature reports of high-throughput platforms that have been used in academia and industry for solid-form screening (Storey et al., 2004; Hilfiker et al., 2003; Almarsson et al., 2003; Morisette et al., 2003; Florence et al., 2006). Driving the concept to even smaller quantities, Lee et al. (2006) have described the technique of "polymorph farming" on a silicon wafer cast, with chitosan pretreated in different ways to affect the surface template properties. Crystallization of solutions of acetaminophen and sulfathiazole gave rise to the different polymorphs, depending upon the level of pretreatment.

The obvious attraction of having a high-throughput system is to conduct many hundreds, if not thousands, of crystallization experiments almost in a random fashion, that is, to throw the net far and wide in the hope of scouring as much of the available space as possible. However, a more rationalized and systematic approach will generally lead to a more fruitful search. Indeed, Stahly (2007), in a note of caution, has stated that these high-throughput methods should be used in conjunction with those more systematic methodologies already in place. The rationale being that high-throughput polymorph screening methodologies using evaporation from well plates tend to induce crystallization of a greater number of metastable phases. This was illustrated by Capes and Cameron (2007) who observed that the metastable form of acetaminophen was preferentially nucleated at the edge of the meniscus and was another explanation for the appearance of metastable forms from these experiments.

While increased effort has been expended into exploring the polymorphic hypersurface of compounds, Jarring et al. (2006) indicated that the actual number of solid-state forms is in fact not terribly important from an industrial point of view. Rather, the effort should be focused on finding those physical forms that have an advantage from a performance, formulation, and large-scale production perspective. Ultimately, the aim is to identify all development suitable forms and potential near-neighbor polymorphs, with the preference for selecting and progressing the form that is the most thermodynamically stable (Miller et al., 2005).

For polymorph screening purposes, Mirmehrabi and Rohani (2005) have proposed a systematic approach to solvent selection on the basis of the hydrogen-bonding propensities of the solute and the solvent molecules. They were able to calculate a polarity index (PI) for a wide range for ICH class 2 and class 3 solvents (also reporting a very useful table of properties such as dielectric constant, solubility parameter, and dipole moments for the solvents). In this case polymorphism of ranitidine was explored, and they were able to conclude that strong H-bond donor solvents lead to the dominant nitronic acid tautomer of form II, while weak H-bond donors or aprotic solvents favored the enamine tautomer found in form I. This approach therefore allowed easy identification of suitable isolation conditions for these polymorphs.

Interconversion of Polymorphs
In addition to recrystallization, solution maturation or slurry studies can be exploited to induce physical form conversions. These experiments are largely thermodynamically (rather than kinetically) driven and result in the conversion of less stable forms into physical forms that are more thermodynamically stable under the slurry conditions. When a mixture of two or more polymorphs (or hydrate and anhydrate) is slurried, it is sometimes known as a bridging experiment (Ticehurst et al., 2002). The solvents that are used can profoundly affect the rate and extent of conversion. For example, Gu et al. (2001) have studied the influence of the solvent on the rate of solvent-mediated transformations, and Mukuta et al. (2005) have reported the role of impurities, which were found to have a profound impact on the conversion. By studying the polymorphs of sulfamerazine, Gu et al. (2001) found that the rate of transformation was faster in a solvent that afforded high solubilities compared with those in which the solubility was lower. Furthermore, the conversion rate was found to be slower in solvents that had a greater H-bond acceptor potential. It was noted that the rate of solution agitation and temperature also affected the speed of the conversion. The more intense the agitation, the quicker the conversion, and since the relationship between these two forms of sulfamerazine is enantiotropic, the rate of conversion to form I was higher at lower temperatures and lower near the transition temperature (50°C). This work also suggested that a solubility of at least 8 mM was needed to ensure that the transformation proceeded satisfactorily. The corollary of this is that the solubility should not be too high, for example, greater than 200 mM to avoid using too much of a limited amount of compound (Miller, 2005).

As touched upon earlier, the role of impurities can also play a crucial role in the formation or conversion of polymorphic forms. For example, Blagden et al. (1998) have explored the role of related substances (as structurally related impurities) in the case of the disappearing polymorphs of sulfathiazole. These studies showed that a reaction by-product from the final hydrolysis stage could stabilize different polymorphic forms of the compound depending on the concentration of this by-product. By using molecular modeling techniques, they were able to show that the by-product, ethamidosulfathiazole, influenced the hydrogen-bonding network and hence polymorphic form and crystal morphology. The presence of impurities can also inhibit solution-mediated phase transformations, and this can be of particular concern for screening for polymorphs at an early stage when perhaps less pure materials are available (Gong et al., 2008). Additionally, changes in the synthetic regime during the progression of the drug compound through development can give rise to significantly different impurities, which even in very minor quantities may affect the appearance or inhibition of specific polymorphs. In this study, it was shown that an acetyl derivative of sulfamerazine inhibited the conversion of form I to form II. An increase in the conversion rate, however, was attributed to a number of factors, namely, (1) increasing the solubility, (2) reducing the level of the impurity causing the problem (possibly by changing the synthetic route), (3) pretreatment of the solid to reach maximum supersaturation, and (4) increased temperature.

While there are a number of ways to screen for polymorphism and related phenomena, Kuhnert-Brandstatter and Gasser (as early as 1971) stated that "investigations of poly-morphism can never be considered to be completely exhaustive in that there is always the possibility that with specific seeding a heretofore unknown crystal modification may appear," adding that "there is always the possibility of finding a new modification from some unique solvent and condition." Although Gavezotti and Filippini (1995) agreed that polymorphism of organic crystals was very frequent at room temperature, the appearance of polymorphs was not as common as it sometimes has been portrayed to be. The most recent data gathered from 245 polymorph screens carried at a contract research organization reported that 90% of the compounds exhibited "multiple and noncrystalline forms," of which only 50% were polymorphic (Stahly, 2007).

Dunitz and Bernstein (1995) have reviewed the appearance of and subsequent disappearance of polymorphs. Essentially this describes the scenario whereupon nucleation of a more stable form, the previously isolated, metastable, form could no longer be made. For example, the orthorhombic polymorph of paracetamol previously prepared by crystallization from solution had proved elusive since it was first discovered in 1974. However, crystallizing a supersaturated solution with seeds obtained from melt crystallization gave rise to a suitable laboratory scale method to obtain this metastable phase (Nichols and Frampton, 1998). A commentary on this phenomenon by Bernstein and Henck (1998) stated that "we believe that once a particular polymorph has been obtained it is always possible to obtain it again; it is only a matter of finding the right experimental conditions."

Yu (2007) has discussed the nucleation behavior of polymorphs and its importance in determining the nature of the polymorph to be isolated, showing that an early nucleating polymorph can generally nucleate a faster-growing polymorph, thus emphasizing the fact that both thermodynamic and kinetic factors have control on the appearance of certain polymorphs. Blagden and Davey (2003) attempted to combine the effect of thermodynamics, kinetics, and nucleation, in conjunction with modeling techniques, to the selection of the polymorphs. However their approach, while showing some success, highlighted the need for an improvement in the prediction of solute-solvent interactions.

In most industries in which polymorphism plays an important role in materials and their properties, there are several business drivers for polymorph characterization and selection. Firstly, there is a need to understand the external effect on structural behavior, enabling the selection of a robust and stable material that will not interconvert to a less desirable polymorph upon storage or processing. Secondly, it is important to have as much of the polymorph "hypersurface" mapped to ensure that all plausible low-energy structures, which could represent developable forms, are isolated and characterized. Information on structural relationships and the ease of interconversion (exploring both kinetics and mechanisms) allow the selection of the most optimum or developable form. Leading on from this is another business driver, which relates to intellectual property. On identifying all possible developable polymorphs, it is important to have patent coverage to protect intellectual property. In the area of pharmaceuticals there have been several important polymorph litigation cases (Bernstein, 2002; Cabri et al., 2007). As a consequence of the foregoing discussion regarding the physicochemical and biopharmaceutical implications of polymorphism, it can be appreciated that it is an extremely important topic from a drug regulatory perspective (De Camp, 2001).

Polymorph Production Methods

A number of protocols exploring both solvent-mediated and nonsolvent-induced poly-morphism can be employed to ensure that as much of the polymorphism hypersurface can be mapped. These are summarized in the following list:

1. Crystallization from different solvents under variable conditions, for example, different agitation speeds and temperatures (as exemplified by Blagden et al., 1998; Threlfall, 2000; Allesø et al., 2008). Therefore, it is important to screen a variety of solvents that cover a diversity of physicochemical parameters (Table 4). Although the solvent of crystallization can be critical in producing a particular polymorph, Getsoian et al. (2008) showed that for carbamazepine varying the crystallization

temperature and level of supersaturation was sufficient to produce three of the four known polymorphs from a single solvent.

2. Precipitation by, for example, addition of an antisolvent to a solution containing the drug or by pH adjustment of solutions of weak acids or bases (Bosch et al., 2004). An interesting example of this phenomenon is the quasi-emulsion precipitation of a number of polymorphic compounds using PEG300 as the solvent and water as the antisolvent (Wang et al., 2005). In this system, the intensity of mixing appeared to control the polymorphic form because of increased viscosity of the PEG300-water solution.

3. Concentration or evaporation. Capes and Cameron (2007) reported that a metastable form was obtained from the periphery of an evaporating solution. The resultant metastable form that was left free of the solvent was unable to transform to the more stable polymorph via a solvent-mediated phase transformation.

4. Formation of polymorphs from solvate desolvation. Nicolai et al. (2007) showed that forms I of spironolactone could be obtained by desolvation of its ethanol solvate.

5. Crystallization from the melt, assuming that melting is not accompanied by thermal degradation. Schmidt et al. (2006) found that modification I of salicaine HCl crystallized from the melt above 110°C and modification II crystallized from the melt below this temperature.

6. Grinding and compression. Trask et al. (2005a) have reported that polymorphic conversions of anthranilic acid (*ortho*-aminobenzoic acid), for example, could be induced by dry grinding (neat powder) and also in the presence of a small amount of solvent. Linol and Coquerel (2007) have also demonstrated that high-energy milling could be used to accelerate (relative to slurry experiments) the polymorphic conversion between the monoclinic and orthorhombic forms of (±) 5-methyl-(4′-methyl phenyl)hydantoin.

7. Lyophilization (freeze-drying) can induce polymorphism, as exemplified by pentamidine isethionate where various polymorphs can be obtained by altering the freeze-drying conditions (Chongprasert et al., 1998). Often, however, the compound is rendered amorphous by the freeze-drying process (Zhu and Sacchetti, 2002).

8. Spray-drying. Amorphous ursodeoxycholic acid can be prepared by spray-drying (Ueno et al., 1998).

9. Crystallization from supercritical fluids. Park et al. (2007) used a supercritical antisolvent (SAS) process to produce different forms of fluconazole.

10. Potentiometric cycling. Llinàs et al. (2007) used this method to produce polymorphic forms of sulindac.

11. High pressure. Piracetam has been crystallized in a number of polymorphic forms using the high pressures (0.07–0.4 GPa) generated using a diamond anvil cell (Fabbiani et al., 2005).

12. Sublimation. Exploiting the vapor phase as a solvent-free method of crystallizing polymorphs, as shown by Liu et al. (2008).

Assessment of the Physical Stability and Assignment of Relative Thermodynamic Stability of Polymorphs

Once polymorphs have been identified, an understanding of the relative stabilities of different polymorphic forms is important, particularly in relation to handling, primary, and secondary processing of the material. A crucial aspect in selecting a physical form (polymorph, hydrate, etc.) is in understanding its relative thermodynamic stability and the stability hierarchy that exists between all isolated physical forms. Ideally a robust and controllable form is chosen for progression, with the thermodynamically stable form representing the safest choice. This is also important from a regulatory perspective with regard to control. In progressing a thermodynamically stable form, it can be largely ensured that there is control on manufacture, storage, formulatability, and performance. Indeed, Brittain (2000a) has advised that, unless there were special circumstances, the stable form of the compound should be developed.

Table 6 Thermodynamic Rules for Polymorphic Transitions

Enantiotropy	Monotropy
Transition < melting 1	Transition > melting I
I stable > transition	I always stable
II stable < transition	–
Transition reversible	Transition irreversible
Solubility I higher < transition	Solubility I always lower
Solubility I lower > transition	–
Transition II → I endothermic	Transition II→I exothermic
$\Delta H_f^I < \Delta H_f^{II}$	$\Delta H_f^I > \Delta H_f^{II}$
IR peak I before II	IR peak I after II
Density I < density II	Density I> density II

Abbreviation: IR, infrared. *Source*: From Giron (1995), with permission from Elsevier.

Furthermore, if polymorphs were known to affect bioavailability, then they needed to be strictly controlled, which of course will need the development and validation of a suitable analytical technique. Typically, this might be an infrared (IR) or XRPD method.

Thermodynamics Related to Polymorphism
In general, true polymorphs can be classified, thermodynamically, into two different types (Giron, 1995):

1. Enantiotropic, in which one polymorph can be reversibly converted into another by varying the temperature and/or pressure.
2. Monotropic, in which the change between the two forms is irreversible.

Several empirical methods exist to assign the relative thermodynamic behavior between polymorphs, and these are summarized in Table 6.

The importance of understanding the control and robustness of polymorphs is illustrated by the ritonavir example. Ritonivir (ABT-538) was approved by the FDA in March 1996 and marketed as a semisolid formulation. In 1998, however, batches began to fail dissolution tests, and investigations revealed that a more stable polymorph was precipitating from the formulation. As a result, Abbot had to withdraw the product from the market. (Chemburkar et al., 2000). Further work (Bauer et al., 2001) showed that the problem arose because of an extreme case of conformational polymorphism (as discussed earlier), which arose because of the presence of a new degradation product providing a molecular template for form II (the more stable form of the compound).

Assigning the relative stability hierarchy of polymorphs, especially over the temperature and pressure space, is important in industries where polymorphism plays an important role in product integrity. The stability hierarchy, defined in terms of enantiotropism or monotropism, is related to the differences in free energy (ΔG) between pairs of polymorphs. Assessing the variation of free energy over temperature and pressure space provides increased confidence that a robust polymorph has been selected, which is stable to both primary and secondary processing (e.g., manufacture, drying, and milling). One way of achieving this is to represent the stability profile of all isolated polymorphs as a function of free energy and temperature in the form of energy-temperature (E/T) and pressure-temperature (P/T) diagrams. These are topological two-dimensional representations of polymorph thermodynamic space utilizing Gibbs fundamental equation shown in equation equation (22).

$$dG = V\,dP - S\,dT + \sum_B \mu_B\,dn_B \tag{22}$$

For polymorphs, the last component of equation (22), relating to changes in chemical composition can be neglected, and hence the topological representations consider the first two terms only.

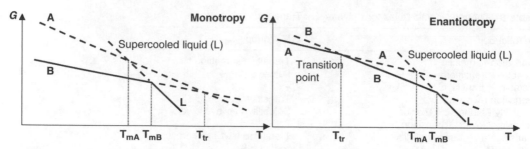

Figure 7   *E/T* diagrams showing monotropy and enantiotropy.

An E/T diagram is a topological representation of enthalpy and free energy of polymorphs as a function of temperature, extracted from DSC data and extrapolated to 0 K. The approach assumes that any contribution of pressure to phase transitions is negligible and solely related to temperature, enthalpy and differences in heat capacity of melting of polymorphs (Yu, 1995). Figure 7 illustrates E/T diagrams for monotropic and enantiotropic dimorphic systems. In the case of enantiotropy, a transition temperature exists below the melting temperatures of the polymorphs evaluated. This transition temperature represents a point at which the difference in free energy between the two forms is equal to zero. It also defines the temperature at which the stability hierarchy changes.

A more rigorous assessment of free energy differences between polymorphs incorporates an assessment not only over temperature but also pressure space (Ceolin et al., 1992; Espeau et al., 2005). A P/T approach is based on the fact that each polymorph is capable of coexisting in the three states of matter, solids, liquid, and vapor. As such, the P/T diagram is composed of triple points representing the equilibrium points of the three states of matter and equilibrium curves that represent the equilibrium boundary between two phases. The diagram is constructed from parameters obtained from melting thermodynamics, temperature-related volume variation in the solid and liquid state, and information on sublimation characteristics.

The number of triple points of a one component system, capable of existing in more than one solid phase, is defined in accordance with the expression shown in equation (23).

$$N = \frac{n \times (n-1) \times (n-2)}{1 \times 2 \times 3} \tag{23}$$

where N represents the number of triple points to be found in the diagram, and n represents the total number of phases (liquid, vapor, and all solids) under consideration.

The slopes of the phase equilibrium curves are obtained from the Clapeyron equation, shown in equation (24).

$$\frac{dp}{dT} = \frac{\Delta H_i}{T \Delta V_i} \tag{24}$$

where ΔH_i represents the change in enthalpy as a function of the phase transition (for instance melting or sublimation), and ΔV_i represents the change in volume, also as a function of the phase transition.

The P/T diagrams are a two-dimensional representation of the three-dimensional assessment of stability assignment, and the continuous three-dimensional surfaces are depicted as phase equilibrium curves that cross at the triple points. The stability hierarchy is assigned on the basis of Ostwald's criteria of positions relative to temperature and pressure, and also on the alternance rule (Ceolin et al., 1992; Espeau et al., 2005).

Sublimation experiments can be utilized to first establish the stability hierarchy and then identify transition temperatures. In this technique, a sample when placed in a sealed tube under vacuum and exposed to a thermal gradient may undergo sublimation, provided that exposure to high temperatures does not induce any thermal decomposition. The sample in the vapor phase will then condense at specific point along the cooler end of the tube dependent on the stability hierarchy. For example, for a monotropic system, sublimation of the more stable

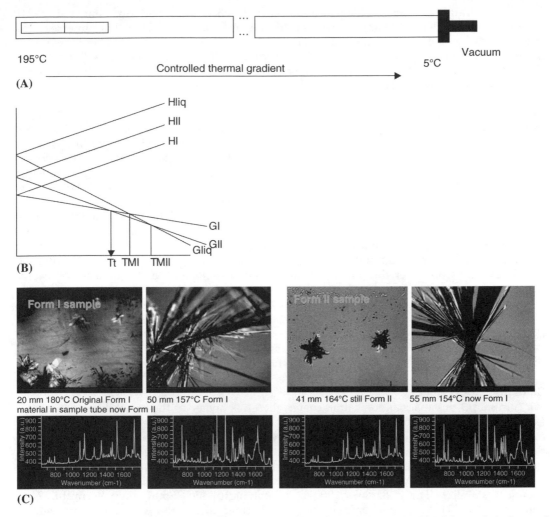

Figure 8 Overview of a sublimation experiment showing (**A**) a schematic representation of the sealed tube used during the sublimation experiment, where the sample is placed at the hot end; (**B**) E/T diagram of a development compound showing an enantiotropic relationship between forms I and II and a transition temperature of ~158°C; and (**C**) the results from the sublimation experiment of this enantiotropic development compound.

phase will give rise to condensation of the same form at the cooler regions of the sublimation tube. On performance of the same experiment with metastable phase of a monotropic system, the condensed material would be expected to be the more thermodynamically stable form. Conversely, for an enantiotropic system, several points of condensed crystalline material would be anticipated, each representing the polymorphic form stable at the temperature at which condensation/crystallization had occurred. An example of an enantiotropic system is illustrated in Figure 8. Here a dimorphic system was shown, from the topological E/T phase diagram, to be enantiotropic with a transition temperature of around 158°C. Form I represented the stable form below, and form II the more stable above this temperature. The sublimation experiment performed using both form I and form II revealed two main regions of condensed crystalline material at the cooler ends, with form II in both cases crystallizing at temperatures of greater than 160°C, while form I crystallized at temperatures of 157°C or below.

By measuring the solubility of different phases, the thermodynamic quantities involved in the transition from a metastable to a stable polymorph can be calculated. Experimentally, the solubilities of the polymorphs are determined at various temperatures and then the log of the solubility is plotted against the reciprocal of the temperature (the van't Hoff method). This results in a straight line (the problem of nonlinearity has been dealt with by Grant et al., 1984), from which the enthalpy of solution can be calculated from the slope. If the lines intersect, this is known as the transition temperature, and one consequence of this is that there may be a transition from one polymorph to another, depending on the storage conditions. For example, the formation of the monohydrate of metronidazole benzoate from a suspension of the anhydrate was predicted from such data (Hoelgaard and Møller, 1983).

Polymorph Prediction

The occurrence of polymorphism can also be explored using computational methodology (Verwer and Leusen, 1998; Beyer et al., 2001; Neumann, 2008), employing ab initio prediction strategies. The basis of these approaches involves in silico generation of all plausible crystal structures, which are subsequently ranked in order of calculated lattice energies or a function of the lattice energy utilizing appropriate force fields to compute and rank each polymorph. Furthermore, Young and Ando (2007) have used analysis of known crystal structures as a starting point to design polymorph prediction strategies. While these methods show applicability for smaller more rigid structures, there are still many limitations in the wider use of these approaches—in particular for structures with significant degree of freedom, for example, polymorphs of salt and those structures that exhibit a certain degree of conformational flexibility. Moreover, the veracity of such approaches depends on the quality of the force fields used to model thermodynamic and kinetic properties satisfactorily (Gavezzotti, 2002), which renders the current approaches applicable only to a small subset of organic structures. However, a few successes for flexible molecules have been reported, for example, a number of polymorphs of 4-amidinoindanone guanylhydrazone (AIGH) were correctly predicted (Krafunkel et al., 1996). Payne et al. (1999) and Hulme (2005) have successfully predicted the polymorphs of primidone, progesterone, and 5-fluorouracil, respectively.

Salts and Cocrystals

If a compound possesses an ionization center, then this opens up the possibility of forming a salt. The majority of drugs administered as medicines are salts of the active pharmaceutical ingredient (Stahl and Wermuth, 2002). Therefore, salt evaluation should be an integral part of the prenomination phase and is usually carried out to modulate the physicochemical properties of the free acid or base. Properties that can be altered by salt formation include solubility, dissolution, bioavailability (Gwak et al., 2005), hygroscopicity, taste, physical and chemical stability (Farag Badawy, 2001), or polymorphism (Stahl and Wermuth, 2002; Serajuddin, 2007). It is not only innovator pharmaceutical companies that investigate alternative salts of compounds, but generic manufacturers are also interested in alternative salts to gain access to the innovator companies business (Verbeek et al., 2006). However, Verbeek concluded that any alternative salt proposed by the generic company may have to undergo toxicological testing in addition to bioequivalence testing before it would be accepted by the regulatory authorities as an acceptable alternative. The intellectual property implications of generic companies' exploitation of alternative salts have been explored by Slowik (2003).

As example of property modulation using salts, Figure 9 shows the bioavailability of a free acid versus that of a sodium salt. Clearly, the sodium salt shows much higher bioavailability than the corresponding free acid. However, salts may not always enhance bioavailability, as shown in the example in Figure 10. The goal in any early development studies is to ensure adequate exposure of the drug in safety or tolerability studies, and thus, if the free acid or base shows sufficient exposure, then this would be used as the primary material of choice.

Gould (1986) has identified a number of pivotal issues with respect to salt selection for basic drugs. These specifically take into consideration the molecular and bulk properties of the material and the impact of the material as a salt form to the pharmacokinetics of the molecule. The range of salts used in drug products is shown in Table 7 (Berge et al., 1977). Haynes et al. (2005) have extended this by an analysis of the CSD. Chloride was found to have the highest number of hits (45.5%), followed by bromide. Another interesting observation was the fact that pharmaceutically acceptable counterions showed a higher level of hydrate formation

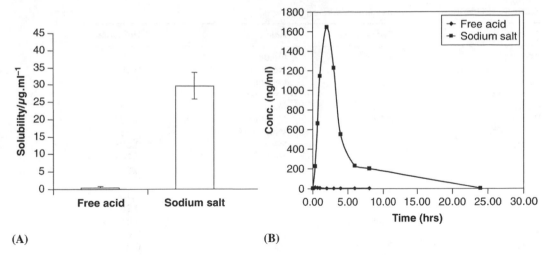

(A)   (B)

Figure 9   Dog bioavailability of a free acid versus its sodium salt (**A**) showing in vitro kinetic solubility data and (**B**) plasma profile following oral administration.

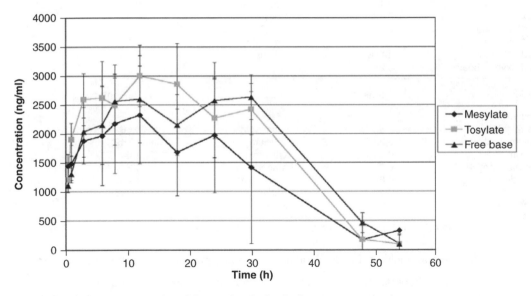

Figure 10   Plasma concentration of three salts of a basic discovery compound.

compared to the CSD as a whole. Table 8 shows the pK_as of some weak acids used in salt formation. Although this is a useful list of salt formers, it can be further classified according to the following four classes (Pfaankuch et al., 2002).

Class 1: Unrestricted use. The counterions in this class typically form ions that are natural in origin. In addition, they must have at least *one example* of a recently approved (last 20 years) product and *no significant* safety concerns. Examples include acetic acid and L-arginine.

Class 2: The counterions in this class, through previous application, have been shown to be *low in toxicity*. They typically have several examples of marketed products; however, unlike class 1, many are *historical in nature* (>20 years since approval). Examples include malonic acid and benzoic acid.

Table 7 FDA-Approved Commercially Marketed Salts

Anion	Percentage	Anion	Percentage
Acetate	1.26	Iodide	2.02
Benzenesulfonate	0.25	Isothionate	0.88
Benzoate	0.51	Lactate	0.76
Bicarbonate	0.13	Lactobionate	0.13
Bitartrate	0.63	Malate	0.13
Bromide	4.68	Maleate	3.03
Calcium edetate	0.25	Mandelate	0.38
Camsylate	0.25	Mesylate	2.02
Carbonate	0.38	Methylbromide	0.76
Chloride	4.17	Methylnitrate	0.38
Citrate	3.03	Methylsulfate	0.88
Dihydrochloride	0.51	Mucate	0.13
Edatate	0.25	Napsylate	0.25
Edisylate	0.38	Nitrate	0.64
Estolate	0.13	Pamoate	1.01
Esylate	0.13	Pantothenate	0.25
Fumarate	0.25	(Di)phosphate	3.16
Gluceptate	0.18	Polygalactoronate	0.13
Gluconate	0.51	Salicylate	0.88
Glutamate	0.25	Stearate	0.25
Glycollylarsinate	0.13	Subacetate	0.38
Hexylresorcinate	0.13	Succinate	0.38
Hydrabamine	0.25	Sulfate	7.46
Hydrobromide	1.90	Teoclate	0.13
Hydrochloride	42.98	Triethiodide	0.13
Hydroxynapthoate	0.25		

Cation	Percentage	Cation	Percentage
Organic		*Metallic*	
Benzathine	0.66	Aluminum	0.66
Chloroprocaine	0.33	Calcium	10.49
Choline	0.33	Lithium	1.64
Diethanolamine	0.98	Magnesium	1.31
Ethyldiamine	0.66	Potassium	10.82
Meglumine	2.29	Sodium	61.97
Procaine	0.66	Zinc	2.95

Source: From Berge et al. (1977), with permission J Wiley and Sons, Inc.

Class 3: The counterions in this class will have limited application, and some may be restricted.

- Typically there is very little safety data and/or regulatory precedent.
- Some counterions in this class may be used to impart a particular property to the resultant salt, restricted to very specific areas.
- Counterions in this class will typically only be considered where no suitable salt is identified from within class 1 or class 2. If considered, further data will be required. Examples include salicylic acid and piperazine.

Class 4: Counterions in this class should not be used to form salts of an active pharmaceutical ingredient (API). Their use is prohibited primarily because of safety/toxicity issues.

Morris et al. (1994) extended the scope of Gould's review and described an integrated approach to the selection of the optimal salt form for new drug candidates. In the first tier of their decision-making process, the salts are evaluated for their hygroscopicity. Those salts that show a greater propensity to sorb moisture are eliminated from consideration. The rationale behind using moisture sorption as the criterion for selection is that excessive moisture by a salt may cause handling, stability (chemical and physical), and manufacturing problems. Furthermore, if the moisture content changes on a batch-to-batch basis, this has the potential

Table 8 Table of Acid pK_as

Name	pK_a
Acetate	4.76
Benzoate	4.20
Oleate	~4.0
Fumarate	3.0, 4.4
Succinate	4.2, 5.6
Ascorbate	4.21
Maleate	1.9, 6.3
Malate	3.5, 5.1
Gluconate	3.60
Tartrate	3.0, 4.3
Citrate	3.13
Napsylate	0.17
Hydrobromide	−8.0
Hydrochloride	−6.1
Sulfate	−3
Phosphate	2.15, 7.20, 12.38
Besylate	2.54
Tosylate	−0.51
Besylate	2.54
Mesylate	1.92

to lead to variation in potency of the prepared dosage forms. Those salts that survive this primary screen proceed to the second tier, whereby any crystal structure changes induced by high levels of moisture are elucidated. In addition, the aqueous solubility of the remaining salts are determined to ascertain whether there may be dissolution or bioavailability problems. In the final tier, the stability of the final candidate salts are then investigated under accelerated conditions, (temperature, humidity, and presence of excipients). If desired, compatibility testing with excipients may be conducted at this stage. Consideration of ease of synthesis, analysis, potential impurities, and so on must also be undertaken. Intimately related to the salt selection procedure is the phenomenon of polymorphism. If a salt has the propensity to form many polymorphs, then, unless production of the desired form can be easily controlled, it should be rejected in favor of one that exhibits less polymorphic behavior.

To comply with the concept that in preformulation studies minimal amounts of compound are used, an in situ salt-screening technique for basic compounds has been developed by Tong and Whitesell (1998). Firstly, the protocol for basic drug compounds is based on only using counterions with a pK_a value that is at least two pH units from that of the drug. Secondly, solubility studies should be performed on the base in solutions of the chosen acid counterions. The concentration of the acid should account for an excess after the formation of the salt. It was recommended that the amount of base added should be accurately recorded because of its effects on the amount of acid consumed in preparing the salt and the pH of the final solution recorded. Finally, the solids formed (both wet and dry) should then be analyzed using the standard techniques, for example, DSC, thermogravimetric analysis (TGA), and XRPD. By using this protocol, there was good agreement between the solubilities of salts prepared by conventional means and the solubility of the base in the in situ technique in all cases except for the succinate. This was probably due to the fact that, as prepared, it was a hydrate and highlighted a potential drawback of the technique. Indeed, it was stated that the in situ technique should not replace traditional salt selection techniques. Rather, it should be used as salt-screening tool to rule out those salts that have poor solubility characteristics, thus obviating the need for their synthesis.

As with polymorphism studies, screening of salts can be conducted using small-scale throughput well-plate methodologies (Kojima et al., 2006). Typically, the protocol for a manual salt selection might follow a protocol such as this:

- Dissolve drug in methanol or other suitable standard solvent
- Add drug solution to 96-well plate using, for example, a multipipette
- Add counterion solutions (2 of each)

- Evaporate slowly, normally subambient
- Select crystalline (crossed polarizers) particles and store their x, y, z coordinates
- Collect Raman spectra (batch job)
- Repeat procedure in different solvents

The hits detected by the polarized microscope and Raman spectroscopy can then be scaled up, and their properties elucidated. In the literature, Ware and Lu (2004) have studied the use of a Biomek 2000 automation workstation for screening the salts of trazodone. Gross et al. (2007) have set out a decision tree–based approach to early-phase salt selection, which allows a more systematic method. Additionally, Guo et al. (2008) have described a 96-well approach to determine the salt solubility parameter (K_{sp}) for weakly basic salts. By using this technique, they claim that as little as 10 mg of compound enables an evaluation of eight different counterions using five acid concentrations. The reported bottleneck for this approach was data analysis resulting in a throughput of approximately 25 per week. One solution to this problem is the use of classification softwares, which have been written to group spectra and diffraction data (Barr et al., 2004; Gilmore et al., 2004; Ivanisevic, et al. 2005).

In contrast to the high-throughput approaches reported by other workers, Black et al. (2007) have presented a systematic investigation into the salt formation of the weak base ephedrine. In this study, they investigated a range of salt formers, including carboxylic acids, dicarboxylic acids, hydroxy acids, inorganics, and sulfonic acids. An important aspect of this study was the effect of the solvent (in the case of this study methanol vs. water) on the apparent pK_a values of the acid and base in solution. The apparent pK_a values of a range of acids and bases in, for example, methanol (Rived et al., 1998, 2001) and THF (Garrido et al., 2006). These studies have highlighted that the pK_a values of weak acids can vary quite markedly between water and methanol. For example, the pK_a of acetic acid in water is 4.8, while in methanol it increases to 9.6. Weak bases, however, appear to be less affected by solvents, as exemplified by ephedrine, where the pK_a decreases from 9.7 to 8.7. The data indicate that in methanol the pK_a values are not sufficiently separated for salt formation to take place. Indeed this was the case for acetic acid and the other weak carboxylic acids used in the study. In contrast, the strong acids (with a pK_a <2) gave salts from both methanol and water. These changes in pK_a will have an obvious affect on salt screening, since alcoholic solvents are often used to dissolve the salt-forming species prior to combining to form the salt. This study indicated that, at least in the case of ephedrine, the salt screen would be unsuccessful if only alcoholic solutions are used.

There are less salt-forming species for weak acids than there are for weak bases, and the available information suggests that, in general, alkali metal salts exhibit greater solubility than the corresponding alkaline earth salts. However, as shown by Chowan (1978) no specific conclusions can be drawn as to which cation will produce the greater solubility. In this paper, an attempt was made to predict solubilities on the basis of lattice and hydration energies, and the ionic radii of the cation. However, there was insufficient agreement between theory and experiment, except in general terms. In the case of amine salts, Anderson and Conradi (1985) were also unable to correlate properties of the amine such as hydrophilicity with the observed solubility order. Solubility did show a good correlation with the melting point of the salts, suggesting that the interactions within the crystal largely dominanted the properties of amine salts. Therefore, attempts to increase solubility through increased hydrophilicity of the amine counterion alone may not be successful. Salt formation may also be useful to modulate processing properties as exemplified by the use of a calcium salt of fenoprofen to overcome the low (40°C) melting point of the free acid (Hirsch, 1978). By increasing the melting point, the problems with frictional heat due to mechanical handling were overcome.

The use of alkali (or alkali-earth) metals is often complicated by the ready formation of hydrates of varying stoichiometries. For example, Rubino (1989) had investigated the solid-state properties of the sodium salts of drugs such as barbiturates, sulfonamides, and hydantoins. When the logarithm of their aqueous solubilities were plotted against their melting points, a reciprocal relationship was found to hold. It was also found that in many cases hydrate formation occurred, and that the stoichiometry differed before and after equilibration. It was concluded that the solubility of the salts was primarily controlled by the properties of the solid, in equilibrium with the solution phase. Rubino and Thomas (1990) followed up this work and examined the influence of solvent composition on the solubility and solid-state properties of these sodium salts. In many cases it was found that the solubility of the salts in the mixed solvent (propylene glycol/water) were lower than that found in water alone. Conversely, several other salts showed an increase in solubility in the solvent mixes. This was shown not to be related to the intrinsic lipophilicity of the acidic form of the drug, but rather to the hydrate formation. Moreover, it was found that those compounds with a low dehydration temperature showed increased solubility in propylene glycol-water and vice versa. Thus, it would appear that crystal hydrate formation plays a significant role in determining whether a cosolvent can be used to enhance the solubility of sodium salts. For hygroscopicity, it is not possible, again, to be specific with regard to the cation.

Modulation of chemical stability can also be a driver for salt formation. For instance, in a study by Cotton et al. (1994), a salt selection procedure was carried out because of the inherent instability of the free acid of L-649,923, an orally active leukotriene D_4 antagonist, which rapidly hydrolyzed to a less active form of the compound. Therefore, to ensure that this did not occur, the compound had to be isolated as a salt. The physical and chemical properties of the sodium, calcium, ethylene diamine, and benzathine salts were evaluated, and the calcium salt was selected as the most pharmaceutically acceptable form of the compound.

In most cases, the salt-forming species shown in Table 7 form the primary list from which salts are selected. In 1987, Gu and Strickley described the physical properties of the tris (hydroxymethyl)aminomethane (THAM) salts of four analgesic/anti-inflammatory agents with sodium salts and free acids. They concluded that the THAM salts had superior hygroscopicity properties compared to the sodium salt and did not show any loss in aqueous solubility or intrinsic dissolution rate. The one exception to this was the THAM salt of naproxen. Ketoralac is now marketed as the tromethamine (THAM) salt. Although in screens tris salts may show better physicochemical properties, this should not be the only consideration. For example, Wu et al. (2003) showed that THAM becomes unstable at temperatures greater than 70°C, and therefore any long-term stability studies involving it should be carefully monitored for degradation.

Fini et al. (1991) have investigated the *N*-(2-hydroxyethyl)-pyrrolidine (epolamine) salt of diclofenac and found that it was more soluble and dissolved more rapidly than diclofenac sodium. Furthermore, studies showed that this salt gave faster plasma levels when administered orally; this has been marketed both for systemic and topical use (Giachetti et al., 1996).

Salts of Weak Bases

As shown in Table 7, there are many more acids that can be used to form salts with weak bases. However, in terms of usage, the hydrochloride is by far the most frequently used, and hence this salt should be used as a benchmark for comparison. Engel et al. (2000) highlighted that of the NCEs approved by the FDA over a five year period, up until 2000, 20% were mesylate salts. However, there has been some concern about sulfonic acids with the production of potential genotoxic impurities (PGIs) in the presence of alcohols (Snodin, 2007). For example, in mid-2007, Roche had to recall nelfinavir mesylate (viracept) tablets because of high levels of methane sulfonic acid ethyl ester produced after cleaning with ethanol (PJ article, 2007).

According to Gould (1986), to form a salt of a basic compound, the pK_a of the salt-forming acid has to be less than or equal to the pK_a of the basic center of the compound. Thus, for very weakly basic compounds having a pK_a of around 2, they will only form salts with strong acids such as hydrochloric, sulfuric, and toluene sulfonic acids. Bases with higher pK_as have a greater range of possibilities for salt formation, as shown by the range of weaker acids in Table 8.

Increasing or decreasing the solubility of a compound are two of the most important reasons for salt selection. One of the major factors determining the solubility of a salt is the pH of the resultant solution. That is, the salts of the stronger acids will produce slurries with a lower pH, thus promoting the dissolution of the base. For example, the pK_a of HCl is –6.1, and so on dissolution of a hydrochloride salt, the resultant low solution pH will promote a high solubility of the basic drug. However, other factors may also play a part in solubility modulation through salt formation. For instance, a reduction in the melting point of the salt, or improved hydrogen bonding, may also contribute to the process. In this respect, hydroxyl groups, for example, in the conjugate acid to increase hydrogen-bonding capacity of the salt can be of use, and it is best to avoid conjugate acids with hydrophobic groups or those that contain long alkyl chains (Gould, 1986).

Salt formation, however, does not always offer a panacea, and may result in causing other issues with the material. For instance, it is not always a successful strategy for increasing the solubility of compounds as exemplified by Miyazaki et al. (1981), who showed that the formation of hydrochloride salts does not always enhance solubility and bioavailabilty due to the common ion effect in gastric fluid, which is rich in chloride ions. Salts can also affect the dissolution properties of a compound, even though solubility characteristics may be similar. This was illustrated by Shah and Maniar (1993), who examined these properties for bupivacaine and its hydrochloride salt. The difference in the intrinsic dissolution behavior was explained as being due to the pH of the diffusion layer, that is, when solid dissolves, there is a stagnant film where the pH is different compared with the bulk dissolution medium. Thus, when the base is dissolved in an acidic medium, for example, pH 1 to 5, the pH will be increased to 6 to 7 because of self-buffering. In alkaline solutions, however, the pH will not change because ionization will be suppressed because of the pK_a of drug being 8.2. In the case of the salt, however, the opposite occurred, that is, in acid the pH remained unchanged and alkaline pHs were reduced to about 5 to 7. The reduction in pH arose because of the release of HCl, as the salt dissolved. Li et al. (2005a) have investigated the effect of chloride ion concentration on the intrinsic dissolution rates of the mesylate, phosphate, and hydrochloride salts of haloperidol and found that the dissolution of the hydrochloride was decreased in the presence of the chloride ion (0.01M HCl). They found that the nonhydrochloride salts converted to hydrochloride salt during dissolution studies with discs, but when experiments were performed using a powder, the dissolution was complete before conversion could take place, suggesting that the nonhydrochloride salts would be better from a dosage form perspective.

Often the solubility modulation of salts is utilized to increase the solubility or dissolution rate of drugs. However, salts with lower solubilities may offer some advantages such as taste masking, slower dissolution, and increased chemical stability. An example of salt formation to decrease dissolution rate is described by Benjamin and Lin (1985) who prepared a range of salts of an experimental antihypertensive. These in vitro tests showed that there were significant differences in the dissolution rate when the experiments were performed in water and buffer. However, the difference in the IDRs of the salts were similar in 0.1M HCl. Hence it was recommended that the ebonate, 3-hydroxynapthoate, or napyslate salts, should be formulated as enteric-coated dosage forms, thus avoiding dissolution in the stomach acid, which could cause local GI irritation and still provide release of the compound.

The results of an investigation into the effect of salt formation on the solubility of a development compound in water and saline is shown in Table 9. Although there was the expected range of solubilities of the free base and the salts in water, the solubility values were reduced when the experiment was conducted in isotonic saline.

Table 9   Solubility of a Free Base and Selected Salts in Water and Isotonic Saline

Salt	Solubility (mM)		Melting point (°C)	pH[a]
	Water	Saline		
Free base	–	0.46		
Hydrochloride	10.9	0.74	201	4.52
		0.66		
Tartrate	23.2	1.34	160	2.95
		1.07		
p-Toluenesulfonate (tosylate)	1.39	1.77	170	5.39
1-Hydroxy-2-napthoate (xinafoate)	0.11	0.14	176	6.00
Hemisuccinate	1.36	2.15	182	5.96
Hexanoate	2.97	3.85	131	5.87

[a]Saturated suspension of compound.

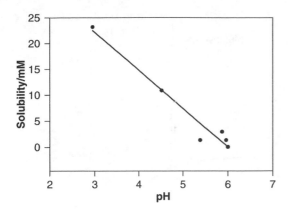

Figure 11 Solubility as a function of suspension pH of the salts shown in Table 9.

The relationship between the pH of the suspensions and the resulting solubility is shown in Figure 11; however, the scatter of results indicated that the solubility was not simply due to pH but was also influenced by the nature of the conjugate base. O'Connor and Corrigan (2001) prepared and characterized a range of basic salts of diclofenac, a nonsteroidal anti-inflammatory drug. With regard to solubility, they found that there was a correlation between the inverse of the melting point of the salt and the log of the aqueous solubility. They concluded from this study that solubility of the salts were a combination of lattice strength and the pH of the saturated salt solution. In saline, the mechanism of the reduction in solubility is less clear. The decrease observed for the hydrochloride salt is most probably due to the common ion effect as noted above.

The possibility of producing slowly dissolving salbutamol salts for delivery to the lung was investigated by preparing its adipic and stearic acid salts (Jashnani et al.,1993). The aqueous solubilities of the adipate and stearate salts were 353 and 0.6 mg/mL compared to the free base and sulfate, which had solubilities of 15.7 and 250 mg/mL, respectively. In terms of the intrinsic dissolution rate, the stearate dissolved much more slowly than the other salts and free base. This was due to the deposition of a stearate-rich layer on the dissolving surface of the compacted salt.

In another study Walkling et al. (1983) found that xilobam, as the free base, was sensitive to high humidity and temperature. In an effort to overcome this problem, the tosylate, 1-napsylate, 2-napsylate, and saccharinate salts were prepared and assessed with respect to their solid-state stability by storing samples at 74% relative humidity (RH) and 70°C for up to seven days. In addition to the stability studies, the dissolution of tablets made from the salts was investigated. These data and the results from the dissolution studies showed that not only was the 1-napsylate most stable it also exhibited faster dissolution properties.

Saesmaa and Halmekoski (1987) have reviewed the slightly water-soluble salts of the β-lactam antibiotics. This paper consists of much information on the early literature of these compounds. As examples, they described the use of the benzathine salts of penicillin G and V for depot injections. The benzathine salt of penicillin V has also been used to mask the taste of the antibiotic for pediatric use. In another example, they quoted a comparison of the napsylate and hydrochloride salts of talampicillin. As a direct consequence of its lower water solubility, the napsylate had more acceptable organoleptic properties (when formulated as a syrup) compared with the hydrochloride salt and had comparable blood levels to a tablet formulation of the hydrochloride.

It is worth adding a note of caution with regard to salt formation. In a series of benzathine and emboate salts of the β-lactam antibiotics, ampicillin, amoxicillin, cephalexin, and talampicillin studied by XRPD (Saesmaa et al., 1990), the results showed that the emboate salts of ampicillin, amoxicillin, and cephalexin were nearly identical in structure with that of the stiochiometric physical mixture of the two starting materials. Furthermore, the XRPD of benzathine amoxicillin and amoxicillin trihydrate were identical. In contrast, the benzathine salts of ampicillin and cephalexin were formed, illustrating that formation of the salt should

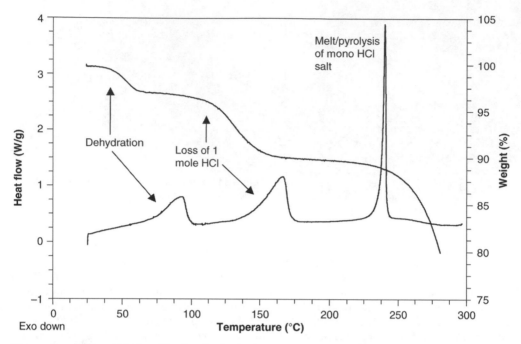

Figure 12   DSC and TGA profile of a dihydrochoride salt illustrating the thermolabile nature of an HCl salt of a very weak base. *Abbreviations*: DSC, differential scanning calorimetry; TGA, thermogravimetric analysis.

always be confirmed by a solid-state characterization technique such as XRPD or Raman spectroscopy.

Stability of the salt could also be an important issue. For example, Nakanishi et al. (1998) found that the hydrochloride of the anticancer drug, NK109, was less stable than the sulfate salt. This was thought to be due to the low pK_a (5.3) of the basic moiety and the volatility of HCl. When NK109 was stressed (at 70°C under reduced pressure), it was found that the chloride changed color from orange to amber and was accompanied by decrease in purity (99.45 to 98.78) compared with the sulfate, which showed no change. Furthermore, salts of weak bases from volatile counterions such as HCl could also result in the possibility of thermally or mechanically induced disproportionation. This phenomenon has been demonstrated by an AstraZeneca development compound, selected as a dihydrochloride salt. The counterion associated with the weaker of the two basic moieties of the drug was shown to be labile to thermal and mechanical stress. Figure 12 illustrates the thermal properties of this dihydrochloride salt, which crystallized as a monohydrate.

Thermal disproportionation of the labile salt was shown to occur at around 70°C (with an associated loss by thermogravimetric analysis of 7.1% w/w HCl corresponding to 1M equivalent) with implications to the robustness of the material. As part of the salt selection process, an assessment into the robustness of the material to manufacture, storage, and processing is important. In this particular example, small-scale assessments on the impact to storage at various elevated temperature conditions and mechanical processing such as grinding or compression showed a variation in the loss of the labile salt, as summarized in Table 10. Analysis of the TGA loss of the labile HCl coupled with total chloride level analysis indicated that thermal and mechanical manipulation resulted in varying degrees of disproportionation, thus indicating that the progression of the dihydrochloride salt was not desirable.

Hydrolysis of a salt back to the free base may also take place if the pK_a of the base is sufficiently weak. As an example, a hydrochloride salt of an investigational compound was prepared from a weak base containing a pyridine moiety with a pK_a of 5.4. When this salt was slurried in water or subjected to high humidity, hydrolysis back to the free base was induced. Figure 13 shows the DSC thermograms of the hydrochloride, the free base, and a sample of the

Table 10 Assessment of the Levels of Labile HCl Following Thermal and Mechanical Treatment of a Dihydrochloride Salt (No Loss Corresponds to the Fact that All the Labile HCl Has Been Removed During the Treatment Process)

Process	TGA loss of labile HCl (% w/w)	Chloride analysis (% w/w)
Recrystallized from water	7.1	13.8
Heated to 80°C for 24 hr	No loss observed	7.7
Heated to 120°C for 24 hr	No loss observed	7.7
Heated to 60°C for 1 hr	5.8	12.9
Ground with 10% H_2O and dried at 80°C for 1 hr	3.7	11.1
Direct compression	~5	12.8

Abbreviation: TGA, thermogravimetric analysis

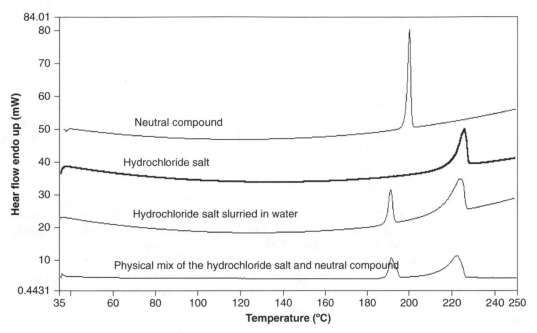

Figure 13 DSC thermograms of a free base, its hydrochloride salt (+ physical mix), and the effect of slurrying in water. *Abbreviation:* DSC, differential scanning calorimetry.

hydrochloride slurried in water. A DSC thermogram of a physical mix of the base and the hydrochloride is also shown.

Hydrochloride salts may also have disadvantages compared to other salts in terms of tablet production. For example, Nururkar et al. (1985) reported that a hydrochloride salt of an investigational compound caused the rusting of tablet punches and dies. Thus, while salts offer the advantage of a simple process to modulate properties, a certain degree of caution needs to be exercised to determine whether material properties will compromise the studies for which it is intended.

Cocrystals

In contrast to salt formation, which is accompanied by proton transfer from an acid to a base, cocrystals are crystalline materials where two or more neutral molecules are hydrogen bonded to each other. Childs et al. (2007) have argued that both salts and cocrystals are both part of a continuum of multicomponent crystals linked by the extent of proton transfer. Indeed there is a gradation of properties such that, for example, norfloxacin forms both salts (succinate, malonate, and maleate) and a cocrystal (isonicotinamide) (Basavoju et al., 2006).

However, as with salt formation, the goal of cocrystal formation is to alter or improve the properties of the parent compound; thus, the choice of whether to take a salt or cocrystal into development should not represent a concern so long as the cocrystal meets the criteria set for selection (Aakeröy et al., 2007). For example, cocrystal formation was used to control the hygroscopicity of caffeine with the oxalic acid cocrystal showing complete stability even at high relative humidities (Trask et al., 2005b). Similarly, the same group showed that the physical stability of theophylline, with regard to moisture uptake, could be enhanced through cocrystal formation (Trask et al., 2006). Moisture uptake as a method of producing co-crystals has been reported by Jayasankar et al. (2007). By using a variety of substances (e.g., carbamazepine—saccharin), they formed the cocrystal by exposing it to very high levels of RH, which caused deliquescence followed by cocrystal formation. Microscopically, it was observed that after excessive moisture uptake the compounds dissolved to form a solution from which the cocrystal underwent nucleation and growth.

In vivo studies comparing the bioavailability of anhydrous carbamazepine with its saccharin cocrystal showed that the cocrystal had the same chemical stability, superior suspension stability, and bioavailability comparable to an immediate-release tablet (Hickey et al., 2007a). A glutaric acid cocrystal with a development compound (a potential sodium channel blocker) was shown to improve its bioavailability (MacNamara et al., 2006). As noted above, cocrystals can contain more than two components, and as an example Karki et al. (2007) have reported the cocrystal between theophylline, citric acid, and water in the ratio 1:1:1.

In production, cocrystals have been produced by a variety of means, for example, dry grinding and solvent-assisted grinding are popular. Zhang et al. (2007) have communicated a slurry/suspension method for screening cocrystal formers. In essence the screen extends that for hydrate screening. The basic equation pertaining to cocrystallization is given below.

$$D_{solid} + nCCF_{solution\ or\ solid} \leftrightarrow CC_{solid} \tag{25}$$

where D is the API, CCF is the cocrystal former, n is the stoichiometry, CC is the cocrystal formed by the reaction, and K_c is the formation constant. As with the hydrate/anhydrate phase transformation, there is a critical CCF (between 0 and 1) where D and CC are in equilibrium. Thus, when the activity of the CCF is higher than the activity of the API, then the cocrystal is more stable than the API and thus will form: if it exists. Clearly, this approach will lend itself to high-throughput techniques and thus allow pharmaceutical scientists other options with respect to solid form selection. Lara-Oochoa and Espinosa-Pérez (2007) have discussed some of the issues surrounding the patentability of cocrystals, and the reader is referred to this paper for further information.

Solvates

Solvates are materials where solvent or water molecules (in either stoichiometric or nonstoichiometric amounts) are incorporated in the crystal lattice or in interstitial voids or channels. It has been described by some authors by the term pseudopolymorphism; however, there has been some debate about whether this is the meaningful description and its use should now be avoided (Desiraju, 2004; Seddon, 2004). Generally speaking, four main roles are fulfilled by solvents in crystal structures (van der Sluis and Kroon, 1989). These are: (1) participation as acceptors and/or donors in hydrogen-bonding schemes, (2) filling void spaces, (3) completing coordination around metal ions, and (4) bridging polar and nonpolar regions in the crystal. Specific interactions can take place through hydrogen bonding, and Bingham et al. (2001) have classified the space filling solvates as inclusion phases and the hydrogen-bonded species as cocrystals. Another type of inclusion solvate, known as clathrate, has been defined where the solvent is located in isolated lattice sites with no significant interaction to the host molecule; for example, Kemperman et al. (2000) have reported the clathrated β-naphthol structures of a range of cephalosporin antibiotics. Furthermore, Sheth et al. (2002) have pointed out that these guest molecules lie trapped in closed, three-dimensional cavities formed by the crystalline structure of the host. By using this definition and a determination of the crystal structure, they showed that the material supplied as "warfarin sodium clathrate" (with 2-propanol) was in fact a solvate.

If the crystal has large empty crystallographic channels or holes, their nature will determine which solvent will be included and the structure of the resulting solvate. From a structural point of view, the inclusion of a variety of solvates can show regularity. For example, Hosokawa et al. (2004) have reported the isostructurality of the 2:1 benzene, cyclohexane, 1,4 dioxin, tetrahydrofuran, tetrachloromethane, and chloroform solvates of phenylbutazone.

In thermodynamic terms, Senthil Kumar et al. (1999) have described the formation of solvates in the following terms: "If solute-solvent interactions are unusually important, say because of multipoint recognition, the entropic advantage associated with solvent expulsion into the bulk may be overridden by these additional enthalpic factors, resulting in retention of some solvent in the crystal."

Although solvates can show higher solubilities and dissolution rates compared to nonsolvated species (Stoltz et al., 1988; Suleiman and Najib, 1989), solvates cannot normally be used in the pharmaceutical arena because of the intrinsic toxicity of the solvent itself.

Görbitz and Hersleth (2000) have mined the CSD for information on the inclusion of solvent molecules in the crystal structures of organic compounds. It should be noted that the crystal lattice can hold more than one solvent (heterosolvates). For example, Shirotani et al. (1988) found that the cell dimensions of griseofulvin 1-bromo-2-chloroethane and bromoethane solvates were almost equal, and when griseofulvin was recrystallized from different molar ratios mix of the two solvents, a mixed solvate resulted. According to Görbitz and Hersleth (2000), the most common heterosolvate is the methanol-dichloromethane combination, with up to four different solvents having been observed in a single structure!

The remarkable capacity of sulfathiazole to incorporate solvent has been reported by Bingham et al. (2001). In this paper, it was claimed that sulfathiazole has the ability to form over 100 solvates, with over 60 crystal structures being solved. Structure property relationships were attempted, and the results indicated that a solvent containing an aromatic carbocyclic group did not give solvates, as did those solvents containing a hydroxy group, with the exception of *n*-propanol, which was unstable. Other solvents were incorporated into the crystal lattice, and on the basis of this study they proposed that two types of structure could be classified. These were (1) clathrates or inclusion phases, where the solvent fills space or is weakly H-bonded in the structure and (2) cocrystals, where the solvent is hydrogen bonded in the structure.

Usually solvates arise in the manufacturing process. Typically, solvates are formed at lower temperatures such that the temperature solubility curves will show temperature regions where solvates and unsolvated species are stable. The number of solvates that can be formed is a matter of experimentation, and clearly, high-throughput crystallization studies now yield many previously undiscovered solvates. Recently, Johnston et al. (2008) have employed a classification technique known as Random Forest classification to target crystallization of novel carbamazepine solvates.

If the solvate cannot be avoided from a process point of view, then it is important that solvates are desolvated before use. Typically, vacuum drying is used; however, it has been noted for several compounds that solvated alcohol can be removed more quickly by exposure of the solvate to water vapor (Pikal et al., 1983). However, in the case of warfarin sodium 2-propanol solvate, this approach was found to be unsuccessful (Sheth et al., 2004). When this solvate was exposed, elevated relative humidities deliquescence took place, which did not change the underlying solvate structure. Associated with the desolvated solvate there may be residual solvent, which must be controlled. Perhaps a more direct and complete method of desolvation is to suspend the solvate in water. For example, Mallet et al. (2001) was able to exchange DMSO for water by suspension in water, which proceeded by way of a destructive-reconstructive mechanism. Similarly, Wang et al. (2007) transformed the acetone solvate of erythromycin to the dihydrate by slurrying the solvate in water.

When the solvent is removed from the crystal lattice, which retains its three-dimensional order, a so-called isomorphic desolvate is created (Stephenson et al., 1998). The desolvated structure is highly energetic and reduces this situation by simply taking up moisture from the atmosphere or undergoing a certain degree of structural collapse to reduce the unit cell volume. Petit et al. (2007) have investigated the mechanism of a range of cortisone acetate solvates. They identified two main mechanisms by which the solvent was lost. The dihydrate and the tetrahydrofuran solvate lost their solvent anisotropically, which was followed by a cooperative structural rearrangement to an anhydrous polymorph. In contrast the dimethylformamide and dimethylsulfoxide solvates desolvated via a partial dissolution of the internal part of the crystals.

Residual solvents have been classified by the ICH into three classes:

Class I solvents: Solvents to be avoided
> Known human carcinogens, strongly suspected human carcinogens, and environmental hazards, for example, benzene, carbon tetrachloride, 1,2 dichloroethane

Class II solvents: Solvents to be limited
> Nongenotoxic animal carcinogens or possible causative agents of other irreversible toxicity such as neurotoxicity or tetrogenicity, for example, acetonitrile, cyclohexane, toluene, methanol, and N,N-dimethylacetamide Solvents suspected of other significant but reversible toxicities

Class III solvents: Solvents with low toxic potential, for example, acetic acid, acetone, ethanol ethyl acetate, and ethyl ether
> Solvents with low toxic potential to man; no health-based exposed limit is needed. Class 3 solvents have PDEs of 50 mg or more a day

While the use of solvates is not usual (because of toxicity), it is interesting to note that according to Glaxo's British patent 1,429,184, the crystal form of beclomethasone dipropionate used in the metered-dose inhaler is the trichlorofluoromethane solvate. By using the solvate, it was found that crystal growth due to solvation of the propellant CFCs was prevented. Of course, CFC12 is now being phased out from use because of their ozone-depleting properties.

Hydrates

The most common case of solvation is the incorporation of water molecules, and they are almost always involved in hydrogen bonding. Indeed, it is the hydrogen-bonding network that contributes to the coherence of the crystal, such that they usually show, for example, slower dissolution rates compared with the corresponding anhydrates. Byrn (1982) has illustrated the importance of this topic by stating that there are more than 90 hydrates listed in the USP. It should be noted that not only the APIs but excipients also have the potential to form hydrates, for example, magnesium stearate (Bracconi et al., 2003). As shown by Salameh and Taylor (2006), excipients can also have an effect on the stability of hydrates. For example, when PVP12 was mixed with theophylline monohydrate and carbamazepine dihydrate, it dehydrated both hydrates.

A full understanding of the hydration state of compounds is not only important from a scientific perspective, it can also be important from an intellectual property point of view. This was exemplified by the case where a generic company, Apotex, which was successful in demonstrating noninfringement of the patent on paroxetine hydrochloride. GSK marketed an anhydrous form of the compound and Apotex came forward with an abbreviated new drug application (ANDA) for a hemihydrate. Without detailing the legal or scientific arguments presented by each side, the final result was the loss of exclusivity by GSK (Gardner et al., 2004).

In a search of structures in the CSD performed in 1999 (Senthil Kumar et al.), only 25% of all reported crystals of small organic molecules were solvates. This observation was attributed in part to the increase in free energy of the structure if solvents were included (as a result of loss of entropy by including solvent molecules), particularly if scope for favorable intermolecular interactions exists in the parent structure. The formation and occurrence of hydrates, as with all other processes, results from a fine thermodynamic balance, that is, compensation between enthalpy and entropy of the system. Generally, the formation of hydrates is governed by a net increase in favorable intermolecular interactions and the requirement of water is to satisfy specific roles to stabilize the crystal structure. Furthermore, the presence of water may serve to increase packing efficiency within the three-dimensional framework, thus maintaining a stable low-energy structure in accordance with the edict on the stability of the structure being related to density (Kitaigorodskii, 1961).

Gillon et al. (2003) have performed a more recent review of the hydration of organic molecular crystals using the CSD. By using the data from 3315 structures, they found that the two most common ways that water interacted was through the formation of three or four H-bonds with neighboring molecules. Infantes et al. (2007) used the CSD in an attempt to define which factors were important in their formation. Statistically, they found the donor/acceptor ratio and the molecular weight of the compounds, proposed earlier as factors, to be predictors of hydrate formation. Rather they found that the total polar surface increased the propensity for hydrate formation. Work has also started in the prediction of organic hydrate crystal structures. For example, Hulme and Price (2007) were successful in predicting the structures within 5 kJ/mol of 5-azauracil monohydrate.

Inclusion of water of crystallization can alter the free energy of a crystal structure and consequently, as with polymorphism, can have a profound impact on physicochemical properties such as solubility, dissolution (and hence bioavailability in the case of pharmaceuticals), and stability. An understanding of the properties and stability of hydrates relative to any parent anhydrate is important to rationalize material selection. Knowledge of the structural disposition to form hydrates would also impact on crystal-engineering developments (i.e., identification of chemistry and isolation procedures to maximize material properties).

In instances for which water plays a crucial role in maintaining the crystal structure via the formation of a hydrogen-bonding network, dehydration can often lead to complete structural collapse, giving rise to an amorphous anhydrate, as observed with eprosartan mesylate dihydrate (Sheng et al., 1999). In this particular case, the water of crystallization forms a hydrogen-bonding framework directly to the parent drug and the salt counterion. Dehydration results in an amorphous material, which becomes annealed upon heating, giving rise to a crystalline hydrate. Such hydrates are considered to be very stable and represent developable materials.

Hydrates in which water acts as a "space filler" occupying voids or crystallographic channels can dehydrate to give isomorphous anhydrates or undergo a change of structure to give a more densely packed arrangement. Examples of these types of hydrates include cephalexin (Kennedy et al., 2003), erythromycin A, and cefaclor (Stephenson et al., 1997), all of which give rise to isomorphous anhydrates as determined by XRPD analysis. Generally, these types of hydrates are nonstoichiometric and the number of equivalent water molecules in the structure is directly related to the water activity (a_w) in the surrounding environment. The geometry and size of the solvent channels in these structures can vary significantly from long, wide rigid structures that are maintained by a robust hydrogen-bonded framework to small interweaving arrangements for which the water may interact with the "host" structure. Dehydration from the long rigid channels results in minimal structural disruption and hence the resultant hydrate is structurally identical to the parent. Instances in which dehydration occurs from interweaving channels can give rise to disruption of the structure, creating a high-energy arrangement that may undergo relaxation in the form of anisotropic contraction of the lattice, evident by a shift in the XRPD lines from larger to smaller *d*-spacings, as observed in cephalexin (Stephenson et al., 2000). In both cases however, the parent anhydrate is regarded as a hygroscopic material. Typically, this category of hydrates is regarded as less stable and less desirable as a developable material.

Authelin (2005) has classified hydrates into two types, stoiochiometric and non-stoichiometric. By definition, stoichiometric hydrates, for example, mono-, di-, and trihydrates have well-defined moisture contents, and their crystal structures are different from the anhydrated form of the compound. Nonstoichiometric hydrates, on the other hand, exhibit a moisture content that is variable in nature. From a structural point of view, any uptake of water is usually accompanied by an anisotropic expansion of the crystal lattice.

Further classifications of hydrates have been described by Morris (1999) and Vippagunta (2001). These are as follows:

1. *Isolated lattice site water*. In this situation, the water molecules are not in contact with each other, that is, they are separated by the drug molecules. These are sometimes termed "pocket hydrates." These are quite stable, unless heated; however, heating

can result in crystal collapse to an amorphous form. These are often stoichiometric in nature. Two isomorphic clathrates of the cephalosporins, cefazolin sodium pentahydrate (α-form) and FK041 hydrates, have been reported by Mimura et al. (2002b).

2. *Lattice channel water.* As can be surmised, the water molecules lie hydrogen bonded in channels and perform a space-filling role and are generally nonstoichiometric. They are frequently unstable, and the water is easily lost on drying. Crystallinity is maintained on drying, however. Indeed, if water is not important to the stability of the crystal lattice, the structure may be the same as the parent hydrate, albeit with some crystal lattice contraction. The isomorphic structures are often very hygroscopic and rapidly rehydrate under ambient relative humidities. An example of a channel hydrate is cephalexin (Kennedy et al., 2003). Mimura et al. (2002a) has further classified the behavior of this type of hydrate:

   i. Class A: Desorption of the water molecules leads to collapse of lattice to yield an amorphous solid. The water molecules show strong interaction with the API.
   ii. Class B: Desorption and/or adsorption of water promotes transition to a new crystal form. As with a class A, there is a strong interaction with the API.
   iii. Class C: As above, but the lattice expands to accommodate the water or contacts when it loses it. Cromolyn sodium is an example of this type of structure (Stephenson and Disroad, 2000).
   iv. Class D: No significant change in the crystal structure takes place when water is adsorbed or desorbed. The water molecules occupy definite positions in lattice channels, but their interactions are rather weak in nature. A number of compounds have been reported to exhibit this type of behavior, for example, dirithromycin (Stephenson et al., 1994).

3. *Metal ion–coordinated water.* This arises in the salts of weak acids, for example, calcium salts where the metal ion coordinates with the water molecules and is included in the growing lattice structure. These show both stoichiometric and nonstoichiometric behavior, for example Fenoprofen sodium is an example of a stoichometric hydrate (Stephenson and Disroad, 2000).

4. In some structures, both (2) and (3) can occur together, for example, nedocromil sodium trihydrate (Freer et al., 1987) and show both metal coordinated water and channel water.

Hydrates can also exhibit polymorphism. For example, amiloride hydrochloride dihydrate is present in two polymorphic forms. By milling or compressing both forms, it was shown that form A was more stable than form B. Moreover, it was shown that the anhydrate rapidly rehydrated to form A dihydrate on exposure to atmospheric RH (Jozwiakowski et al., 1993). Niclosamide also exists as two monohydrated forms and an anhydrated phase (van Tonder et al., 2004). It was found that suspension formulations of the anhydrate readily converted to thick suspensions of monohydrate. Rapid solution-mediated conversion to a hydrate can often result in the formation of an unusable thixotropic formulation. In addition to this complication, in situ formation of a hydrated phase may modify dissolution and hence bioavailability of the material. For these reasons, it is important to assess the propensity for hydrate formation in formulation vehicles as part of the material selection program. In another instance, during prenomination studies of one of the MCT-1 compounds reported by Guile et al. (2005), a compound was undergoing safety studies as a suspension formulation. The integrity of the suspension formulation showed a high degree of variability, with some aliquots of this formulation (when stored at subambient temperatures from a chemical stability perspective) giving rise to the formation of a thixotropic gel. Analysis of the resultant gel-like material revealed the presence of an interweaving network of crystals that were thin and fibrous in nature (as illustrated in Fig. 14), which were later identified as a hydrated form of the anhydrous starting material. Rapid solution-mediated conversion to a hydrated phase can also be illustrated by caffeine, which almost immediately converts to its monohydrate when suspended in water (Fig. 15).

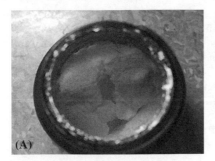
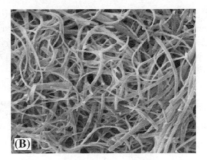

Figure 14 Pictures of a suspension formulation following rapid solution-mediated transformation of an anhydrate to an hydrate showing (**A**) visual image of the integrity of the formulation and (**B**) scanning electron micrograph of the material showing formation of a dense network of fine crystals.

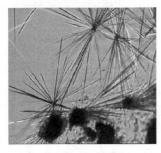

Figure 15 Conversion of caffeine to caffeine hydrate by suspension in water.

For the selection of the best form to progress into development, Bray et al. (1999) have described experiments suitable to characterize the properties of a number of hydrates based on the example of the fibrinogen antagonist L-738,167. Four solid-state forms of the compound were identified using XRPD, DSC, and moisture uptake studies. The four forms were a pentahydrate, a trihydrate, and two others where the stoichiometry was determined to be 2.41 and 0.59. The trihydrate was shown to convert to the pentahydrate above 50% RH and hence was rejected as a candidate. From suspension studies it was found that the 0.59 hydrate converted to the pentahydrate; however, the 2.41 hydrate did not. Thus, the pentahydrate and 2.41 hydrate were recommended with the caveat that additional formulation and processing experiments should be carried out to choose which of these hydrates should be used in a solid-dosage form.

The hydration state of a hydrate depends on the a_w in the crystallization medium, as shown by Zhu et al. (1996), using theophylline and its hydrate (as crystallized from organic solvent-water mixtures). However, the relative amount of water to water-miscible organic solvent is critical and is often only assessed in a semiempirical way. Results obtained using methanol-water and isopropyl alcohol (IPA)-water mixtures showed that the anhydrate was obtained at a_w values of less than 0.25, independent of whether the solid was anhydrate or the hydrated form of the drug. The monohydrate was obtained at a_w values of 0.25. As an extension of this type of approach, Variankaval et al. (2007) showed that the phase boundary between the anhydrate and the hydrate was independent of the nature of the cosolvent such that it was not necessary to determine the phase equilibria in each cosolvent system.

Polymorphic hydrates add a further complexity to the isolation procedure, as exemplified, for instance, by talterelin, a compound that exhibits two polymorphic forms of a tetrahydrate (Maruyama and Ooshima, 2000). Although the α-form of the compound showed good isolation behavior, the β-form was the thermodynamic stable form of the compound, especially in the presence of methanol. At low-methanol concentrations (0–10% w/w methanol), there was a conformational change that led to crystallization of the α-form, even though the crystallization may have been seeded with the stable β-form. At 30% methanol, crystallization of the β-form dominated to the extent that it grew on the surface of the α-form. Llinàs et al. (2008) have described the situation where two polymorphic trihydrate have crystallized concomitantly from solution. Often a larger degree of prework is required to evaluate the conditions that represent the stability domains of the anhydrate and hydrated phases, as described by Sacchetti (2004), who used a slurry equilibration method to determine under which conditions the anhydrate and monohydrate of GW2016 were stable (between 0.04 and 0.11 mole fraction water in methanol or 7% and 15% RH).

Li et al. (2008) have examined the a_w on the transformation between the anhydrate and hydrate of carbamazepine, and Qu et al. (2007) have examined the effect of additives on the conversion. It was found that hydroxypropyl methylcellulose (HPMC) had a strong inhibitory effect on transformation, and this property might be useful from an early safety assessment point of view where compounds may be formulated using HPMC as a suspending agent.

Amorphous Phases

Amorphous phases are noncrystalline materials that possess no long-range order, but can exhibit a certain degree of short-range order (Yu, 2001; Bhugra and Pikal, 2008). Amorphous phases represent highly energetic, unstable materials largely because of this lack of three-dimensional or long-range order found in crystalline materials. This lack of three-dimensional periodicity is reflected in the materials' inability to diffract X rays constructively; as such analysis of an amorphous sample by XRPD gives rise to a diffuse profile devoid of the characteristic peaks observed for crystalline phases. However, it must be borne in mind that there are some samples that when analyzed by XRPD also give rise to a diffuse profile, but are shown by other methods (such as the presence of a discrete melting event) to be crystalline. Such phases are termed X-ray amorphous and represent micro- or nanocrystalline structures.

The amorphous phase can be thought of as a frozen or supercooled liquid, but with the thermal fluctuations present in a liquid frozen to a greater or lesser extent, leaving only largely static structural disorder (Elliot et al., 1986). According to the USP, the degree of crystallinity depends on the fraction of crystalline material in the mixture, and this is termed the two-state model. Another way of viewing this situation is that the crystallinity can have a value that ranges from 100% for perfect crystals (0 entropy) to 0% (noncrystalline or amorphous); this is known as the one-state model. Yu (2001) has reviewed the characteristics and significance of the amorphous state with regard to pharmaceuticals.

The amorphous state can be characterized by the glass transition temperature (T_g), where the molecular motion is faster above and slower below this transition (Zhou et al., 2002). The T_g can be thought of as similar to a second-order phase transition, but the glassy state is regarded as far from being in thermal equilibrium. In their paper, Hancock and Shamblin (2001) addressed the question of how the molecular mobility of the material influences its performance. By using DSC, they argued that most pharmaceutical glasses should have a similar relaxation time around the T_g.

The T_g can probably be best visualized through its thermal behavior and can be measured using DSC as a second-order transition, as shown in Figure 16. Furthermore, it can also be assessed in terms of impact to volume or density as a function of temperature, as illustrated in Figure 17.

One consequence of heating through the glass transition is that the sample, as the density and viscosity become reduced, may have sufficient mobility to crystallize, and then when heated further may show complex polymorphic transitions induced by heating (Bhugra and Pikal, 2008). In general, for chemical and physical stability, a high T_g is preferred ($>100°C$). Amorphous materials typically exhibit a higher degree of hygroscopicity, and the glass transition is sensitive to moisture. An increase in moisture content tends to lower the T_g and has the potential to render the material more chemically and physically unstable.

It should be noted that the glass transition is variable in nature and is a function of the preparation conditions of the amorphous phase and any subsequent pretreatment to analysis. Since salt evaluation is an integral part of the pharmaceutical material selection process, it is interesting to note that Tong et al. (2002) examined the influence of the alkali metal counterion on the T_g of amorphous indomethacin salts. They found that there was as an increase in the T_g that was inversely proportional to the ionic radius of the cation. The Li salt had the highest T_g; however, this is not used in pharmaceutical formulations and hence only the sodium and potassium salts would normally be considered in this series.

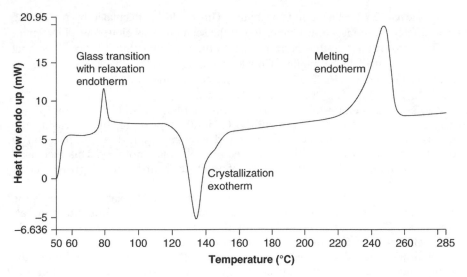

Figure 16   DSC second-order transition (glass transition). *Abbreviation*: DSC, differential scanning calorimetry.

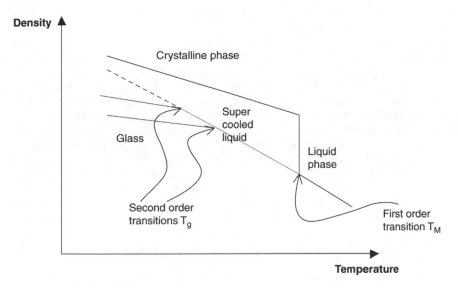

Figure 17   Schematic showing the density relationship as a function of temperature of some equilibrium and nonequilibrium phases.

Fragility (defined by equation 26) is a term that has been used to describe temperature dependence of the molecular motions in the region of the glass transition (Hancock et al., 1998), and is also considered an important measure that reflects the stability of the amorphous phase in relation to short- and intermediate-range order (Moura Ramos, et al. 2002).

$$m = \frac{\Delta H}{2.303 R T_g} \tag{26}$$

where ΔH is the activation energy for the molecular motions at T_g and R the gas constant. Thus, if m has a large value, this corresponds to a change of molecular motion of 10 times for every 10 K change in temperature, the glass can be considered fragile. Smaller values of m correspond to stronger glasses. For example, sorbitol, with a value of $m = 95$, was considered to be fragile, while zinc chloride, with $m = 30$, was considered to be a strong glass. In the latter case the molecular motion was calculated to change by 10 times for every 25 K change in temperature. This could be calculated by performing DSC experiments at different scan rates in which the log of the scan rate was plotted as a function of the reciprocal T_g. The slope of the line thus corresponded to the activation energy, ΔH^{DSC}, so that equation (26) can be used to calculate the fragility. Crowley and Zografi (2001) have reported the use of the Vogel–Tammann–Fulcher (VTF) fragility parameters for a range of pharmaceuticals, and proposed D values from 7 to 15 covered the majority glass formers.

Numerous studies have been undertaken to correlate the physical stability of amorphous materials with the prevalence of molecular mobility. Generally speaking, by increasing the temperature, there is a decrease in molecular density and viscosity (that does not necessarily follow Arrhenius's behavior), allowing a higher degree of molecular mobility. This increased level of mobility is associated with the occurrence of nucleation and crystal growth at or around the T_g (Sun et al., 2008). Interestingly, there have been several reports of crystallization of amorphous phases at temperatures significantly lower than the T_g. An example of this is the assessment of the crystallization of amorphous indomethacin following different pretreatments (Carpentier et al., 2006). Rapid quenching of the amorphous state to below the T_g resulted in the crystallization of the metastable α-phase, while slow cooling close to the T_g resulted in the formation of the more stable γ-phase. Evaluating the molecular mobility of the different phases by dielectric and ^{1}H NMR spectroscopy showed variation in the mobility of the glassy states obtained by the different pretreatment processes. The investigations demonstrated that in each case the subsistence of molecular mobility and relaxation processes to a differing extent led to the formation of precursor molecular self-assemblies, which resulted in the crystallization of different polymorphs.

The existence of multiple amorphous states has been discussed extensively (Shalaev and Zografi, 2002; Hancock et al., 2002; Hedoux et al., 2004). The term polyamorphism has been used to describe systems that possess multiple supercooled liquid states, representing different and discrete phases that are thermodynamically separated by distinct phase transitions (Hancock et al., 2002). Such discrete phases are thought to possess different physical and chemical properties in accordance with the conditions of isolation and pretreatment. However, glassy amorphous states that have discrete properties, but are not related by discrete transitions between one state and another, have been referred to as "pseudopolyamorphs."

Methods for the production of the amorphous state include quenching the melt of a compound, rapid precipitation from solution by, for example, addition of an antisolvent, freeze and spray-drying (Ueno et al., 1998), dehydration of crystalline hydrates, and grinding/milling (Wildfong et al., 2006; Chieng et al., 2008). One consequence of a disordered structure is that amorphous phases are thermodynamically unstable, and, therefore, they are the most energetic forms of a compound. The tendency of amorphous phases is thus to revert to a more stable, crystalline form. According to Bhugra and Pikal (2008), the predisposition to crystallize appears to be related to the degree of similarity between any short-range order in the amorphous phase and a crystalline phase (Hancock and Shamblin, 2001). However, the crystallization kinetics may be reasonably slow at room temperature, and it is the average rate of molecular motion that is the most important aspect of an amorphous solid, and this can be used to explain and predict the stability of an amorphous phase. By utilizing this knowledge, storage conditions can be selected to prevent degradation (Crowley and Zografi, 2001). For a material to progress into development, the robustness in the mode of preparation or manufacture, storage, formulatability, and performance needs to be demonstrated. The inherent physical and chemical instability associated with amorphous phases renders them less desirable. The main issues surrounding instability arise from spontaneous crystallization upon storage of the drug (e.g., especially if there are fluctuations in temperature and moisture content), crystallization or chemical instability in formulations, and secondary processing. As such, attempts should be made to find a crystalline form of the compound through crystallization experiments or salt formation. One consequence for some compounds with a low degree of crystallinity is a decrease in stability, and this is particularly true for freeze-dried materials. In the case of the antibiotic imipenem, a method of freeze crystallizing the compound was developed, thus avoiding the problems induced by the amorphous nature of the compound after freeze-drying (Connolly et al., 1996). As an exception, it has been reported that amorphous insulin is more stable than the corresponding crystalline state (Pikal and Rigsbee, 1997).

In spite of the inherent stability issues, it should be borne in mind that amorphous phases, where kinetic stability has been demonstrated, can offer some advantages over the crystalline phase. For example, a stabilized amorphous form of novobiocin was found to be 10 times more soluble and therapeutically active compared with the crystalline form (Haleblian, 1975). However, for amorphous material, it is often difficult to obtain a measure of the true solubility. Attempts have been made to correlate predicted thermodynamic solubility data with actual solubility data, treating the amorphous state as a pseudoequilibrium solid (Hancock and Parks, 2000). From this study it was found that the predicted solubility ratio between crystalline and amorphous states ranged from 10-fold up to approximately 1700. However, the observed solubility ratio was closer to the range 4 to 25. The competition between solubility and crystallization during the solubility measurements is thought to largely describe this discrepancy. That having been said, the increase in in vivo exposure for some drugs is attributed to the advantages obtained in terms of dissolution kinetics rather than solubility. For example, it has been found that MK-0591 was poorly absorbed when administered as the crystalline sodium salt. However, the freeze-dried form, which was amorphous, showed a much higher aqueous solubility and was very well absorbed and found to be stable over a long period of time, for example, no crystallization was observed after six months' storage at 30°C at 75% RH (Clas et al., 1996). The lack of crystallization was attributed to two factors: (1) the high glass transition of the compound (~125°C) and (2) the formation of liquid crystals in solution at concentrations greater than 60 mg/mL. Thus, because of its high glass transition, its liquid crystalline properties indicated that this compound, in its lyophilized state, would be suitable for an oral formulation. Lyophilized amorphous acadesine, however, has been found to crystallize when exposed to water vapor (Larsen et al., 1997). By using isothermal calorimetry, they showed that below 40% RH crystallization never occurred. However, above 50% RH samples always crystallized after 1.5 hours. Interestingly, the crystalline phase obtained was anhydrous, but was produced via a metastable hydrate, which apparently decomposed to give the crystalline anhydrate.

ASSESSMENT OF THE ORGANIC SOLID STATE

There are many analytical techniques available to characterize the salts and polymorphs of CDs (Threlfall, 1995; Clas, 2003; Giron, 2003; Giron et al., 2004). Indeed, in polymorphism studies it is particularly advisable to analyze the modifications by more than one technique. The principal physicochemical techniques that could be used to characterize the compounds are:

- X-ray diffraction (XRD) (powder and single crystal) (Stephenson, 2005)
- Microscopy [optical (Nichols, 1998); electron (Tian et al., 2006); and atomic force (Hooton, et al. 2006)]
- Thermal analytical techniques, for example, DSC, TGA [with MS or Fourier transform infrared (FTIR) for effluent gas analysis (Rodriguez and Bugey, 1997)], and hot-stage microscopy (HSM) (Vitez et al., 1998)
- Isothermal microcalorimetry (Phipps and Mackin, 2000)
- Solution calorimetry (Gu and Grant, 2001)
- Mid- and near-IR spectroscopies (Threlfall and Chalmers, 2007)
- Raman spectroscopy (Fini, 2004)
- Cross polarization magic angle spinning (CP MAS) solid-state NMR (Harris, 2007)
- Hygroscopicity measurements (Kawakami et al., 2005)
- Phase solubility analysis (Sheikhzadeh et al., 2007)
- Intrinsic dissolution rates (Pereira et al., 2007)

Byrn et al. (1995) have proposed a strategic conceptual approach to the regulatory considerations regarding the characterization of pharmaceutical solids. This is based on flow charts for (1) polymorphs, (2) hydrates, (3) desolvated solvates, and (4) amorphous forms. Figure 18

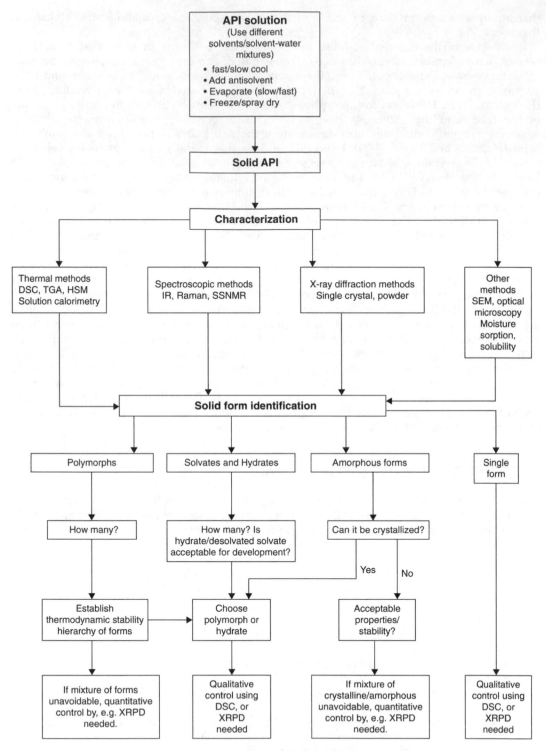

Figure 18   Flow diagram regarding polymorph, etc. Production and characterization.

shows a simplified flow diagram illustrating a solid-state form generation, assessment and control procedure. A few examples are given here to show the utilization of these techniques:

- Exploring long-range order
- XRD methods

Single Crystal Structure Determination

The crystal structure of a compound is regarded as the "gold standard" for all solid-state studies, since this provides the following information:

- Molecular identity
- Basic crystal information such as bond lengths and angles and space group
- Molecular conformations
- Absolute configuration of chiral molecules (R or S)
- Molecular disorder
- Hydrogen-bonding motifs

Other data can be derived from single-crystal data, such as the true density, the calculated XRPD pattern and the morphology. Together these data provide an absolute proof of structure that can be presented in investigational new drug (IND) and new drug applications (NDAs).

Brittain (2000b) has presented an introductory paper on the use of single-crystal XRD (SXRD) to study polymorphism and psuedopolymorphism, and a good introductory text is that by Glusker et al. (1994). Clegg's (1998) primer on the subject is also a good starting place for the novice. Datta and Grant (2004) have reviewed the advances in the determination, prediction, and engineering of crystal structures.

X rays are short wavelength, high-energy beams of electromagnetic radiation between 0.1 and 100 Å. X rays are generated when a beam of electrons are accelerated against (usually) a copper target (anode) where the electrons are stopped by the electrons of the target element and a broad band of continuous radiation is emitted (bremsstrahlung—braking radiation-white radiation), superimposed on which are discrete wavelengths of varying intensity (X rays). The former is due to collisions between the electrons and the target, and the latter is due to ionization of the metal atoms, which lose an inner shell electron. The Cu $K_{\alpha1}$, $K_{\alpha2}$ doublet has an energy of approximately 8.05 keV, which is equivalent to a wavelength of 1.541 Å. For high-resolution work, the K_{α} radiation should be monochromatized to use only the $K_{\alpha1}$ radiation. Needless to say, white radiation is of little value and needs to be eliminated or reduced. Other anodes can be used, for example, cobalt, which has a $K_{\alpha1}$ wavelength of 1.788965 Å.

For laboratory single-crystal structure determinations, a good quality crystal of a suitable size, for example, $0.1 \times 0.1 \times 0.1$ mm^3, and perfection is required (De Ranter, 1986). However, larger crystals can also be used, for example, Görbitz (1999) used a single crystal of the glycl-L-serine with dimensions $2.2 \times 2.0 \times 0.8$ mm^3 and found that with a CCD diffractometer a complete and good-quality data set was obtained in less than 25 minutes. Very small crystals, on the other hand, usually need synchrotron radiation for their solution. For example, Clegg and Teat (2000) were able to determine the structure of tetracycline hydrochloride with a crystal of size $0.04 \times 0.03 \times 0.02$ mm^3 with synchrotron radiation with wavelength $\lambda = 0.6883$ Å. van der Sluis and Kroon (1989) have described some general strategies to obtain suitable single crystals of low-molecular-weight compounds for X-ray structure determination. These methods include evaporation, batch crystallization, liquid-liquid diffusion, sublimation, gel crystallization, etc.

The structure determination is a two-step procedure, including an experimental and computational part. For laboratory determinations, a suitable well-diffracting single crystal must be available. The best size is about 0.1 to 0.2 mm in 3D with smaller single crystals, synchrotron radiation can be used. The crystal is mounted on a goniometer head and placed in the X-ray beam of the single-crystal X-ray diffractometer. The unit cell parameters are deduced from the scattering that is, the diffraction pattern. These parameters describe the dimensions of the repetitive unit in the crystal. The reflection intensities are measured using a CCD area detector.

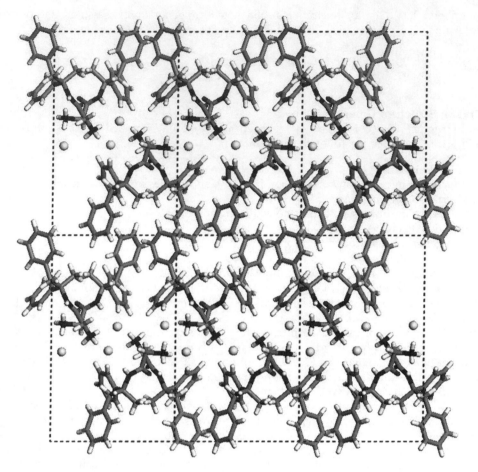

Figure 19 Crystal structure of remacemide HCl.

After the experiment, the intensity data are processed and reduced. The structure is solved using various mathematical and statistical relationships ("direct methods") to produce a structure model. Subsequent refinement of the structure model against the observed diffraction data gives a measure (reliability index or R factor) of how well the model agrees with the experimental data. A low R factor of say 0.1 is desired. After the refinement has converged and the structure seems reasonable, the geometrical parameters can be calculated and interpreted and graphical illustrations of the molecule and its crystal packing can be produced. Figure 19 shows the crystal structure some crystal data for remacemide HCl (Lewis et al., 2005).

Visualization of crystal structures held in the CSD, which contains in excess of a quarter of a million crystal structures (Allen, 2002), can be implemented using free software (Mercury) that can be downloaded from the Internet (Bruno et al., 2002). The powder pattern can, of course, be calculated from the single-crystal data (normally an R of <5% is required). This can be done using the SHELXTL-PLUS program. If additional peaks are found in the experimental diffraction pattern, this may indicate the presence of other solid phases, for example, polymorphs that have nucleated and grown from solution (Coquerel, 2006).

XRPD

The book by Jenkins and Synder (1996) is particularly recommended as an excellent introduction to the science of XRPD. Some of the salient points made in this book and other sources are presented later in the chapter.

X rays are part of the electromagnetic spectrum lying between UV and γ rays, and they are expressed in angstrom units (Å). Diffraction is a scattering phenomenon, and when X rays are incident on crystalline solids, they are scattered in all directions. Scattering occurs due to the radiation wavelength being in the same order of magnitude as the interatomic distances within the crystal structure.

Bragg's law describes the conditions under which diffraction will occur. Diffraction will occur if a perfectly parallel and monochromatic X-ray beam of wavelength λ is incident on a crystalline sample at an angle θ that satisfies the Bragg equation (equation 27),

$$n\lambda = 2d \sin \theta \qquad (27)$$

where n is the order of reflection (an integer, usually 1), λ the wavelength of X ray, d the distance between planes in crystal (d-spacings), and θ the angle of incidence/reflection.

An X-ray diffractometer is made up of an X-ray tube generating X rays from, for example, Cu K$_\alpha$ or Co source and a detector. The most common arrangement in pharmaceutical powder studies is the Bragg—Bentano reflection θ-θ or θ-2θ configurations (Fig. 20). These arrangements are summarized in Table 11.

The powder pattern consists of a series of peaks that have been collected at various scattering angles, which are related to d-spacings such that unit cell dimensions can be determined. In most cases, measurement of the d-spacings will suffice to positively identifying a crystalline material. If the sample does not show long-range order, that is, it is amorphous, the X rays are incoherently scattered leading to the so-called halo pattern. Figure 21 shows an example of a crystalline, amorphous and a partially crystalline phase. In addition to amorphous phases of a compound, the existence of disordered nanocrystalline phase should be included (Bates et al., 2006). Those samples that exhibit continuous peak broadening are nanocrystalline in contrast to amorphous phases that do not show this effect. The observation of glass transition during DSC analysis of a sample would be sufficient confirmation to distinguish it from a nanocrystalline sample.

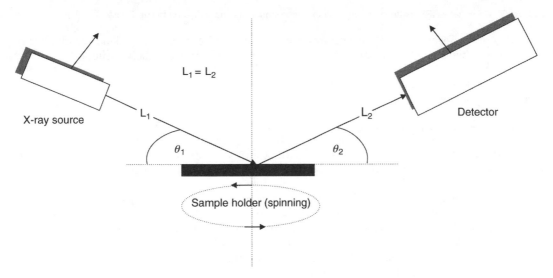

Figure 20 Bragg–Bentano geometry used in XRPD experiments. *Abbreviation*: XRPD, X-ray powder diffraction.

Table 11 X-Ray Tube and Detector Arrangements

Type	Tube	Specimen	Receiving slit	L$_1$	L$_2$
Bragg–Bentano θ-2θ	Fixed	Varies as θ	Varies as 2θ	Fixed	=L$_1$
Bragg–Bentano θ-θ	Varies as θ	Fixed	Varies as θ	Fixed	=L$_1$

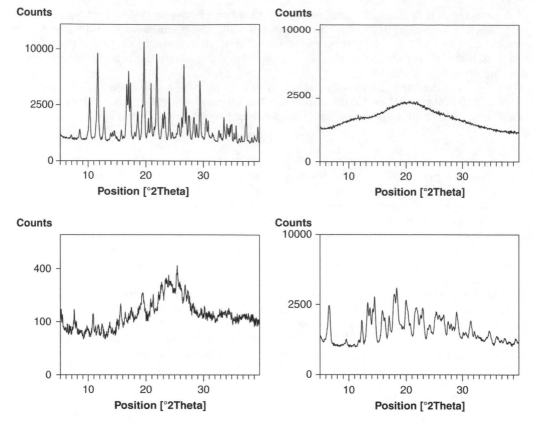

Figure 21 Typical XRPD patterns of crystalline, amorphous, and partially crystalline forms.

It is often observed that the diffraction peaks obtained are not sharp. This broadening is due to a number of factors. Coquerel (2006) has exemplified these as being due to:

- Poor long-range order
- Very small particles
- The presence of solid solutions
- Disorder, for example, static and dynamic

Although XRPD analysis is a relatively straightforward technique for the identification of solid-phase structures, there are a number of sources of error. These include the following:

1. *Variations in particle size.* Large anisotropic particles can lead to nonrandom orientation and so particles less than 10 μm should be used, that is, the sample should be *carefully* ground. However, if the size is too small, for example, 1 μm, this may lead to broadening of the diffraction peaks (known as the Scherrer effect). Indeed, if the crystal sizes are sufficiently small, then the sample may appear to be amorphous (as discussed earlier).
2. *Preferred orientation* (Davidovich et al., 2004). If a powder consists of anisotropic polycrystalline materials, for example, needle- or plate-shaped particles, these tend to become aligned parallel to the specimen axis, and thus certain planes have a greater chance of reflecting the X rays. To reduce the errors due to this source, the sample should be lightly ground in a mortar and pestle to ensure a more random-shaped sample, which is then rotated in situ to increase the randomness of the sample (Campbell Roberts et al., 2002b; Cheung et al., 2003). Alternatively, the sample can be packed into a capillary. Figure 22 shows some examples of preferred orientation. As noted by Stephenson (2005), poor particle statistics and preferred orientation effects are

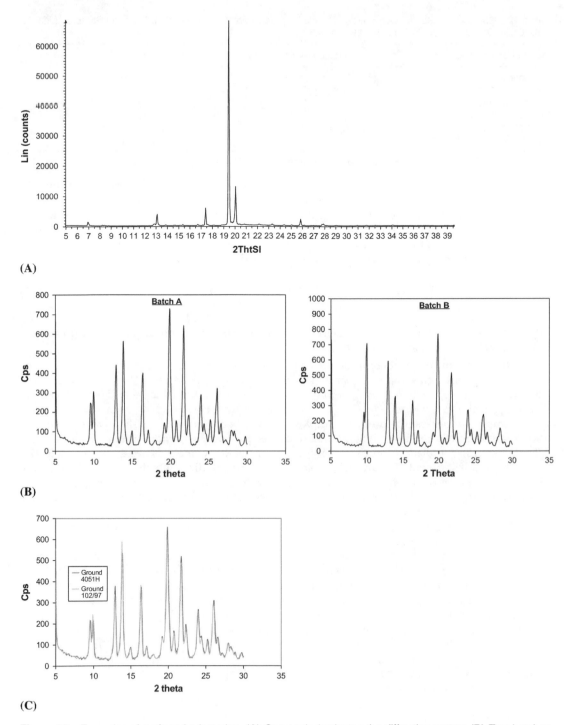

Figure 22 Examples of preferred orientation: (**A**) One peak dominates the diffraction pattern.(**B**) Two batches have apparently different XRPD patterns.(**C**) Effect of grinding both samples in (**B**). *Abbreviation*: XRPD, X-ray powder diffraction.

probably at their worst from samples obtained from high-throughput crystallization experiments, and this should be borne in mind when analyzing these data.

The magnitude of statistical errors depends on the number of photons counted. To keep these small, scanning should be carried out at an appropriately slow speed.

Table 12 Possible Causes for Compositional Variations Between "As-Received" and Ground Samples (JCPDS Data Collection and Analysis Subcommittee, 1986)

Induced by grinding	Induced by irradiation	Special problems
Amorphism	Polymerization	Hydration, carbonization
Strain	Decomposition	Loss of water in vacuum
Decomposition		Decomposition at high temperature
Polymorphic change		
Solid-state reactions		
Contamination by the mortar		

Source: From Jenkins et al., 1986, with permission from Powder Diffraction.

3. *Sample height*. The literature states that a thick sample with random orientation will produce less accurate peak positions, but more reliable intensities. Samples should be prepared at the correct height, that is, level with the top of the holder, since the diffraction peaks will shift on the 2θ scale. Thus, if the sample is too low, the pattern shifts down the 2θ scale and vice versa. It should be remembered that the shift is not linear and increases with decreasing 2θ, as described by equation (28).

$$\Delta 2\theta = \left(\frac{2s \cos \theta}{R} \right) \tag{28}$$

where $\Delta 2\theta$ is the change in displacement (in radians), s the specimen displacement (in mm), θ the angle (in degrees), and R the radius of goniometer.

This is one of the most common errors in XRPD experiments, and every effort should be to eliminate it through sample preparation. The sample should be at level with the top of the holder. If the sample height is too low, the pattern shifts down the 2θ scale, and if it is too high, it moves up the 2θ scale.

Sample preparation procedures for XRPD have been reported (JCPDS Data Collection and Analysis Sub-committee, 1986). Possible causes for compositional variations between as-received samples and those prepared (by grinding) for X-ray analysis are given in Table 12.

The greatest potential source of problems is due to grinding, which can introduce strain, amorphism, and polymorphic changes. Furthermore, the atmosphere surrounding the sample can create problems because of loss or gain of moisture or carbon dioxide. This is particularly true if a heating stage is used.

As already mentioned, the limited availability of compounds in early development can be problematic. However, modern powder diffractometers can use so-called zero-background holders (ZBH). These are made from a single crystal of silicon that has been cut along a nondiffracting plane and then polished to an optically flat finish (Misture et al., 1994). Thus, X rays incident upon this surface will be negated by Bragg extinction. By using this technique, a thin layer of grease is placed on the ZBH surface, and the sample of ground compound is placed on the surface. The excess is removed such that only a monolayer is examined. The total thickness of the sample and grease should be of the order of a few microns. According to Misture et al. (1994), it is important that the sample is deagglomerated so that the monolayer condition is met. By using this technique, the diffraction pattern of approximately 10 mg of compound can be obtained. One disadvantage of the ZBH is that any weak reflections may not be readily detectable because of the small sample size used.

The XRPD can be calibrated using a variety of standards. These are available from the Laboratory of the Government Chemist (LGC) in the United Kingdom or National Institute of Standards and Technology (NIST) in the United States. The types of standards used in XRPD are shown in Table 13 (Jenkins and Snyder, 1996).

Analyzing one or two peaks of LaB_6, at least weekly, should give confidence in the diffractometer performance and alert the user to any problems that may be developing.

Nonambient studies with XRPD
In addition to collecting and analyzing data at ambient temperature for phase identification, XRPD can be used be used to determine a variety of phenomena under nonambient conditions,

Table 13 Standards Used in X-Ray Diffraction Studies

Type	Use	Standard
External 2θ standards		Silicon
		α-Quartz
		Gold
Internal d-spacing standards	Primary	Silicon
	Primary	Fluorophlogopit
	Secondary	Tungsten, silver, quartz, and diamond
Internal intensity standards	Quantitative	Al_2O_3
	Intensity	α- and β-silicon nitride
	Respirable	Oxides of Al, Ce, Cr, Ti, and Zn
	Quartz	α-Silicon dioxide
		Cristobalite
External sensitivity standards		Al_2O_3
Line profile standards	Broadening calibration	LaB_6

Source: From Jenkins and Snyder (1996).

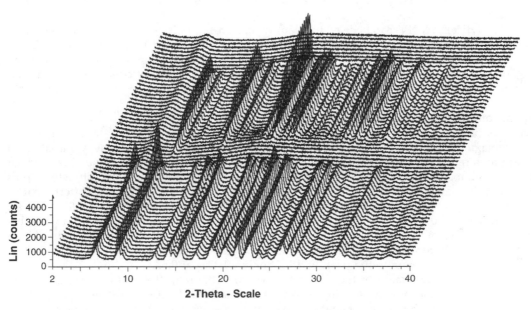

Figure 23 Temperature-XRPD pattern of a compound undergoing a polymorphic change. *Abbreviation*: XRPD, X-ray powder diffraction.

for instance, phase transformations (Evans and Radosavljević, 2004). A heating stage may be of value for investigating thermal events detected during DSC experiments (Krajalaininen et al., 2005). By using the Anton Parr TTK temperature attachment, the compound can be investigated between subambient temperatures and several hundred degrees. Figure 23 shows the diffraction patterns obtained on heating a sample (obtained by desolvating a methanol solvate followed by micronization). The accompanying DSC thermograms show the corresponding sequence investigated in the temperature XRPD experiment. Prior to the start of the XRPD experiment, the compound was partially amorphous due to desolvation and micronization. However, as the sample was heated, the XRPD peaks became sharper and stronger, indicating an increase in crystallinity; this corresponds to the annealing exotherm observed in the DSC thermogram. This DSC experiment showed a melt-recrystallization-melt polymorphic transformation, which is also shown by the XRPD, whereby a change in crystal structure was evident as the sample was heated, followed by a diffuse pattern from the final melt. These data were collected using a position-sensitive detector (PSD). The PSD collects data simultaneously over all angles, which allows a higher count rate, enabling significantly faster data acquisition. This type of attachment is well suited for high-throughput crystallization screening, as described by Florence et al. (2003). Kishi et al. (2002) have described a combined XRPD-DSC, which they used to study the dependence of thermal dehydration behavior of nitrofurantoin monohydrate on humidity.

In a similar way the sample can be exposed to varying degrees of humidity in situ and the diffraction pattern determined using, for example, an Anton Parr TTK-450 variable temperature/humidity stage (Vogt et al., 2006; Linnow et al., 2007). The mechanism of dehydration of theophylline monohydrate using a two-dimensional XRPD and synchrotron radiation has been reported by Nunes et al. (2006).

Reutzel-Edens et al. (2003) found three dehydrates of olanzapine, which could be produced from a "fragile" higher hydrate that was only observed in wet cakes of the compound. According to Storey et al. (2003), this behavior is typical when the solvent or water occupies positions in the crystal lattice without any significant hydrogen bonding. As the solvent evaporates, this loosely bound solvent is lost and hence the lattice contracts so as to fill the space left by the departed solvent/water. This phenomenon can be easily followed by allowing a wet cake to dry in air on an XRPD plate and assessing the change in the diffraction pattern with time.

Analytically, XRPD can be used to quantify mixtures of polymorphs (Iyengar et al., 2001; Byard et al., 2005) and amorphous in crystalline (and vice versa) (O'Sullivan et al., 2002); Sarsfield et al., 2006). Operationally, it appears to be difficult to obtain accurate results below 5% amorphous content; however, a 1.8% limit of quantitation (LOQ) of crystallinity with limit of detection (LOD) of 0.9% has been reported for sucrose (Surana and Suryanaryanan, 2000).

Synchrotron Radiation
Synchrotrons utilize accelerated electrons traveling close to the speed of light to generate electromagnetic radiation. This radiation has the advantage of high-intensity radiation, a continuous range of wavelengths (radio frequency, but also in the IR, UV, and X ray, which means a monochromator is needed), and low divergence, which gives sharp diffraction spots and intensity data. This leads to greatly enhanced resolution in the diffraction pattern, that is, narrow peak widths and highly accurate measurements of peak positions and intensities. As an example of the power of a synchrotron source, it has been calculated that the Grenoble facility in France produces X rays that are one trillion times brighter than those produced by a laboratory diffractometer. Furthermore, there is a very high resolution in 2θ, with an instrumental contribution to the peak width of only ~0.006° at 0.6Å.

Because of the quality of the diffraction pattern, obtaining the unit cell parameters by indexing, using the common indexing programs such as ITO, TREOR, and DICVOL, is easier when compared to laboratory data, where peak overlap is common. Very small crystals can be examined. Figure 24 shows the synchrotron data obtained from a sibenedit hydrochloride at two temperatures and the corresponding laboratory data. The superior peak resolution afforded by the synchrotron data is evident.

Although data collection using synchrotron radiation perhaps offers a greater opportunity for solving the structure from powder data, the solution of structures from laboratory-generated X rays is not unknown. For example, Johnston et al. (2004) solved the structure of AR-C69457CC from powder data (using DASH) collected on a laboratory diffractometer using the powder contained in borosilicate glass capillary.

Ab Initio Crystal Structure Solution From XRPD Data
As discussed previously, it is recognized that single-crystal data are one of the most powerful solid-state analytical techniques available to pharmaceutical scientists. However, one limitation is the availability of single crystals of suitable size and perfection. Additionally, it can be almost impossible to obtain and analyze crystals of metastable phases at ambient temperature. A further advantage of obtaining the crystal structure directly from the polycrystalline sample is that it is representative of the powder rather than of one specific single crystal selected for analysis.

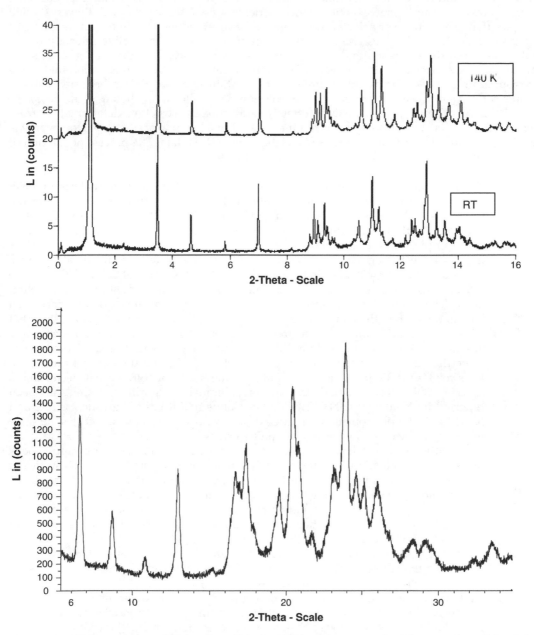

Figure 24 XRPD synchrotron data for sibenedit hydrochloride and corresponding laboratory data. *Abbreviation*: XRPD, X-ray powder diffraction.

The protocol used to establish the crystal structure (either directly from single crystals or from powder data methods) involves data collection from a good-quality sample, followed by unit cell determination, space group assignment, and structure solution, and finally, structure refinement. In the case of SXRD, the structural information is distributed in three-dimensional space, whereas for XRPD, the three-dimensional diffraction data are compressed into one-dimensional space (i.e., the powder pattern). As a consequence, the powder diffraction pattern often has severe peak overlap, leading to difficulties in reliable peak intensity (I_{hkl}) extraction. Furthermore, peak overlap may also give rise to ambiguities in indexing the powder pattern (to define the unit cell parameters), and space group assignment. The data should be collected from a powder sample that exhibits random orientation of the crystallites. Polycrystalline samples that exhibit plate or acicular morphologies have a tendency to align with the plane of the sample holder. This gives rise to a disproportionate increase in relative intensity of the reflections from these orientations, an occurrence known as preferred orientation effects. To ensure that the collected data are devoid of preferred orientation effects, it is important to take appropriate measures. The extent of preferred orientation in a sample can be tested using a simple diffraction procedure prior to high-resolution data collection (Cheung et al., 2003).

While synchrotron X-ray analysis offers one avenue for structure determination from very small crystals, it is not suitable for routine use within a laboratory situation. However, it is now possible to solve crystal structures from laboratory XRPD data. The process of solution of crystal structures from XRPD data can be described as follows:

1. Determination of the unit cell parameters (a, b, c, α, β, γ) from analysis of peak positions in the powder diffraction pattern. The pattern can be indexed using the programs such as DICVOL91 (Boultif and Louer, 1991), TREOR (Werner et al., 1985), and ITO. All these techniques measure the peak positions of about the first 20 peaks; for example, TREOR searches for solutions in index space by varying the Miller indices. It has been noted that ITO and TREOR need accurate low-angle data because of the use of the first 20 lines in the indexing routine (Werner, 2002). DICVOL, on the other hand, is less sensitive since the data errors are independent of the diffraction angle. Therefore, it makes sense to use more than one indexing program since each has its own strengths and weaknesses. For example, Werner (2002) suggested that ITO would find it impossible to index a pattern, which had many nonsystematic absences. Another point made in this paper was that it would be a mistake to use more than 20 to 25 lines when using DICVOL and TREOR; the optimal number of lines for ITO is 35. In terms of computing, time speed of solution has been ranked as ITO <TREOR90 < DICVOL91. A newer indexing algorithm, X-Cell, has been reported by Neumann (2003). This author claims that it has a high success rate and handles all the phenomena encountered, for example, peaks from other solid-state forms, peak overlap, and peak-positioning errors.

   Difficulties in indexing can arise from a number of sources, for example, peak overlap, contamination by another polymorph, poor crystallinity, or insufficient instrumental resolution. On a practical note, monochromatic $K_{\alpha 1}$ X rays should be used to index the pattern using the compound packed into a capillary or using a θ-2θ reflection stage. Indexing is a most important step in the structure determination process, that is, if the diffraction pattern cannot be indexed, then any subsequent structure solution will be impossible (Florence et al., 2003).

   From experimental $2\theta_{hkl}$ values, we can obtain d_{hkl} from which we must determine the lattice parameters. However, the relationship is usually expressed in terms of the reciprocal lattice parameters a^*, b^*, c^*, α^*, β^*, γ^*.

2. Unit cell refinement, intensity extraction, and space group determination. There are two approaches that have been developed for this purpose: Pawley (1981) and Le Bail (1988) fitting methods. The least squares refinement procedure involves assessment of cell parameters, position of the zero point, peak shapes, and areas (the Le Bail method extracts peak area data by accounting for the contribution of structural factors). In the first instance, the space group is assigned manually on the basis of systematic absences. The final discrimination and assignment involves least squares refinement and assessment of the goodness of fit of the extracted powder pattern, and the newly calculated cell is then assessed against the experimental data. The problem of peak overlap can limit unambiguous assignment. Consequently, several space groups may have to be considered in the structure solution calculations.

3. Structure solution.

4. Structure refinement.

However, there are a number of problems associated with the use of XRPD data, and these are as follows:

- Information from XRPD results from three-dimensional information being compressed into one dimension. The net effect of this operation is that the peaks severely overlap at high 2θ angle, which leads to a loss of information.
- Preferred orientation effects; however, this can be overcome by performing data collection experiments with a capillary instead of a flat plate.
- Fall off intensity, that is, the scattering intensity falls off at higher 2θ values. This can be overcome by counting for longer at the higher angles.

The crystal structure is defined by a series of structure factors (which are proportional to the electron density), F_{hkl}, of each atom or molecule type in the unit cell. F_{hkl} can be split into two components: the factor amplitude $|F_{hkl}|$ and the phase component α_{hkl}. The amplitude values can be obtained form the powder diffraction data, but the phase data are not so readily attainable. This is known as the phase problem and, as such, direct solutions of the crystal structure are not possible. Several methodologies exist that allow structure solution from powder data to be performed. These encompass traditional approaches and direct-space methods. The traditional approaches, such as Patterson or direct methods, involve extraction of the intensities of individual reflections I_{hkl} directly from the powder diffraction pattern. These methods then use algorithms to calculate and refine an electron density map using either Fourier summation or probability distribution-based logic (Christensen et al., 1985; McCusker, 1991; Cheetham et al., 1991; Harris and Tremayne, 1996).

Direct-space methods involve the generation of trial structures in direct space, and using the extracted powder patterns of these trial structures, a goodness of fit against the experimental powder pattern is assessed (Harris and Cheung, 2004). This protocol bypasses the need to use the diffraction-integrated intensities and the phase problem on the basis that from any trial structure the diffraction pattern (the $|F_{hkl}|$ data) can always be determined accurately. Algorithms that utilize the direct-space approach include the entropy maximization method and the likelihood ranking (Gilmore et al., 1993), simulated annealing (Newsam et al., 1992), Monte Carlo (Harris et al., 1994; Harris and Tremayne, 1996) and combined Monte-Carlo/simulated annealing (Engel et al., 1999; David et al., 1998), and a genetic algorithm method (Harris et al., 1998; Kariuki et al., 1999). A number of software packages are commercially available. One is now commercially available from the CSD and marketed as DASH (David et al., 2002, 2006). Another is marketed by Accelrys Inc. and is known as Reflex, which is part of their Materials Studio package. Harris and Cheung (2004) have also described the procedure. Notwithstanding these limitations, XRPD allows assessment of structures for which growth of a suitable single crystal is not feasible.

EXPLORING SHORT- AND MEDIUM-RANGE ORDER SPECTROSCOPIC TECHNIQUES

Mid-Infrared Spectroscopy

In addition to being used as a chemical identification technique, mid-IR spectroscopy can also be used to distinguish different solid-state structures of compounds. It is complementary to XRD; but in contrast to XRD, it provides short-range information. Vibrational spectroscopy techniques such as Fourier transform infrared (FTIR) spectroscopy provide information on quantized vibrational energy levels in a molecule. Subjecting a sample to monochromatic incident radiation (of frequency v_0) results in a perturbation of the system, for example, by absorption of the incident radiation. The absorption spectrum arises from the coupling of the incident radiation with a specific type of motion associated with the bonds in a molecule. For a vibration to be IR active (i.e., for a strong absorption band to be observed), the vibration must produce an oscillating dipole moment, which interacts with the oscillating electric field of the incident radiation, provided the frequency of the incident radiation equals that of the vibration. Homo-atomic bonds (such as C–C bonds) possess a poor dipole moment and hence either give rise to a weak absorption band or are IR inactive. This technique therefore provides information on mainly hetero-atomic interactions and is useful in extracting details such as hydrogen-bonding arrangements. IR spectroscopy using standard FTIR spectrometers allows information to be extracted from 4000 to 500 cm^{-1}. Variations in the spatial arrangement of atoms in the solid state will lead to differences in local symmetry, and this in turn leads to different stretching frequencies useful in distinguishing polymorphic forms of a compound. In addition, the inclusion of solvent or water can be detected using this technique, for example, the broad –OH stretch associated with water will be seen as will the stretch of the carbonyl group at around 1700/cm. Because of its ability to probe the structural configuration of the molecules in the solid state, it is a routine tool in the study of polymorphism; for example, Ayala et al. (2006) characterized the polymorphs of olanzapine using IR and Raman spectroscopy. Among other techniques, Zupančic et al. (2005) used IR spectroscopy to characterize the hydrates of pantoprazole sodium.

Experimentally, IR spectroscopy can be performed in a number of ways, by Nujol mull, KBr disk, or the diffuse or total reflectance technique. The KBr diskc technique is a transmission method in which the compound (1–3 mg) is mixed with the KBr (~350 mg) and compressed into a disk (at around 12,000 psi) using a press and die. This can be a disadvantage if the compound undergoes a polymorphic transformation under pressure (Chan and Doelker, 1985). However, in some cases extremes of pressure may have little or no impact on phase transitions as exemplified by the polymorphs of famotidine, which were not affected by pressurization when subjected to up to 106 kN in an IR hydraulic press (Német et al., 2005). One way to overcome this problem is to use the diffuse reflectance infrared Fourier transform (DRIFT) technique, whereby a few milligrams of compound are dispersed in approximately 250 mg of KBr and the spectrum obtained by reflection from the surface.

Increasingly, the attenuated total reflectance (ATR) technique is used, whereby the sample is gently ground and the spectrum is collected via a diamond sensor element. The principle of ATR is based on measuring the changes, which occur in totally internally reflected IR when it comes into contact with the sample. The IR beam is focused onto an optically dense crystal with high refractive index, which gives way to a so-called evanescent wave. This wave only protrudes approximately 0.5 to5 μm from the diamond surface so that a good contact between the crystal and the sample is essential. Other materials are also available for ATR measurements, for example, zinc selenide and germanium; however, diamond has the best durability and chemical resistance. In summary, the ATR technique offers faster sampling, improved inter-sample reproducibility, etc.

The FTIR spectra of two polymorphs, an amorphous form and a methanol solvate of AR-C69457AA, are shown in Figure 25. As can be seen, the spectrum of the amorphous form of the compound is less well defined and reflects the multitude of molecular environments present in this form of the compound.

Variable temperature experiments are also possible using IR spectroscopy. Bartolomei et al. (1997) used variable temperature IR spectroscopy to confirm that a solid-solid transition took place on heating two forms of fluocinolone acetonide. The spectrum at 230°C showed frequency shifts characteristic of form A transforming into form B. However, these did not match the frequencies of form B. The analytical potential of FTIR thermo-microscopy of sulfaproxiline and diflupredate has been studied by Ghetti et al. (1994). Spectra were recorded for every 2°C increase of temperature, and in case of sulfaproxiline, for example, between 184°C and 186°C, the NH bands at 3140 and 2870 per cm disappeared and a broadband at 3280/cm appeared. This is characteristic of the melt phase of this polymorph. At 190°C this band was replaced by a strong band at 3300/cm that was distinctive of form I of the compound. Chan et al. (2007) have described experiments using an FTIR-imaging system with respect to temperature and humidity in a high-throughput situation. This system utilized a focal plane detector (FPA), which consisted of 4096 small detector elements, which captures an IR spectrum from different locations of the sample. This has obvious advantages with respect to screening purposes.

The quantitative analysis of polymorphs using FTIR has been reported by Kipouros (2006). In essence characteristic bands are necessary, which should not overlap between the polymorphs or solvated/hydrated species. Like all analytical investigations sample preparation is key, this being particularly true for the calibration samples.

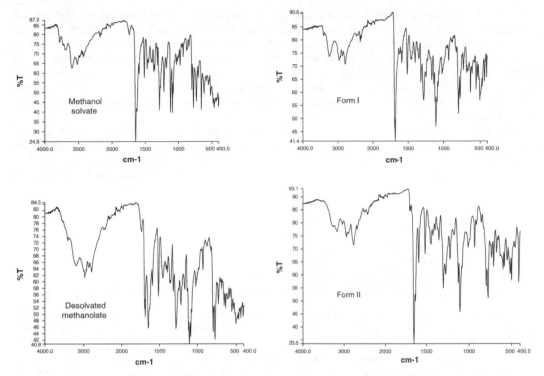

Figure 25 IR spectra of a number of solid-state forms of AR-C69457AA. *Abbreviation*: IR, infrared.

Near-IR Spectroscopy

Dziki et al. (2000) used near-IR spectroscopy (NIR) to distinguish sarafloxacin hydrate batches that exhibited differences in granulation processability. These differences were not evident using conventional solid-state analytical techniques. Since the XRPD patterns were identical, the batches were structurally identical; however, the NIR was able to show that the samples subtly differed in how the molecules were held in the lattice, which in turn, resulted in differences in wetting.

Terahertz Spectroscopy

Terahertz-pulsed spectroscopy works in the 0.1 to 3.0 THz region of the electromagnetic spectrum (Taday, 2004), and the main information gleaned from spectrum is rotational. It has been used by a number of authors to examine polymorphs (Strachan et al., 2005) and hydrates (Zeitler et al., 2007).

Solid-State Raman Spectroscopy

Raman spectroscopy, as with IR spectroscopy, provides information on quantized vibrational energy levels in a molecule, with subjected incident radiation being scattered by the sample. Raman spectroscopy relies on molecular polarizability; a bond must be anisotropically polarizable for the vibration of the bond to be Raman active. The distortion of a bond in an electric field gives rise to an induced dipole, the magnitude of which is determined by the extent of polarizability. As this polar state is more energetic than the relaxed state, spontaneous relaxation is accompanied by a release of energy. It is this relaxation or emission of radiation that is termed scattering. A high degree of polarizability (such as that found in most homo-atomic bonds) gives rise to Raman active bands. Furthermore, the Raman spectrometer design allows information to be obtained in the frequency region 4000 to 100 per cm, thus allowing lattice vibrational modes (i.e., translation and rotation motions of the entire molecule within the crystalline lattice) to be evaluated (Bugay, 2001).

As with IR spectroscopy, the Raman spectrum provides a unique fingerprint of the compound being studied. Since the method is based on the vibrations of the molecule, it is sensitive to small changes in the molecular structure (such as conformations) that affect vibrational behavior. As an example of its use, Variankaval et al. (2000) examined the polymorphs of β-estradiol. A and B were easily distinguishable; however, C and D were almost identical. Maherns et al. (2005) have provided a method of analysis based on descriptive statistics and analysis of variance (ANOVA) methods to address these subtle differences in the Raman spectra of polymorphs.

Low-wavelength Raman spectroscopy in the region of 10 to 150 cm^{-1} can also be used to detect molecular skeletal deformations, libations, and translations (Ayala, 2007). From an experimental viewpoint it has some advantages over more conventional methods of polymorph analysis. Usually the Raman spectrum is obtained by collecting backscattered laser light from a powder or formulation. Bolton and Prasad (1981) listed the advantages (griseofulvin and its chloro- and bromoform solvates) as follows:

1. No special sample preparation is involved.
2. Small amounts of material are required.
3. Short data collection time period is required.
4. Thermal, for example, desolvation studies can be carried out.
5. Low-level laser light can be used that permits work on highly colored species.

Like many other techniques used in the analysis of the organic solid state, heating experiments can be conducted (Gamberini et al., 2006). In addition, Raman spectroscopy has been used to measure the transition temperature and conversion kinetics for the enantiotropic polymorphic transitions for flufenamic acid slurries (Hu et al., 2007). As with the other solid-state analytical techniques, Raman spectroscopy can be used for quantifying mixtures of polymorphs. For example, Kachrimanis et al. (2007) have described the quantitative analysis of polymorphs of paracetamol in powder mixtures using multivariate calibration techniques. An earlier paper by Campbell Roberts et al. (2002a) used a more conventional method of peak intensity ratios to determine the relative concentrations of the polymorphs of mannitol.

Solid-State NMR

NMR spectroscopy was invented in the 1940s and, within 10 years of the first detection of signals, became established as a crucial technique for chemical structure analysis (Abraham et al., 1988). Notwithstanding the fact that NMR spectroscopy is most familiar as a high-resolution spectroscopic technique for the study of liquids and solutions, primarily to determine molecular structure, solid-state NMR has seen a steady increase in use. The initial lack of utility of solid-state NMR was attributed to an inherent deficiency in spectral resolution of a solid sample placed in a conventional high-resolution spectrometer suitable for liquids. The onset of ancillary techniques and subroutines enabled higher resolution to be achieved, resulting in a proportional increase in the use and application of solid-state NMR (SSNMR) spectroscopy (Duer, 2002). However, SSNMR spectra are composed of broader lines, that is, ^{13}C NMR line broadening is still typically of the order of 30 to 60 Hz for a crystalline organic solid, as compared with typical solution ^{13}C NMR line widths of only a few Hertz. Nevertheless, it remains a very powerful technique for investigating the solid state, and the resulting spectra are, in principle, far more information rich than those of solutions (Harris, 2006).

In addition to gleaning information on molecular structure, SSNMR is recognized as an important adjunct to powder diffraction studies in the elucidation of crystal structure from powder data. For instance, this technique can be used to provide insights into the number of molecules present in the asymmetric unit and also information on site symmetry within the crystal structure. Furthermore, SSNMR can be used to assess the incidence and mechanism of dynamic disorder within the ordered solid state—a property that is not amenable to exploration using diffraction studies (data from which indicate a time-averaged representation). Dynamic processes can be studied by SSNMR using, among other methods, the measurement of relaxation times as a function of temperature.

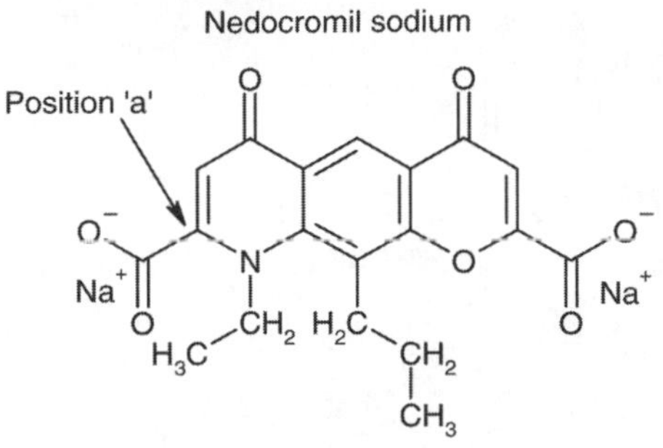

Nedocromil sodium

Figure 26 Structure of nedocromil dianion.

In the case of SSNMR it is necessary to consider certain important interactions encountered by a nuclear spin within a solid. These include dipole-dipole and quadrupolar interactions together with chemical shift anisotropy. These interactions, while also being present in the solution state, are either averaged to zero (for the direct dipole-dipole and quadrupolar interactions) or averaged to their isotropic value (for the chemical shift and indirect spin-spin interaction). The reduction or complete elimination of these anisotropic interactions in the solution state is due to rapid isotropic molecular motion, which is restricted or absent in the solid state. In pharmaceutical R&D, there are a number of nuclei that can be used to probe the solid-state chemistry of drugs, for example, ^{13}C, ^{31}P, ^{15}N, ^{25}Mg, and ^{23}Na. Geppi et al. (2008) have provided an excellent review on the applications of various SSNMR investigations on pharmaceutical systems, using both low- and high-resolution techniques to explore structure, dynamics, and morphological aspects of various solid-state materials.

As an example of structural assessment, Chen et al. (2000) have reported the SSNMR and IR analyses of the hydrates of nedocromil sodium (Fig. 26). In this paper they reported the spectra of the amorphous phase, heptahemihydrate, trihydrate, monohydrate, and a previously unreported methanol/water-mixed solvate. The spectra were significantly different, allowing identification of each phase.

The chemical shift of the carbon atom at position "a" atom appears to be sensitive to the conformation of the left-sided carboxylate group, that is, when the left-sided carboxylate carbon is out of the tricyclic plane, the position "a" carbon is shifted upfield. This is also linked to the color of nedocromil sodium such that when it is in plane, nedocromil sodium heptahemihydrate is intensely yellow, whereas the trihydrate is pale yellow (out of plane). In the trihydrate, the C_{21} and C_{81} resonances show two peaks indicating that there is more than one molecule in the asymmetric unit. In the heptahemihydrate, however, all carbon atoms have one resonance, indicating the likelihood of only one molecule in the asymmetric unit. The methanol/water solvate has three molecules per assymetric unit, which leads to the observation of multiple resonances. The monohydrate is only slightly changed from the trihydrate spectrum.

Cosgrove et al. (2005) reported the crucial role SSNMR played in the understanding of dynamic disorder, leading to polymorphism, in the structure of sibenidet hydrochloride before the crystal structure was determined using synchrotron radiation. As shown in Figure 27, sibenidet has a long chain structure, and using various SSNMR techniques [variable temperature NQS, spin-lattice (T1) relaxation] the polymorphism was shown to be associated with variations in local symmetry around the C_{18} and C_{20} atoms. In addition, the terminal phenyl group was shown to be dynamically disordered, undergoing, most probably, ring flipping.

Figure 28 shows the SSNMR spectra of a number of phases of AR-C69457AA—a potential D_2/β_2 agonist from the same series of compounds that generated sibenidet hydrochloride. These spectra show that the spectra for forms I and II are significantly different. In particular, the spectrum of form II shows that the resonances are doubled indicating the presence of more than one molecule in the asymmetric unit. It has been estimated that between 8% and 11% of organic solids exhibit this phenomenon (Steiner, 2000). The amorphicity introduced by desolvating the methanolate gives rise to much broader resonance peaks.

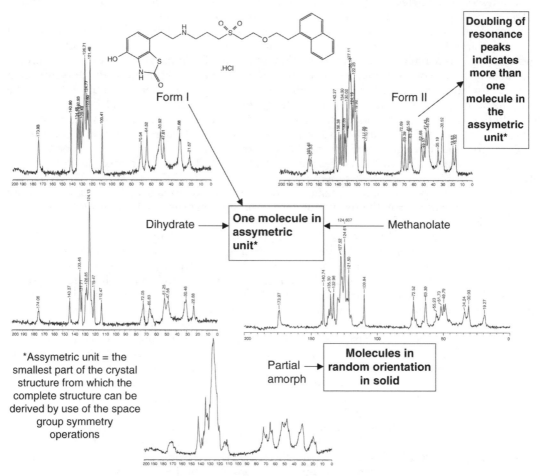

Figure 27 Structure of sibenidit HCl and the ^{13}C SSNMR spectra of forms I and II. *Abbreviation*: SSNMR, solid state nuclear magnetic resonance.

Figure 28 Solid-state NMR spectra of a number of solid-state forms of AR-C69457AA. *Abbreviation*: NMR, nuclear magnetic resonance.

In terms of using SSNMR in a quantitative manner, Apperley et al. (2003) have described its use with the system formoterol anhydrate and dihydrate. Using relaxation time measurements they were able to build a quantitative analytical method for their determination in mixtures with lactose (formoterol fumarate is delivered in dry powder inhalation devices where lactose is an excipient) down to a mass ratio of 0.45%.

INITIAL SOLID-STATE STABILITY

The solid-state degradation of CDs, particularly in the candidate selection phase, is an important consideration since degradation rates as slow as 0.5% per year at 25°C may affect the development of the compound. Monkhouse and van Campen (1984) have reviewed solid-state reactions and highlighted that decomposition in the solid state will be different from that in a liquid insofar that the concepts of concentration and order of reaction are less applicable. Moreover, solid-state degradation reactions can be complex and can involve both oxidation and hydrolysis together. As with solutions, solids can also exhibit instability due to light. This is further complicated by the fact that in solids these reactions usually occur only on the surface. Hickey et al. (2007b) surveyed the solid-state reactivity of the hydrates of the β-lactam antibiotics and concluded that the rate of their hydrolysis diminished quickly because the reaction was diffusion limited—the water molecules are required to diffuse through the layer that has already reacted before they could promote further decomposition.

Figure 29 shows a potential scheme for the solid-state degradation of a drug. Šimon et al. (2004) have published a screening method for the determination of the oxidative stability of pharmaceuticals using a nonisothermal DSC methodology, which relies on an induction period for the decomposition. Since this accelerated test takes approximately two days, this improves on the conventional stability testing protocol usually performed.

Three phases have been identified: the lag, acceleration, and deceleration. Depending on the conditions of temperature and the humidity to which the solid is exposed, the acceleration phase may follow zero, first, or higher orders. A general equation (the Ng equation) has been proposed to describe the decomposition process (equation 29).

$$\frac{d\alpha}{dt} = k\alpha^{1-x}(1 - \alpha)^{1-y} \tag{29}$$

where α is the fraction of the reaction that has occurred at time t, such that $\alpha = 0$ when $t = 0$, and $\alpha = 1$ at $t = \infty$; k is the rate constant; and x and y are constants characteristic of the reaction rate law, that is, when $x = y = 1$, the reaction is zero order; if, however, $x = 1$ and $y = 0$, the reaction is first order. If x and y have fractional values, the reaction will be autocatalytic.

To accelerate the degradation so that the amount degraded becomes quantifiable in a shorter period of time, elevated temperatures are used, and the amount of degradation is typically calculated using the Arrhenius equation. The assumption made during these studies is that the mechanism of degradation is constant over a wide temperature range. However, this need not be the case, and a nonlinear Arrhenius plot may be an indication of change of mechanism as a function of temperature. Furthermore, many compounds that exist as hydrates dehydrate at higher temperatures, which can change the degradation mechanism in the solid state.

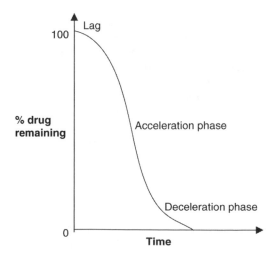

Figure 29 Typical solid-state decomposition curve.

In terms of the chemical stability of compounds with respect to moisture uptake, the following descriptions have been used to describe classes of surface moisture (Cartensen and Li Wan Po, 1992).

- Limited water: The water is used up during the degradation reaction, and there is not enough present to degrade the compound completely.
- Adequate water: Sufficient water is present to decompose the compound completely.
- Excess water: This is an amount of water equal to or greater than the amount of moisture necessary to dissolve the drug. As such, this may develop as the mass of intact drug that decomposes with time.

In terms of crystallinity, it should be noted that amorphous materials are generally less stable than the corresponding crystalline phase. For amorphous solids the net effect of water sorption is to lower the T_g and hence plasticize the material. In turn this increases molecular mobility and therefore increases the potential for chemical reactivity (Ahlneck and Zografi, 1990). Often, amorphous phases crystallize with exposure to moisture. In prenomination studies a useful protocol to assess the effects of these factors is as follows:

The compound is accurately weighed into each of six open glass vials. These are then placed (in duplicate if possible) under the following conditions: Light stress (5000 lux, 25°C) and conditions of 40°C/75% RH and 30°C/60% RH. Typically materials would be sampled at regular intervals up to a three-month time point to determine its stability. After each time point all samples are assessed visually and with a suitable HPLC (or LC-MS) method that can detect degradation products. In addition, DSC and XRPD can be used to detect phase changes.

Photostability

As illustrated in the book *Drugs Photochemistry and Photostability*, edited by Albini and Fasani (1998), a wide range of drug types can undergo photochemical degradation. Theoretically, CDs with absorption maxima greater than 280 nm may decompose in sunlight. However, instability due to light will probably only be of concern if it significantly absorbs light with a wavelength greater than 330 nm and, even then, only if the reaction proceeds at a significant rate (Albini and Fasani, 1998). Light instability is a problem in both the solid and solution state and if highlighted would mean that formulations therefore need to be designed to protect the compound from its deleterious effects. Like many aspects of pharmaceutical discovery and development, the photostability of pharmaceuticals is covered by the ICH guideline Q1B (Aman and Thoma, 2003).

The number of compounds showing photo-instability is large; for example, Tønnesen (2001) has stated that more than 100 of the most commonly used drugs are unstable with respect to light. There are a number of chemical groups that might be expected to give rise to decomposition. These include the carbonyl group, the nitroaromatic group, the N-oxide group, the C=C bond, the aryl chloride group, groups with a weak C–H bond, and sulfides, alkenes, polyenes, and phenols (Albini and Fasani, 1998).

It is therefore important to establish the propensity of a CD to decompose due to light as soon as possible in preformulation studies, since this can have ramifications for its formulation and packaging (Tønnesen, 2001). The first evidence that compounds are light sensitive is usually discovered during LO studies. CDs should therefore be assessed in the prenomination phase with respect to light stability to alert the formulation experts as to whether precautionary measures are needed to protect the drug from light. Indeed, this could be used as a selection criterion in many cases to reject unsuitable compounds as potential CDs.

A guideline for the photostability testing of new drug substances and products has been published in the European pharmacopeia (1996) and the ICH. This states that photostability testing should consist of forced degradation and confirmatory testing. The forced degradation experiments can involve the CD alone, in solution or in suspension using exposure conditions that reflect the nature of the compound and the intensity of the light sources used. The samples are then analyzed at various time points using appropriate techniques, for example, HPLC. In addition, changes in physical properties such as appearance and clarity or color should be noted. Confirmatory studies involve exposing the compound to light whose total output is not less than 1.2 million lux hours and has a near-UV energy of not less than 200 W hr/m^2. Light sources for testing the photostability include artificial daylight tubes, xenon lamps, tungsten-mercury lamps, laboratory light, and natural light (Anderson et al., 1991). According to Aman and Thoma (2003), natural light varies between 389 and 500 W/m^2 on a sunny day and 50 and 120 W/m^2 on a cloudy day.

In terms of the kinetics, light degradation in dilute solution is first order; however, in more concentrated solution decomposition approaches pseudo–zero order (Connors et al., 1986). The reason for this observation is that as the solution becomes more concentrated, degradation becomes limited because of the limited number of incident quanta and quenching reactions between the molecules. It should be noted that ionizable compounds, for example, ciprofloxacin, showed large differences in photostability between the ionized and unionized forms (Torniainen et al., 1996). The extent of the photodegradation can also be influenced by the solvent.

Solids can undergo photolysis and oxidation (Glass et al., 2004). For example, de Villiers et al. (1992) showed that form II of furosemide was less stable to light than form I, particularly in the presence of oxygen. As noted earlier the decomposition showed more complex behavior. The reaction consisted of a number of steps. The first occurred on the surface, which was followed by a gas phase mass transfer step. After this the reaction proceeded by diffusion via a porous-reacted zone and chemical reaction at the boundary. Investigations by Aman and Thoma (2002) into the light stability of nifedipine and molsidomine showed that particle size had a considerable effect on their photostability. It was found that after two hours of irradiation, decomposition was approximately 5% to 10% higher in the smaller-size ranges of the compounds.

The Hanau sun test is a constant intense light source, thus using 10 µM of the CD in pH 7.4 at room temperature, the degradation is measured. Under these conditions if the compound shows a half-life of greater than five hours, it is classified as stable. If the compound has a half-life of less than five minutes, it is classified as very photolytically unstable.

Solution Calorimetry

Solution calorimetry provides a direct measure of the thermodynamics (and kinetics) of dissolution. On mixing a material with an appropriate solvent, heat flow is measured (Royall and Gaisford, 2005) as a function of time and integrated to give the molar enthalpy of solution ($\Delta_{sol}H$). The cumulative enthalpy of solution encompasses a measure of the energy associated with wetting, breaking of lattice bonds, and solvation. Classification of thermodynamic stability by solution calorimetry relies upon the energetics of wetting and solvation across polymorphs to be constant, thereby providing a measure of lattice "strength" or energy. While the component associated with heat of solvation may be correctly regarded as constant between polymorphs, the heat of wetting may vary as a function of crystal habit and changes in surface characteristics, thus giving rise to some variability.

There are two types of solution calorimetry systems: isoperibol and isothermal. In the former technique, the heat change caused by dissolution of the solute results in a change in temperature of the solution. This results in a temperature-time plot from which the heat of solution is calculated. By contrast, in isothermal solution calorimetry (where, by definition, the temperature is maintained constant) any heat change is compensated by an equal, but opposite, energy change, which is then the heat of solution (Gu and Grant, 2001). Furthermore, microsolution calorimetry can be used with as little as 3 to 5 mg of compound. Experimentally the sample is introduced into the equilibrated solvent system, and the heat flow is measured by a heat conduction calorimeter such as thermal activity monitor (TAM).

The relative stability of polymorphs can be investigated by assessing the magnitude and sign (endothermic/exothermic) of the enthalpy of dissolution. For instance, a more endothermic (or less exothermic) response indicates that the energy of solvation of the solute does not compensate for the breaking of lattice bonds, and it is therefore the more stable solid or polymorph (Goa and Rytting, 1997). Solution calorimetry was used by Pikal et al. (1978) to determine the heats of solution of different forms of some β-lactam antibiotics. It has also been used to quantitate binary mixtures of three crystalline forms of sulfamethoxazole (Guillory and Erb, 1985). Solution calorimetry, in conjunction with thermal analysis, was used by Wu et al.

(1993), to examine the two polymorphs of losartan. The heats of solution for polymorphs I and II were measured in water and N,N-dimethylformamide. However, the heats of transitions were insignificant ($\Delta H_T = 1.72$ kcal/mol). Gu and Grant (2001) used isoperibol solution calorimetry (in addition to solubility measurements) to estimate the transition temperature of the polymorphs of sulfamerzine at any one temperature. They validated their method by a bracketing technique for assessing the solution-mediated transition of the polymorphs around the predicted transition temperature.

One problem commonly encountered with lipophilic drug molecules is around wettability in aqueous media. Poor wettability often leads to a broadening of the dissolution process to such an extent that, in some cases, integration of the data to determine the enthalpy of dissolution becomes intractable. To deal with this problem surfactants can be used, as exemplified by the solution calorimetry assessment of cimetidine polymorphs (Souillac et al., 2002). The surfactants sodium dodecyl sulfate (1% w/v) and polysorbate 80 (3% w/v) were used at concentrations significantly above their critical micelle concentrations (cmcs) to aid the wetting process. Positive results were obtained with regard to wettability, and they were able to demonstrate that form A of cimetidine was the most stable polymorph.

Hendriksen (1990) used solution calorimetry to investigate the crystallinity of calcium fenoprofen samples. The more perfect the crystals, the higher the heat of solution. Lattices with higher levels of disruption, conversely, gave lower heats of solution. Coquerel (2006) has discussed the issue of structural purity and the range of analytical techniques (including solution calorimetry) used to assess the aspect of the organic solid state. Solution calorimetry can also be used to evaluate amorphous-crystalline compositions in binary mixtures.

Solution calorimeters are calibrated using KCl in water (for endothermic processes) and tris-HCl in 0.01M HCl (for exothermic processes) standards. For example, the heat of solution (ΔH^s) of KCl at 25°C (298.15 K) is 235.86 ± 0.23 J/g. Similarly, the ΔH^s for tris-HCl at 25°C is -29.80 kJ/mol (Kilday, 1980). Further work by the NIST has examined the enthalpy of solution of sodium chloride and reported further work on KCl as a standard (Archer and Kirklin, 2000). Yff et al. (2004) have investigated a number of methods used for solution calorimetry calibration. In this study, experiments were performed using 50, 100, and 200 mg of KCl in water, tris, and sucrose as calibrants. They found that 200 mg of KCl gave the best results and that although the tris data was more variable, it was still acceptable. Similarly, sucrose was found to be acceptable although less robust than KCl.

Intrinsic Dissolution

During the preformulation stage, an understanding of the dissolution rate of a drug candidate is necessary, since this property of the compound is recognized as a significant factor involved in drug bioavailability. Dissolution of a solid usually takes place in two stages: solvation of the solute molecules by the solvent molecules followed by transport of these molecules from the interface into the bulk medium by convection or diffusion. The major factor that determines the dissolution rate is the aqueous solubility of the compound; however, other factors such as particle size, crystalline state (polymorphs, hydrates, etc.), pH, and buffer concentration can affect the rate. Moreover, physical properties such as viscosity and wettability can also influence the dissolution process.

Ideally dissolution should simulate in vivo conditions. To do this it should be carried out in a large volume of dissolution medium, or there must be some mechanism whereby the dissolution medium is constantly replenished by fresh solvent to mimic the dynamic in vivo state. Provided this condition is met, the dissolution testing is defined as taking place under sink conditions. Conversely, if there is a concentration increase during dissolution testing, such that the dissolution is retarded by a concentration gradient, the dissolution is said to be nonsink. While the use of the USP paddle dissolution apparatus, for example, is mandatory when developing a tablet, the rotating disc method has great utility with regard to preformulation studies. The intrinsic dissolution rate is the dissolution rate of the compound under the condition of constant surface area. The rationale for the use of a compressed disk of pure material is that the intrinsic tendency of the test material to dissolve can be evaluated without formulation excipients.

Intrinsic dissolution rates of compounds obtained from rotating disks have been theoretically reported by Levich. Under hydrodynamic conditions, the intrinsic dissolution rate is usually proportional to the solubility of the solid. However, as predicted by Levich, the dissolution rate obtained will be dependent on the rotation speed. Jashnani et al. (1993) have reported the validation of an improved rotating disk apparatus after finding that the original apparatus gave nonzero intercepts when the experiments of albuterol disks were conducted at various rotation speeds.

In the Wood's dissolution apparatus experiments, a disk is prepared by compression of ~200 mg of the CD in a hydraulic press—an IR press is ideal, and this gives a disk with a diameter of 1.3 cm. It should be noted that some compounds do not compress well and may exhibit elastic compression properties, that is, the disk may be very weak, might cap and laminate, rendering the experiment impossible. In addition to poor compression properties, another complication is that some compounds can undergo polymorphic transformations due to the application of pressure. This should therefore be borne in mind if there is insufficient compound to perform post-compaction investigations such as by XRPD. Persson et al. (2008) has described the design and characterization of a miniaturized intrinsic dissolution apparatus. The disks in this apparatus amount to 5 mg, which makes them amenable for screening purposes in early development.

If the disk has reasonable compression properties, it is then attached to a holder and set in motion in the dissolution medium (e.g., water, buffer, or simulated gastric fluid) at rotation speeds of around 100 rpm. A number of analytical techniques can be used to follow the dissolution process; however, UV-visible spectrophotometry and HPLC with fixed or variable wavelength detectors (or diode array) appear to be the most common. The UV system employs a flow-through system and does not require much attention; however, if HPLC is used, then any aliquot taken should be replaced by an equal amount of solvent. The intrinsic dissolution rate is given by the slope of the linear portion of the concentration versus time curve and has the units of $mg/min \, cm^2$. The use of ATR UV-visible spectrophotometry has also been used by Florence and Johnston (2005). The advantage of the ATR technique is that the measurements can be done in situ in the dissolution flask. This relies on the occurrence of a short-lived wave in the suspension medium compared with crystals where the radiation is propagated due to internal reflection. Since the penetration of this wave is of the order of the wavelength of the radiation (d_p), then it is supposed that there is no interaction with the particles and hence can be used to measure the, much higher, solution concentration of the solute (Schlemmer and Katzer, 1987).

Figure 30 shows the increase in absorbance due to dissolution of approximately 200 mg of the sodium and calcium salts of nedocromil in water. The sodium salt, which is soluble to approximately 300 mg/mL, dissolved much more rapidly than the calcium salt, whose solubility is only 1.4 mg/mL. Similarly, Li et al. (2005b) compared the intrinsic dissolution profiles of haloperidol and its hydrochloride and mesylate salts. They found that the dissolution rates (at constant pH) of the mesylate were much higher than either the freebase or hydrochloride (except at pH <2). At higher pH values the HCl salt showed a higher rate such that a diffusion layer pH effect could be used to explain the rank order of dissolution. With respect to the presence of water in the crystal lattice, Pereira et al. (2007) showed that the intrinsic dissolution rate of the anhydrate of nevirapine was 1.5 times faster than that of the hemihydrate in 0.01M HCl.

Yu et al. (2004) have investigated the feasibility of using this technique to determine the BCS solubility class of drugs. They determined the intrinsic dissolution rates of six low solubility and nine high solubility model drugs at three pHs (1.2, 4.5, and 6.8) under a variety of experimental conditions, for example, compression force and dissolution medium volume. Since these parameters had no effect on the dissolution rates of the test compounds, they recommended that investigations be carried out at 2000 psi (compression), 900 mL (dissolution medium volume), 0.5 in. (die position), and 100 rpm (rotation speed). Although the test compounds gave rise to a good correlation between the dissolution rate and the BCS solubility classification, the authors highlighted that further work was needed before it could be utilized as a regulatory test.

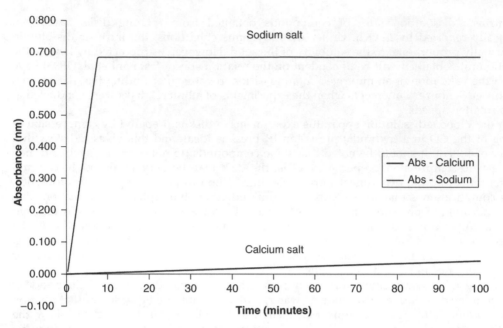

Figure 30   Plot of increase in absorbance versus time for a sodium and calcium salt of nedocromil undergoing intrinsic dissolution in water.

CRYSTAL MORPHOLOGY ASSESSMENT

The external shape or morphology of a crystal is termed the crystal habit, and a variety of shapes have been defined in the USP. These include acicular, which are needlelike crystals, whose width and thickness are similar and is typical of that crystallized by many pharmaceutical compounds (Puel et al., 2008). Needlelike crystals present many difficulties in both the primary and secondary manufacturing arenas. For example, they may be difficult to filter and dry once crystallized and in formulation terms may have poor bulk densities and flow properties (Variankaval et al., 2008). Other morphologies defined are columnar, flake, plate, lath, and equant. In addition to the habit of individual crystals, the crystals may come together in aggregates or agglomerates where they either adhere or fuse together. The habit of a crystal is determined by the way in which the solutes orientate themselves during crystallization and growth (Gadewar et al, 2004). Therefore, the general shape of a crystal is the result of the way individual faces grow, and during growth the fastest growing faces are usually eliminated.

Crystal morphology or habit is important, since it can influence a number of formulation properties of the compound (Tiwary, 2003). For example, powder flow properties (Banga et al., 2007), compaction (Rasenack and Müller, 2002) and stability have all been found to be largely dependent on crystal morphology. As another example of the effect of the crystal habit on a formulation, Tiwary and Panpalia (1999) examined the effect of the crystal habit on the suspension stability and pharmokinetics of trimethoprim. They found that crystals (produced under different crystallization conditions) with the most anisotropic shape exhibited the best physical stability; however, the pharmacokinetics of each crystal habit examined showed equivalent pharmacokinetics.

Since solvents can preferentially adsorb to crystal faces during the growth process, crystals of a substance produced under different crystallization conditions may exhibit an entirely different physical appearance, even though they still belong to the same crystal system (Stoica et al., 2004). This arises due to the fact that strong solvent-solute interactions inhibit the development of specific faces of the growing crystal leading to a different morphology. Of course polymorphs can exhibit different morphologies (Coombes et al., 2002). Figure 31 shows

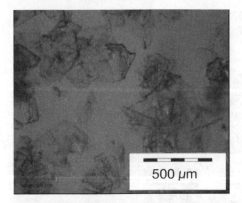

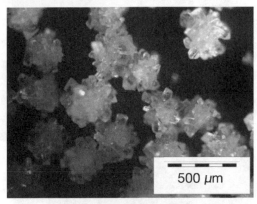

Figure 31 Morphologies of two polymorphs of a development compound.

two morphologies obtained after crystallization from IMS-water and heptane. The sample obtained from heptane exhibited a platelike morphology, and the second sample, more tabular and agglomerated, was obtained from an IMS-water mixture.

If a compound exhibits a particular morphology that may cause formulation problems, it is worthwhile investigating ways in which to change the habit via crystallization from different solvents (Winn and Doherty, 2000). Additionally, the effect of impurities or additives on the crystal habit should not be overlooked, as these can act as crystal poisons or promote growth in a particular crystallographic direction. Figure 32 shows some scanning electron micrographs of a variety of crystal habits found for some CDs.

The most accurate way of determining the symmetry of a crystal is to use an optical goniometer to measure the angles between the crystal faces (Lechuga-Ballesteros and Rodriguez-Hornedo, 1995). However, this technique requires a good-quality crystal of adequate size, typically greater than 0.05 mm in each direction.

The Materials Studio software (Accelrys) can be used to model the morphology of crystals as well as the effect of additives on morphology. Both the BFDH (Bravais, Friedel, Donnay, and Harker) and attachment energy models, in conjunction with force field methods, are used in the morphology prediction. The attachment energy approach gives the growth morphology of the crystal studied, but it is also possible to calculate the shape of a small particle in equilibrium with its growth environment by computing the surface energy of each relevant face. Figures 33 and 34 show the predicted morphologies of α- and γ-indomethacin using the attachment energy models. Although reasonable comparison can be made it is clear that for γ-indomethacin, the crystals are less elongated than predicted by the model and points to an interaction between the crystal and solvent of crystallization.

Deij et al. (2008) has presented a comparison of the morphology prediction methods of the polymorphs of venlafaxine. In addition to the BFDH and attachment energy methods, they also used a kinetic Monte Carlo growth simulation, which was compared to experimental

Form I

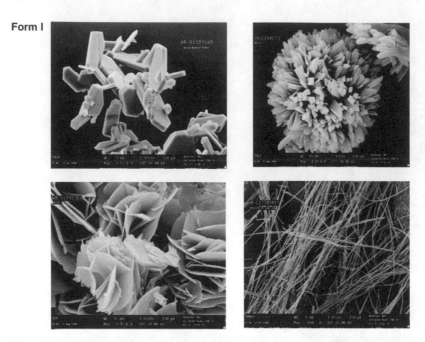

Figure 32 SEM micrographs of some crystal morphologies. *Abbreviation*: SEM, scanning electron microscopy.

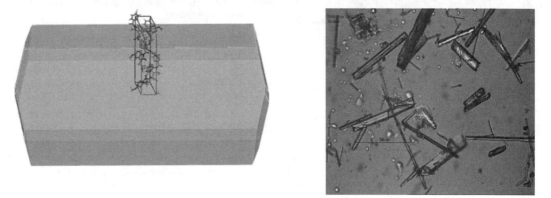

Figure 33 Attachment energy morphology prediction α-indomethacin.

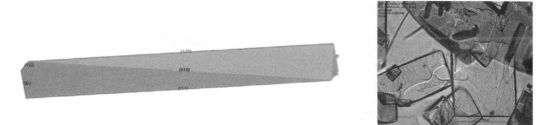

Figure 34 Attachment energy model morphology prediction γ-Indomethacin.

observations of morphology. They showed that for three polymorphs the BFDH methodology did not give good results. The attachment energy method showed better results, but still was not in good agreement with those observed experimentally. In contrast the Monte Carlo method showed much better concordance with the habits except for form III of this compound.

Surface interactions between solvent molecules and growing faces can also be modeled. It is well known that the stronger the solvent binds to a particular face, the more it will inhibit the growth of that face so that morphology will be affected. This can be computationally simulated, for example, the interaction of paracetamol with ethanol has been reported (Green and Meenan, 1996). The ability to predict crystal morphology, that is, to identify key growth faces, combined with the ability to analyze the surface chemistry of each of the faces in detail (including interactions with solvent molecules, excipients, and impurities) enables rational control of morphology and crystal growth, for example, an undesirable morphology (a plate) can be transformed into a more isometrical shape.

MICROSCOPY

Optical Microsocopy

The optical microscope is a powerful analytical technique (Cooke, 2000). Direct observation can allow the investigating scientist to evaluate such things as, for example, crystal size, shape, and birefringence. Often different polymorphs can have very different shapes, and this might be the first clue that a change in crystallization conditions has produced another polymorph. For example the α- and β-indomethacin polymorphs show needle- and platelike habits, respectively (Figs. 33 and 34). In addition to morphological assessments of crystals, optical microscopy can be used to measure their refractive indices. Watanabe et al. (1980) have shown that to identify the crystal it is not necessary to measure the principal refractive indices. By simply measuring two indices that are unique and reproducible is sufficient. These were termed the key refractive indices that, according to these workers, are all that are needed to identify any particular compound.

Birefringence is a phenomenon whereby polarized light is refracted through the crystal. It occurs when a crystal separates a beam of light into two unequally refracted, polarized beams because the velocity of the light beam through the crystal is not the same in all directions. If crystals exhibit birefringence, this is a good indicator that the sample is crystalline and thus is a quick and easy check if a crystallization process has been successful.

Different polymorphs have different internal structures so that they belong to different crystal systems. Therefore, theoretically, polymorphs can be distinguished using polarized light and a microscope. The crystals can be either isotropic or anisotropic. In the case of isotropic crystals the velocity of light is the same in all directions, while anisotropic crystals have two or three different light velocities or refractive indices. The refractive indices, along with some other optical properties, of form I and II of paracetamol have been reported by Nichols (1998). From these data it was concluded that form I of paracetamol could be optically distinguished from form II due to its lower birefringence and strongly dispersed extinction. Its morphology was also shown to be different.

Scanning Electron Microscopy

Often crystal sizes are so small that they cannot be seen easily using an optical microscope. Under these circumstances scanning electron microscopy (SEM) becomes the method of choice for imaging. An SEM is composed of a tungsten filament (the electron source), a column (which contains a number of electromagnetic lenses), and a sample chamber. Since it uses electrons as the source of illumination, far higher magnifications and resolutions can be obtained.

After production, the electrons are accelerated along the path of the column, pass through the electromagnetic lenses to give a fine beam of electrons, which impact the surface of the sample. The sample is mounted on a stage contained in the chamber area, which can be under high or low vacuum depending on the design of the microscope. The electron beam rasters (scans) across to produce the image from the electrons generated at the surface

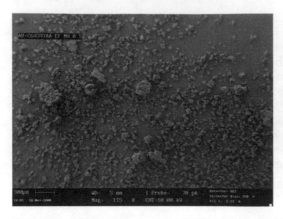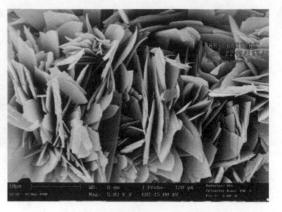

Figure 35 SEM images of sibenadit HCl and low and high magnification. *Abbreviation*: SEM, scanning electron microscopy.

(secondary electrons) or from deeper down in the sample (backscattered). Both secondary and backscattered electrons arise from electrons being knocked out of orbit from the impact of the accelerated electrons from the filament. Traditionally, to prevent charge build up on nonconductive particles, samples need to be coated with gold or palladium and run under high vacuum. However, over the last decade environmental scanning electron microscopy (ESEM) allows the examination of samples surrounded by a low vacuum gaseous environment, that is, high vacuum is not required and the specimen does not need to be conductive. These microscopes are designed so that the electron gun and electron optical system are maintained under high vacuum, while the sample chamber is maintained at a lower vacuum. A small aperture connecting the two parts allows this differential pressure to be maintained.

In ESEM mode the primary electron beam on bombarding the specimen results in secondary electrons being produced, which are attracted to the positively charged detector. However, as the secondary electrons travel toward the detector, they collide with the nitrogen molecules in the atmosphere, resulting in more electrons causing an amplification of signal and ionization of the gas molecules. The positively charged gas ions are attracted to negatively charged samples, neutralizing the charge. Likewise water vapor can be introduced into the sample chamber, allowing wet samples to be examined.

These signals can provide information not only about the surface appearance or topography of the sample but also its composition and microstructure. To obtain good images the user needs to identify the optimum combination of accelerating voltage, spot size, vapor pressure, and working distances, especially for small particles. Often, in such cases faster turnaround times can be obtained using coated samples. Figure 35 shows two images obtained of sibenadit HCl at low and high magnification. In the first image, obtained at a magnification of 115×, only clusters of crystals are observable. However, when the magnification was increased to 12000×, the clusters were seen to be composed of very fine thin plates. The second example (Fig. 36) shows a wet sample obtained using ESEM fresh from a filter cake after deliquoring—this was an example of a fragile hydrate where the water content was greater than 80%.

Atomic Force Microscopy

Atomic Force Microscopy (AFM), a high-resolution scanning probe microscope instrument, operates by measuring attractive or repulsive forces between a cantilevered tip and the sample. In its repulsive "contact" mode, the instrument lightly touches the end of a leaf spring or cantilever to the sample. As a raster scans and drags the tip over the sample, a detection apparatus measures the vertical deflection of the cantilever, which indicates the height of the local sample. AFMs can achieve a resolution of 10 pm and, unlike electron microscopes, can image samples in air or under water.

AFM has numerous uses including, for example, the characterization of polymorphs (Muster and Prestidge, 2002; Danesh et al., 2001). The fact that AFM measurements can be

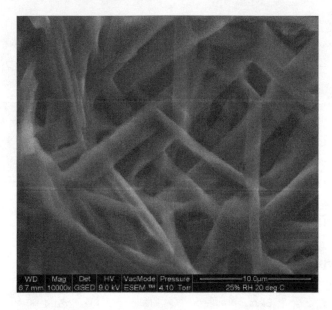

Figure 36 ESEM of a fragile hydrate.
Abbreviation: ESEM, environmental scanning electron microscopy.

performed under aqueous conditions allows both crystallization and dissolution processes to be studied (Danesh et al. 2001, Wilkins et al. 2002). The AFM can also be combined with thermal analysis. Known as scanning thermal microscopy (SThM), it has been used to distinguish the polymorphs of cimetidine (Sanders et al., 2000).

HYGROSCOPICITY

Hygroscopicity is the interaction of a material with moisture in the atmosphere (Reutzel-Edens and Newman, 2006 and Newman et al., 2007). The propensity of a compound to sorb moisture is an important aspect to consider during the selection of a CD. Properties such as the crystal structure, powder flow, compaction, lubricity, dissolution rate, and polymer film permeability can be affected by moisture adsorption (Ahlneck and Zografi, 1990). As an example of its importance in the inhalation area, Young et al. (2003) reported the effect of humidity level on the aerosolization behavior of micronized sodium cromoglycate, salbutamol sulfate, and triamcinolone acetonide. They found that the fine particle and delivered dose for both salbutamol sulfate and sodium cromoglycate decreased with increasing relative humidities.

Moisture is also an important factor that can affect the stability of CDs and their formulations. Sorption of water molecules onto a CD (or excipient) can often induce hydrolysis (Yoshioka and Cartensen, 1990). The influence that moisture has on stability depends on how strongly it is bound, that is, it depends on whether the moisture is free or bound moisture. Generally, degradation arises as a function of free water, which may be due to its ability to change the pH of the surfaces of CD and excipient (Monkhouse, 1984). The sorption of moisture onto drug excipient mixtures may result in surface dissolution and alteration of the pH. This in turn has the possibility of inducing degradation. For example, when remacemide HCl salt was mixed with lactose, it was apparently stable even when stored at 90°C for 12 weeks. However, when the experiment was carried out in the presence of moisture, extensive degradation by way of the well-known Maillard reaction took place (Table 14).

The measurement of free water is expressed as a_w or equilibrium relative humidity (ERH). The a_w of a substance is thus defined as the ratio of the vapor pressure of water due to the substance (P_{sub}) to the vapor pressure of pure water (P_{H_2O}) at a given temperature (equation 30).

$$a_w = \frac{P_{sub}}{P_{H_2O}} \qquad (30)$$

Table 14 Compatibility Study Between Remacemide HCl and Lactose

Water added (µL)	Storage temperature (°C)	Storage time (wk)	Color	Moisture by TGA	Percent of drug recovered
0	25	1	White	2.6	101.2
		4	White	2.6	99.4
		12	White	2.6	102.8
	70	1	White	2.6	105.0
		4	White	2.6	101.8
		12	Off-white	2.5	100.3
	90	1	White	2.6	102.5
		4	White	2.6	98.5
		12	Off-white	2.2	100.2
25	25	1	White	2.6	93.6
		4	White	6.8	102.6
		12	White	5.0	88.4
	70	1	Brown	3.2	91.4
		4	Brown/black	N/I[a]	99.7
		12	Brown/black	N/I	74.4
	90	1	Brown	4.0	98.5
		4	Brown/black	N/I	90.0
		12	Black	N/I	51.4

[a]Themogram not interpretable due to extensive sample degradation.

ERH is a_w expressed as a percentage (equation 31).

$$ERH = a_w \times 100 \qquad (31)$$

Numerically ERH equals the RH generated by a substance in a closed system.

The ambient moisture level in the atmosphere will vary with time as shown by Figure 37; these data were recorded in Loughborough, United Kingdom, in February 2001. As can be seen, the temperature was relatively constant in the laboratory at around 22°C; however, the RH varied from ~20% to 60% RH. Thus, information on the sensitivity of compounds and their formulations to ambient RH is needed and indeed can be critical for the selection of compound from the discovery phase.

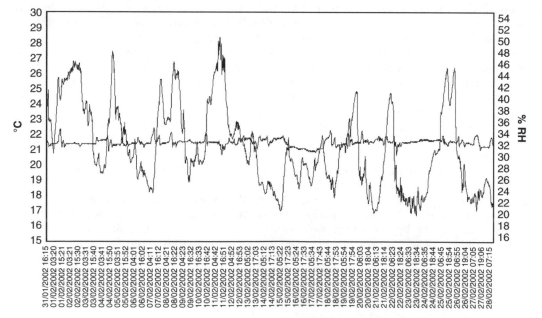

Figure 37 Temperature and laboratory relative humidity levels in Loughborough, United Kingdom, in winter.

Table 15 Hygroscopicity Classification

Class 1: Nonhygroscopic	Essentially no moisture increases occur at relative humidities below 90%
Class 2: Slightly hygroscopic	Essentially no moisture increases occur at relative humidities below 80%
Class 3: Moderately hygroscopic	Moisture content does not increase more than 5% after storage for 1 wk at relative humidities below 60%
Class 4: Very hygroscopic	Moisture content increase may occur at relative humidities as low as 40–50%

Source: From Callaghan (1982).

When compounds interact with moisture, they retain the water by either bulk or surface adsorption, capillary condensation, chemical reaction, and, in extreme cases, formation of a solution (deliquescence). It has been shown that when moisture is absorbed to the extent that deliquescence takes place at a certain critical relative humidity (CRH), the liquid film surrounding the solid is saturated. This process is dictated by vapor diffusion and heat transport rates (Kontny et al., 1987). The converse of deliquescence is efflorescence, and this occurs when the crystal loses water of crystallization below a critical water vapor pressure. For example, Griesser and Burger (1995) found that caffeine hydrate lost its water of crystallization even at 61% RH. It has also been observed that the three known polymorphs of oxytetracycline have different hygroscopicity profiles (Burger et al., 1985). Bound water is not available if it is (1) a crystal hydrate, (2) hydrogen bonded, or (3) sorbed or trapped in an amorphous structure. Callaghan et al. (1982) have classified the degree of hygroscopicity of some excipients into four classes (Table 15). Another classification system has been proposed by the European pharmacopeia (1999).

Visalakshi et al. (2005) used the same approach to examine a range of 30 drugs. Using RH conditions between 11% and 93%, they found that 23 were class I, 4 were class II, and 3 were class III (which exhibited deliquescence). The same group also reported the apparent increased uptake of moisture in the presence of light (Kaur et al., 2003). While the basis of these observations was not explored, they concluded that this phenomenon should be borne in mind for those products developed and packaged for countries with high levels of intense daylight.

If a CD or salt is moderately or very hygroscopic, it would normally be rejected. However, the decision to proceed with a compound that takes up less water should be taken on a case-by-case basis: experience indicates that around 2% to 3% is a sensible cutoff. However, a compound may take up to 5% moisture and not be accompanied by any serious effects, that is, may remain stable and free flowing despite a high level of surface moisture. Moreover, there may be phase change to a hydrate, which may be beneficial in some circumstances. For inhalation compounds, however, moisture sorption and desorption can have serious deleterious effects on the formulation, and lower limits of moisture can be tolerated. This is particularly true if the compound is a hydrate that takes up water from the atmosphere nonstoichiometrically.

Hygroscopicity—Methods

Gravimetric Vapor Sorption

Measurement of the hygroscopic properties of a compound can be carried out on small quantities of compound using, for example, a gravimetric vapor sorption (GVS) analyzer (Roberts, 1999). The RH is generated by bubbling nitrogen through a water reservoir where it is saturated with moisture. Using a mixing chamber the moist nitrogen is mixed with dry nitrogen in a fixed ratio, thus producing the required RH. The moist nitrogen is then passed over the sample, and the instrument is programmed such that the increase in weight due to moisture is monitored with time using an ultrasensitive microbalance. The compound takes up moisture and reaches equilibrium, at which point the next RH stage is programmed to start. The sorption and desorption of moisture can be studied using this instrument, and, in addition, the effect of temperature can be investigated. Using this technique, a quantity as small as 1 mg can be assessed. As an extension to the use of this instrument to investigate the propensity of compounds to from hydrates, it can also be used to determine whether compounds form solvates. As example of this analogous behavior, Burnett et al. (2007)

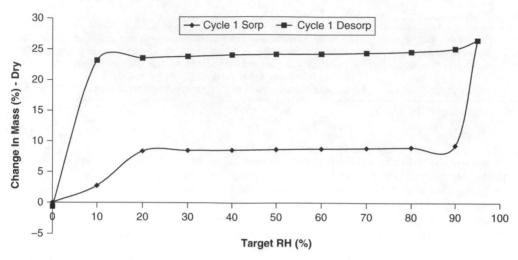

Figure 38   Moisture sorption-desorption profile of nedocromil sodium.

reported formation and desolvation of the acetone solvate of carbamazepine when subjected to increasing or decreasing partial pressures of acetone.

Normally the moisture sorption-desorption profile of the compound is investigated. From a practical point of view, we have found that a two-cycle regime starting at 40% RH, increasing to 90% RH, decreasing to 0% RH, and then repeating the cycle can reveal a range of phenomena associated with the solid. Starting the experiment at 0% RH is not recommended since hydrates or solvates that are prone to desolvation at low RHs will proceed to dehydrate before the start of the experiment proper and therefore may mislead the operator.

Alternatively there may be a larger uptake of moisture, which can indicate a phase change. In this case, the desorption phase is characterized by only small decreases in the moisture content (depending on the stability of the hydrate formed) until at a certain RH the moisture is lost. In some cases, hydrated amorphous forms are formed on desorption of the hydrate formed on the sorption phase. Figure 38 shows the moisture sorption-desorption profile of nedocromil sodium (Khankari et al., 1998).

The crystal structure of nedocromil sodium (discovered and developed at AstraZeneca's R&D site in Loughborough, U.K.) shows that it is a stoichiometric channel hydrate [the crystal structures of the trihydrate (Freer et al., 1987) and a heptahemihydrate (Khankari et al., 1995) have been reported]. Figure 39 shows the crystal structure (viewed along the *a*-axis, with sodium ions and oxygen atoms of the water molecules highlighted) obtained from the CSD (code FUFJUL).

At ambient RH the compound exists as a trihydrate, which changes to a heptahemihydrate (7.5 mole equivalent H_2O) when the RH exceeds 90%. The higher hydrate was found to be stable to decreasing RH conditions until less than 10% RH was achieved, resulting in the loss of all the sorbed moisture to generate a partially amorphous phase. Nedocromil sodium proceeds from one hydrate to another at a defined RH and can be classified as a stoichiometric hydrate. The uptake of moisture to form hydrates is a relatively common phenomenon observed for sodium salts, and in some circumstances, the free acid or another salt may be preferred. Figure 40 shows the moisture sorption-desorption profiles of the sodium salt and free acid of a development compound. The sodium salt forms a dihydrate and tetrahydrate on exposure to increasing relative humidities, whereas the free acid sorbs much less moisture from the atmosphere and thus, from a development point of view, is the more attractive option.

In contrast, a compound in the MCT-1 series reported by Guile et al. (2006) exhibited a number of polymorphic forms with very different moisture sorption and desorption profiles. For example form I, which was obtained from ethyl acetate, showed low moisture uptake; however, form III crystallized from water and formed a stoichiometric channel hydrate (shown

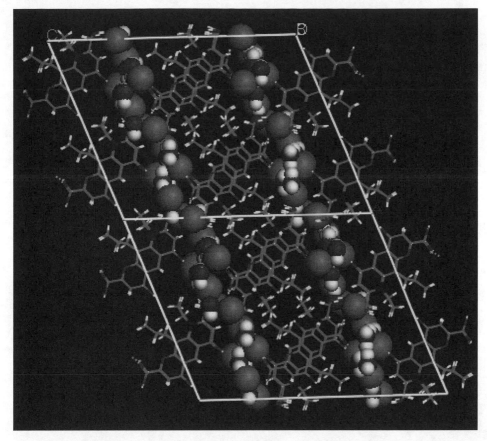

Figure 39 Crystal structure of nedocromil sodium trihydrate. *Source*: 3D Search and Research Using the Cambridge Structural Database, Allen, F. H. and Kennard O. Chemical Design Automation News, 8 (1) pp 1 & 31–37, 1993.

in Fig. 41) with a very narrow stability window between an anhydrated phase and a tetrahydrate. The consequence of this behavior was that because of atmospheric RH changes, the moisture content form could change from day to day, making form III a very unattractive solid form.

In terms of salt selection procedures, the CRH of each salt should be identified. This is defined as the point at which the compound starts to sorb moisture (Cartensen et al., 1987). Clearly, compounds or salts that exhibit excessive moisture uptake should be rejected. The level of this uptake is debatable, but those that exhibit deliquescence (where the sample dissolves in the moisture that has been sorbed) should be automatically excluded from further consideration.

One unusual case that is worth sharing is that of *tert*-butylhydroxylamine acetate. This compound showed variable moisture content, but when investigated by GVS, in an attempt to understand its moisture sorption properties, gave very strange mass change versus RH plots as shown in Figure 42.

It was observed that the compound had an unusually high vapor pressure, which meant that when subjected to the nitrogen flow in the GVS, it disappeared from the sample pan! To overcome the tendency of this compound to evaporate, the flow rate of the nitrogen was reduced from 120 to 5 cc/min: the temperature was also reduced from 25°C to 5°C in an effort to control the mass loss due to the nitrogen flow. Even with these measures in place some weight loss was noted; however, the results did point to the formation of a stoichiometric hydrate (Fig. 43).

The automation of moisture sorption measurements is now a routine method of characterizing the moisture sorption properties of compounds. Prior to this advance, moisture

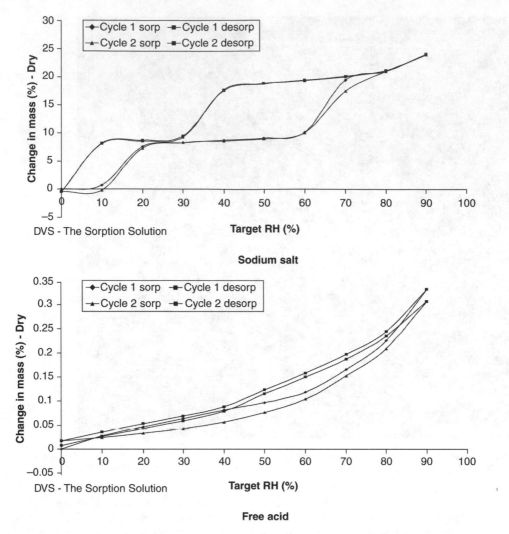

Figure 40 Moisture sorption and desorption properties for the sodium salt and free acid of a development compound.

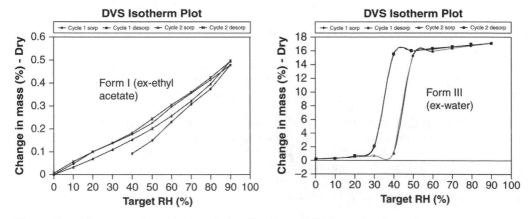

Figure 41 Moisture sorption and desorption profiles for an MCT-1 compound.

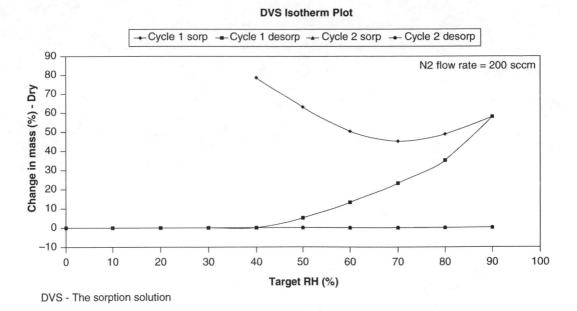

DVS - The sorption solution

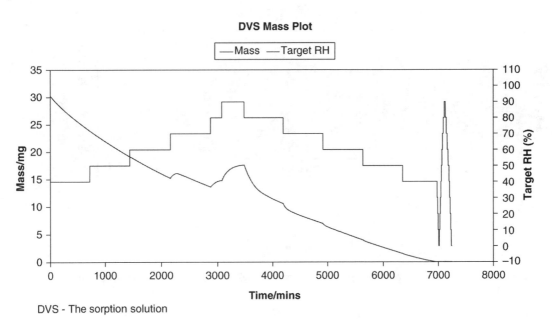

DVS - The sorption solution

Figure 42 Moisture sorption and desorption profile for *tert*-butylhydroxylamine acetate under normal operating conditions.

sorption of compounds (~10 mg) was done by exposing weighed amounts of compound in dishes placed in sealed desiccators containing saturated salt solutions. Saturated solutions of salts that give defined RHs (as a function of temperature) have been reported by Nyqvist (1983). A typical range at 25°C is given in Table 16. The samples are then stored at a selected temperature and analyzed at various time points for moisture and stability usually by TGA and HPLC, respectively.

When conducting these experiments it is wise to analyze the solid phase during or after the experiments to ascertain the effect of the moisture sorption and desorption process. For example, Gift and Taylor (2007) modified their moisture sorption instrument to accommodate

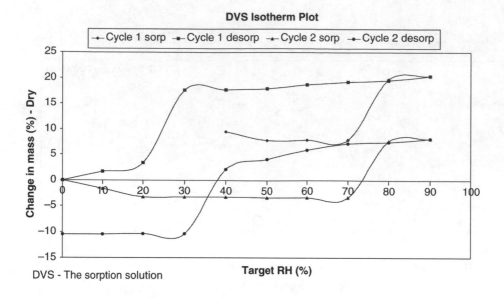

DVS - The sorption solution

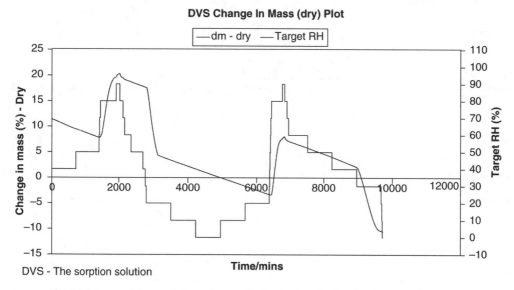

DVS - The sorption solution

Figure 43   Moisture sorption and desorption profile for *tert*-butylhydroxylamine acetate under reduced operating conditions.

Table 16   Relative Humidities Generated by Various Saturated Salt Solutions

Salt solution	Percent of relative humidity at 25°C
Silica gel	0
Potassium acetate	20
Calcium chloride	32
Sodium bromide	58
Potassium bromide	84
Dipotassium hydrogen phosphate	92
Water	100

Source: From Nyqvist (1983).

a Raman spectrometer. Using this combination of techniques, they were able to follow the mechanism of a number of moisture sorption processes, for example, hydrate formation and amorphous to crystalline transitions. Off-line analysis should also be undertaken; for example, SEM, DSC, and XRPD can be used to examine whether a sample has changed after hygroscopicity experiments.

While most companies use GVS as a compound classification technique for screening purposes and selection, Willson and Beezer (2003) have explored the thermodynamic aspects of the sorption process.

THERMAL ANALYSIS

There are a number of interrelated thermal analytical techniques that can be used to characterize the salts and polymorphs of CDs. As noted earlier, the melting point of a salt can be manipulated to produce compounds with desirable physicochemical properties for specific formulation types. Giron (1995) has reviewed thermal analytical and calorimetric methods used in the characterization of polymorphs and solvates. Of the thermal methods available for investigating polymorphism and related phenomena, DSC, TGA, and HSM are the most widely used. The combination of thermal analysis with other techniques has been described by Giron (2001).

Differential Scanning Calorimetry

There are two basic types of DSC. The first is the heat flux type (e.g., Mettler and du Pont), where sample and reference cells are heated at a constant rate, and thermocouples are used to detect the extent of the differential heat transfer between the two pans. The other DSC system is the power compensation type (e.g., Perkin–Elmer). With this type of calorimeter, if an exothermic or endothermic event occurs when a sample is heated, the power added or subtracted to one or both of the furnaces to compensate for the energy change occurring in the sample is measured. Thus, the system is maintained in a thermally neutral position at all times, and the amount of power required to maintain the system at equilibrium is directly proportional to the energy changes that are occurring in the sample. In both instruments, a few milligrams of the compound under study are weighed into an aluminum pan that can be open, hermetically sealed, or pierced to allow the escape of water, solvent, or decomposition products from pyrolysis reactions. The third type of DSC is the T_{zero} DSC marketed by TA instruments, which is a hybrid of the power compensation and heat flux instruments (Dallas et al., 2001). The T_{zero} accounts for the differences between the two types of instruments such that the sensitivity and resolution is improved on a very flat baseline, which can be a disadvantage of the power-compensated machines. In addition to these advantages, direct measurement of heat capacity can be obtained.

There are a number of variables that can affect DSC results (van Dooren, 1982). These include the type of pan, heating rate, the nature and mass of the compound, the particle size distribution, packing and porosity, pretreatment, and dilution of the sample. Normally experiments are carried out under a nitrogen atmosphere. Phenomena that can be detected using this technique include melting (endothermic), solid-state transitions (endothermic), glass transitions, crystallization (endothermic), decomposition (exothermic), and dehydration or desolvation (endothermic). DSC can also be used for purity analysis (Giron and Goldbronn, 1995). However, this is restricted to those compounds that are greater than 98% pure. It may be appropriate, if HPLC methods are not available, to use DSC to estimate purity, but it should be emphasized that DSC is much less accurate than HPLC in this respect.

A heating rate of 10°C/min is a useful compromise between speed of analysis and detecting any heating rate–dependent phenomena. If any heating rate–dependent phenomena are evident, experiments should be repeated varying the heating rate to attempt to identify the nature of the transition(s). These may be related to polymorphism, discussed earlier in this chapter, or to particle size. Roy et al. (2002) have produced a paper regarding the establishment of an experimental design for DSC experiments. Using benzoic acid and vanillin they examined the effect of sample size, heating rates, atmosphere, crucible type, and RH. Their

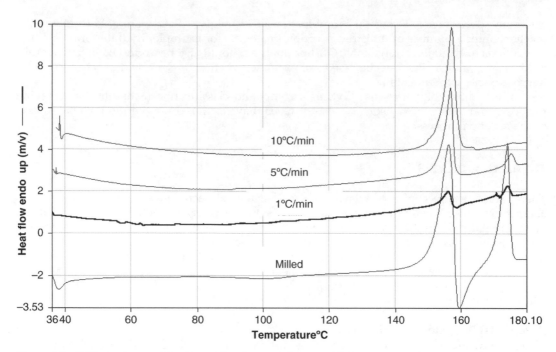

Figure 44 DSC showing particle size and heating rate effects on AR-C69457AA. *Abbreviation*: DSC, differential scanning calorimetry.

study concluded that a small sample size (3–5 mg), a low-heating rate (2°C/min), a nitrogen atmosphere, and a crimped crucible without a pinhole were the preferred experimental conditions. Figure 44 shows the effect of particle size and heating rate on the polymorphic transition of AR-C69457AA.

At 10°C/min the sample showed a single endotherm; however, when the sample was milled, it gave a thermogram that showed a melt-recrystallization-melt transformation. By reducing the heating rate it can be seen that rather than being due to a polymorphic transformation induced by the milling process, the transformation was due to a reduction in particle size.

There are a number of parameters that can be measured from the various thermal events detected by DSC. For example, for a melting endotherm the onset, peak temperatures, and enthalpy of fusion can be derived. The onset temperature is obtained by extrapolation from the leading edge of the endotherm to the baseline. The peak temperature is the temperature corresponding to the maximum of the endotherm, and enthalpy of fusion is derived from the area of the thermogram. It is the accepted custom that the extrapolated onset temperature is taken as the melting point; however, some users report the peak temperature in this respect. We tend to report both for completeness.

Recycling experiments can also be conducted whereby a sample is heated and then cooled. The thermogram may show a crystallization exotherm for the sample, which on subsequent reheating may show a different melting point to the first run. In a similar way amorphous forms can be produced by cooling the molten sample to form a glass.

Figure 45 shows the DSC behavior of the methanolate, the desolvated solvate, and two polymorphs of AR-C69457AA. These thermograms are quite complicated and would be difficult to interpret in the absence of other measurements and observations using TGA, HSM, and XRPD.

1. This is the methanol solvate, which showed a desolvation endotherm between 75°C and 100°C: TGA recorded a weight loss of 4.5%. A second much smaller endotherm

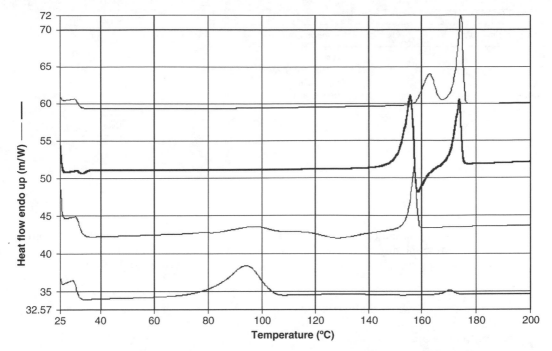

Figure 45 DSC thermograms of a number of forms of the hydrochloride salt of AR-C69457AA. *Abbreviation*: DSC, differential scanning calorimetry.

was detected at ~170°C; however, no thermal events at this temperature were noted using HSM.

2. This thermogram was obtained after the methanol solvate was desolvated in an oven. As can be seen, the thermogram contained a number of thermal events. The first, at ~100°C corresponded to small weight loss (residual solvent) detected by TGA. An exotherm corresponding to crystallization was noted at ~125°C, which indicated that desolvation produced an amorphous form which on heating crystallized. The noncrystalline nature of this phase was confirmed by XRPD. The crystalline material produced by this heating process melted at ~160°C.

3. This is the DSC thermogram of the first polymorph of the compound, which consisted of an endotherm corresponding to the melting followed by an exotherm due to immediate recrystallization to form a higher melting form of the compound.

4. The second polymorphic form of the compound consisted of two thermal events. The first of which was a solid-state transition, that is, a transformation without a melt. The second was confirmed by HSM to be the melting endotherm.

In an interesting extension of using DSC for polymorph investigations, Park et al. (2003) have developed a DSC technique for determining the solubility of forms I and III of carbamazepine, α and β-glycine and forms I and III of mefenamic acid. The small amount of compound required is attractive—especially when it is in short supply during prenomination studies. Ledru et al. (2007) have used a high-pressure DSC pressured up to 450 MPa to investigate the pressure dependence of the melting of forms I and II of paracetamol. This work experimentally confirmed the topological P/T diagrams used by Espeau et al. (2005) to determine the I-II-liquid triple point for these polymorphs.

This clearly shows that DSC can be an extremely informative technique, but it should not be used in isolation, that is, additional information from other techniques is almost always required for complete interpretation of the results.

Table 17 Standards for Thermal Analysis

Temperature (°C)	Substance
0	Water
26.87	Phenoxybenzene
114.2	Acetanilide
151.4	Adipic acid
156.6	Indium
229	Tin
232	Caffeine
327.5	Lead
419.6	Zinc

Source: From Giron-Forest et al. (1989), with permission from Elsevier.

DSC Calibration

The goal is to match the melting onset temperatures indicated by the furnace thermocouple readout to the known melting points of standards and should be calibrated as close as possible to the desired temperature. The standards should have the following properties:

- High purity
- Accurately known enthalpies
- Thermally stable
- Nonhygroscopic
- Unreactive pan atmosphere

The calibration of a DSC employs the use of standards, and Giron-Forest et al. (1989) have listed a number of materials that can be used (Table 17). In this respect ultrapure indium and lead traceable standards are probably the most convenient for a two-point calibration. The relevant data are

indium	onset temperature = 156.61 ± 0.25°C, ΔH = 28.45 ± 0.50 J/g
lead	onset temperature = 327.47 ± 0.50°C, ΔH = 23.01 ± 1.0 J/g

Archer (2006) has reported a number of new traceable NIST Standard Reference Materials (SRMs) for DSC measurements, that is, SRMs 2234 (gallium) and 2235 (bismuth).

Hyper-DSC™

Recently the use of Hyper-DSC (McGregor et al., 2004) or fast-scan DSC (FSDSC) (Riga et al., 2007) has been advocated as a method to investigate polymorphic transitions and other thermal phenomena. Riga et al. (2007) showed that for a range of standard pharmaceuticals FSDSC caused little or no variation in the melting temperature and heat of fusion values. One advantage of increased heating rate is obviously a shorter analysis time and increased throughput.

Modulated DSC

In modulated DSC (MDSC) experiments the heating program is applied sinusoidally such that any thermal events are resolved into reversing and nonreversing components. This allows complex and even overlapping processes to be deconvoluted (Coleman and Craig, 1996). The heat flow signal in conventional DSC is a combination of "kinetic" and heat capacity responses, and FT techniques are used to separate the heat flow component from the underlying heat flow signal. The cyclic heat flow part of the signal (heat capacity, C_p × heating rate) is termed the reversing heat flow component. The nonreversing part is obtained by subtracting this value from the total heat flow curve: It is important to note that all of the noise appears in the nonreversing signal.

In MDSC experiments there are a number of experimental conditions that need to be optimized.

Samples should be small, thin, and completely encapsulated in the DSC pan. This minimizes temperature gradients and maximizes conductivity during the heating and cooling cycles. Good thermal contact must also be ensured between the pans and the DSC head.

The heat capacity heat flow contribution during the heating and cooling cycles is completely reversible.

The limitations of MDSC have been described as follows (Craig and Royall, 1998).

The sample does not follow the heating signal. There needs to be a sufficient number of cycles to cover the thermal event under investigation. Some samples may fluctuate in temperature during the sinusoidal ramp in temperature.

Royall et al. (1998) have described its use in the characterization of amorphous saquinavir. Using this technique the glass transition could be separated from a relaxation endotherm that appeared as part of the transition. Although it is useful in this respect the measurements can be affected by such instrumental parameters as temperature cycling and modulation period.

Rabel et al. (1999) have investigated the use of MDSC in preformulation studies. Its use in investigating glass transitions was discussed; however, this was extended to consider its use with regard to desolvation and degradation. For example, they showed that MDSC could deconvolute concomitant melting and degradation thermal events. The events were separated as melt (endothermic), which was reversible, and decomposition, which was nonreversible. Polymorphic transformations were also investigated. The solid-state transformation of losartan was subjected to the MDSC program, and in this case the transition was seen in the nonreversible heat flow, and almost no reversible transition was detected.

Manduva et al. (2008) have extended the technique by describing a quasi-isothermal modulated temperature differential scanning calorimetric (QI-MTDSC) analysis of the polymorphs of caffeine. It differs from the conventional MDSC experiments described above whereby the temperature of the sample is modulated around a constant underlying temperature for a specified time. After this the temperature is moved up or down to produce a set of quasi-isothermal steps. The net effect of this procedure is to eliminate the effect of heating programs and thus obtain heat capacity data.

Microthermal Analysis

Microthermal analysis (μTA) is the combination of scanning probe microscopy with thermal analysis (Craig et al., 2002). Using this technique, a sample can be scanned for not only thermal conductivity but also topography, allowing thermal analysis to be performed on specific regions of a sample.

Thermogravimetric Analysis

TGA is a thermal analytical technique that can be used to detect the weight lost on heating solvates and hydrates as well as for determining thermal stability (Czarnecki and Šesták, 2000). It is based on a sensitive balance that records the weight of the sample as it is heated. Typically 5 to 10 mg of compound is examined, and, like DSC, the experiments are normally conducted under flowing nitrogen.

As an example, Figure 46 shows the TGA profile of nedocromil sodium trihydrate. It can be seen from this figure that the water is lost in two steps. The first two-thirds of the water is lost relatively easily on heating and corresponds to "loosely bound" hydrogen-bonded channel water. The remaining one-third of the weight loss clearly represents water held more tightly in the structure and is the water associated with a sodium ion in the crystal lattice. Thus, TGA can detect that water or solvent is held in different locations in the crystal lattice and therefore has the advantage over Karl Fischer titrations or loss on drying experiments that can only measure the total amount of moisture present.

When conducting TGA experiments, it is a good practice not to use too small a sample weight in the analysis, as this may give rise to inaccuracies due to buoyancy and convection current effects. The total amount of moisture lost in TGA experiments is not affected by the heating rate; however, the temperature at which it occurs may vary (Fig. 47). In addition, the dehydration mechanism and activation of the reaction may be dependent on the particle size and sample weight (Agbada and York, 1994). Galway (2000) has comprehensively reviewed the dehydration

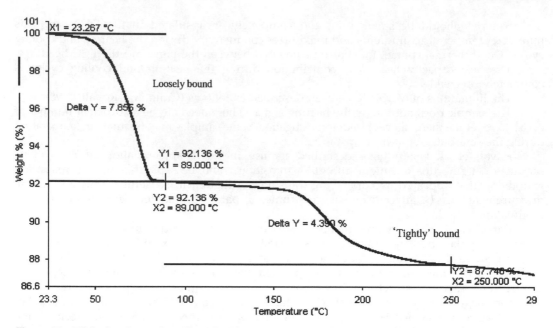

Figure 46 TGA of nedocromil sodium trihydrate. *Abbreviation*: TGA, thermogravimetric analysis.

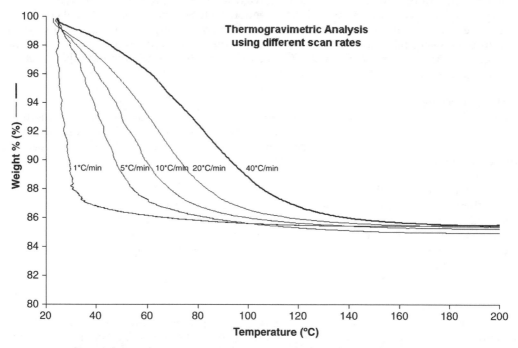

Figure 47 Effect of heating rate on the weight loss during a TGA experiment. *Abbreviation*: TGA, thermogravimetric analysis.

mechanisms of hydrates in general, and Gillon et al. (2005) have examined the mechanism of water loss from inosine dihydrate. Reddy et al. (2007) have described a TGA method for quantifying the amount of sodium pantoprazole monohydrate in the sesquihydrate.

To identify the effluent gases and vapors that are evolved during TGA experiment it needs to be coupled to another analytical instrument such as an FTIR or mass spectrometry [e.g., Pan et al. (2005) for a gas chromatography-mass spectrometry (GC-MS) study of the succinate salt of a CD].

The TGA can be calibrated using magnetic standards (e.g., alumel, cobalt, nickel, and three alloys of nickel and cobalt) (Gallagher et al., 2003). If sublimation studies are being undertaken, benzoic acid has been proposed as a calibration standard (Wright et al., 2002).

Hot-Stage Microscopy

HSM is a thermal analytical technique whereby a few milligrams of material is spread on a microscope slide, which is then placed in the hot stage and heated. The hot stage consists of a sample chamber with windows that allows the light from the microscope to pass through the sample. The sample can be heated at different rates in the sample chamber, and the atmosphere can be controlled. Subambient work can also be carried out using liquid nitrogen as a coolant. Thermal events can be observed using a microscopy; however, it is more usual to record digital images as stills or movies. HSM is usually carried out in conjunction with DSC and TGA to assist with the interpretation of the thermograms obtained from these experiments (Vitez et al. 1998).

As an example, the DSC thermogram for carbamazepine (Fig. 48) shows a number of thermal events that, without the aid of HSM, might be difficult to interpret.

Figure 48 shows the sequence of events that were recorded on heating a sample of carbamazepine. It shows that on heating the carbamazepine sample melted, which corresponded to the first endotherm recorded in the DSC thermogram. As the sample was heated further, a second form of the compound recrystallized from the melt as acicular crystals; however, this event was not detected by DSC analysis. The acicular crystals continued to grow until the second crystal form of the compound melted, corresponding to the second, large endotherm on the DSC thermogram (Fig. 49).

Isothermal microcalorimetry can also be used be to determine, among other things, the stability and hygroscopicity of substances (Beezer et al, 2004, Yang and Wu, 2008). When investigating hygroscopicity two ways of determining the moisture uptake can be used. For example, in the ramp mode this technique can be used, like DVS, to examine milligram quantities of compound. This instrument utilizes a perfusion attachment with a precision flow-switching valve. The moist gas is pumped into a reaction ampoule through two inlets, one that delivers dry nitrogen at 0% RH, and the other delivers nitrogen that has been saturated by passing it through two humidifier chambers maintained at 100% RH. The required RH is then achieved by the switching valve that varies the proportion of dry to saturated gas. The RH can then be increased or decreased to determine the effect of moisture on the physicochemical

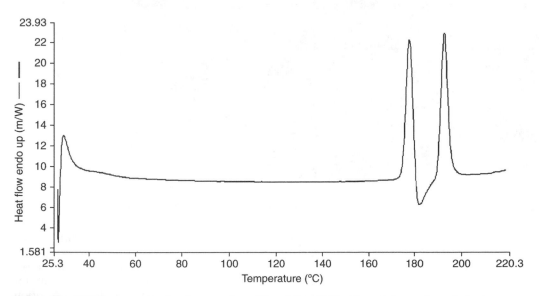

Figure 48 DSC thermogram of carbamazepine. *Abbreviation*: DSC, differential scanning calorimetry.

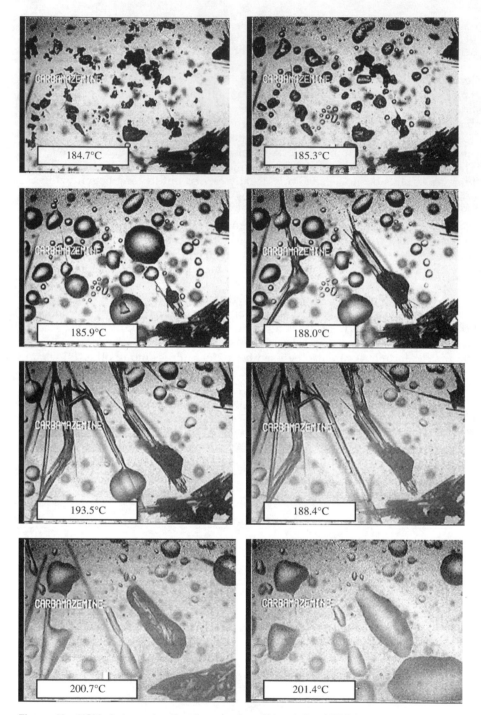

Figure 49   HSM photographs of carbamazepine. *Abbreviation*: HSM, hot-stage microscopy.

properties of the compound. In addition to examining the effect of moisture on compounds, organic vapors can also be used (Samra and Buckton, 2004).

It is probably more popular to perform microcalorimetry in the static mode. In the so-called internal hygrostat method described by Briggner et al. (1994), the compound under investigation is sealed into a vial with an open pipette tip containing the saturated salt solution chosen to give the required RH. This is shown in Figure 50.

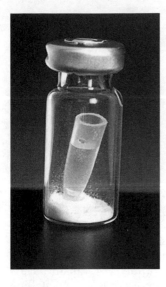

Figure 50 Internal hygrostat for microcalorimetry experiments.

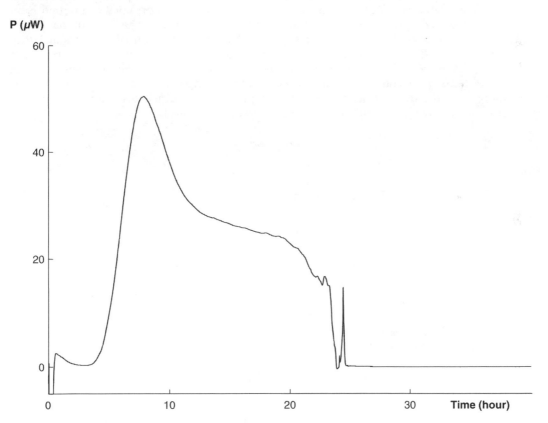

Figure 51 Microcalorimetric output for the hydration of nedocromil sodium using internal hygrostat experiment.

Figure 51 shows the heat output recorded when using an 84% RH internal hygrostat for nedocromil sodium whose GVS isotherm is shown in Figure 38. In this example, there was a transformation from a crystalline trihydrate to a heptahemihydrate.

Other examples of use include the stability testing of enalapril maleate and its tablets (Simoncic et al., 2007). The data showed very good agreement of that obtained using HPLC from which they concluded that microcalorimetry was a fast, predictive method of assessing

Table 18 Heat of Solution for an Amorphous and Crystalline Substance

Determination	Amorphous $\Delta_{sol}H^{\infty}$ (kJ/mol)	Crystalline $\Delta_{sol}H^{\infty}$ (kJ/mol)
1	−9.92	37.59
2	−11.60	37.89
3	−10.42	37.47
4	−11.53	37.32
Mean	−10.87	37.57
SD	0.72	0.21
C of V/%	6.60	0.56

stability at the preformulation stage of development and could be used to accelerate CDs to market. Hamedi and Grolier (2007) have used isothermal microcalorimetry to determine the solubility in a solvent-antisolvent system whereby the heat of dissolution of the compound under investigation is measured after the addition of a solvent. It can also be used to characterize polymorphs and related polymorphs via solution calorimetry (Urakami et al., 2005). For example, Table 18 shows the enthalpy of solution of the amorphous and crystalline forms of a compound (Fig. 52). The enthalpy of solution for the amorphous compound is an exothermic event, while that of the crystalline hydrate is endothermic. The order of magnitude of $\Delta_{sol}H^{\infty}$ for the crystalline compound suggests that the disruption of the crystal lattice predominates over the heat of solvation. In addition, the ready solubility of the compound in aqueous media is probably governed by entropy considerations. Furthermore, assessments of the heat flow as a function of amorphous-crystalline composition ratios is based on the assumption that the dissolution kinetics of both phases was sufficiently similar (at infinite dilution), thus allowing one cumulative thermal event to manifest.

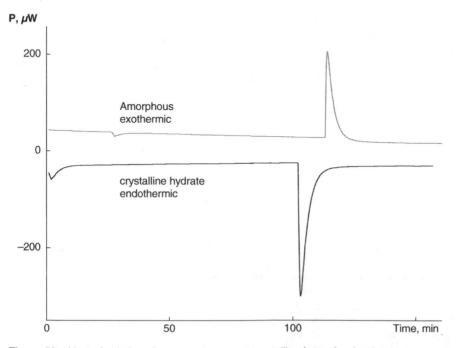

Figure 52 Heat of solution of an amorphous and crystalline form of a development compound.

HIGH-PERFORMANCE LIQUID CHROMATOGRAPHY

HPLC is now considered to be an established standard technique in most preformulation and formulation laboratories. We use HPLC to assess the degradation of the compound in the solid or solution state and, from our measurements, we should be able to determine, for example, the kinetics of degradation. Furthermore, if we can identify the degradation products of the reaction by combining this technique with mass spectroscopy, then it may also be possible to elucidate the degradation mechanism. The advantages of HPLC lie in the combination of sensitivity, efficiency, reliability, and speed of analysis of the technique. A brief guidance is presented here—a more detailed discussion of HPLC methodology and applications are beyond the scope of this book. For a recent review of up-to-date HPLC method development methodologies in the early phases of pharmaceutical development (Rasmussen et al., 2007). Prior to developing a HPLC method, its intended use must be carefully considered. For example, if the analysis is required to obtain an approximate value for the amount of CD such as for a solubility experiment, a "crude" method may be acceptable. Alternatively, if the HPLC method is to separate and determine related substances, that is, synthesis intermediates and degradation products, from the compound of interest, a more robust method will have to be developed. Other considerations will include the amount of compound to be determined, from what type of matrix (e.g., formulation, reaction mixture, drug substance), and how quickly and the number of analyses to be performed.

For most assays, where the compound is easily detected and there are relatively high concentrations in a simple matrix, isocratic elution is usually preferred, since it is simple and no post-equilibration phase is required prior to the next analysis. However, where degradation products (products of side reactions), excipients or synthetic intermediates of differing lipophilicities are likely to be encountered a gradient elution may be used.

Gradient elution offers the advantage of sharper peaks, increased sensitivity, greater peak capacity, and selectivity (increased resolving power). On the other hand, gradient elution may lead to an extended analysis time due to post-run equilibration. In addition, the system dwell times of different HPLC configurations may result in major differences in retention times and selectivity.

The type of detector to be used is usually dictated by the chemical structure of the compound under investigation. Since most compounds of pharmaceutical interest contain aromatic rings, UV detection is the most common detection method. When using this technique, the most appropriate wavelength is selected from the UV spectrum of the pure compound and that of the system suitability sample. Usually, the λ_{max} is chosen; however, to remove unwanted interference, it may be necessary to move away from this value. Where possible, the use of wavelengths less than 250 nm should be avoided because of the high level of background interference and solvent adsorption. In practical terms this requires the use of far-UV grade solvents and avoidance of organic buffers.

Other types of detection include refractive index, fluorescence or mass selective detectors. The use of other types of detector, such as those based on fluorescence, can be used for assay of compounds that can be specifically detected at low concentrations in the presence of nonfluorescent species. However, since few compounds are naturally fluorescent, they require to be chemically modified, assuming they have a suitable reactive group, to give a fluorescent derivative.

During the early stages of development, the amount of method validation carried out is likely to be limited due to compound availability. At the very least, a calibration curve should be obtained using either an internal standard or external standard procedure. The latter procedure is commonly employed by injecting a fixed volume of standard samples containing a range of known concentrations of the compound of interest. Plots of peak height and/or area versus concentration are checked for linearity by subjecting the data to linear regression analysis. Other tests such as the limit of detection, precision of the detector response, accuracy, reproducibility, specificity, and ruggedness may be carried out if more extensive validation is required.

CONCLUDING REMARKS

The preformulation phase is a critical phase in establishing the properties of CDs that will allow suitable risk assessment for development. Typically it begins during the lead optimization phase, continues through prenomination, and on into the early phases of development. Decisions made on the information generated during this phase can have a profound effect on the subsequent development of those compounds. Therefore, it is imperative that preformulation should be performed as carefully as possible to enable rational decisions to be made. The quantity and quality of the drugs can affect the data generated as well as the equipment available and the expertise of the personnel conducting the investigations.

In some companies there are specialized preformulation teams, but in others the information is generated by a number of other teams. Whichever way a company chooses to organize its preformulation information gathering, one of the most important facets is the close communication between its various departments. Preformulation studies should not be conducted on a checklist basis. Rather, they should form the basis of a controlled investigation into the physicochemical characteristics of CDs.

ACKNOWLEDGMENTS

We would like to recognize the contributions of David O'Sullivan, Phil Plumb, Clare Westwood, Steve Cosgrove, and Rob Whittock made to the science of preformulation and early development at AstraZeneca R&D Charnwood. Special thanks also to Arvind Varsani, Alan Tatham, Will Barton, Gavin Gunn, and Dee Patel, students from Loughborough University, who have also contributed to our work.

REFERENCES

Aakeröy CB, Fasulo ME, Desper J. Cocrystal or salt: does it really matter? Mol Pharm 2007; 4:317–322.

Abraham RJ, Fisher J, Loftus P. Introduction to NMR Spectroscopy. New York: Wiley, 1988.

Agbada CO and York P. Dehydration of theophylline monohydrate powder—effects of particle size and sample weight. Int J Pharm 1994; 106:33–40.

Ahlneck C, Zografi G. The molecular basis of moisture effects on the physical and chemical stability of drugs in the solid-state. Int J Pharm 1990; 62:87–95.

Albert A, Sargeant E P. The Determination of Ionization Constants: A Laboratory Manual. 3rd Ed. London: Chapman & Hall, 1984.

Allen FH. The Cambridge Structural Database: a quarter of a million crystal structures and rising. Acta Crystallogr 2002; B58:380–388.

Allesø M, Berg FVD, Cornett C, et al. Solvent diversity in polymorph screening. J Pharm Sci 2008; 97: 2145–2159.

Almarsson Ö, Hickey MB, Peterson ML, et al. High-throughput surveys of crystal form diversity of highly polymorphic pharmaceutical compounds. Crystal Growth Des 2003; 3:927–933.

Alsenz J, Kansy M. High throughput solubility measurement in drug discovery and development. Adv Drug Deliv Rev 2007; 59:546–567.

Alverez Núñez FA, Yalkowsky SH. Foaming activity and pKa of some surface active compounds. Int J Pharm 1997; 151:193–199.

Aman W, Thoma K. The influence of formulation and manufacturing process on the photostability of tablets. Int J Pharm 2002; 243:33–47.

Aman W, Thoma K. ICH Guideline for photostability testing: aspects and directions for use. Pharmazie 2003; 58:877–880.

Amidon GL, Lennernäs H, Shah VP, et al. A theoretical basis for a Biopharmaceutic Drug Classification: the correlation of in vitro drug product dissolution and in vivo bioavailability. Pharm Res 1995; 12:413–420.

Anderson BD, Conradi RA. Predictive relationships in the water solubility of salts of a nonsteroidal anti-inflammatory drug. J Pharm Sci 1985; 74:815–820.

Andricopulo AD, Montanari CA. Structure-activity relationships for the design of small-molecule inhibitors. Mini Rev Med Chem 2005; 5:585–593.

Apperley DC, Harris RK, Larsson T, et al. Quantitative nuclear magnetic resonance analysis of solid formoterol fumarate and its dihydrate. J Pharm Sci 2003; 92:2496–2503.

Archer DG, Kirklin DR. NIST and standards for calorimetry. Thermochim Acta 2000; 347:21–30.

Archer DG. New NIST-traceable standards for calibration and validation of DSC. J Therm Biomed Anal 2006; 85:131–134

Asuero AG, Navas MJ, Herrador MA, et al. Spectrophotometric evaluation of acidity constants of isonicotinic acid. Int J Pharm 1986; 34:81–92.

Austin RP, Davis AM, Manners CN. Partitioning of ionizing molecules between aqueous buffers and phospholipid vesicles. J Pharm Sci 1995; 84:1180–1183.

Authelin JR. Thermodynamics of non-stoichiometric pharmaceutical hydrates. Int J Pharm 2005; 303: 37–53.

Avdeef A, Berger CM, Brownell C. H-metric solubility. 2. Correlation between the acid-base titration and the saturation shake–flask solubility–pH methods. Pharm Res 2000; 17:85–89.

Avdeef A. Physicochemical profiling (solubility, permeability and charge state). Curr Top Med Chem 2001, 1:277–351.

Avdeef A, Box KJ, Comer JEA, et al. H-metric log P 11. pKa determination of water-insoluble drugs in organic-solvent mixtures. J Pharm Biomed Anal 1999; 20:631–641.

Ayala AP. Polymorphism in drugs investigated by low wavenumber Raman scattering. Vib Spec 2007; 45:112–116.

Ayala AP, Siesler HW, Boese R, et al. Solid-state characterization of olanzapine polymorphs using vibrational spectroscopy. Int J Pharm 2006; 326:69–79.

Azibi M, Draguet-Brughmans M, Bouche R, et al. Conformational study of two polymorphs of spiperone: possible consequences on the interpretation of pharmacological activity. J Pharm Sci 1983; 72: 232–235.

Balbach S, Korn C. Pharmaceutical evaluation of early development candidates "the 100 mg approach". Int J Pharm 2004; 275:1–12.

Banga S, Chawla G, Varandani D, et al. Modification of the crystal habit of celecoxib for improved processability. J Pharm Pharmacol 2007; 59:29–39.

Barbeto F, di Marino G, Grumetto L, et al. Prediction of drug-membrane interactions by IAM-HPLC: effects of different phospholipid stationary phases on the partition of bases. Eur J Pharm Sci 2004; 22:261–269.

Barr G, Dong W, Gilmore CJ. PolySNAP: a computer program for analyzing high throughput powder diffraction data. J Appl Crystallogr 2004; 37:658–664.

Bartolomei M, Ramusino MC, Ghetti P. Solid-state investigation of flucinolone acetonide. J Pharm Biomed Anal 1997; 15:1813–1820.

Basavoju S, Boström D, Velaga SP. Pharmaceutical cocrystal and salts of norfloxacin. Cryst Growth Des 2006; 6:2699–2708.

Bates S, Zografi G, Engers D, et al. Analysis of amorphous and nanocrystalline solids from their X-ray diffraction patterns. Pharm Res 2006; 23:2333–2349.

Bauer J, Spanton S, Henry R, et al. Ritonavir: an extraordinary example of conformational polymorphism. Pharm Res 2001; 18:859–866.

Baxter A, Cooper A, Kinchin E, et al. Hit-to-lead studies: the discovery of potent, orally bioavailable thiazolopyrimidine CXCR2 receptor antagonists. Bioorg Med Chem Lett 2006; 16:960–963.

Beall HD, Getz JJ, Sloan KB. The estimation of relative water solubility for prodrugs that are unstable in water. Int J Pharm 1993; 93:37–47.

Beezer AE, O'Neill MAA, Urakami K, et al. Pharmaceutical microcalorimetry: recent advances in the study of solid-state materials. Thermochim Acta 2004; 420:19–22.

Benjamin EJ, Lin LH. Preparation and in vitro evaluation of salts of an antihypertensive agent to obtain slow release. Drug Dev Ind Pharm 1985; 11:771–790.

Berge SM, Bighley LD, Monkhouse DC. Pharmaceutical salts. J Pharm Sci 1977; 66:1–18.

Bergström CAS, Luthman K, Artursson P. Accuracy of calculated pH-dependent aqueous solubility. Eur J Pharm Sci 2005; 22:387–398.

Bernstein J. Polymorphism in Molecular Crystals. IUCr monographs on Crystallography 14. Oxford: Clarendon Press, 2002.

Bernstein J, Henck JO. Disappearing and reappearing polymorphs-an anathema to crystal engineering? Cryst Eng 1998; 1:119–128.

Beyer T, Lewis T, Price SL. Which organic crystal structures are predictable by lattice energy minimization? CrystEngComm 2001; 44:178–212.

Bhal SK, Kassam K, Peirson IG, et al. The rule of five revisited: applying log D in place of log P in drug likeness filters. Mol Pharm 2008; 4:556–560.

Bhatt PM, Desiraju GR. Tautomeric polymorphism in omeprazole. Chem Commun (Camb) 2007; 2057–2059.

Bhattachar SN, Deschenes LA, Wesley JA. Solubility: it's not just for physical chemists. Drug Disc Today 2006; 11:1012–1018.

Bhugra C, Pikal MJ. Role of thermodynamic, molecular, and kinetic factors in crystallization from the amorphous state. J Pharm Sci 2008; 94:1329–1349.

Bingham AL, Hughes DS, Hursthouse MB, et al. Over one hundred solvates of sulfathiazole. Chem Commun (Camb) 2001; 603–604.

Black SN, Collier EA, Davey RJ, et al. Structure, solubility, screening and synthesis of molecular salts. J Pharm Sci 2007; 96:1053–1068.

Blagden N, Davey RJ. Polymorph selection: challenges for the future. Cryst Growth Des 2003; 3: 873–885.

Blagden N, Davey RJ, Lieberman HF, et al. Crystal chemistry and solvent polymorphic systems– sulphathiazole. J Chem Soc Faraday Trans 1998; 94:1035–1044.

Blanco LH, Sanabrai NR, Dávila MT. Solubility of 1,3,5,7-tetratricyclo[3.3.1.1^{3,7}]decane (HMT) in water from 275.15K to 313.15K. Thermochim Acta 2006; 450:73–75.

Bolton BA, Prasad PN. Laser Raman investigation of pharmaceutical solids: griseofulvin and its solvates. J Pharm Sci 1981; 70:789–793.

Borka L, Haleblian JK. Crystal polymorphism of pharmaceuticals. Acta Pharm Jugosl 1990; 40:71–94.

Bosch HW, Škapin SD, Matijević E. Preparation and characterization of finely dispersed drugs. 5,Ethyl 3, 5-di (acetylamino)-2,4,6 triiodobenzoate. Coll Surf Physicochem Eng Aspects 2004; 250:43–50.

Boultif A, Louer D. Indexing of powder diffraction patterns for low-symmetry lattices by the successive dichotomy method. J Appl Crystallogr 1991; 24:987–993.

Box K, Bevan C, Comer J, et al. High-throughput measurement of pKa values in a mixed buffer linear pH gradient system. Anal Chem 2003; 75:883–892.

Box K, Völgyi G, Baka E, et al. Equilibrium versus kinetic measurements of aqueous solubility, and the ability of compounds to supersaturate in solution—a validation study. J Pharm Sci 2006; 95:1–10.

Box K, Völgyi G. Ruiz R, et al. Physicochemical properties of a new multicomponent cosolvent system for the pKa determination of poorly soluble pharmaceutical compounds. Helv Chim Acta 2007; 90:1538–1553.

Bracconi P, Andrès C, Ndiaye A. Structural properties of magnesium stearate pseudopolymorphs: effect of temperature. Int J Pharm 2003; 262:109–124.

Bray ML, Jahansouz H, Kaufman MJ. Selection of optimal hydrate/solvate forms of a fibrinogen receptor antagonist for solid dosage development. Pharm Dev Technol 1999; 4:81–87.

Briggner LE, Buckton G, Bystrom K, et al. Use of isothermal microcalorimetry in the study of changes in crystallinity induced during the processing of powders. Int J Pharm 1994; 105:125–135.

Brittain HG. The impact of polymorphism on drug development: a regulatory viewpoint. Am Pharm Rev 2000a; 67–70.

Brittain HG. X-ray diffraction II: using single-crystal X-ray diffraction to study polymorphism and solvatomorphism. Spectroscopy 2000b; 15:34–39.

Bruno IJ, Cole JC, Edgington PR, et al. New software for searching the Cambridge Structural Database and visualizing crystal structures. Acta Crystallogr Sect 2002; B58:389–397.

Bugay DE. Characterization of the solid-state: spectroscopic techniques. Adv Drug Deliv Rev 2001; 48: 43–65.

Burger A, Brox W, Ratz AW. Polymorphie und pseudopolymorphie von celiprololhydrochlorid. Acta Pharm Technol 1985; 31:230–235.

Burnett DJ, Thielmann F, Sokoloski TD. Investigating carbamazepine-acetone solvate formation via gravimetric vapor sorption. J Therm Anal Calorim 2007; 89:693–698.

Busetta B, Courseille C, Hospital M. Crystal and molecular structure of three polymorphous forms of estrone. Acta Cryst 1973; B29:298–313.

Byard SJ, Jackson SL, Smail A, et al. Studies of the crystallinity of a pharmaceutical development drug substance. J Pharm Sci 2005; 94:1321–1335.

Byrn SR. Solid-State Chemistry of Drugs. New York: Academic Press, 1982.

Byrn SR, Pfeiffer R, Ganey M, et al. Pharmaceutical solids: a strategic approach to regulatory considerations. Pharm Res 1995; 12:945–954.

Byrn SR, Pfeiffer RR, Stowell JG. Solid-State Chemistry of Drugs. SSCI Inc.

Cabri W, Ghetti P, Pozzi G, et al. Polymorphisms and patent, market, and legal battles: cefdinir case study. Org Proc Res Dev 2007; 11:64–72.

Callaghan JC, Clearly GW, Elefant M, et al. Equilibrium moisture content of pharmaceutical excipients. Drug Dev Ind Pharm 1982; 8:355–369.

Campbell Roberts SN, Williams AC, Grimsey IM,et al. Quantitative analysis of mannitol polymorphs. FT-Raman spectroscopy. J Pharm Biomed Anal 2002a; 28:1135–1147.

Campbell Roberts SN, Williams AC, Grimsey IA, et al. Quantitative analysis of mannitol polymorphs. X-ray powder diffractometry—exploring preferred orientation effects. J Pharm Biomed Anal 2002b; 28:1149–1159.

Capes JS, Cameron RE. Contact line crystallization to obtain metastable polymorphs. Cryst Growth Des 2007; 7:108–112.

Cardew PT, Davey RJ. The kinetics of solvent-mediated phase transformations. Proc R Soc 1985; A398:415–428.

Carpentier L, Decressain R, Desprez S, et al. Dynamics of the amorphous and crystalline α-, γ- phases of indomethacin J Phys Chem 2006; B 110:457–464.

Carstensen JT, Danjo K, Yoshioka S, et al. Limits to the concept of solid-state stability. J Pharm Sci 1987; 76:548–550.

Carstensen JT, Li Wan Po A. The state of water in drug decomposition in the moist solid-state: description and modelling. Int J Pharm 1992; 83:87–94.

Carstensen JT. Pharmaceutical Preformulation 2002, CRC Press, New York.

Ceolin R, Toscani S, Agafonov V, et al. Phenomenology of polymorphism. I. Pressure–temperature representation of trimorphism: general rules; application to the case of dimethyl 3,6-dichloro-2, 5-dihydroxyterephthalate. J Solid State Chem 1992; 98:366–378.

Chan HK, Doelker E. Polymorphic transformation of some drugs under compression. Drug Dev Ind Pharm 1985; 11:315–332.

Chan KLA, Kazarian SG, Vassou D, et al. In situ high throughput study of drug polymorphism under controlled temperature and humidity using FT-IR spectroscopic imaging. Vib Spec 2007; 43: 221–226.

Chaubal MV. Application of formulation technologies in lead candidate selection and optimization. Drug Discov Today 2004; 9:603–609.

Cheetham AK, Wilkinson AP. Structure determination and refinement with synchrotron X-ray powder diffraction data. J Phys Chem Solids 1991; 52:1199–1208.

Chemburkar SR, Bauer J, Deming K, et al. Dealing with the impact of ritonavir polymorphs on the late stages of bulk drug process development. Org Proc Res Dev 2000; 4:413–417.

Chen LR, Padden BE, Vippagunta SR, et al. Nuclear magnetic resonance and infrared spectroscopic analysis of nedocromil hydrates. Pharm Res 2000; 17:619–624.

Chen CC, Song Y. Solubility modelling with a nonrandom two-liquid segment activity coefficient model. Ind Eng Chem Res 2004; 43:8354–8362.

Chen XQ, Venkatesh S. Miniature device for aqueous and non-aqueous solubility measurements during drug discovery. Pharm Res 2004; 21:1758–1761.

Cheung EY, Harris KDM, Foxman BM. A straightforward and effective procedure to test for preferred orientation in polycrystalline samples prior to structure determination from powder diffraction data. Cryst Growth Des 2003; 3:705–710.

Chieng N, Rades T, Saville D. Formation and physical stability of the amorphous phase of ranitidine hydrochloride polymorphs prepared by cryo-milling. Eur J Pharm Biopharm 2008; 68:771–780.

Childs SL, Stahly P, Park A. The salt–cocrystal continuum: the influence of crystal structure on ionization state. Mol Pharm 2007; 4:323–338.

Chongprasert S, Griesser UJ, Bottorff AT, et al. Effects of freeze-dry processing conditions on the crystallization of pentamidine isethionate. J Pharm Sci 1998; 87:1155–1160.

Chowan ZT. pH solubility profiles of organic carboxylic acids and their salts. J Pharm Sci 1978; 67: 1257–1260.

Christensen AN, Lehmann MS, Nielsen M. Solving crystal structures from powder diffraction data. Aust J Phys 1985; 38:497–505.

Clas SD. The importance of characterizing the crystal form of the drug substance during drug development. Curr Opin Drug Discov Devel 2003; 6:550–560.

Clegg W. Crystal Structure Determination. Oxford: Oxford Science Publications, University Press, 1998.

Clegg W, Teat SJ. Tetracycline hydrochloride: a synchrotron microcrystal study. Acta Crystallogr C 2000; C56:1343–1345.

Cohen MD, Green BS. Organic chemistry in the solid state. Chem Brit 1973; 9:490–497.

Coleman NJ, Craig DQM. Modulated temperature differential scanning calorimetry: a novel approach to pharmaceutical thermal analysis. Int J Pharm 1996; 135:13–29.

Connors KA, Amidon GL, Stella VJ. Chemical Stability of Pharmaceuticals. A Handbook for Pharmacists. 2nd ed. New York: Wiley, 1986.

Cooke, Peter M. Chemical microscopy. Anal Chem 2000; 72:169–188.

Coombes DS, Catlow RA, Gales JD, et al. Theoretical and experimental investigations on the morphology of pharmaceutical crystals. J Pharm Sci 2002; 91:1652–1658.

Coquerel G. The 'structural purity' of molecular solids–an elusive concept? Chem Eng Proc 2006; 45: 857–862.

Cosgrove SD, Steele G, Plumb AP, et al. Understanding the polymorphic behaviour of sibenadit hydrochloride through detailed studies integrating structural and dynamical assessment. J Pharm Sci 2005; 94:2403–2415.

Cotton ML, Lamarche P, Motola S, et al. L-649,923–the selection of an appropriate salt form and preparation of a stable oral formulation. Int J Pharm 1994; 109:237–249.

Craig DQM, Royall PG. The use of modulated temperature DSC for the study of pharmaceutical systems: potential uses and limitations. Pharm Res 1998; 15:1152–1153.

Craig DQM, Vett VL, Andrews CS, et al. Pharmaceutical applications of microthermal analysis. J Pharm Sci 2002; 91:1201–1213.

Crowley KJ, Zografi G. The use of thermal methods for predicting glass-former fragility. Thermochim Acta 2001; 380:79–93.

Czarnecki J, Šesták J. Practical thermogravimetry. J Therm Anal Calorim 2000; 60:759–778.

Dallas G, Groh J, Kelly T, et al. A new technology to improve DSC performance. Am Lab 2001; 33: 26–29.

Danesh A, Connell SD, Davies MC, et al. An in situ dissolution study of aspirin crystal planes (100) and (001) by atomic force microscopy. Pharm Res 2001; 18:299–303.

Datta S, Grant DJW. Crystal structures of drugs: advances in determination, prediction and engineering. Nat Rev Drug Disc 2004; 3:42–57.

Davey RJ, Cardew PT, McEwan D, et al. Rate controlling processes in solvent-mediated phase transformations. J Cryst Growth 1986; 79:648–653.

David WIF, Shankland K, McCusker LB, et al. Structure Determination from Powder Diffraction Data IUCr Monographs on Crystallography 13. Oxford: Oxford University Press, 2002.

David WIF, Shankland K, Shankland N. Routine determination of molecular crystal structures from powder diffraction data. Chem Commun 1998; 931–932.

David WIF, Shankland K, van de Streek J, et al. DASH: a program for crystal structure determination from powder diffraction data. J Appl Crystallogr 2006; 39:910–915.

Davidovich M, Gougoutas JZ, Scaringe RP, et al. Detection of polymorphism by powder X-ray diffraction: interference by preferred orientation. Am Pharm Rev 2004; 7:10–16, 100.

Davis AM, Keeling DJ, Steele J, et al. Components of successful lead generation. Curr Top Med Chem 2005; 5:421–439.

Dearden JC, Bresnen GM. The measurement of partition coefficients. Quant Struct Act Relat 1988; 7: 133–144.

De Camp. The impact of polymorphism on drug development: a regulator's viewpoint Am Pharm Rev 2001; 4:70–77.

De Ranter CJ. Applications of X-ray diffractometric techniques in the analysis of drugs. J Pharm Biomed Anal 1986; 4:747–754.

Deij MA, van Eupen J, Meekes H, et al. Experimental and computational morphology of three polymorphs of the free base of venlafaxine: a comparison of morphology of prediction methods. Int J Pharm 2008; 353:113–123.

Desiraju GR. Counterpoint: what's in a name? Cryst Growth Des 2004; 4:1089–1090.

Desrosiers PJ. The potential of preform. Mod Drug Disc 2004; 40–43.

De Villiers MM, van der Watt JG, Lötter AP. Kinetic study of the solid-state photolytic degradation of two polymorphic forms of furosemide. Int J Pharm 1992; 88:275–283.

Duchowicz PR, Talevi A, Bellera C, et al. Application of descriptors based on Lipinski's rules in the QSPR study of aqueous solubilities. Bioorg Med Chem 2007; 15:3711–3719. [Epub 2007, Mar 18].

Duer MJ. Solid State NMR Spectroscopy Principles and Applications. Oxford: Blackwell Science, 2002.

Dunitz JD, Bernstein J. Disappearing polymorphs. Acc Chem Res 1995; 28:193–200.

Dziki W, Bauer JF, Szpylman JJ, et al. The use of near-infrared spectroscopy to monitor the mobility of water within the sarafloxacin crystal lattice. J Pharm Biomed Anal 2000; 22:829–848.

El-Tayar N, Tsai RS, Testa B, et al. Partitioning of solutes in different solvent systems: contribution of hydrogen-bonding capacity and polarity. J Pharm Sci 1991; 80:590–598.

Elliot SR, Rao CNR, Thomas JM. The chemistry of the non-crystalline state. Angew Chem Int Ed Engl 1986; 25:31–46.

Engel GL, Farid NA, Faul MM, et al. Salt form selection and characterization of LY333531 mesylate monohydrate. Int J Pharm 2000; 198:239–247.

Engel GE, Wilke S, König O. et al. PowderSolve—a complete package for crystal structure solution from powder diffraction patterns. J Appl Crystallogr 1999; 32:1169–1179.

Espeau P, Céolin R, Tamarit JL, et al. Polymorphism of paracetamol: relative stabilities of the monoclinic and orthorhombic phases inferred from topological pressure-temperature and temperature-volume phase diagrams. J Pharm Sci 2005; 94:524–539.

Evans JSO, Radosavljević Evans I. Beyond classical applications of powder diffraction. Chem Soc Rev 2004; 33:539–547.

Fabbiani FPA, Allan DR, Parsons S, et al. An exploration of the polymorphism of piracetam using high pressure. CrystEngComm 2005; 7:179–186.

Faller B, Ertl P. Computational approaches to determine drug solubility. Adv Drug Deliv Rev 2007; 59:533–545.

Faller B, Grimm HP, Loeuillet-Ritzler F, et al. High–throughput lipophilicity measurement with immobilized artificial membranes. J Med Chem 2005; 48:2571–2576.

Farag Badawy SI. Effect of salt form on chemical stability of an ester prodrug of a glycoprotein IIb/IIIa receptor antagonist in solid dosage forms. Int J Pharm 2001; 223:81–87.

Federsel HJ. Facing chirality in the 21st century: approaching the challenges in the pharmaceutical industry. Chirality 2003; 15:S128–S142.

Fini G. Applications of Raman spectroscopy to pharmacy. J Raman Spectrosc 2004; 35:335–337.

Fini A, Fazio G, Orienti I, et al. Chemical properties-dissolution relationship. Part 4. Behaviour in solution of the diclofenac N-(2-hydroxyethyl) pyrrolidine salt (DHEP). Pharm Acta Helv 1991; 66:201–203.

Florence AJ, Baumgartner, Weston C, et al. Indexing powder patterns in physical form screening: instrumentation and data quality. J Pharm Sci 2003; 92:1930–1938.

Florence AJ, Johnstone A. Applications of ATR UV/vis spectroscopy in physical form characterisation of pharmaceuticals. Spectrosc Eur 2005; 16:24–27.

Florence AJ, Johnstone A, Price SL, et al. An automated parallel crystallization search for predicted crystal structures and packing motifs of carbamazepine. J Pharm Sci 2006; 95:1918–1930.

Franks NP, Abraham MH, Lieb WR. Molecular organization of liquid n-octanol: an X-ray diffraction analysis. J Pharm Sci 1993; 82:466–470.

Frantz S. Pharma faces major challenges after a year of failures and heated battles. Nat Rev Drug Discov 2007; 6:5–7.

Freer AA, Payling DW, Suschitzky JL. Structure of nedocromil sodium: a novel anti-asthmatic agent. Acta Cryst Sect C: Cryst Struct Comm 1987; C43:1900–1905.

Gadewar SB, Hofmann HM, Doherty MF. Evolution of crystal shape. Cryst Growth Des 2004; 4:109–112.

Gallagher PK, Blaine R, Charsley EL, et al. Magnetic temperature standards for TG. J Therm Anal Calorim 2003; 72:1109–1116.

Galway AK. Structure and order in thermal dehydrations of crystalline solids. Thermochim Acta 2000; 355:181–238.

Gamberini MC, Baraldi C, Tinti A, et al. Solid-state characterization of chloramphenicol palmitate. Raman spectroscopy applied to pharmaceutical polymorphs. J Mol Struct 2006; 785:216–224.

Gardner CR, Walsh CT, Almarsson ö. Drugs as materials: valuing physical form in drug discovery. Nat Rev Drug Discov 2004; 3:927–934.

Garrido G, Koort E, Ràfols C,et al. Acid-base equilibrium non-polar media. Absolute pKa scale of bases in tetrahydrofuran. J Org Chem 2006; 71:9062–9067.

Gavazotti A. A solid-state chemist's view of the crystal polymorphism of organic compounds. J. Pharm Sci 2007; 96:2232–2241.

Gavezzotti A, Filippini G. Polymorphic forms of organic crystals at room conditions–thermodynamic and structural implications. J Am Chem Soc 1995; 117:12299–12305.

Gavezzotti A. Ten years of experience in polymorph prediction: what next? CrystEngComm 2002; 4: 343–347.

Geppi M, Mollica G, Borsacchi S, et al. Solid–state NMR studies of pharmaceutical systems. Appl Spectrosc Rev 2008; 43:202–302.

Getsoian A, Lodaya RM, Blackburn AC. One solvent polymorph screen of carbamazepine. Int J Pharm 2008; 348:3–9.

Ghetti P, Ghedini A, Stradi R. Analytical potential of FT-IR microscopy. I. Applications to the drug polymorphism study. Boll Chim Farm 1994; 133:689–697.

Giachetti C, Assandri A, Mautone G, et al. Pharmacokinetics and metabolism of N-(2-hydroxyethyl)-2,5-[^{14}C]-pyrolidine (HEP, Epolamine) in male healthy volunteers. Eur J Drug Met Pharmcokinet 1996; 21:261–268.

Gift AD, Taylor LS. Hyphenation of Raman spectroscopy with gravimetric analysis to interrogate water-solid interactions in pharmaceutical systems. J Pharm Biomed Anal 2007; 43:14–23.

Gillon AL, Davey RJ, Storey R, et al. Solid-state dehydration processes; mechanism of water loss from crystalline inosine dihydrate. Phys Chem 2005; 109:5341–5347.

Gillon AL, Feeder N, Davey RG, et al. Hydration in molecular crystals–a Cambridge structural analysis. Cryst Growth Des 2003; 3:663–673.

Gilmore CJ, Barr G, Paisley J. High-throughput powder diffraction pattern analysis using full pattern profiles. J Appl Crystallogr 2004; 37:231–242.

Gilmore CJ, Shankland K, Bricogne G. Applications of the maximum entropy method to powder diffraction and electron crystallography. Proc R Soc 1993; A442:97–111.

Giron D. Thermal analysis and calorimetric methods in the characterization of polymorphs and solvates. Thermochim Acta 1995; 248:1–59.

Giron D. Investigations of polymorphism and psuedopolymorphism in pharmaceuticals by combined thermoanalytical techniques. J Therm Anal Calorim 2001; 64:37–60.

Giron D. Characterisation of salts of drug substances. J Therm Anal Calorim 2003; 73:441–457.

Giron D, Goldbronn C. Place of DSC purity analysis in pharmaceutical development. J Thermal Anal 1995; 44:217–251.

Giron-Forest D, Goldbronn C, Piechon P. Thermal analysis methods for pharmacopeial materials. J Pharm Biomed Anal 1989; 7:1421–1433.

Giron D, Mutz M, Garnier S. Solid-state of pharmaceutical compounds. Impact of the ICH Q6 Guideline on Industrial Development. J Therm Anal Calorim 2004; 77:709–747.

Glass BD, Novák CS, Brown ME. The thermal and photostability of solid pharmaceuticals. J Therm Anal Calorim 2004; 77:1013–1236.

Glomme A, März J, Dressman JB. Comparison of a miniaturized shake-flask solubility method with automated potentiometric acid/base titrations and calculated solubilities. J Pharm Sci 2005; 94:1–16.

Glusker JP, Lewis M, Rossi M. Crystal Structure Analysis for Chemists and Biologists. New York: VCH, 1994.

Goa D, Rytting JH. Use of solution calorimetry to determine the extent of crystallinity of drugs and excipients. Int J Pharm 1997; 151:183–192.

Gong Y, Collman BN, Mehrens SM, et al. Stable-form screening: overcoming trace impurities that inhibit solution–mediated phase transformation to the stable polymorph of sulfamerazine. J Pharm Sci 2008; 97:2130–2144.

Görbitz CH. What is the best crystal, size for collection of X-ray data? Refinement of the structure of glycyl-L-serine based on data from a very large crystal. Acta Cryst Sect B–Struct Sci 1999; 55:1090–1098.

Görbitz CH, Hersleth HP. On the inclusion of solvent molecules in the crystal structures of organic compounds. Acta Cryst 2000; B56:526–534.

Gould PL. Salt selection for basic drugs. Int J Pharm 1986; 33:201–217.

Gracin S, Rasmuson Å. Solubility of phenylacetic acid, p-hydroxyphenyl acetic acid, p-aminophenylacetic acid, p-hydroxybenzoic acid, and ibuprofen in pure solvents. J Chem Eng Data 2002; 47:1379–1383.

Granberg RA, Rasmuson ÅC. Solubility of paracetamol in binary and ternary mixtures of water + acetone + toluene. J Chem Eng Data 2000; 45:478–483.

Grant DJW, Mehdizadeh M, Chow AHL, et al. Nonlinear van't Hoff solubility-temperature plots and their pharmaceutical interpretation. Int J Pharm 1984; 18:25–38.

Green DA, Meenan P. Crystal Growth of Organic Materials. In: Myerson AS, Green DA, Meenan P, eds. ACS Conference Proceedings;p 78.

Griesser UJ, Burger A. The effect of water vapor pressure on desolvation kinetics of caffeine 4/5-hydrate. Int J Pharm 1995; 120:83–93.

Gross TD, Schaab K, Quellette M, et al. An approach to early-phase salt selection: application to NBI-75043. Org Proc Res Dev 2007; 11:365–377.

Gu CH, Grant DJW. Estimating the relative stability of polymorphs and hydrates from heats of solution and solubility data. J Pharm Sci 2001; 90:1277–1287.

Gu CH, LiH, Gandhi RB, et al. Grouping solvents by statistical analysis of solvent property parameters: implication to polymorph screening. Int J Pharm 2004; 283:117–125.

Gu L, Strickley RG. Preformulation salt selection-physical property comparisons of the tris(hydroxymethyl)aminomethane (THAM) salts of four analgesic/anti-inflammatory agents with the sodium salts and the free acids. Pharm Res 1987; 4:255–257.

Gu CH, Young V, Grant DJW. Polymorph screening: influence of solvents on the rate of solvent-mediated polymorphic transformation. J Pharm Sci 2001; 90:1878–1890.

Guile SD, Bantick JR, Cheshire DR, et al. Potent blockers of monocarboxylate transporter MCT1: novel immunomodulatory compounds. Bioorg Med Chem Lett 2006; 16:2260–2265.

Guillory JK, Erb DM. Using solution calorimetry to quantitate binary mixtures of three forms of sulfamethoxazole. Pharm Manufacturing 1985; 2:30–33.

Guo J, Elzinga PA, Hageman MJ, et al. Rapid throughput screening of apparent K_{sp} values for weakly basic drugs using a 96-well format. Pharm Sci 2008; 97:2080–2090.

Gustavo González A. Practical digest for the evaluation of acidity constants of drugs by reversed phase high performance liquid chromatography. Int J Pharm 1993; 91:R1–R5.

Gwak HS, Choi JS, Choi HK. Enhanced bioavailability of piroxicam via salt formation with ethanolamines. Int J Pharm 2005; 297:156–161.

Haleblian JK. Characterization of habits and crystalline modification of solids and their pharmaceutical applications. J Pharm Sci 1975; 64:1269–1288.

Hamedi MH, Grolier JPE. Solubility diagrams in solvent-antisolvent systems by titration calorimetry. J Therm Anal Calorim 2007; 89:87–92.

Hancock BC, Parks M. True solubility advantage for amorphous pharmaceuticals. Pharm Res 2000; 17:397–404.

Hancock BC, Dalton CR, Pikal MJ, et al. A pragmatic test of a simple calorimetric method for determining the fragility of some amorphous pharmaceutical materials. Pharm Res 1998; 15:762–767.

Hancock BC, Shalaev EY, Shamblin SL. Polyamorphism: a pharmaceutical perspective. J Pharm Pharmacol 2002; 54:1151–1152.

Hancock BC, Shamblin SL. Molecular mobility of amorphous pharmaceuticals determined using differential scanning calorimetry. Thermochim Acta 2001; 380:95–107.

Harris RK. NMR studies of organic polymorphs & solvates. Analyst 2006; 131:351–373.

Harris KDM, Cheung EY. How to determine structures when single crystals cannot be grown: opportunities for structure determination of molecular materials using powder diffraction data. Chem Soc Rev 2004; 33:526–538.

Harris KDM, Johnston RL, Kariuki BM. The genetic algorithm: foundations and applications in structure solution from powder diffraction data. Acta Cryst 1998; A54:632–645.

Harris KDM, Tremayne M. Crystal structure determination from powder diffraction data. Chem Mater 1996; 8:2554–2570.

Harris RK. Applications of solid-state NMR to pharmaceutical polymorphism and related matters. J Pharm Pharmacol 2007; 59:225–239.

Harris KDM, Tremayne M, Lightfoot P, et al. Crystal structure determination from powder diffraction data by Monte Carlo methods. J Am Chem Soc 1994; 116:3543–3547.

Haynes DA, Jones W, Motherwell WDS. Occurrence of pharmaceutical acceptable anions in the Cambridge Structural Database. J Pharm Sci 2005; 94:2111–2120.

Hedoux A, Guinet Y, Derollez P, et al. A contribution to the understanding of the polyamorphism situation in triphenyl phosphate. Phys Chem Chem Phys 2004; 6:3192–3199.

Hendriksen BA. Characterization of calcium fenoprofen. 1. Powder dissolution rate and degree of crystallinity. Int J Pharm 1990; 60:243–252.

Hickey MB, Peterson ML, Manas ES, et al. Hydrates and solid-state reactivity: a survey of β-lactam antibiotics. J Pharm Sci 2007b; 96:1090–1099.

Hickey MB, Peterson ML, Scoppettuolo LA, et al. Performance comparison of a co-crystal of carbamazepine with marketed product. Eur J Pharm Biopharm 2007a; 67:112–119.

Hilfiker R, Berghausen J, Blatter F, et al. Polymorphism-integrated approach from high-throughput to crystallization optimization. J Therm Anal Calorim 2003; 73:429–440.

Hirsch CA, Messenger RJ, Brannon JL. Fenoprofen: drug form selection and preformulation stability studies. J Pharm Sci 1978; 67:231–236.

Hitchingham L, Thomas VH. Development of a semi-automated chemical stability system to analyze solution based formulations in support of discovery candidate selection. J Pharm Biomed Anal 2007; 43:522–526.

Hoelgaard A, Møller N. Hydrate formation of metronidazole benzoate in aqueous suspensions. Int J Pharm 1983; 15:213–221.

Hooton JC, German CS, Davies MC, et al. A comparison of morphology and surface energy characteristics of sulfathiazole polymorphs based upon single particle studies. Eur J Pharm Sci 2006; 28: 315–324.

Hörter D, Dressman JB. Influence of physicochemical properties on dissolution of drugs in the gastrointestinal tract. Adv Drug Deliv Rev 1997; 25:3–14.

Hosokawa T, Datta S, Sheth AR, et al. Isostructurality among Five Solvates of phenylbutazone. Cryst Growth Des 2004; 4:1195–1201.

Hosokawa K, Goto J, Hirayama N. Prediction of solvents suitable for crystallization of small organic molecules. Chem Pharm Bull (Tokyo) 2005; 53:1296–1299.

Hu Y, Wikström H, Byrn SR, et al. Estimation of the transition temperature for an enantiotropic polymorphic system from the transformation kinetics monitored using Raman spectroscopy. J Pharm Biomed Anal 2007; 45:546–551.

Hulme AT, Price SL. Toward the prediction of organic hydrate crystal structures. J Chem Theory Comput 2007; 3:1597–1608.

Hulme AT, Price SL, Tocher DA. A new polymorph of 5-fluorouracil found by following computational crystal structure predictions. J Am Chem Soc 2005; 127:1116–1117.

Infantes L, Fábián L, Motherwell SDS. Organic crystal hydrates: what are the important factors for formation? CrystEngComm 2007; 9:65–71.

Ivanisevic I, Bugey DE, Bates S. On pattern matching of X-ray powder diffraction data. J Phys Chem 2005; B109:7781–7787.

Iyengar SS, Phadnis NV, Suryanarayanan R. Quantitative analyses of complex pharmaceutical mixtures by the Rietveld method. Powder Diffr 2001; 16:20–24.

James KC. Solubility and Related Phenomena. New York: Mercel Dekker Inc., 1986.

Jarring K, Larsson T, Ymén I. Thermodynamic stability and crystal structures for polymorphs and solvates of formoterol fumarate. J Pharm Sci 2006; 95:1144–1161.

Jashnani RK, Byron PR, Dalby RN. Validation of an improved Wood's rotating disk dissolution apparatus. J Pharm Sci 1993; 82:670–671.

Jayasankar A, Good DJ, Rodriguez-Hornedo N. Mechanisms by which moisture generates cocrystals. Mol Pharm 2007; 4:360–372.

Jenkins R, Fawcett T.G, Smith DK, Visser JW, Morris MC, Frevel LK JCPDS - International Center for Diffraction Data Sample Preparation Methods in X-ray Powder Diffraction. Powder Diff 1986; 1:51–63.

Jenkins R, Snyder RL. Introduction to X-Ray Powder Diffractometry. New York: Wiley, 1996.

Johnston A, Florence AJ, Shankland K, et al. Powder study of (N-[2-(4-hydroxy-2-oxo-2,3-dihydro-1,3-benzothiazol-7-yl)ethyl]-3-[2-(2-napthalen-1-ylethoxy)ethylsulfonyl]propylaminium benzoate. Acta Cryst 2004; E60:1751–1753.

Johnston A, Johnston BF, Kennedy AR, et al. Targeted crystallization of novel carbamazepine solvates based on a retrospective random forest classification. CrystEngComm 2008; 10:23–25.

Joshi HN. Drug development and imperfect design. Int J Pharm 2007; 343:1–3.

Jozwiakowski MJ, Williams SO, Hathaway RD. Relative physical stability of the solid forms of amiloride hydrochloride. Int J Pharm 1993; 91:195–207.

Kachrimanis K, Braun DE, Griesser UJ. Qunatitaive analysis of paracetamol polymorphs in polymorphs in powder mixtures by FT-Raman spectroscopy and PLS regression. J Pharm Biomed Anal 2007; 43:407–412.

Kariuki B, Calcagno P, Harris KDM, et al. Evolving opportunities in structure solution from powder diffraction data-crystal structure determination of a molecular system with twelve variable torsion angles. Angew Chem Int Ed 1999; 38:831–835.

Kariuki BM, Psallidas K, Harris KDM, et al. Structure determination of a steroid directly from powder diffraction data. Chem Commun 1999; 1677–1678.

Karjalainen M, Airaksinen S, Rantanen J, et al. Characterization of polymorphic solid-state changes using variable temperature X-ray powder diffraction. J Pharm Biomed Anal 2005; 39:27–32.

Karki S, Friščić T, Jones W, et al. Screening for pharmaceutical cocrystals hydrates via neat and liquid-assisted grinding. Mol Pharm 2007; 4:347–354.

Kaur H, Mariappan TT, Singh S. Behaviour of moisture by drugs and excipients under accelerated conditions of temperature and humidity in the absence and the presence of light. Part III. Various drug substances and excipients. Pharm Tech 2003; 52–56.

Kawakami K, Ida Y, Yamaguchi T. Effect of salt type on hygroscopicity of a new cephalosporin S-3578. Pharm Res 2005; 22:1365–1373.

Kemperman GJ, De Gelder R, Dommerholt et al. Induced fit phenomena in clathrate structures of cephalosporins. J Chem Soc Perkin 2000; 2:1425–1429.

Kennedy AR, Okoth MO, Sheen DB, et al. Cephalexin: a channel hydrate. Acta Cryst 2003; C59:650–652.

Kerns EH. High throughput physicochemical profiling for drug discovery. J Pharm Sci 2001; 90:1838–1858.

Khankari RK, Ojala WH, Gleason WB, et al. Crystal structure of nedocromil sodium heptahemihydrate and comparison with that of nedocromil sodium trihydrate. J Chem Cryst 1995; 25:863–870.

Khankari RK, Chan L, Grant DJW. Physical characterization of nedocromil sodium hydrates. J Pharm Sci 1998; 87:1052–1061.

Kilday MV. The enthalpy of solution of SRM 1655 potassium chloride in water. J Res Natl Bur Stand 1980; 85:467–481.

Kim S, Lotz B, Lindrud M, et al. Control of the particle properties of a drug product by crystallization engineering and the effect on drug product formulation. Org Proc Res Dev 2005; 9:894–901.

Kimura K, Hirayama F, Uekama K. Characterization of tolbutamide polymorphs (Burger's forms II and IV) and polymorphic transition behavior. J Pharm Sci 1999; 88:385–391.

Kipouros K, Kachrimanis K, Nikolakakis I, et al. Simultaneous quantification of carbamazepine crystal forms in ternary mixtures (I, III, and IV) by diffuse reflectance FTIR spectroscopy (DRIFTS) and multivariate calibration. J Pharm Sci 2006; 95:2419–2431.

Kishi A, Otsuka M, Matsuda Y. The effect of humidity on dehydration behaviour of nitrofurantoin monohydrate studied by humidity controlled simultaneous instrument for X-ray diffractometry and differential scanning calorimetry (XRD-DSC). Colloids Surf B Biointerfaces 2002; 25:281–291.

Kitaigorodskii AI. Organic Chemical Crystallography. New York: Consultants Bureau, 1961.

Kojima T, Onoue S, Murase N, et al. Crystalline form information from multiwell plate salt screening by use of Raman microscopy. Pharm Res 2006; 23:806–812.

Kokitkar PB, Plocharczyk E, Chen CC. Modeling drug solubility to identify optimal solvent systems for crystallization. Org Proc Res Dev 2008; 12:249–256.

Kola I, Landis J. Can the pharmaceutical industry reduce attrition rates? Nat Rev Drug Discov 2004; 3: 711–715.

Kong X, Zhou T, Liu Z, et al. pH indicator titration: a novel fast pKa determination method. J Pharm Sci 2007; 96:2777–2783.

Kontny MJ, Grandolfi GP, Zografi G. Water vapor sorption of water-soluble substances: studies of crystalline solids below their critical relative humidities. Pharm Res 1987; 4:104–112.

Krafunkel HR, Wu ZJ, Burkhard A, et al. Crystal packing calculations and rietveld refinement in elucidating the crystal structures of two modifications of 4-amidoindanone guanylhydrazone. Acta Cryst 1996; B52:555–561.

Kramer JA, Sagartz JE, Morris DL. The application of discovery toxicology and pathology towards the design of safer pharmaceutical lead candidates. Nat Rev Drug Discov 2007; 6:636–649.

Kuhnert-Brandstatter M, Gasser P. Polymorphic modifications and solvates of fluocortolone pivalate. Arch Pharm Ber Dtsch Pharm Ges 1971; 304:926–932.

Lara-Oochoa F, Espinosa-Pérez G. Cocrystals and patents. Cryst Growth Des 2007; 7:1213–1215.

Larsen MJ, Hemming DJB, Bergstrom RG, et al. Water-catalyzed crystallization of amorphous acadesine. Int J Pharm 1997; 154:103–107.

Larsen SW, Østergaard J, Poulsen SV, et al. Difunisal salts of bupivacaine, lidocaine and morphine. Use of the common ion effect for prolonging the release of bupivacaine from mixed salt suspensions in an in vitro model. Eur J Pharm Sci 2007; 31:172–179.

Le Bail A, Duroy H, Fourquet JL. Ab-initio structure determination of LiSbWO$_6$ by x-ray Powder diffraction. Mater Res Bull 1998; 23:447–452.

Lechuga-Ballesteros D, Rodriguez-Hornedo N. Effects of molecular structure and growth kinetics on the morphology of L-alanine crystals. Int J Pharm 1995; 115:151–160.

Ledru I, Imrie CT, Pulham CR, et al. High pressure differential scanning calorimetry investigations on the pressure dependence of the melting of paracetamol polymorphs I and II. J Pharm Sci 2007; 96: 2784–2794.

Ledwidge MT, Corrigan OI. Effects of surface active characteristics and solid-state forms on the pH—solubility profiles of drug-salt systems. Int J Pharm 1998; 174:187–200.

Lee T, Hung ST, Kuo CS. Polymorph farming of acetaminophen and sulfathiazole on a chip. Pharm Res 2006; 23:2542–2555.

Leeson PD, Davis AM. Time-related differences in the physical property profiles of oral drugs. J Med Chem 2004; 47:6338–6348.

Leeson PD, Davis AM, Steele J. Drug-like properties: guiding principles for design—or chemical prejudice? Drug Discov Today 2004; 189–195.

Leeson P, Springthorpe B. The influence of drug-like concepts on decision-making in medicinal chemistry. Nat Rev Drug Discov 2007; 6:881–890.

Leo A, Hansch C, Elkins D. Partition coefficients and their uses. Chem Rev 1971; 71:525–616.

Lewis GR, Steele G, McBride L, et al. Hydrophobic vs. hydrophilic: ionic competition in remacemide salt structures. Cryst Growth Des 2005; 5:427–438.

Li AP. A comprehensive approach for drug safety assessment. Chem Biol Interact 2004; 150:27–33.

Li Y, Chow PS, Tan RBH, et al. Effect of water activity on the transformation between hydrate and anhydrate of carbamzepine. Org Proc Res Dev 2008; 12:264–270.

Li S, Doyle P, Metz S, et al. Effect of chloride ion on dissolution of different salt forms of haloperidol, a model basic drug. J Pharm Sci 2005a; 94:2224–2231.

Li S, Wong S, Sethia S, et al. Investigation of solubility and dissolution of a free base and two different salt forms as a function of pH. Pharm Res 2005b; 22:628–635.

Lin CH, Deng YJ, Liao WS, et al. Electrophoretic behavior and pKa determination of quinolones with a piperazinyl substituent by capillary zone electrophoresis. J Chromatogr A 2004; 1051:283–290.

Linnow K, Steiger M. Determination of equilibrium humidities using temperature and humidity controlled x-ray diffraction (RH-XRD). Anal Chim Acta 2007; 583:197–201.

Linol J, Coquerel G. Influence of high energy milling on the kinetics of the polymorphic transition from the monoclinic form to the orthorhombic form of (±) 5-methyl-5-(4′-methyl-phenyl)hydantoin. J Ther Anal Calorim 2007; 90:367–370.

Lipinski CA, Lombardo F, Dominy BW, et al. Experimental and computational approaches to estimate solubility and permeability in drug discovery and development settings. Adv Drug Deliv Rev 1997; 23:2–25.

Liu Z, Zhong L, Ying P, et al. Crystallization of metastable γ-glycine from gas phase via the sublimation of α or γ form in vacuum. Biophys Chem 2008; 132:18–22.

Llinàs A, Box KJ, Burley JC, et al. A new method for the reproducible generation of polymorphs: two forms of sulindac with very different solubilities. J Appl Crystallogr 2007; 40:379–381.

Llinàs A, Burley JC, Prior TJ, et al. Concomitant hydrate polymorphism in the precipitation of sparfloxacin from aqueous solution. Cryst Growth Des 2008; 8:114–118.

Machatha SG, Yalkowsky SH. Comparison of the octanol/water partition coefficients calculated by ClogP®, ACDlogP and KowWin® to experimentally determined values. Int J Pharm 2005; 294:185–192.

MacNamara DP, Childs DP, Giordanao J, et al. Use of a glutaric acid cocrystal to improve oral bioavailability of a low solubility API. Pharm Res 2006; 23:1888–1897.

Maherns SH, Kale UJ, Qu X. Statistical analysis of differences in the Raman spectra of polymorphs. J Pharm Sci 2005; 94:1354–1366.

Mallet F, Petit S, Petit MN, et al. Solvent exchange between dimetthylsulfoxide and water in the dexamethasone acetate. J Phys IV 2001; 11:253–259.

Manduva R, Kett VL, Banks SR, et al. Alorimetric and spatial characterization of polymorphic transitions in caffeine using quasi-isothermal MTDSC and localized thermochemical analysis. J Pharm Sci 2008; 97:1285–1300.

Mansky P, Dai WG, Li S, et al. Screening method to identify preclinical liquid and semi-solid formulations for low solubility compounds: miniaturization and automation of solvent casting and dissolution testing. J Pharm Sci 2007; 96:1548–1563.

Maruyama S, Ooshima H. Crystallization behavior of taltirelin polymorphs in a mixture of water and methanol. J Cryst Growth 2000; 212:239–245.

Mayers CL, Jenke DR. Stabilization of oxygen-sensitive formulations via a secondary oxygen scavenger. Pharm Res 1993; 10:445–448.

McCrone WC. Fusion Methods in Chemical Microscopy. New York: Interscience Publishers Inc., 1965.

McCusker LB. Zeolite crystallography. Structure determination in the absence of conventional single-crystal data. Acta Cryst 1991; A47:297–313.

McGregor C, Saunders MH, Buckton G, et al. The use of high-speed differential scanning calorimetry (Hyper-DSC™) to study the thermal properties of carbamazepine polymorphs. Thermochim Acta 2004; 417:231–237.

Meloun M, Bordovská S. Benchmarking and validating algorithms that estimate pKa values of drugs based on their molecular structures. Anal Bioanal Chem 2007; 389:1267–1281.

Miller JM, Collman BM, Greene LR, et al. Identifying the stable polymorph early in the drug discovery—development process. Pharm Dev Technol 2005; 10:291–297.

Mimura H, Gato K, Kitamura S, et al. Effect of water content on the solid-state stability in two isomorphic clathrates of cephalosporin: cefazolin sodium pentahydrate (alpha form) and FK401 hydrate. Chem Pharm Bull (Tokyo) 2002a; 50:766–770.

Mimura H, Kitamura S, Kitagawa T, et al. Characterization of the non-stoichiometric and isomorphic hydration and solvation in FK401 clathrate. Colloids Surf B 2002b; 26:397–406.

Mirmehrabi M, Rohani S. An approach to solvent screening for crystallization of polymorphic pharmaceuticals and fine chemicals. J Pharm Sci 2005; 94:1560–1576.

Misture ST, Chatfield L, Snyder RL. Accurate powder patterns using zero background holders. Powder Diffr 1994; 9:172–179.

Miyazaki S, Oshiba M, Nadai T. Precaution on the use of HCl salts in pharmaceutical formulation. J Pharm Sci 1981; 70:594–596.

Monkhouse DC. Stability aspects of preformulation and formulation of solid pharmaceuticals. Drug Dev Ind Pharm 1984; 10:1373–1412.

Monkhouse DC, Van Campen L. Solid state reactions—theoretical and experimental aspects. Drug Dev Ind Pharm 1984; 10:1175–1276.

Morisette SL, Soukasene S, Levinson D, et al. Elucidation of crystal form diversity of the HIV protease inhibitor ritonavir by high throughput crystallization. PNAS 2003; 100:2180–2184.

Morris K. Structural aspects of hydrates and solvates In: Brittain HG, ed.Polymorphism in Pharmaceutical Solids. New York: Marcel Dekker, 1999:125–226.

Morris KR, Fakes MG, Thakur AB, et al. An integrated approach to the selection of optimal salt form for a new drug candidate. Int J Pharm 1994; 105:209–217.

Moura Ramos JR, Correia NT, Taveira-Marques R, et al. The activation energy at Tg and the fragility index of indomethacin, predicted from the influence of the heating rate on the temperature position and on the intensity of the thermally stimulated depolarization current peak. Pharm Res 2002; 19:1879–1884.

Mukuta T, Lee AY, Kawakami T, et al. Influence of impurities on the solution-mediated phase transformation of an active pharmaceutical ingredient. Cryst Growth Des 2005; 5:1429–1436.

Muster TH, Prestidge CA. Face specific surface properties of pharmaceutical crystals. J Pharm Sci 2002; 91:1432–1444.

Nakanishi T, Suzuki M, Mashiba A, et al. Synthesis of NK109, an anticancer benzo[c]phenanthridine alkaloid. J Org Chem 1998; 63:4235–4239.

Nangia A. Conformational polymorphism in organic crystals. Acc Chem Res 2008; 41:595–604.

Német Z, Hegedüs B, Száantay CJr., et al. Pressurization effects on the polymorphic forms of famotidine. Therochim Acta 2005; 430:35–41.

Neumann MA. X-cell: a novel indexing algorithm for routine tasks and difficult cases. J Appl Crystallogr 2003; 36:356–365.

Neumann MA. A major advance in crystal structure prediction. Agnew Chem Int Ed 2008; 47:2427–2430.

Newman AW, Reutzel-Edens SM, Zografi G. Characterization of the "hygroscopic" properties of active pharmaceutical ingredients. J Pharm Sci 2007; 97: 1047–1059.

Newsam JM, Deem MW, Freeman CM. Direct space methods of structure solution from powder diffraction data. Accuracy in Powder Diffraction II. NIST Spec Publ 1992; 846:80–91.

Nichols G. Optical properties of polymorphic forms I and II of paracetamol. Microscope 1998; 46: 117–122.

Nichols G, Frampton CS. Physicochemical characterization of the orthorhombic polymorph of paracetamol crystallized from solution. J Pharm Sci 1998; 87:684–693.

Nicolai B, Espeau P, Céolin R, et al. Polymorph formation from solvate desolvation. Spironolactone forms I and II from the spironolactone-ethanol solvate. J Therm Anal Calorim 2007; 90:337–339.

Niedzialek N, Urbanczyk-Lipowska Z. New crystalline form of 7-amino-4-methylcoumarin (Coumarin 120)—a polymorph with 1:1 valance tautomers. CrystEngComm 2007; 9:735–739.

Nunes C, Mahendrasingam A, Suryanarayanan R. Investigation of the multi-step dehydration reaction of theophylline monohydrate using 2-dimesional powder x-ray diffractometry. Pharm Res 2006; 23:2393–2404.

Nururkar AN, Purkaystha AR, Sheen PC. Effect of various factors on the corrosion and rusting of tooling material used in tablet manufacturing. Drug Dev Ind Pharm 1985; 11:1487–1495.

Nyqvist H. Saturated salt solutions for maintaining specified relative humidities. Int J Pharm Tech Prod Mfr 1983; 4:47–48.

O'Connor KM, Corrigan OI. Preparation and characterisation of a range of diclofenac salts Int J Pharm 2001; 226:163–179.

O'Sullivan D, Steele G, Austin TK. Investigations into the amorphous and crystalline forms of a development compound. In: Levine H,ed. Amorphous Food and Pharmaceutical Systems. Cambridge: Royal Society of Chemistry, Special Publication No. 281, 2002:220–230.

Ottaviani G, Martel S, Escarala C, et al. The PAMPA technique as a HTS tool for partition coefficients determination in different solvent/water systems. Eur J Pharm Sci 2008; 35:68–75.

Palmer DS, Llinàs A, Morao I, et al. Predicting intrinsic aqueous solubility by a thermodynamic cycle. Mol Pharm 2008; 5:266–279.

Pan C, Liu F, Sutton P, et al. The use of thermal desorption GC/MS to study weight loss in thermogravimetric analysis of di-acid salts. Thermochim Acta 2005; 435:11–17.

Pardillo-Fontdevila E, Acosta-Esquijarosa J, Nuevas-Paz L, et al. Solubility of cefotaxime sodium salt in seven solvents used in the pharmaceutical industry. J Chem Eng Data 1998; 43:49–50.

Park K, Evans JMB, Myerson AS. Determination of solubility of polymorphs using differential scanning calorimetry. Cryst Growth Des 2003; 3:991–995.

Park HJ, Kim MS, Lee S, et al. Recystallization of fluconazole using the supercritical antisolvent (SAS) process. Int J Pharm 2007; 328:152–160.

Pawley GS. Unit—cell refinement from powder diffraction scans. J Appl Crystallogr 1981; 14:357–361.

Payne RS, Roberts RJ, Rowe RC, et al. Examples of successful crystal structure prediction: polymorphs of primidone and progesterone. Int J Pharm 1999; 177:231–245.

Pereira B, Fonte-Boa FD, Resende JALC, et al. Pseudopolymorphs and intrinsic dissolution of nevirapine. Cryst Growth Des 2007; 7:2016–2023.

Persson AM, Baumann K, Sundelöf, LO, et al. Design and characterization of a new miniaturized rotating disk equipment for in vitro dissolution rate studies. J Pharm Sci 2008; 97:3344–3355.

Petit S, Mallet F, Petit MN, et al. Role of structural and macrocrystalline factors in the desolvation behavior of cortisone acetate solvates. J Therm Anal Calorim 2007; 90:39–47.

Petrillo EW. Lean thinking for drug discovery—better productivity for pharma. Drug Disc World 2007: 9–14.

Pfaankuch F, Rettig H, Stahl PH. Biological effects of the drug salt form. In: Stahl PH, Wermuth CG, eds. Handbook of Pharmaceutical Salts. Zurich: Wiley-VCH, 2002.

Phipps MA, Mackin LA. Application of isothermal microcalorimetry in solid state drug development. Pharm Sci Techolo Today 2000; 3:9–17.

Pikal MJ, Lang JE, Shah S. Desolvation kinetics of cefamandole sodium methanolate: the effect of water vapor. Int J Pharm 1983; 17:237–262.

Pikal MJ, Lukes AL, Lang JE, et al. Quantitative crystallinity determinations for β-lactam antibiotics by solution calorimetry: correlations with stability. J Pharm Sci 1978; 67:767–773.

Pikal MJ, Rigsbee DR. The stability of insulin in crystalline and amorphous solids: observation of greater stability for the amorphous form. Pharm Res 1997; 14:1379–1387.

PJ article. Viracept recall resulted from cleaning errors. Pharm J 2007; 278:728.

Pudipeddi M, Serajuddin ATM. Trends in solubility of polymorphs. J Pharm Sci 2005; 94:929–939.

Puel F, Verurand E, Taulelle P, et al. Crystallization mechanisms of acicular crystals. J Cryst Growth 2008; 310:110–115.

Qing-Zhu J, Pei-Sheng M, Huan Z, et al. The effect of temperature on the solubility of benzoic acid derivatives in water. Fluid Phase Equilib 2006; 250:165–172.

Qu H, Louhi-Kultan M, Kallas J. Additive effects on the solvent-mediated anhydrate/hydrate phase transformation in a mixed solvent. Cryst Growth Des 2007; 7:724–729.

Quarterman CP, Banham NM, Irwan AK. Improving the odds—high throughput techniques in new drug selection. Eur Pharm Rev 1998; 3:27–31.

Rabel SR, Jona JA, Maurin MB. Applications of modulated differential scanning calorimetry in preformulation studies. J Pharm Biomed Anal 1999; 21:339–345.

Rasenack N, Müller BW. Crystal habit and tabletting behavior. Int J Pharm 2002; 244:45–57.

Rasmussen HT, Swinney KA, Gaiki S. HPLC method development in early phase pharmaceutical development. In: Ahuja S, Rasmussen H,eds. HPLC Method Development for Pharmaceuticals. Vol 8. (Separation Science and Technology). San Diego, CA: Elsevier, 2007:353–371.

Reddy VR, Rajmohan MA, Shilpa RL, et al. A novel quantification method of pantaprazole sodium mononohydrate in sesquihydrate by thermogravimetric analyzer. J Pharm Biomed Anal 2007; 43:1836–1841.

Reutzel-Edens SM, Bush JK, Magee PA, et al. Anhydrates and hydrates of olanzapine: crystallization, solid-state characterization, and structural relationships. Cryst Growth Des 2003; 3:897–907.

Reutzel-Edens SM, Newman AW. Physical characterization of hygroscopicity in pharmaceutical solids. In: Hilfiker R, ed. Polymorphism in the Pharmaceutical System. Weinham: Wiley-VCH Verlag GmbH & Co. KGaA, 2006.

Riga AT, Golinar M, Alexander KS. Fast scan differential scanning calorimetry distinguishes melting-degradation/sublimation and thermal stability of drugs. J ASTM Int 2007; 4:1–8.

Rived F, Canals I, Bosch E, et al. Acidity in methanol-water. Anal Chim Acta 2001; 439:315–333.

Rived F, Rosés M, Bosch E. Dissociation constants of neutral and charged acids in methyl alcohol. Anal Chim Acta 1998; 374:309–324.

Roberts A. The design of an automatic system for the gravimetric measurement of water sorption. J Therm Anal Calorim 1999; 55:389–396.

Rodriguez C, Bugey DE. Characterization of pharmaceutical solvates by combined thermogravimetric and infrared analysis. J Pharm Sci 1997; 86:263–266.

Rosenberg LS, Wagenknecht DM. pKa determination of sparingly soluble compounds by difference potentiometry. Drug Dev Ind Pharm 1986; 12:1449–1467.

Roy S, Aitipamula S, Nangia A. Thermochemical analysis of venlafaxine hydrochloride polymorphs 1–5. Cryst Growth Des 2005; 5:2268–2276.

Roy SD, Flynn GL. Solubility behavior of narcotic analgesics in aqueous media: solubilities and dissociation constants of morphine, fentanyl and sufentanil. Pharm Res 1989; 6:147–151.

Roy S, Riga AT, Alexander KS. Experimental design aids the development of a differential scanning calorimetry standard test procedure for pharmaceuticals. Thermochim Acta 2002: 392–393, 399–404.

Royall PG, Craig DQM, Doherty C. Characterization of the glass transition of an amorphous drug using modulated DSC. Pharm Res 1998; 15:1117–1130.

Royall PG, Gaisford S. Application of solution calorimetry in pharmaceutical and biopharmaceutical research. Curr Pharm Biotechnol 2005; 6:215–222.

Rubino JT. Solubilities and solid-state properties of the sodium salts of drugs. J Pharm Sci 1989; 78: 485–489.

Rubino JT, Thomas E. Influence of solvent composition on the solubilities and solid-state properties of the sodium salts of some drugs. Int J Pharm 1990; 65:141–145.

Sacchetti M. Determining the relative physical stability of anhydrous and hydrous crystal forms of GW2016. Int J Pharm 2004; 273:195–202.

Saesmaa T, Halmekoski J. Slightly water-soluble salts of *β*-lactam antibiotics. Acta Pharm Fenn 1987; 96:65–78.

Saesmaa T, Makela T, Tannienen VP. Physical studies on the benzathine and embonate salts of some β-lactam antibiotics. Part 1. X-Ray Powder Diffractometric Study. Acta Pharm Fenn 1990; 99:157–162.

Salameh AK, Taylor LS. Physical stability of crystal hydrates and their anhydrates in the presence of excipients. J Pharm Sci 2006; 95:446–461.

Samra RM, Buckton G. The crystallization of a model hydrophobic drug (terfenadine) following exposure to humidity and organic vapors. Int J Pharm 2004; 284:53–60.

Sanders GHW, Roberts CJ, Danesh A, et al. Discrimination of polymorphic forms of a drug product by localized thermal analysis. J Microsc 2000; 198:77–81.

Sarsfield BA, Davidovich M, Desikan S, et al. Powder x-ray diffraction detection of crystalline phases in amorphous pharmaceuticals. Adv X-Ray Diffr 2006; 49:322–327.

Schlemmer H, Katzer J. ATR technique for UV/visible analytical measurements. Fresenius Z Anal Chem 1987; 329:435–439.

Schmid EF, Smith DA. R&D technology investments: misguided and expensive or a better way to discover medicines. Drug Discov Today 2006; 11:775–784.

Schmidt AC, Schwarz I, Mereiter K. Polymorphism and pseudopolymorphism of salicaine and salicaine hydrochloride. Crystal polymorphism of local anesthetic drugs, Part V. J Pharm Sci 2006; 95: 1097–1113.

Seadeek C, Ando H, Bhattchar SN, et al. Automated approaches to couple solubility with final pH and crystallinity for pharmaceutical discovery compounds. J Pharm Biomed Anal 2007; 43:1660–1666.

Seddon KR. *Pseudo*polymorph: a polemic. Cryst Growth Des 2004; 6:1087.

Senthil Kumar VS, Kuduva SS, Desiraju GS. Pseudopolymorphs of 3,5-dinitrosalicylic acid. J Chem Soc Perkin Trans 2 1999; 6:1069–1073.

Serajuddin AT. Salt formation to improve drug solubility. Adv Drug Deliv Rev 2007; 59:603–616.

Serajuddin AT, Mufson D. PH—solubility profiles of organic bases and their hydrochloride salts. Pharm Res 1985; 2:65–68.

Shah JC, Maniar M. pH-dependent solubility and dissolution of bupivacaine and its relevance to the formulation of a controlled release system. J Control Release 1993; 23:261–270.

Shalaev E, Zografi G. The concept of "structure" in amorphous solids from the perspective of the pharmaceutical sciences. In: Levine H, ed. Amorphous Food and Pharmaceutical Systems. Cambridge, UK: The Royal Society of Chemistry, 2002:11–30.

Sheikhzadeh M, Rohani S, Taffish M. Solubility analysis of buspirone hydrochloride polymorphs: measurements and prediction. Int J Pharm 338: 55–63.

Sheng J, Venkatesh GM, Duddu SP, et al. Dehydration behavior of eprosartan mesylate dihydrate. J Pharm Sci 1999; 88:1021–1029.

Sheth AG, Brennessel WW, Young VG Jr., et al. Solid-state properties of warfarin sodium 2-propanol solvate. J Pharm Sci 2004; 93:2669–2680.

Sheth AR, Young VG Jr., Grant DJW. Warfarin sodium 2—propanol solvate. Acta Cryst 2002; E58:197–199.

Shirotani KI, Suzuki E, Morita Y, et al. Studies on methods of particle size reduction of medicinal compounds. Part XXVI. Solvate formation of griseofulvin with alkyl halide and alkyl dihalides. Chem Pharm Bull 1988; 36:4045–4054.

Šimon P, Veverka M, Okuliar J. New screening method for the determination of stability of pharmaceuticals. Int J Pharm 2004; 270:21–26.

Simoncic Z, Zupancic P, Roskar R, et al. Use of microcalorimetry in determination of stability of enalapril maleate and enalapril maleate tablet formulations. Int J Pharm 2007; 342:145–151.

Slowik H. The battle for IP. In Vivo 2003; 1–8.

Snodin DJ. Residues of genotoxic alkyl mesylates in mesylate salt drug substances: real or imaginary problems? Regul Toxicol Pharmacol 2006; 45:79–90.

Souillac PO, Dave P, Rytting JH. The use of solution calorimetry with micellar solvent systems for the detection of polymorphism. Int J Pharm 2002; 231:185–196.

Stahl PH, Wermuth CG. eds. Handbook of Pharmaceutical Salts: Properties, Selection and Use. Chichester: Wiley-VCH, 2002.

Stahly GP. Diversity in single- and multiple-component crystals. The search for and prevalence of polymorphs and cocrystals. Cryst Growth Des 2007; 6:1007–1026.

Stegmann S, Levellier F, Franchi D, et al. When poor solubility becomes an issue: from early stage to proof of concept. Eur J Pharm Sci 2007; 31:249–261.

Steiner T. Frequency of Z' values in organic and organometallic crystal structures. Acta Cryst 2000; B56:673–676.

Stephenson GA. Application of x-ray powder diffraction in the pharmaceutical industry. Rigaku J 2005; 22:2–15.

Stephenson GA, Diseroad BA. Structural relationship and desolvation behavior of cromolyn, cefazolin and fenoprofen sodium hydrates. Int J Pharm 2000; 198:167–177.

Stephenson GA, Groleau EG, Kleemann RL, et al. Formation of isomorphic desolvates: creating a molecular vacuum. J Pharm Sci 1998; 87:536–542.

Stephenson GA, Stowell JG, Toma PH, et al. Solid-state analysis of polymorphic, isomorphic, and solvated forms of dirithromycin. J Am Chem Soc 1994; 116:5766–5773.

Stephenson GA, Stowell JG, Toma PH, et al. Solid-state investigations of erythromycin A dihydrate: structure, NMR spectroscopy, and hygroscopicity. J Pharm Sci 1997; 86:1239–1244.

Stewart PJ, Tucker IG. Prediction of drug stability-Part 2: hydrolysis. Aust J Hosp Pharm 1985; 15:11–16.

Stoica C, Verwer P, Meekes H, et al. Understanding the effect of a solvent on the crystal habit. Cryst Growth Des 2004; 4:765–768.

Stoltz M, Lötter AP, van der Watt JG. Physical characterization of two oxyphenbutazone pseudopolymorphs. J Pharm Sci 1988; 77:1047–1049.

Storey RA, Docherty R, Higginson PD. Integration of high throughput screening methodologies and manual processes for solid form selection. Am Pharm Rev 2003; 6:100, 102, 104–105.

Storey RA, Docherty R, Higginson P, et al. Automation of solid form screening procedures in the pharmaceutical industry—how to avoid the bottlenecks. Cryst Rev 2004; 10:45–56.

Strachan CJ, Taday PF, Newnham DA, et al. Using terahertz pulsed spectroscopy to quantify pharmaceutical polymorphism and crystallinity. J Pharm Sci 2005; 94:837–846.

Stuart M, Box K. Chasing equilibrium: measuring the intrinsic solubility of weak acids. Anal Chem 2005; 77:983–990.

Suleiman MS, Najib NM. Isolation and physicochemical characterization of solid forms of glibenclamide. Int J Pharm 1989; 50:103–109.

Sun Y, Xi H, Chen S, et al. Crystallization near glass transition: transition from diffusion controlled to diffusionless crystal growth studied with seven polymorphs. J Phys Chem B 2008; 112:5594–5601.

Surana R, Suryanaryanan R. Quantitation of crystallinity in substantially amorphous pharmaceuticals and study of crystallization kinetics by x-ray powder diffractometry. Powder Diffr 2000; 15:2–6.

Taday PF. Application of terahertz spectroscopy to pharmaceutical sciences. Philos Trans R Soc Lond A 2004; 362:351–364.

Takács-Novák K, Box KJ, Avdeef A. Potentiometric pKa determination of water-insoluble compounds: validation study in methanol/water mixtures. Int J Pharm 1997; 151:235–248.

Tetko IV, Bruneau P. Application of ALOGPS to predict 1-octanol/water distribution coefficients, logP and logD of AstraZeneca in-house database. J Pharm Sci 2004; 93:3103–3110.

Thomas E, Rubino J. Solubility, melting point and salting-out relationships in a group of secondary amine hydrochloride salts. Int J Pharm 1996; 130:179–185.

Threlfall TL. The analysis of organic polymorphs. Analyst 1995; 120:2435–2460.

Threlfall TL. Crystallization of polymorphs: thermodynamic insight into the role of the solvent. Org Proc Res Dev 2000; 4:384–390.

Threlfall TL. Structural and thermodynamic explanations of Ostwald's rule. Org Proc Res Dev 2003; 7:1017–1027.

Threlfall TL, Chalmers JM. Vibrational spectroscopy of solid-state form—introduction, principles and overview. In: Pivonka DE, Chalmers JM, Griffiths PR, et al., ed. Application of Vibrational Spectroscopy in Pharmaceutical Research and Development. Hoboken, NJ, U.S.A.: Wiley, 2007.

Tian F, Sandler N, Gordon KC, et al. Visualizing the conversion of carbamazepine in aqueous suspension with and without the presence of excipients: a single crystal study using SEM and Raman microscopy. Eur J Pharm Biopharm 2006; 64:326–335.

Ticehurst M, Docherty R. From molecules to pharmaceutical products—the drug substance/drug product interface. Am Pharm Rev 2006; 9:32–36.

Ticehurst MD, Storey RA, Watt C. Application of slurry bridging experiments at controlled water activities to predict solid-state conversion between anhydrous and hydrated forms using theophylline as a model drug. Int J Pharm 2002; 247:1–10.

Tiwary AK. Crystal habit changes and dosage form performance. Drug Dev Ind Pharm 2003; 65–79.

Tiwary AK, Panpalia GM. Influence of crystal habit on trimethoprim suspension formulation. Pharm Res 1999; 16:261–265.

Tong P, Taylor LS, Zografi G. Influence of alkali metal counterions on the glass transition temperature of amorphous indomethacin salts. Pharm Res 2002; 19:649–654.

Tong WQ, Whitesell G. In situ salt screening—a useful technique for discovery support and preformulation studies. Pharm Dev Technol 1998; 3:215–223.

Tønnesen HH. Formulation and stability testing of photolabile drugs. Int J Pharm 2001; 225:1–14.

Torniainen K and Tammilehto S. The effect of pH, buffer type and drug concentration on the photodegradation of ciprofloxacin. Int J Pharm 1996; 132:53–61.

Trask AV, Motherwell WDS, Jones W. Pharmaceutical cocrystallization: engineering a remedy for caffeine hydration. Cryst Growth Des 2005b; 5:1–9.

Trask AV, Motherwell WDS, Jones W. Physical stability enhancement of theophylline via cocrystallization. Int J Pharm 2006; 320:114–123.

Trask AV, Shan N, Motherwell WD, et al. Selective polymorph transformation via solvent—drop grinding. Chem Commun (Camb) 2005a; 880–882.

Tsung HH, Tabora J, Variankaval N, et al. Prediction of pharmaceutical solubility via NRTL-SAC and COSMO-SAC. J Pharm Sci 2008; 97:1813–1820.

Ueno Y, Yonemochi E, Tozuka Y, et al. Characterization of amorphous ursodeoxycholic acid prepared by spray-drying. J Pharm Pharmacol 1998; 50:1213–1219.

Urakami K. Characterization of pharmaceutical polymorphs by isothermal microcalorimetry. Curr Pharm Biotechnol 2005; 6:193–203.

Valkó K. Application of high-performance liquid chromatography based measurements of lipophilicity to model biological distribution. J Chromatogr A 2007; 1037:299–310.

van der Sluis P, Kroon J. Solvents and X-ray crystallography. J Cryst Growth 1989; 97:645–656.

Van Dooren AA. Effects of heating rates and particle sizes on DSC peaks. Anal Proc 1982; 554–555.

Van Tonder EC, Maleka TSP, Liebenberg W, et al. Preparation and physicochemical properties of niclosamide anhydrate and two monohydrates. Int J Pharm 2004; 269:417–432.

Variankaval N, Cote AS, Doherty MF. From form to function: crystallization of active pharmaceutical ingredients. AIChE J 2008; 54:1682–1688.

Variankaval NE, Jacob KI, Dinh SM. Characterization of crystal forms of b- estradiol – thermal analysis, Raman microscopy, X-ray analysis and solid-state NMR. J Cryst Growth 2000; 217:320–331.

Variankaval N, Lee C, Xu J, et al. Water activity-mediated control of crystalline phases of an active pharmaceutical ingredient. Org Proc Res Dev 2007; 11:229–236.

Venkatesh S, Lipper RA. Role of the development scientist in compound lead selection and optimization. J Pharm Sci 2000; 89:145–154.

Verbeek RK, Kanfer I, Walker RB. Generic substitution: the use of medicinal products containing different salts and implications for safety and efficacy. Eur J Pharm Sci 2006; 28:1–6.

Verwer P, Leusen FJJ. Computer simulation to predict possible crystal polymorphs. Rev Comput Chem 1998; 12:327–365.

Vieth M, Siegel MG, Higgs RE, et al. Characteristic physical properties and structural fragments of marketed oral drugs. J Med Chem 2004; 47:224–232.

Vippagunta SR, Brittain HG, Grant DJW. Crystalline solids. Adv Drug Deliv 2001; 48:3–26.

Visalakshi NA, Mariappan TT, Bhutani H, et al. Behaviour of moisture gain and equilibrium moisture contents (EMC) of various drug substances and correlation with compendial information on hygroscopicity and loss on drying. Pharm Dev Technol 2005; 10:489–497.

Vitez IM, Newman AC, Davidovich M, et al. The evolution of hot-stage microscopy to aid solid-state characterizations of pharmaceutical solids. Thermochim Acta 1998; 324:187–196.

Vogt FG, Brum J, Katrincic LM, et al. Physical, crystallographic and spectroscopic characterization of a crystalline pharmaceutical hydrate: understanding the role of water. Cryst Growth Des 2006; 6:2333–2354.

Volgyi G, Ruiz R, Box K, et al. Potentiometric and spectrophotrometric pKa determination of water-insoluble compounds: validation study in a new cosolvent system. Anal Chim Acta 2007; 583:418–428.

Walkling WD, Reynolds BE, Fegely BJ, et al. Xilobam: effect of salt form on pharmaceutical properties. Drug Dev Ind Pharm 1983; 9:809–819.

Wan H, Holmén AG, Wang Y, et al. High-throughput screening of pKa values of pharmaceuticals by pressure assisted capillary electrophoresis and mass spectrometry. Rapid Commun Mass Spectrom 2003; 17:2639–2648.

Wang X, Ponder CS, Kirwan DJ. Low molecular weight poly(ethylene glycol) as an environmentally benign solvent for pharmaceutical crystallization and precipitation. Cryst Growth Des 2005; 5: 85–92.

Wang Z, Wang J, Dang L, et al. Crystal structures and the solvent-mediated transformation of erythromycin acetone solvate to dihydrate during batch crystallization. Ind Eng Chem Res 2007; 46:1851–1858.

Ward MD, Bobafede SJ, Hillier AC. Michl J. ed. Modular Chemistry. Boston: Kluwer Academic Publishers, 1997.

Ward GH, Schultz RK. Process-induced crystallinity changes in albuterol sulfate and its effect on powder physical stability. Pharm Res 1995; 12:773–779.

Ware EC, Lu DR. An automated approach to salt selection for new unique trazodone salts. Pharm Sci 2004; 21:177–184.

Watanabe A, Yamaoka Y, Kuroda K. Study of crystalline drugs by means of polarizing microscope. III. Key refractive indices of some crystalline drugs and their measurement using an improved immersion method. Chem Pharm Bull (Tokyo) 1980; 28:372–378.

Waterman KC, Adami RC. Accelerated ageing: prediction of chemical stability of pharmaceuticals. Int J Pharm 2005; 293:101–125.

Wells JI. Pharmaceutical Preformulation. The Physicochemical Properties of Drug Substances. Chichester, UK: Ellis Horwood Ltd, 1988:219.

Werner PE. Autoindexing in structure determination from powder diffraction data. In: David WIF, Shankland K, McCusker LB, et al., eds. IUCr Monographs on Crystallography 13. Oxford: Oxford University Press, 2002:118–135.

Werner PE, Eriksson L, Westdhal M. TREOR, a semi-exhaustive trial-and-error powder indexing program for all symmetries. J Appl Crystallogr 1985; 18:367–370.

Wildfong PLD, Hancock BC, Moore MD, et al. Towards an understanding of the structurally based potential for mechanically activated disordering of small molecule organic crystals. J Pharm Sci 2006; 95:2645–2656.

Wildfong PLD, Morley NA, Moore MD, et al. Quantitative determination of polymorphic composition in intact compacts by parallel-beam x-ray powder diffractometry II. Data correction for analysis of phase transformations as a function of pressure. J Pharm Biomed Anal 2005; 39:1–7.

Williams-Seton L, Davey RJ, Lieberman HF. Solution chemistry and twinning in saccharin crystals: a combined probe for the structure and functionality of the crystal-fluid interface. J Am Chem Soc 1999; 121:4563–4567.

Willson RJ, Beezer AE. The determination of equilibrium constants, ΔG, ΔH and ΔS for vapor interaction with a pharmaceutical drug using gravimetric vapor sorption. Int J Pharm 2003; 258:77–83.

Wilson D M, Wang X, Walsh E, et al. High throughput log D determination using liquid chromatography-mass spectrometry. Comb Chem High Throughput Screen 2001; 4:511–519.

Winn D, Doherty MF. Modelling crystal shapes of organic materials grown from solution. AIChE J 2000; 46:1348–1367.

Wright JD. Molecular Crystals. Cambridge: Cambridge University Press, 1995.

Wright SF, Phang P, Dollimore D, et al. An overview of calibration materials used in thermal analysis-benzoic acid. Thermochim Acta 2002; 392–393:251–257.

Wu LS, Gerard C, Hussain MA. Thermal analysis and solution calorimetry studies on losartan polymorphs. Pharm Res 1993; 10:1793–1795.

Wu Y, Hwang TL, Algayer K, et al. Identification of oxidative degradates of the TRIS salt of a 5,6,7, 8-tetrahydro-1,8-naphthyridine derivative by LC/MS/MS and NMR spectroscopy-interactions between the active pharmaceutical ingredient and its counterion. J Pharm Biomed Anal 2003; 33:999–1015.

Wunderlich B. A classification of molecules, phases, and transitions as recognized by thermal analysis. Thermochim Acta 1999; 340–341:37–52

Wyttenbach N, Alsenz J, Grassmann O. Miniaturized assay for solubility and residual solid-screening (SORESOS) in early drug development. Pharm Res 2007; 24:888–818.

Xu D, Redman-Furey N. Statistical cluster analysis of pharmaceutical solvents. Int J Pharm 2007; 339: 175–188.

Yalkowsky SH, Banerjee S. Aqueous Solubility. Methods for Estimation for Organic Compounds. New York: Marcel Dekker Inc., 1992.

Yang W, Wu D. The role of isothermal microcalorimetry in solid-state characterization and formulation screening in pharmaceutical development. Am Pharm Rev 2008; 11:119–120, 122–125.

Yff BTS, Royall PG, Brown MB, et al. An investigation of calibration methods for solution calorimetry. Int J Pharm 2004; 269:361–372.

Yoshioka S, Cartensen JL. Nonlinear estimation of kinetic parameters for solid-state hydrolysis of water-soluble drugs. Part 2. Rational presentation mode below the critical moisture content. J Pharm Sci 1990; 79:799–801.

Young PH, Ando HY. Analysis of known crystals to design polymorph prediction strategies. J Pharm Sci 2007; 96:1203–1236.

Young PM, Price R, Tobyn MJ, et al. Effect of humidity on aerolization of micronized drugs. Drug Dev Ind Pharm 2003; 29:959–966.

Yu L. Inferring thermodynamic stability relationship of polymorphs from melting data. J Pharm Sci 1995; 84:966–974.

Yu L. Amorphous pharmaceutical solids: preparation, characterization and stabilization. Adv Drug Deliv Rev 2001; 48:27–42.

Yu L. Color changes caused by conformational polymorphism: optical crystallography, single-crystal spectroscopy, and computational chemistry. J Phys Chem A 2002; 106:544–550.

Yu L. Survival of the fittest polymorph: how fast nucleater can lose to fast grower. CrystEngComm 2007; 9:847–851.

Yu LX, Carlin AS, Amidon GL, et al. Feasibility studies of utilizing disk intrinsic dissolution rate to classify drugs. Int J Pharm 2004; 270:221–227.

Yu L, Stephenson GA, Mitchell CA, et al. Thermochemistry and conformational polymorphism of a hexamorphic crystal system. J Am Chem Soc 2000; 122:585–591.

Yuchun X, Huizhou L, Jiayong Chen. Kinetics of base catalyzed racemization of ibuprofen enantiomers. Int J Pharm 2000; 196:21–26.

Zeitler JA, Kogermann K, Rantanen J, et al. Drug hydrate systems and dehydration processes studied by terahertz pulsed spectroscopy. Int J Pharm 2007; 334:78–84.

Zhang GGZ, Henry RF, Borchardt TB, et al. Efficient co-crystal screening using solution-mediated phase transformation. J Pharm Sci 2007; 96:990–995.

Zhou D, Schmitt EA, Zhang GGZ, et al. Model-free treatment of the dehydration kinetics of nedocromil sodium trihydrate. J Pharm 2003; 92:1367–1376.

Zhou D, Zhang GGZ, Law D, et al. Physical stability of amorphous pharmaceuticals: importance of configurational thermodynamic quantities and molecular mobility. J Pharm Sci 2002; 9: 1863–1872.

Zhu M. Solubility and density of the disodium salt hemiheptahemihydrate of cetriaxone in water + ethanol mixtures. J Chem Eng Data 2001; 46:175–176.

Zhu H, Sacchetti M. Solid-state characterization of a neuromuscular blocking agent-GW280430A. Int J Pharm 2002; 234:19–23.

Zhu H, Yuen C, Grant DJW. Influence of water activity in organic solvent + water mixtures on the nature of the crystallizing drug phase. 1. Theophylline. Int J Pharm 1996; 135:57–65.

Zimmermann I. Determination of pK_a values from solubility data. Int J Pharm 1982; 13:57–65.

Zimmermann I. Determination of overlapping pK_a values from solubility data. Int J Pharm 1986; 31:69–74.

Zupančic V, Orgrajšek N, Kotar-Jordan B, et al. Physical Characterization of Pantoprazole Sodium Hydrates. Int J Pharm 2005; 291:59–68.

4 | Biopharmaceutical Support in Candidate Drug Selection

Anna-Lena Ungell and Bertil Abrahamsson
AstraZeneca, Mölndal, Sweden

INTRODUCTION

Administration via the oral route has been, and still is, the most popular and convenient route for patient therapeutics. However, even though it is the most convenient route, it is not the simplest route, as the barriers of the gastrointestinal (GI) tract are in many cases difficult to circumvent. The main barriers of the GI tract to systemic delivery are the environment in the stomach and intestinal lumen, the presence of different enzymes, the physical barrier of the epithelium, and the liver extraction. These barriers are of functional importance for the organism in controlling intake of water, electrolytes, and food constituents, and still remain a complete barrier to harmful organisms such as bacteria, viruses, and toxic compounds.

Generally, drug absorption from the GI tract requires that the drug is brought into solution in the GI fluids and that it is capable of crossing the intestinal membrane into the systemic circulation. It has therefore been suggested that the drug must be in its molecular form before it can be absorbed. Therefore, the rate of dissolution of the drug in the GI lumen can be a rate-limiting step in the absorption of drugs given orally. Particles of drugs, for example, insoluble crystalline forms or specific delivery systems such as liposomes, are generally found to be absorbed to a very small extent. The cascade of events from the release of the drug from its dosage form, that is, *dissolution* of the drug in the gut lumen, *interactions* and/or degradation within the lumen, and the *uptake* of its molecular form across the intestinal membrane into the systemic circulation, is schematically shown in Figure 1. For rapid and effective design and development of new drug products, methods for drug absorption are required that describe the different steps involved before and during the absorption process. The need for such specific methods is determined by the information on the rate-limiting step in the cascade of events (e.g., solubility, permeability, or metabolic instability limited). The results from these methods act as a guide to a more efficient discovery process in which resources are given to optimizing structures that lead to the selection of a good drug candidate with well-defined pharmacokinetic and physicochemical properties. Multivariate analysis for analyzing large data sets is nowadays used to obtain trends in a given parameter. Screening and optimization of several parameters in parallel, for example, permeability, metabolic stability, solubility, potency, duration, and toxicity, represent also a growing area for rationalizing drug discovery using multivariate statistical models (Eriksson et al., 1999). The importance of this is obvious: there is no point in using resources to increase the potency of an oral drug candidate if the drug is not predicted to be orally bioavailable.

The dissolution rate and/or the aqueous solubility of the drug will also affect the outcome of studies using biological methods, in very early phases of screening. If not dissolved in the test system, low-solubility drugs will not appear on the receiver side/blood side of a membrane or will show incomplete absorption in vivo. Consequently, the drug will be considered a low-permeability drug and be discarded as being of no potential use as a systemically active drug. The situation is even more complex, since there are also mechanistic membrane processes that can give the same result. Such processes include drug efflux systems that transport the drug from inside the epithelial cell to the lumen of the intestine [e.g., efflux proteins (Hunter and Hirst, 1997)] or metabolism during transport and adhesion to plastics in the test system (Table 1). The evaluation of the reason for low transport is therefore crucial for the design of proper screening procedures.

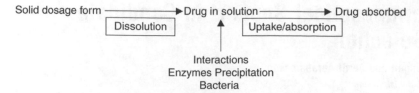

Figure 1 Drawing showing the different steps in the absorption process including the dissolution of the compound from the solid dosage form, interactions with the dissolved material in the gastrointestinal lumen, and the uptake of the compound through the epithelial membrane.

Table 1 Suggested Reasons for Low Permeability Values During Transport Studies with In Vitro Models

Adhesions to plastics
Low solubility
Complexation with ions in the buffer
Metabolism in the lumen or in the intestinal segment
Low activity/viability of the tissue (active transport)
Analytical problems (analytical response limited)
Large unstirred water layer or mucus layer (unstirred models)
True low permeability

In the drug discovery process, the selection of a suitable drug candidate is the milestone for continuing into a costly development and clinical phase. Some *optimal absorption criteria* from a biopharmaceutical point of view are shown below:

- High-permeability coefficient (determined using in vitro assays such as Caco-2 cell monolayers, Ussing chambers, intestinal perfusions, etc.; see below) throughout the GI tract [extended release (ER) formulation]
- Passive diffusion–directed transport or known mechanism for carrier-mediated transport or interaction
- High solubility in aqueous media and over a wide pH range (e.g., pH 1–7)
- No or low degradation/metabolism in intestinal luminal fluids, intestinal homogenates, and/or microsomal preparations from the intestine and liver (i.e., low first-pass metabolism)
- Complete absorption in the GI tract in vivo in several animal species

These criteria are usually difficult to achieve, and the relationship between the in vitro *effect of the drug* (potency/concentration needed), *therapeutic effect and index* (acceptable variation in plasma concentration from safety and efficacy point of view), and the *rate and extent of absorption* must therefore be evaluated carefully for each project and drug. Furthermore, the physicochemical characteristics (e.g., the ability of the drug to be formulated into a relevant delivery system) of the drug as determined in preformulation studies also guide the selection of a potential drug candidate.

The biopharmaceutical information gathered in the candidate drug selection process regarding the characteristics of the drug molecule (e.g., dissolution, solubility, stability in fluids at the site of administration, enzymatic stability, membrane transport, and bioavailability) is also very useful as input to the subsequent formulation development. This information is important, for example,

- to determine suitable formulation types and technologies, to set biopharmaceutical targets for formulation development,
- to define initial biopharmaceutical test methods and studies needed to reach the targets, and
- as background data for interpretation of different studies used in the development of a formulation.

Thus, a well-performed drug substance characterization minimizes the risk of a suboptimal final formulation as a result of neglecting important biopharmaceutical prerequisites for a certain drug substance. Furthermore, such information also allows an efficient development process based on science, while trial-and-error approaches are avoided.

The ideal model for the biopharmaceutical assessment of drug transport, metabolism, and dissolution should have certain characteristics, that is, should represent the main physiological or physicochemical barrier as relevantly as possible to the human in vivo situation. No single method can represent all barriers and at the same time give information about the mechanisms underlying the absorption process. Furthermore, no single method can provide all the information needed, from the synthesis of a series of compounds in the screening phase (discovery) to the development of the specific formulation intended for human use. Many different methods have been developed over the last 20 years for use in different phases of drug discovery and development. This chapter will deal with some of these techniques to gain a basic knowledge of drug absorption. Also, it will give a description of related methods, and the functional use of the information provided by these methods to aid in the selection of a candidate drug and the development of formulations intended for use in humans.

DRUG DISSOLUTION AND SOLUBILITY

Drug dissolution is a prerequisite for oral absorption. Thus, a drug that is not fully dissolved cannot be completely absorbed through the GI epithelium. It is thus extremely important to understand drug dissolution and solubility in aqueous media, both in early drug discovery studies and as a prerequisite for the subsequent formulation development. More specifically, drug dissolution/solubility data give important information that provides answers to the following biopharmaceutical questions during the discovery phase:

- Will the drug absorption be limited by the drug dissolution/solubility?
- Will the drug dissolution/solubility limit the bioavailability to an extent that endangers the clinical usefulness of the drug?
- Which types of vehicles are needed in preclinical studies to provide the desired drug exposure?
- Should the substance form be changed to improve dissolution (e.g., salt, polymorph, particle size)?

After the choice of a candidate drug, solubility and dissolution data are used for guidance in the following:

- Should dissolution rate–enhancing principles be applied in the formulation development (e.g., wetting agents, micronization, solubilizing agents, solid solutions, emulsions, and nanoparticles)?
- In the case of modified release formulations, which formulation principles are suitable and which release mechanisms can be expected?
- Which test conditions should be used for in vitro dissolution testing of solid formulations?

It should be emphasized that *dissolution* is the dynamic process by which a material is dissolved in a solvent and is characterized by a rate (amount dissolved per time unit), while *solubility* is the amount of material dissolved per volume unit of a certain solvent. Solubility is often used as a short form for "saturation solubility," which is the maximum amount of drug that can be dissolved at equilibrium conditions. Finally, the term *intrinsic solubility* is sometimes used as well, which is the solubility of the neutral form of a proteolytic drug.

Theoretically, the dissolution rate is most often described by the Noyes–Whitney equation (equation 1)

$$\frac{dm}{dt} = \left(\frac{D \times A}{h}\right) \times (C_s - C_t) \tag{1}$$

where D is the diffusion coefficient of the drug substance in a stagnant water layer around each drug particle with a thickness h, A is the drug particle surface area, C_s is the saturation solubility, and C_t is the drug concentration in the bulk solution. If C_t in equation (1) is negligible as compared with C_s, the dissolution rate is not affected by C_t. This state is denoted a "sink condition" and is often assumed to be the case in vivo, owing to the continuous removal of a drug from the intestine due to the absorption over the intestinal wall. A, C_t, and h in equation (1) will be time dependent, whereas the other variables are constants at a certain test condition. The surface area (A) of a dissolving particle will be constantly reduced by time (provided that no precipitation occurs); the thickness of the diffusion layer (h) is dependent on the radius of the particle size; and the bulk solution will increase toward its maximum when the total amount has been dissolved. In addition, no solid drug powder is monodisperse, that is, the starting material will consist of a dispersion of different particle sizes with different surface areas (A). Extensions of equation (1) have therefore been derived that take into account some or all of these factors. A full review of such equations and underlying assumptions and a presentation of some other less used theories for dissolution can be found elsewhere (Abdou, 1989). A modification of equation (1) was recently presented, which takes into account all time-dependent factors that can be useful for predictions of the dissolution rate (Hintz and Johnson, 1989).

Basic theoretic considerations and experimental methods regarding solubility are reviewed in more detail in chapter 3.

The present chapter focuses on aspects of drug solubility/dissolution of specific relevance for biopharmaceutical support in candidate drug selection and preformulation. These aspects include solubility in candidate drug screening, physiological aspects of test media, solubility of amphiphilic drugs, and substance characterization prior to solubility/dissolution tests.

Aspects of Solubility in Candidate Drug Screening

Although drug solubility is an important factor in drug absorption in the GI tract, it has not been extensively screened for as a barrier to absorption. Drug solubility should, however, be complementary to models predicting drug permeability through the lipid membrane. Solubility as a high-throughput screening (HTS) parameter has therefore been discussed rather intensively. However, the importance of solubility as a selective tool during early screening of hundreds of compounds, to choose a drug with a potential to be absorbed in vivo in humans has not been fully evaluated. Several drugs that are very useful in the clinical situation have very low water solubility. For example, candesartan cilexetil, an effective and well-tolerated antihypertensive drug, has a water solubility of about 0.1 µg/mL. On the other hand, more soluble drugs will minimize the risk of failure during the subsequent development phase and may avoid delays, increased costs, or discontinuation of the project.

Another aspect of solubility is seen during screening for good pharmacokinetic properties of candidate drugs. The HTS systems or in vitro assays are the critical point for most drugs insoluble in water. This means that if the drug is not soluble in the buffer solution used in the in vitro system, it cannot be properly experimentally evaluated. The most common negative effect of this is that the concentration needed to induce transport across the epithelial membrane in the in vitro model is too low to be detected on the receiver side (Table 1). For this reason, vehicles known to increase the solubility of sparingly soluble compounds are used (see section "Vehicles for Absorption Studies"). However, since these vehicles are based on surfactant systems, toxic effects may be seen on the membrane (Oberle et al., 1995; Ingels et al., 2007), and the permeability values obtained may be overestimated. New methods are now available for screening large numbers of compounds for determining solubility in small volumes [e.g., the nephelometer (BMG Lab Technologies GmbH)]. This method is based on turbidimetric determinations and is therefore not an exact tool. It can, however, contribute substantially as a first estimate of solubility of sparingly soluble compounds and make it possible to understand the results of the screening methods and to design specific experiments using vehicles.

Determinations of Drug Dissolution Rate

The dissolution rate, rather than the saturation solubility, is most often the primary determinant in the absorption process of a sparingly soluble drug. Experimental determinations of the dissolution rate are therefore of great importance. The main area for dissolution rate studies is evaluation of different solid forms of a drug (e.g., salts, solvates, polymorphs, amorphous, stereoisomers) or effects of particle size. The dissolution rate can either be determined for a constant surface area of the drug in a rotating disk apparatus or as a dispersed powder in a beaker with agitation.

The *rotating disk method* is in most cases the technique of choice for determining the drug dissolution rate of drug substances. Compressed disks of the pure drug without any excipients are placed in a holder (Fig. 2A, B). The disk is immersed in a dissolution medium and rotated at a high speed (e.g., 300–1000 rpm). The disk may be centrally or excentrally mounted to the stirring rod. The dissolution process is preferably monitored by online measurements of the dissolved drug. A more detailed description of the application of the rotating disk method in a preformulation program can be found elsewhere (Niklasson et al., 1985).

The dissolution rate is determined by linear regression from the slope of the initial linear part of the dissolution time curve. It is often expressed as the amount of drug dissolved per time and surface area unit (G), for example, mg/cm^2·s, by dividing the rate by the surface area of the disk. This dissolution rate is specific for the rotational speed (ω) of the disk and is linearly related to the square root of the rotational speed of the disk according to hydrodynamic theories that have been experimentally verified (Levich, 1962). Thus, if experiments are performed at several rotational speeds and the dissolution rate at each speed is plotted versus the square root of the rotational speed, a linear relationship should be obtained. It should be noted that this determination of dissolution rate is still dependent on other experimental hydrodynamic conditions, such as positioning of the disk, shape of the vessel, and viscosity. An equation has therefore been derived that allows for determination of an "intrinsic dissolution rate" (k_1) that is independent of the drug diffusion in the boundary layer (Niklasson and Magnusson, 1985)

$$\frac{1}{G} = \frac{1}{k_1} + \frac{k'}{R \times \omega^{0.5}} \tag{2}$$

where k' is a proportionality constant. The rotating disk must be mounted eccentrically at a certain distance (R) from the center of the stirring rod to perform this evaluation. A plot is made between $1/G$ and ($R \times \omega^{0.5}$) at different agitation rates, which should yield a straight line. The reciprocal of

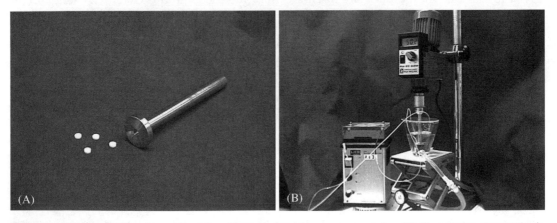

Figure 2 **(A)** The rotating disc method: the disc holder and the compressed disc. **(B)** The rotating disc method: experimental setup for the rotating disc.

the intrinsic dissolution rate $(1/k_1)$ is determined by extrapolating the line to the y-axis. If G is determined at different speeds, and laminar flow along the disk can be assumed, other theoretical evaluations of the data can be made, such as determination of the diffusion coefficient of the drug in the boundary layer around the solid particles and the thickness of the diffusion boundary layer (Levich, 1962).

The main merits of the rotating disk apparatus are the well-defined hydrodynamic conditions and constant surface area. These reduce the risk of artifacts in dissolution rate determinations caused by nonideal test conditions. Furthermore, it is possible to determine an intrinsic dissolution rate and to perform other mechanistic evaluations of the dissolution process. The main limitation of the method is that it is not suitable for drugs that form fragile or porous disks, since it is not possible to maintain a constant surface area.

The drug dissolution rate of powder may be determined by methods such as in a beaker with appropriate agitation, as described in the pharmacopoeial methods. The dissolution rate determined by such approaches will be method dependent, and it will not be possible to derive an intrinsic value of the dissolution rate. The main reason for using this type of experimental approach can be understood when the effect of the drug particle size must be considered. Experimental errors and uncontrollable variations may occur for hydrophobic drugs because of agglomeration in the test medium or because of floating. The use of a wetting agent in the test medium [such as a surfactant in concentrations well below the critical micelle concentration (CMC)] may be needed to avoid such undesired effects.

Biopharmaceutical Interpretation of Dissolution/Solubility Data

It is desirable to predict the influence of drug dissolution on oral absorption on the basis of measurements of dissolution or solubility, both before the selection of a candidate drug, to obtain a drug molecule with acceptable properties, and in the preformulation phase, to determine the need for solubility-enhancing formulation principles. The primary variable for judgments of in vivo absorption is the dissolution rate rather than the solubility. Drug dissolution will limit the bioavailability when the dissolution rate is too slow to provide complete dissolution in the part of the intestine where it can be absorbed. In addition, the drug concentration in the intestinal fluids will be far below the saturation solubility, under the assumption that "sink conditions" in the GI tract will be obtained because of absorption of the drug. However, most often, solubility data are more readily available than dissolution rates for a drug candidate, especially in early phases when the amount of drug available does not allow for accurate dissolution rate determinations. Predictions of in vivo effects on absorption caused by poor dissolution must thus often be made on the basis of solubility data rather than dissolution rate. This can theoretically be justified by the direct proportionality between dissolution rate and solubility under sink conditions according to equation (1). A list of proposed criteria to be used to avoid a reduction in absorption caused by poor dissolution is given in Table 2. These criteria are discussed in further detail in this chapter. A solubility in water of ≥ 10 mg/mL in pH range 1 to 7 has been proposed as an acceptable limit to avoid absorption problems, while another suggestion is that drugs with water solubility less than 0.1 mg/mL often lead to dissolution limitations to absorption (Kaplan, 1972; Hörter and Dressman, 1997). It should be noted that these limits may be conservative, especially in the context of screening and selection for candidate drugs. For example, a drug with much lower solubility, such as felodipine (0.001 mg/mL), provides complete absorption when administered in an appropriate solid dosage form (Wingstrand et al., 1990). This may be explained

Table 2 Proposed Limits of Drug Dissolution on Solubility to Avoid Absorption Problems

Factor	Limit	References
Solubility in pH 1–7	>10 mg/mL at all pH	Kaplan (1972)
Solubility in pH 1–8 and dose	Complete dose dissolved in 250 mL at all pH	Amidon et al. (1995)
Water solubility	>0.1 mg/mL	Hörter and Dressman (1997)
Dissolution rate in pH 1–7	>1 mg/min/cm^2 (0.1–1 mg/nm/cm^2 borderline) at all pH	Kaplan (1972)

Table 3 Biopharmaceutical Classification System

Class	Solubility	Permeability
I	High	High
II	Low	High
III	High	Low
IV	Low	Low

both by successful application of dissolution-enhancing formulation principles and by more favorable drug solubility in vivo owing to the presence of solubilizing agents such as bile acids.

Another model for biopharmaceutical interpretation based on solubility data is found in the biopharmaceutical classification system (BCS) (Amidon et al., 1995). Four different classes of drugs have been identified on the basis of drug solubility and permeability as outlined in Table 3. If the administered dose is completely dissolved in the fluids in the stomach, which is assumed to be 250 mL (50 mL basal level in stomach plus administration of the solid dose with 200 mL of water), the drug is classified as a "high-solubility drug." Such good solubility should be obtained within a range of pH 1 to 8 to cover all possible conditions in a patient and exclude the risk of precipitation in the small intestine due to the generally higher pH there than in the stomach. Drug absorption is expected to be independent of drug dissolution for drugs that fulfill this requirement, since the total amount of the drug will be in solution before entering the major absorptive area in the small intestine and the rate of absorption will be determined by the gastric emptying of fluids. Thus, this model also provides a very conservative approach for judgments of dissolution-limited absorption. However, highly soluble drugs are advantageous in pharmaceutical development since no dissolution-enhancing principles are needed and process parameters that could affect drug particle form and size are generally not critical formulation factors. Furthermore, if certain other criteria are met, in addition to favorable solubility, regulatory advantages can be gained. Bioequivalence studies for bridging between different versions of clinical trial material and/or of a marketed product can be replaced by much more rapid and cheaper in vitro dissolution testing (FDA, 1999; EMEA, 1998).

The assumption of sink condition in vivo is valid in most cases when the permeability of the drug over the intestinal wall is fast, which is a common characteristic of lipophilic, poorly soluble compounds. However, if such a drug is given at a high dose in relation to the solubility, C_t (see equation 1) may become significant even if the permeation rate through the gut wall is high. If the drug concentration is close to C_s (see equation 1) in the intestine, the primary substance-related determinants for absorption are the administered dose and C_s rather than the dissolution rate. It is important to identify such a situation, since it can be expected that the dissolution rate–enhancing formulation principle will not provide any benefits and that higher doses will provide only a small increase in the amount of absorbed drug. As a rough estimate for a high-permeability drug, it has been proposed that this situation can occur when the relationship between the dose (mg) and the solubility (mg/mL) exceeds a factor of 5000 if a dissolution volume of 250 mL is assumed (Amidon, 1996). For example, if the solubility is 0.01 mg/mL, this situation will be approached if doses of about 50 mg or more are administered. It should, however, be realized that this diagnostic tool is based on theoretical simulations rather than in vivo data. For example, physiological factors that might affect the saturation solubility are neglected (described in more detail below).

To predict the fraction absorbed (F_a) in a more quantitative manner, factors other than dissolution, solubility, or dose must be taken into account, such as regional permeability, degradation in the GI lumen, and transit times. Several algorithms with varying degrees of sophistication have been developed that integrate the dissolution or solubility with other factors. A more detailed description is beyond the scope of this chapter, but a comprehensive review has been published by Yu et al. (1996). Computer programs based on such algorithms are also commercially available and permit simulations to identify whether the absorption is limited by dissolution or solubility (GastroPlus™, Simulations Plus, Inc., California, U.S.; Simcyp™, Simcyp Limited, Sheffield, U.K.). As an example, Figure 3 shows simulations performed to investigate the dependence of dose, solubility, and particle radius on the *Fa* for an aprotic, high-permeability drug.

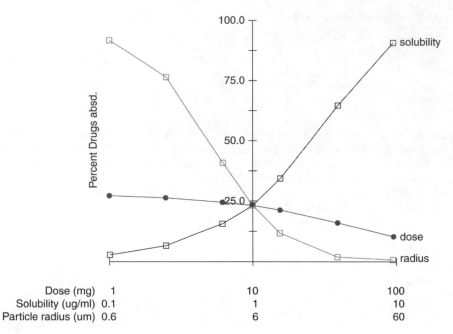

Figure 3 Simulations of fraction of drug absorbed after oral administration for a high-permeability drug ($P_{eff} = 4.5 \times 10^{-4}$ cm/s) for doses 1 to 100 mg, water solubilities 0.1 to 10 g/mL, and radius of drug particles 0.6 to 60 μm. During the variations of one variable, the others are held constant at the midpoint level (dose 10 mg, solubility 1 μg/mL, and particle radius 6 μm).

Physiological Aspects of Dissolution and Solubility Test Conditions

The dissolution of a drug in the gut lumen will depend on luminal conditions, for example, pH of the luminal fluid, volume available, lipids and bile acids, and the hydrodynamic conditions produced from the GI peristaltic movements of the luminal content toward the lower bowel. Such physiological factors influence drug dissolution by controlling the different variables in equation (1) that describe the dissolution rate. This is summarized in Table 4 adapted from Dressman et al. (1998).

The test media used for determining solubility and dissolution should therefore ideally reflect the in vivo situation. The most relevant factors to be considered from an in vivo perspective are

- pH (for proteolytic drugs),
- ionic strength and composition,
- surface-active agents, and
- temperature.

Table 4 Physicochemical and Physiological Parameters Important to Drug Dissolution in the Gastrointestinal Tract

Factor	Physicochemical parameter	Physiological parameter
Surface area of drug (A)	Particle size, wettability	Surfactants in gastric juice and bile
Diffusivity of drug (D)	Molecular size	Viscosity of lumenal contents
Boundary layer thickness (h)		Motility patterns and flow rate
Solubility (C_s)	Hydrophilicity, crystal structure, solubilization	pH, buffer capacity, bile, food components
Amount of drug already dissolved (C_t)		Permeability
Volume of solvent available (C_t)		Secretions, coadministered fluids

Source: From Dressman et al. (1998).

Table 5 The pH and Concentration of Most Dominant Ions in Different Parts of the Gastrointestinal Tract in Humans

	pH		Ionic concentrations (nM)		
	Fasting	Fed	Na$^+$	HCO$_3^-$	Cl$^-$
Stomach	1–2	2–5[a]	70	<20	100
Upper small intestine	5.5–6.5		140	50–110	130
Lower small intestine	6.5–8				
Colon	5.5–7				

[a]Dependent on volume, pH, and buffer capacity of the food.
Source: From Charman et al. (1997) and Lindahl et al. (1997).

The pH varies in the GI tract from 1 to 8 (Table 5), and the dissolution properties should therefore be known over this pH range for orally administered drugs. A more thorough review of intestinal pH conditions can be found elsewhere (Charman et al., 1997; Fallingborg et al., 1989).

It may be argued that, for immediate release formulations intended to quickly dissolve in the stomach, only the more acidic pH levels are of relevance. However, dissolution may occur at higher pH levels for several reasons, for example, concomitant food intake, comedication, diseases, or instant tablet emptying to the small intestine. In addition, since drug absorption over the gastric wall is negligible, the drug will always enter the more neutral conditions in the intestine.

Dissolution studies at pH 1 are generally performed in HCl, which is also present in the stomach. However, to perform studies over the entire pH interval, different buffers are needed to control the pH. In the intestine, pH is controlled by bicarbonate, which is not practical to use in vitro because of the need for continuous bubbling with CO_2. Non-physiological buffer systems, such as phosphates, acetates, or citrates, are therefore often used. It is important to note that the solubility may vary for different buffers at the same pH, because of different "salting in" and "salting out" effects or differences in solubility products (chapter 3) when the drug and buffer component are of opposite charges. If such effects occur, the solubility parameters will also be dependent on the concentration of the buffer system, and the influence of the buffer will increase at higher concentrations. Excessive buffer concentrations beyond what is needed to control the pH should therefore be avoided.

The dominant ions in the GI tract are sodium, chloride, and bicarbonate (Table 5), and their concentrations vary between luminal sites along the GI tract (Lindahl et al., 1997). The total concentration of these ions, expressed as ionic strength, has been determined to be 0.10 to 0.16 and 0.12 to 0.19 in the stomach and small intestine, respectively. The presence of such ions may affect solubility, especially by the common ion effect (chapter 3).

The presence of physiological surface-active agents in the stomach and small intestine will influence the solubility and the dissolution of sparingly soluble drugs by improved wetting of solid particle surface areas and by micellar solubilization. This has been reviewed in more detail by Gibaldi and Feldman (1970) and Charman et al. (1997).

The main endogenous surfactants are the bile acids, which are excreted into the upper jejunum by the bile flow. The bile acids—cholic acid, chenodeoxycholic acid, and deoxycholic acid—are present as conjugates with glycine and taurine as the sodium salts. The total concentrations of bile acids in the upper small intestinal tract are 4 to 6 mM in the fasting state and 10 to 40 mM after ingestion of a meal. The bile acids are reabsorbed in the terminal small intestine (terminal ileum) by active uptake. During normal physiological conditions, micelle formation and solubilization may already occur at the lower bile acid concentrations in the fasting state. The micelles formed not only contain bile acids but are a mixture with endogenous phospholipids excreted by the bile (lecithin) and products from the digestion of dietary fat, such as monoglycerides. The saturation solubility of a sparingly soluble drug has, in some cases, been increased by several orders of magnitude by the addition of physiological amounts of lecithin to a bile salt solution, whereas no solubility improvements are obtained by

(A)

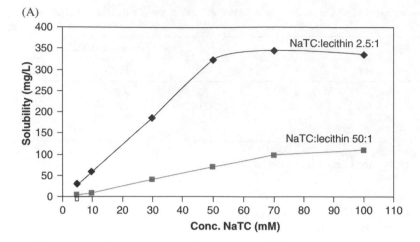

(B)

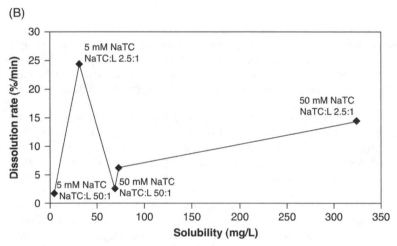

Figure 4 **(A)** The solubility of a poorly soluble compound (water solubility <1 μg/mL) at different concentrations of sodium taurocholate (NaTC) mixed with lecithin in two different ratios, 2.5:1 and 50:1. **(B)** The dissolution rate of a poorly soluble compound (water solubility <1 μg/mL) versus the saturation solubility obtained by testing in different concentrations of NaTC mixed with lecithin at two different ratios, 2.5:1 and 50:1.

the formation of mixed micelles for others. It should also be noted that while the solubility of a very sparingly water-soluble drug is increased by the formation of a mixed micelle, the rate of dissolution might be decreased. This is exemplified in Figure 4A, B showing the saturation solubility and the dissolution rate at different concentrations of lecithin in a bile acid solution for a compound that has a water solubility of less than 1 μg/mL.

Bile acids not only affect the solubility by solubilization of sparingly soluble compounds, they may also decrease the solubility by forming sparingly soluble salts or complexes with drugs. Indications of such phenomena have been shown for a variety of drugs such as pafenolol, tubocurarine, neomycine, kanamycine, nadolol, atenolol, and propranolol (Yamaguchi et al., 1986a,b,c; Grosvenor and Löfroth, 1995).

Solubility or dissolution studies in the presence of physiological surfactants may provide important information with respect to the in vivo absorption process of sparingly soluble compounds, although it is hardly possible to reconstitute the full complexity and dynamics of the in vivo situation in an in vitro model. While bile acids and lecithin are available in purified forms, their use is somewhat limited by their high price. Much less well-defined ox bile preparations are also available, which contain a mixture of conjugated bile acids and other

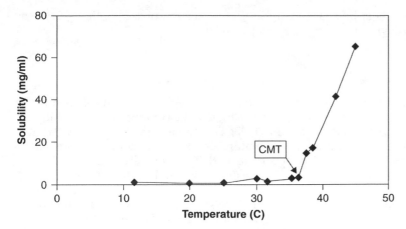

Figure 5 Solubility of an amphiphilic drug at different temperatures in a phosphate buffer, illustrating the effect on solubility at the critical micelle temperature.

bile components. The closest test media to mimic the in vivo lumenal content have been the suggested systems by Dressman et al., the FaSSIF and FeSSIF systems (Dressman et al., 2007, and references therein).

The temperature in dissolution and solubility tests should preferably be identical to the in vivo temperature at the site of administration, since the solubility is dependent on the temperature. The most suitable temperature depends on the intended administration route. For oral administration, testing at 37°C is the obvious choice.

Special Considerations for Surface-Active Drugs

Many drugs consist of both hydrophobic and hydrophilic structural groups, since these are often needed to optimize oral absorption. It is therefore not surprising that surface-active properties have been identified for a large number of drugs. Such drugs may provide unexpected dissolution and solubility properties, owing to the formation of micelles or other forms of self-aggregation. This is exemplified in Figure 5, which shows the solubility of an amphiphilic drug at different temperatures in a phosphate buffer solution. The saturation solubility is drastically increased at about 37°C because of the formation of micelles. The temperature at which micelles are formed in a certain test medium is called the critical micelle temperature (CMT).

If the drug substance is suspected to be surface active, which will be indicated by the molecular structure, the surface-active properties should be further investigated during the biopharmaceutical preformulation phase. The potential for micelle formation should be investigated and, if relevant, the CMC and the CMT should be determined. CMC is determined by measuring a colligative property such as conductivity, surface tension, or osmotic pressure in water solutions of the drug in different concentrations. Typically, for all methods, an increase or decrease is seen in the measured variable at increasing drug concentrations, which is followed by a plateau level. The inflection point between the two phases is the CMC. It should be noted that CMC and CMT are dependent on the composition of the test medium. For example, salts, buffers, and the presence of other amphiphilic compounds affect the micelle formation and thereby the solubility of an amphiphilic compound.

Substance Characterization Prior To Biopharmaceutical Solubility/Dissolution Tests

Several substance properties can affect dissolution and/or solubility, such as purity; particle size and distribution; surface area; and the presence of polymorphs, hydrates or other solvates, or amorphous forms. To avoid misleading or inconclusive results in extensive solubility or dissolution studies, it is important to characterize the drug substance form with respect to such properties, especially in the later biopharmaceutical preformulation phase. Methods for such characterization are described in more detail in chapters 3 and 7.

LUMINAL INTERACTIONS

The rate and extent of drug absorption can be affected by degradation, metabolism, and complex binding in the GI lumen. There is a general change in the composition of the luminal fluid along the GI tract (Hörter and Dressman, 1997; Dressman and Yamada, 1991). The differences are mainly in the concentration and nature of ions, bile, proteins, osmolality, surface tension, and lipids. The interaction of a drug with the luminal content can induce precipitation of the drug with ions to form insoluble salts (Dakas and Takla, 1991; Hörter and Dressman, 1997) or binding to enzymes or proteins (Sjöström et al., 1999) or simply a partition of the drug into luminal compartments (micelles, cell debris). This will result in a reduction of the effective concentration of the drug at the absorption site and will thus lower the flux of the drug across the membrane. For instance, pH in lumen changes along the GI tract and is different before and after a meal (Table 5), starting at pH 1 to 2 during fasting conditions in the stomach, rising to 5 to 6.5 in the duodenum, and going slowly up to 7 to 8 in the ileum region. It then decreases to 6 to 7 in the proximal colon and approaches 7 to 8 in the rectum (Fallingborg et al., 1989). This luminal pH is especially important for the release of the drug from the dosage form or the dissolution in the luminal media. The predicted absorption, based on pH partition hypothesis, of some ionizable drugs was originally based on this luminal pH, and actual values of absorption obtained from in vivo animal studies differed markedly. The reason for this pH shift has been explained in different ways over the years but has been accepted to be an acidic "microclimate region" adjacent to the mucosal membrane (McEwan and Lucas, 1990). The pH during the actual transport of a drug through the epithelial membrane in the intestinal mucosa is therefore approximately one pH unit lower. This microclimate pH favors absorption of weak acids and weak bases (Fig. 6). This means that, for an ionizable drug, the luminal pH is the most important pH for the release of the drug from the dosage form and for dissolution/solubility. However, the pH at the surface of the membrane (i.e., microclimate) will determine the rate of absorption of this drug through the membrane. Both of these pH values vary along the GI tract.

A common phenomenon for drugs is decomposition at acidic pH. The drug stability should therefore be investigated along the entire physiological range (pH 1–8) if such degradation can be expected. Typically, the percentage of drug that remains is determined at different times, and a first-order rate constant or half-life is determined for the degradation process. This is exemplified in Figure 7 for omeprazole in a range of different pH values (Pilbrant and Cederberg, 1985).

Complexation
Complexation of drugs in the GI tract can occur with the luminal content. Any nonmetallic atom, whether free or contained in a neutral molecule, or an ionic compound that can donate

Bulk
pH 6.5

Acid microclimate
pH 5.5

Epithelial cell

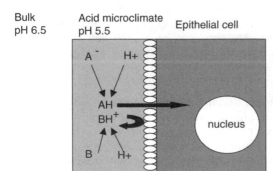

Figure 6 Surface pH hypothesis for weak acids and bases. A model for the influence of the microclimate pH in rat proximal jejunum on weak electrolyte permeation. The weak acid A^- is converted to neutral by the presence of H^+ in the microclimate. The undissociated form can easily be absorbed through the mucosa. In contrast, the weak base B is protonated by the H^+ to BH^+, which is less absorbed through the membrane. *Source*: From McEwan and Lucas (1990).

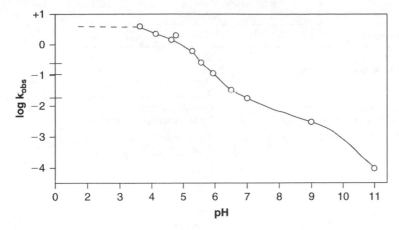

Figure 7 Omeprazol stability as a function of pH. Logarithm of the observed rate constant (k_{obs} 1/h) for the initial, pseudo-first-order degradation of omeprazole in water solution at constant pH plotted as a function of pH. *Source*: From Pilbrant and Cederberg (1985).

an electron pair, may serve as a donor. The acceptor is frequently a metal ion. In general, complexes can be divided into two classes, depending on whether the acceptor component is a metal ion or an organic molecule (Dakas and Takla, 1991; Hörter and Dressman, 1997). Complex formation with components of food, such as milk, can give precipitation of the drug compound and reduce the bioavailability and fraction of the dose absorbed. Complex formation of peptide-like compounds and enzymes in the GI tract lumen has also recently been reported (Sjöström et al., 1999), and a reduced bioavailability was observed.

The complex formation of a coumarin derivative with magnesium ions present in antacid formulations has also been reported (Ambre and Fuher, 1973). The formation of a more absorbable species of the coumarin derivative was found, that is, magnesium bishydroxycoumarin (Dakas and Takla, 1991). Complex formation is therefore not just negative for drug absorption but can also be used positively in formulation development for increasing the solubility of a drug, for example, the use of cyclodextrins.

The composition and concentration of bile acids are different in different species and also vary along the GI tract (Lindahl et al., 1997; Dressman and Yamada, 1991). The composition will affect the wetting ability of the bile and may also give variations in interactions. Drug interactions with bile have been reported (e.g., β-blockers) (Yamaguchi et al., 1986a,b,c; Grosvenor and Löfroth, 1995) and involve binding to the bile acid dimers or micelles or precipitation, which causes an unexpectedly low absorption in the GI tract.

Degradation and Metabolism

The gastric and intestinal fluids contain a multitude of different enzymes that can potentially metabolize different drugs (Table 6). In addition, the microflora, being most significant in the colon, also have a significant metabolizing capacity. A list of such metabolic reactions is shown in Table 7.

Interaction with the luminal content may be a *chemical or enzymatic/microbial degradation*. The chemical degradation is usually related to pH changes in the gut lumen but can also be a result of the reductive environment (redox potential negative) produced by the presence of anaerobic bacteria (Shamat, 1993).

Enzymes are present throughout the GI tract, both within the brush-border membrane and in the lumen. The general gradient is decreased luminal degradation aborally to the small intestine and increased brush-border and intracellular degradation. The main enzymes include proteases, peptidases, esterases, cytochrome P(CYP) 450 enzymes, and conjugating enzymes (Table 6). Some enzymes, such as CYP 450 isoforms, are especially involved in the biotransformation of lipophilic compounds of both endogenous and exogenous origin, such as steroids, bile acids, fatty acids, and prostaglandins (Arlotto et al., 1991). CYP 450 3A4 is

Table 6 Enzymes Found in the Gastrointestinal Tract

Source	Enzyme	Substrate
Salivary glands	Amylase	Starch
Stomach	Pepsinogens/pepsins	Proteins and polypeptides
	Trypsin	Proteins and polypeptides
	Chymotrypsin	Proteins and polypeptides
	Elastase	Elastin and other proteins
	Carboxypeptidase A, B	Proteins and polypeptides
Exocrine pancreas	Pancreatic lipase	Triglycerides
	Pancreatic amylase	Starch
	Ribonuclease	RNA
	Deoxyribonuclease	DNA
	Phospholipase A	Lecithin
	Enterokinase	Trypsinogen
	Aminopeptidases	Polypeptides
	Dipeptidases	Dipeptides
	Maltase	Maltose, maltotriose
Intestinal mucosa	Lactase	Lactose
	Sucrase	Sucrose
	Isomaltase	α-Limit dextrins
	Nuclease and related enzymes	Nucleic acids
	Intestinal lipase	Monoglycerides
	Cytochrome P450	Steroids
	Esterases	Esters of prodrugs

Source: Adapted from Ganong (1975).

Table 7 Some Metabolic Reactions of the Intestinal Microflora

Reactions	Example
Reductions	
Nitro compounds	Clonazepam
Sulfoxides	Sulinac
21-Hydroxycorticoids	Aldosterone
Double bonds	Digoxin
Azo compounds	Prontosil
Hydrolysis	
Nitrate esters	Glyceryl trinitrate
Sulfate esters	Sodium picosulfate
Succinate esters	Carbenoxolone
Amides	Methotrexate
Glucuronides	Morphine glucuronide
Glucosides	Sennosides
Removal of functional groups	
N-dealkylation	Methamphetamine
Deamination	Flucytosine
Other reactions	
Heterocyclic ring fission	Levamisole
Side-chain cleavage	Steroids

Source: From Shamat (1993).

present mainly in the upper GI tract and is concentrated primarily at the villus tips (Paine et al., 1997; Pascoe et al., 1983). CYP 3A is the most abundant isoform in the human intestine (Paine et al., 1997), and among the CYP 3A, CYP 3A4 is often found in coexistence with the MDR1 gene product, the efflux protein, and P-glycoprotein, and shares a significant substrate specificity overlap (Wacher et al., 1998). The main CYP 450 isoforms in the intestine vary with animal species and the intestinal region.

Techniques for studying enzymatic degradation of compounds include

- homogenized intestinal segments, sometimes centrifuged into different subcellular fractions after high-speed centrifugation [crude homogenates, S9 (supernatant fraction constituting the cell plasma content), microsomal fraction (ER and other membrane fractions)];
- degradation in luminal perfusates or fluids (chyme) and identification of metabolites after transport across the intestinal membrane, as in the Ussing chamber model (Ungell et al., 1992); and
- cell monolayers such as Caco-2 cells (Delie and Rubas, 1997; Ungell and Karlsson, 2003).

Caco-2 cells express the main enzymes involved in drug metabolism (Delie and Rubas, 1997; Artursson and Borchardt, 1997; Ungell and Karlsson, 2003) in quantities similar to those in the human small intestine rather than as is present in colonocytes. However, the very important CYP 450 3A family, which is the main CYP 450 in the human intestine, is absent in the Caco-2 cell monolayers, a fact that can explain differences in permeability between this model and intestinal tissues for drugs that are substrates to this enzyme family. The existence of metabolism can also be evaluated by incubation of the drug using pure enzyme preparations.

The *bacterial* content in the lumen of the GI tract varies with the region, starting with approximately 102 organisms in the mouth and increasing to as much as 10^{12} in the colon. Microbial degradation, therefore, increases aborally to the stomach and largely takes place in the colon (Shamat, 1993). Illing (1981) and Coates et al. (1988) reviewed the techniques employed for studying the role of the gut flora in drug metabolism. In general, incubations are made with the drug and the gut content of an animal, or human, in a suitable medium under anaerobic conditions. The degradation pathways are mainly reductive (of nitro compounds, sulfoxides, corticoids, doubles bonds, and azo bonds), hydrolysis (of esters, amides, glucoronides, and glucosides), N-dealkylations, and N-deamination (Shamat, 1993). Anaerobic metabolism can also affect the formulation components, giving false release rates of the drug. This mechanism has been used for targeting drugs to the colon using azopolymer bonds (Saffran et al., 1986; van den Mooter et al., 1997). The degradation of compounds by the gut flora in vitro seems not always to be correlated to the in vivo situation, and so in vivo measurements must be performed (Shamat, 1993).

Enzymatic *degradation of prodrugs* to the active drug can occur in the intestinal lumen (by the gut flora or by luminal or brush-border enzymes) or during transport across the intestinal membrane (intracellular enzymes). Where the prodrug is degraded depends on the nature of the prodrug bond, and the in vitro assay is very important for establishing optimal biotransformation rates and regional absorption/degradation. In general, the most commonly used in vitro models for the biotransformation of prodrugs are incubation with intestinal fluids, liver or intestinal microsomal incubations, and plasma/blood incubations. It is also very important to consider species differences in metabolic activity for prodrug activation. Permeability models, such as Caco-2 cell monolayers, have also been used to evaluate the importance of ester hydrolysis of prodrugs in parallel with transport (Narawane et al., 1993; Augustijns et al., 1998). Care should be taken to study esterase-dependent prodrug activation using the Caco-2 cell monolayers because of differences in substrate specificity of the expressed carboxyl esterase in these cells compared with the intestinal cells in vivo. A report by Imai et al. (2005) indicates that in the case of Caco-2 cells, the main carboxyl esterase is identified as the hCE-1 and corresponds to the hepatic variant, while in the human intestine, the most abundant carboxyl esterase is the hCE-2.

ABSORPTION/UPTAKE OVER THE GI MEMBRANES

Mechanisms of Drug Absorption

Several factors originating from the chemical structure and property of the drug molecule and from the physiology within the environment in the GI tract affect the flow of molecules across the intestinal membrane. These factors include solubility, partition coefficient, pK_a, molecular

Table 8 Physicochemical and Physiological Factors That Influence Drug Bioavailability After Oral Administration

Physicochemical	Physiological
Hydrophobicity	Surface area at the site of administration
Molecular size	Transit time and motility
Molecular conformation	pH in the lumen and at surface
pK_a	Intestinal secretions
Chemical stability	Enzymes
Solubility	Membrane permeability
Complexation	Food and food composition
Particle size	Disease state
Crystal form	Pharmacological effect
Aggregation	Mucus and unstirred water layer
Hydrogen bonding	Water fluxes
Polar surface area	Blood flow
	Bacteria
	Liver uptake and bile excretion

Source: From Ungell (1997).

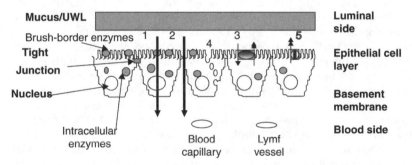

Figure 8 Schematic drawing of the mechanisms and routes of drug absorption across intestinal epithelia. Drugs can be absorbed transcellularly (1) and paracellularly (2) by passive diffusion or transcellularly via carrier-mediated transport (3) or endocytosis (4). Enzymes in the brush-border region or intracellular enzymes and the efflux proteins, for example, P-glycoprotein (5), contribute to the elimination of harmful compounds.

weight, molecular volume, aggregate, particle size, pH in the lumen and at the surface of the membrane, GI secretions, absorptive surface area, blood flow, membrane permeability, and enzymes (for more factors, see Ungell, 1997, and Table 8). Complete absorption occurs when the drug has a maximum permeability coefficient and maximum solubility at the site of absorption (Pade and Stavchansky, 1998).

The uptake of drugs across the intestinal membrane can occur transcellularly across the lipid membrane or paracellularly between the epithelial cells in the tight junctional gap (Fig. 8) (Ungell, 1997). The transcellular route is generally via carrier proteins or by passive diffusion. In addition, the transport across the cell membrane can be via endocytotic processes. Efflux proteins carrying the drug from the inside back into the lumen (e.g., P-glycoprotein, MRP1–6, etc.) have been proposed to be important for the overall absorption of drugs in the GI tract (Saitoh and Aungst, 1995; Hunter and Hirst, 1997; Makhey et al., 1998; Döppenschmitt et al., 1998; Anderle et al., 1998). Models have now been developed for specific studies of the mechanism behind low permeability or active transport via carrier systems, such as oligopeptide transporters, dipeptide transporters, amino acid transporters, and monocarboxylic transporters (Tsuji and Tamai, 1996).

Apart from permeability of the intestine to molecules, the time the molecule spends in the region of absorption, that is, transit time, becomes important. Generally, transit times in humans are seconds in the esophagus, 0.5 to 1.5 hours in the stomach, 3 to 4 hours in the small intestine, and 8 to 72 hours in the colon.

Regionally, the different physiological factors will change, and thereby the potential impact on the drug molecule will also change (Dressman and Yamada, 1991; Hörter and Dressman, 1997; Ungell et al., 1997). For developing extended oral drug release dosage forms, knowledge of the regional differences in the absorption pattern becomes very important in evaluation and success (Thomson et al., 1986; Ungell et al., 1997; Kararli, 1995; Pantzar et al., 1993; Narawane et al., 1993). In addition, these mechanisms are also species different (Kararli, 1995) and must be correlated to the human situation. If the regional difference in absorption probability of the drug is known (regional permeability and interactions), increased absorption can be achieved by the use of an absorption window, for example, targeting the drug to a specific region to avoid critical regions of enzymes or low permeability.

MODELS FOR STUDYING THE ABSORPTION POTENTIAL OF DRUGS

Models for studying drug absorption that are available in industry and at universities and contract organizations are mainly (Hillgren et al., 1995; Ungell, 1997; Borchardt et al., 1996; Stewart et al., 1995)

- computational methods,
- partitioning between water and oil,
- cell cultures,
- membrane vesicles,
- intestinal rings or sacs,
- excised segments from animals in the Ussing chamber,
- in vitro and in situ intestinal perfusions,
- in vivo cannulated or fistulated animals, and
- in vivo gavaged animals.

All of these models have values that must be correlated to human data, mainly F_a (fraction absorbed) (Ungell, 1997; Lennernäs et al., 1997; Artursson et al., 1993; Lennernäs et al., 1996; Artursson and Karlsson, 1991; Ungell and Karlsson, 2003) (Fig. 9). Correlations have been

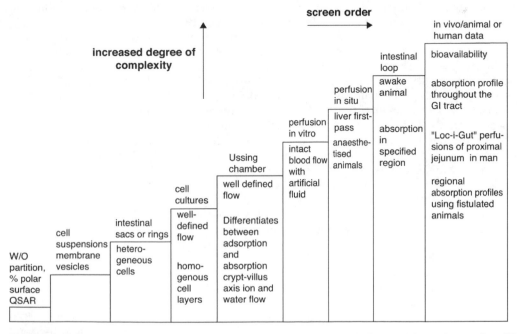

Figure 9 Schematic drawing of a screen ladder. The screen ladder can be used for understanding different complexities in the results, using different screening models. *Source*: From Ungell (1997).

made in different laboratories using different models (Ussing, perfusion, and Caco-2) (Matthes et al., 1992; Rubas et al., 1993; Tanaka et al., 1995; Lennernäs et al., 1997; Fagerholm et al., 1996) and in different laboratories using the same model (Caco-2) (Artursson et al., 1996; Hayeshi et al., 2008).

Methods to describe the process of transport over the GI membrane must describe different mechanisms of absorption for a wide variety of molecules and must be predictive of the absorption process in human. If a new chemical entity (NCE) cannot penetrate the intestinal epithelium, it will not be successfully developed as a pharmaceutical product. This also means that if the rate-limiting step in the absorption process of the drug molecule is not described in the model, the result will be a false positive.

The literature mentions numerous nonbiological (biophysical and computational) and biological in vitro and in vivo methods for screening barriers of absorption (for more information see Borchardt et al., 1996; Kararli, 1989; Ungell, 1997; Hillgren et al., 1995; Lipinski et al., 1996; Lundahl and Beigi, 1997; Yang et al., 1997; Hjort-Krarup et al., 1998; Quilianova et al., 1999; Stewart et al., 1997; Lee et al., 1997; Altomare et al., 1997; van der Waterbeemd et al., 1996; Winiwarter et al., 1998; Oprea and Gottfries, 1999). Each method describes a part of the absorption process, mainly the transport through the lipid membrane. However, it is clear that for drug discovery and rational drug development, there is no single ultimate method, but instead, there is a need for more than one of these screening methods. It is also evident from the literature that we need more information regarding the absorption mechanisms of the particular drug entity and its analogues to be able to obtain structure/absorption relationships and to design the most proper method for screening, for example, HTS. Below is a short review of the different methods available for studying drug absorption.

Nonbiological Methods for the Prediction of Oral Drug Absorption

Passive diffusion through the lipid membrane of the GI tract is considered to represent one of the main drug absorption mechanisms. This is a process generally thought to be governed by physicochemical factors of the drug molecule, such as lipophilicity, surface charges, molecular volume/molecular weight, and conformational flexibility (Navia and Chaturvedi, 1996). The size of the molecule and the charge will also govern whether the molecule can passively pass across the epithelium via the paracellular pathway and between the cells via the tight junctional complex. However, it has been argued that the paracellular route is almost nonexistent and seems to be important only for drugs with molecular weights below 200 g/mol and for nonionic or cationic molecules (Karlsson et al., 1999, 1994; Lennernäs, 1997).

The nonbiological models describing the transmembrane process are very rapid and involve no use of animals. Computer-based models of structure/absorption relationships belong to this group. They have recently become increasingly popular because of the use of chemical libraries and possibilities for testing large sets of biological data, with multivariate analysis models such as partial least squares (PLS) and principal component analysis (PCA) (Eriksson et al., 1999). In fact, the nonbiological methods can, in many cases, replace the biological methods and can be used in an HTS manner. The most challenging ideas for industry today involve trying to avoid time and resource consuming synthesis of structural analogues with no potential of being developed as pharmaceutical products; they therefore focus more on the analogues that have such potential.

The most widely accepted parameter for predicting drug absorption is the *partition coefficient* reflecting partitioning of the drug only into a lipid phase (e.g., octanol/water), the log P (or log D) value (see chapter 3), and general rule-of-thumb models such as the Lipinski rule (Lipinski et al., 1996). This rule states that molecules with a molecular weight of less than 500 g/mol, with a clog P of less than 5, with hydrogen donors fewer than 5, and acceptors fewer than 10 will have greater possibilities for being orally available, and violation of at least two of these rules will lower the potential for the drug to be absorbed. This rule is based on historical data (up to 1997) from a vast number of drugs entering the investigational new drug application (IND) phase, including drugs that fulfilled the criteria of pharmacological activity. The rule is also based on several other assumptions: that the transcellular transport is molecular weight dependent, the drug is *only* absorbed through passive diffusion, the four parameters describe the molecular structure correctly, and the drug is not solubility restricted.

Only the high value of the limit is set; the lower limit of, for instance, clog P is not within the rule. In addition, the parameters in the Lipinski rule describe the two-dimensional structure of the molecule but do not take into account the three-dimensional structure and the true conformation of the molecule. However, regardless of the restrictions of the rule, it can be used as a rule of thumb in the same way as log P or log D is being used, but is a better predictor than lipophilicity alone.

The optimal range in *lipophilicity* that would reflect a good absorption potential has been suggested to be a log P value between 0 and 3 (Navia and Chaturvedi, 1996) or above 3 (Wils et al., 1994a), depending on the method used. This is a general rule of thumb because it means that very hydrophilic drugs (log $P < -3$) and very lipophilic drugs (log $P > 6$) are often associated with incomplete absorption in vivo (Navia and Chaturvedi, 1996; Wils et al., 1994a). Drugs with log P values between -3 and 0 and a log P between 3 and 6 often give varying results (Navia and Chaturvedi, 1996). However, the prediction of incomplete absorption for hydrophilic and very lipophilic drugs has been argued. Hydrophilic drugs, such as atenolol and sotalol, are absorbed from the GI tract, although their partition coefficients are low, and very lipophilic drugs, such as fluvastatin, are completely absorbed (Lindahl et al., 1996). The lack of correlation and the varying results obtained by this method are understandable, since lipophilicity is far from being the only determinant of drug absorption.

Today, however, there is a more complex view of the factors governing the partitioning into a lipid phase, for example, multiple molecular structure descriptors, including a number of hydrogen bonds (acceptors and donors) (Burton et al., 1992), polar surface area (Palm et al., 1996), polarity, integy moments, polarizability, and distances between functional groups of importance (Oprea et al., 2000; Zamora et al., 2003; Norinder et al., 1997; Palm et al., 1997; Cruciani et al., 2000; Goodford, 1985). Future quantitative structure activity relationship (QSAR) models will therefore be based more on multivariate analysis, analyzing a complex set of molecular descriptors.

Below is a short description of some of the nonbiological methods that can be used to predict drug absorption. For more detailed information, see, for example, Ungell (1997), Lipinski et al. (1996), Palm et al. (1997), Burton et al. (1992), Norinder et al. (1997), van der Waterbeemd et al. (1996), and Cruciani et al. (2000).

Computer-Based Prediction Models

A good relationship has been established between the number of *hydrogen bonds* of small model peptides and their permeability coefficients, determined using Caco-2 cell monolayers (Burton et al., 1992). The method reflects the ability of the molecule to form hydrogen bonds with the surrounding solvent. The more bonds the molecule forms with water (luminal fluid), the less potential it has to diffuse into a lipid phase of a membrane.

The total number of hydrogen bonds in the molecule can easily be calculated, including the bonds the molecule can form internally. This may be one of the reasons for the lack of correlation seen for the drug fluvastatin, a very lipophilic drug (log P 3.8) that has a total of eight hydrogen bonds (Lindahl et al., 1996), whereof several are internal within the drug molecule. The total number of hydrogen bonds that should be the limit is five, according to the Lipinski rule (Lipinski et al., 1996), if the drug is to be completely absorbed in the GI tract in human (Lindahl et al., 1996).

Polar surface area is another important determinant of drug absorption, as first proposed by Palm et al. (1996). The method was described as dynamic molecular surface properties. These were calculated with consideration of all low-energy conformations of some β-blockers, and the water-accessible surface areas, which were calculated and averaged according to a Boltzmann distribution. They found a linear relationship between permeability coefficients, measured both with Caco-2 cells and excised segments from the rat intestine, and percentage polar surface area of β-blockers with different lipophilicity. According to the calculated values of log D_{oct} at pH 7.4, there was not as good a relationship, with some additional impaired ranking order between the substances [calculated according to the method of Hansch and coworkers (Palm et al., 1996)]. Polar surface area has also recently been proposed to explain why drugs with very high log D values are not absorbed (Artursson et al., 1996). The authors suggest that these very lipophilic drugs, instead, show a high degree of polar surface area toward the environment, which will reduce their ability to diffuse through a lipid phase. This was shown by a bell-shaped correlation between permeability coefficients determined in HT-29 (18-C) monolayers and log D and, in contrast, a linear relationship between permeability coefficients and calculated polar surface area (Artursson et al., 1996). A good correlation between the fraction absorbed, and the polar surface area of a variety of drugs, as well as for hydrogen acceptors and donors, has been proposed to exist (Palm et al., 1997).

QSAR Models

Several theoretical models attempting to predict the absorption properties from molecular descriptors have been published in the last few years (Palm et al., 1996; Oprea and Gottfries, 1999; Norinder et al., 1997; Hjort-Krarup et al., 1998; Winiwarter et al., 1998). These theoretical models can be based on several different experimental data sets from various absorption models, such as Caco-2 cells, Ussing chambers, in vivo fraction absorbed, and permeability in humans (Palm et al., 1996; Palm et al., 1997; Artursson et al., 1996; Norinder et al., 1997; Winiwarter et al., 1998; Oprea and Gottfries, 1999). There are several new, recently published approaches in this area for creating predictive models for drug absorption properties, the MolSurf™ methodology (Norinder et al., 1997) being one. Another approach is to use the Grid™ methodology, a strategy designed by Goodford (1985) to study interaction fields of a molecule, the target, with a small chemical group, the probe. The Grid™ methodology has been successfully applied in the receptor-substrate interaction analysis. The VolSurf™ program analyzes these interaction fields and obtains different surface properties and volumes to describe the interaction (Zamora et al., 2003). Until recently, it was believed that computer-based methods were only to be used for passive transcellular diffusion. Data have been presented that also indicate the use of these methods for active transport and efflux via carrier systems (Neuhoff et al., 1999; Ekins et al., 2001). The average time for the calculation of each compound is, at the least, seconds, but this differs between models. The more complex and flexible the structure becomes, the more time is required for the calculation. All of the methods described above are computer-based models and do not require any synthesis of compounds. This means that if they can be used in the early screening of thousands of compounds, the time required for evaluating these compounds will be reduced enormously, compared with the synthesis and determination of absorption by biological methods and difficult analytical procedures.

Extraction into a Lipid Phase

Measurement of log P (or log D) usually uses a determination of a drug molecule extracted into the lipid phase of an octanol/water or octanol/buffer extraction system (Palm et al., 1996; Leahy et al., 1989; Mannhold et al., 1990; Leo et al., 1975). The predictive value of log P or log D has been questioned. First, octanol is not the ideal lipid phase because of its own hydrogen bonding capacity. A δlog P, determined between two lipid phases, has instead been suggested, for example, between octanol/water and isooctane/water (Kim et al., 1993). Second, Leahy et al. (1989) showed that there is no simple relationship between log P and drug absorption. The curve is represented by a sigmoidal shape with a plateau (or even reported as a bell-shaped form) (Wils et al., 1994a; Yodoya et al., 1994). The reason for this is not known, but it is suggested to be a consequence of decreased aqueous solubility (Navia and Chaturvedi, 1996), uncertainty in the evaluation of the value of log P (Palm et al., 1996), or a high degree of polar surface area (Artursson et al., 1996).

Measurements of partitioning of drugs into *lipid vesicles, liposomes, or cell membranes* as predictive models for drug absorption are also described in the literature (Hillgren et al., 1995; Balon et al., 1999; Stewart et al., 1997). This may be due to the similarity of these systems to biological membranes and the wish for a "pure membrane system" with the correct lipid and protein composition, but without enzymes and carrier proteins.

Chromatography

Retention time measurements, k', through different types of *chromatographic systems* have recently become very popular, for example, immobilized artificial membrane (IAM) columns, reversed-phase C18 columns, and liposome columns. IAM columns show a good correlation to the determined log D values and drug absorption in vivo in mice for a group of cephalosporins. IAMs also predicted drug permeability through Caco-2 cells. The method is based on the retention of molecules on a column consisting of a solid phase of immobilized phospholipids tethered to a hydrocarbon string onto a silica column. In between the phospholipid strings, C_{10} and C_3 alkyl groups are bound to the column. The mobile phase is 100% aqueous. The substance is thought to be retained on the column mainly in the ranking order of lipophilicity. The molecule interacts more with the polar head groups of the phospholipids, which reflects the biological membrane, than in a separation on a HPLC column would (Pidgeon et al., 1995; Yang et al., 1997).

The method is reported to be very simple and may be used for fast screening of a large quantity of compounds. A good correlation has been reported between IAM chromatography and the membrane partition coefficient for structurally related hydrophobic drugs, but not for non-related compounds (Pidgeon et al., 1995).

The IAM method is similar to a separation on a HPLC column, which has been used for screening substances for drug absorption (Pidgeon et al., 1995; Merino et al., 1995). The method of Merino et al. (1995) is based on a fluorimetric reversed-phase HPLC method for quantification of quinolones in absorption and partition samples. The retention times of two of the quinolones correlated well with data obtained in vivo. The results of this type of separation also reflect the membrane partition coefficient of drugs and can therefore be used when the ranking order of related compounds is evaluated. However, drugs with a very large gap between their lipophilicity will require a gradient system for elution, which can mislead the interpretation. Non-related compounds will give different correlation lines with membrane permeability and partitioning coefficients because of the different mobile phase polarity and differences in the chemical structure (Rathbone and Tucker, 1991).

The chromatographic systems (as for log D or log P calculations or measurements) must be correlated to a biological parameter, for example, permeability over Caco-2 cells or intestinal segments in the Ussing chamber, for a better correlation to the absorption process. However, if this can be done with a wide range of molecules, as was reported for IAM chromatography (Pidgeon et al., 1995), before starting a large synthesis strategy, it might improve, in terms of time and effectiveness, the finding of a drug with good absorption potential.

Liposome chromatography has also recently been used as a tool for predicting permeability (Lundahl and Beigi, 1997; Beigi et al., 1998). For most drugs tested, the method does not predict drug absorption better than other chromatographic methods, such as reversed-phase columns, but some additional knowledge can nevertheless be gathered. The interaction between the drug and the lipophilic phase can be studied with this method, which may play an important role in the determination of the retention factor. This was especially evident when ionizable drugs were studied. Further evaluation is needed to understand whether this information can also contribute to the overall understanding of the process of drug transport across the lipid membrane.

Another method that should be mentioned here is capillary electrophoresis, which has recently been reported as a new tool for predicting drug absorption using β-blockers (Örnskov et al., 2001). This method can very easily be used as an HTS instrument if it can also be proved useful for other types of drug structures.

In Vitro Biological Methods

Many drugs will not perform only according to physicochemical rules, and their absorption cannot be predicted properly using biophysical methods. These are the drugs that are susceptible to any of the carrier-mediated processes (both in absorptive and secretory directions) or the molecules that are degraded during transport. The transport processes used by these drugs must be studied by biological methods, and information is also needed regarding cofactors and scaling factors to predict the fraction absorbed in humans.

Biological methods are therefore used when the mechanisms of absorption (paracellular, transcellular, or carrier mediated) and the enzymatic degradation or regional difference in permeability are to be evaluated. A short description of the best-known biological in vitro methods follows, and more detailed information on each of the methods can be found in, for example, Ungell (1997), Stewart et al. (1997), Hillgren et al. (1995), Borchardt et al. (1996), and Kararli (1995, 1989).

Methods Describing Drug Uptake
Membrane Vesicles and Intestinal Rings

As a group of methods, membrane vesicles and intestinal rings are technically quick and easy to use, even for persons not very skilled in using biological material. They represent the uptake of a drug into the enterocytes. These two methods are mainly used for evaluation of mechanisms of absorption and are not so frequently used in the industry to delineate drug absorption in general.

The use of brush-border *membrane vesicles* (BBMV) in the discovery or development of drugs is usually restricted to mechanistic studies of enzyme interactions or ion transport–coupled processes. The method is based on a homogenization of an inverted frozen intestine to give a purified fraction of the apical cell membranes from a chosen part of the GI tract (Kararli, 1989; Kessler et al., 1978). The method can frequently be used for isolated studies of the brush-border membrane transport characteristics without any basolateral membrane influence. It has been used for studies concerning the intestinal peptide carrier system (Yuasa et al., 1993) to clarify the mechanism of absorption of fosfomycin (Ishizawa et al., 1992), glucose, amino acids, and salicylate uptake (Osiecka et al., 1985). Membrane vesicles have been isolated from numerous animals, including human (Hillgren et al., 1995). The functionality of the preparation (i.e., whether the membrane is closed) is assessed by using substrates to specific carriers, such as glucose, phosphate, or amino acids, and the orientation of the membrane, that is, right side or inside out, is assessed by enzyme markers. Recently, BBMV was tested as a screening model for a large number of compounds using 96-well multiscreen filtration plates (Quilianova et al., 1999). After correction for unspecific binding to the tissue, the permeability values were found to show a good correlation to the in vivo human fraction absorbed. Generally, membrane vesicles used today are vesicles obtained from cells transfected with a certain transporter protein.

Vesicles represent a method of lipid membrane extraction and can be used in drug absorption studies for evaluation of a biological log D value (see the above section on nonbiological methods). This was actually first used for measurements of the lipid composition (Hillgren et al., 1995). Different regions of the GI tract can be used, evaluating the influence of regional differences in lipid composition on the permeability of drugs, as has been suggested by Thomson et al. (1986), Ungell et al. (1997), and Kim et al. (1994). The major disadvantage of the method is that these processes represent only a fraction of the complete absorption process into the cell. No paracellular process can be studied, nor can processes that need the basolateral membrane and its function for absorption, for example, processes linked to the active transport of Na^+ by the basolateral Na^+/K^+ adenosine triphosphatase (ATPase) (Kararli, 1989). There may be a day-to-day variation in vesicle preparation and a leakage of drugs from the vesicles during washing and filtration, which can affect the drug concentration (Osiecka et al., 1985). However, despite these drawbacks, it can be used for mechanistic studies of the drug absorption process, although there are only data on a direct correlation to human in vivo absorption values.

The second method in this group is the *intestinal rings or slices*. This method for studying drug absorption has been used extensively in the early 90s for kinetic analysis of carrier-mediated transport of glucose, amino acids, and peptides (Kararli, 1989; Osiecka et al., 1985; Porter et al., 1985; Kim et al., 1994; Leppert and Fix, 1994). The method is easy to use; the intestine of the animal is cut into rings or slices of approximately 30 to 50 mg (2 to 5 mm in width), which are put into an incubation medium for a short period of time (often up to one minute) with agitation and oxygenation. Samples of the incubation medium and rings are analyzed for drug content after the incubation. The intestine is sometimes everted on a glass rod before cutting, and different regions of the intestinal tract can be used.

The main advantage of this method is its ease of preparation. As in the BBMV, this method can also frequently be used for testing many different drugs simultaneously. However, the intestinal rings have several disadvantages. Diffusion into the tissue slices takes place on the side of the tissue (not only through the lipid membrane), as the connective tissue and muscle layers are exposed to the incubation solution. Correction is not always made for the adsorption of a drug on the surface of the tissue, and the slices do not maintain their integrity for more than 20 to 30 minutes (Osiecka et al., 1985; Levine et al., 1970). The method is also restricted by the limits of the analytical methods. Nevertheless, good mechanistic correlation to in vivo measurements has been achieved with the method in kinetic studies of carrier-mediated mechanisms of peptides (Kim et al., 1994). The method was evaluated for the prediction of in vivo absorption potential (Leppert and Fix, 1994), and it was shown that, under appropriate conditions, uptake into everted intestinal rings closely paralleled known in vivo bioavailability. The method has also recently been experimentally improved for better hydrodynamics and a requirement for lower volumes during the incubation period (Uch and Dressman, 1997; Uch et al., 1999).

Methods with Well-Defined Transport Direction
Cell Cultures
The Caco-2 cell monolayers and other cell cultures (HT-29, IEC-18) from human carcinoma have become increasingly popular as permeability methods in the past few years (Artursson, 1990; Hidalgo et al., 1989; Ma et al., 1992; Wils et al., 1994b; Ungell and Karlsson, 2003). Recently, cell lines such as Madin-Darby canine kidney (MDCK) have also received attention, especially for screening large numbers of compounds. The cell monolayers consist of polarized cells grown onto a filter support. When fully differentiated, the cells express the transport characteristics of mature cells (Fig. 10). Caco-2 cells (Artursson, 1990) and HT-29 (18-C1) (Wils et al., 1994b) grow into tight epithelia extremely useful for the measurement of permeability coefficients of various molecules.

The Caco-2 cell monolayer shows an epithelium membrane barrier function similar to the colon of human (Artursson et al., 1993; Lennernäs, 1997) but has carrier-mediated systems similar to the small intestine (e.g., bile acid transporter, dipeptide carrier, glucose carriers, drug efflux carriers, and vitamin B_{12}) (for references, see Borchardt, 1991; Walter et al., 1995; Ungell and Karlsson, 2003). The transport of pharmaceutical drugs is studied using 6-, 12-, and 25-well systems and side-by-side diffusion cells as in the Ussing chamber. The cells have also been used for culturing cocultures with lymphocytes for studying the transport of particles through lymphoid tissues (M cells) (Kerneis et al., 1997; Delie and Rubas, 1996) and have also been grown upside down to study transport in the opposite direction (Garberg et al., 1999).

Much is known about the performance of this method in predicting the absorption of drugs in humans (Ungell and Artursson, 2009). A good correlation is seen especially for lipophilic high-permeability drugs using the transcellular pathway and the in vivo permeability coefficients measured by perfused human jejunum (Loc-i-Gut® technique) (Lennernäs et al., 1996). Apart from studies of passive transcellular transport (Artursson, 1990; Artursson and Karlsson, 1991), the Caco-2 cell method has also been used for studying mechanisms of

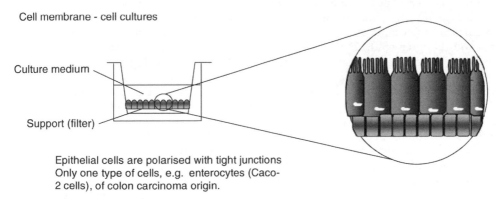

Cell membrane - cell cultures

Culture medium

Support (filter)

Epithelial cells are polarised with tight junctions
Only one type of cells, e.g. enterocytes (Caco-2 cells), of colon carcinoma origin.

Figure 10 Schematic drawing of a cell culture model, Caco-2 cells. Cells are seeded on filter support and are left to differentiate for one to three weeks before the transport experiments. Experiments are started by adding the compound to the donor side and taking out samples from the receiver side at times up to two hours. The incubation with the compound is done with good stirring and at 37°C.

passive paracellular transport (Artursson et al., 1993), carrier-mediated (peptidomimetics and antibiotics) (Walter et al., 1995), oligopeptide transporter (Hidalgo et al., 1995), monocarboxylic acid transporters (Tsuji and Tamai, 1996), efflux systems (P-glycoprotein and other efflux systems) (Kuo et al., 1994; Delie and Rubas, 1996; Döppenschmitt et al., 1998; Anderle et al., 1998), the effect of enhancers (Surendran et al., 1995; Lindmark et al., 1997; Anderberg and Artursson, 1994), and, recently, also cloned Caco-2 cells with specific carrier systems (Wenzel et al., 1996; Artursson and Borchardt, 1997). The importance of the unstirred water layer for the transport of very lipophilic drugs has also been studied (Karlsson and Artursson, 1991), and the HT-29 cell lines have been used for predicting drug absorption and investigating the mechanisms of mucus as a barrier to absorption (Wikman et al., 1993; Wils et al., 1994b; Matthes et al., 1992; MacAdam, 1993). There are also numerous studies of the metabolic capacity of the Caco-2 cells and possible induction of enzyme expression and carrier proteins (Delie and Rubas, 1997; Artursson and Borchardt, 1997; Korjamo et al., 2005).

The advantages of the cell culture method are many, that is, good performance on frequent use, both for the prediction of drug absorption in humans and mechanistic studies, and probably the best potential for use in HTS strategies. The monolayers are extremely useful in automated systems, and to speed up this automation, very young cells, three days old, have been evaluated for drug absorption studies (BioCoat system, BD Vlasante™) (Chong et al., 1997; Artursson and Tavelin, 2003). The experiments are rapid, have good precision, are less time consuming, and are less controversial than, for instance, in vivo animal studies. In addition, cell culture allows evaluation of drug transport under very controlled conditions and offers the major advantage that the cells are derived from humans. The MDCK cell line is, however, an easy cell line to cultivate, although it is derived from dogs instead of humans, which may give species-different results. The disadvantages of cell lines in culture are the tightness of the epithelium (although this can probably be regulated), showing a more colon-like system and giving extremely low-permeability coefficients for hydrophilic drugs. Further disadvantages include the unknown quantity and predictive value of the different carrier-mediated systems (Lennernäs et al., 1996; Lennernäs, 1997), and the unknown composition of the lipid membrane and its lack of crypt-villus axis, which is important for fluid and ion transport in vivo. There are also differences in results from laboratories using this method for establishing a relationship between the permeability coefficients of compounds and the values of the F^a, as reported in the literature (Ungell and Karlsson, 2003). The reason for the differences has not been fully evaluated but may have to do with the cultivation procedure, which can affect enzyme and carrier expressions, cell density, and passage number, and may have to do with differences in the experimental setup (e.g., stirred or unstirred, concentration of compounds tested, etc.) (Delie and Rubas, 1997; Anderle et al., 1998).

Excised Intestinal Segments
The *everted sac* (everted intestine) method is based on the preparation of a 2- to 3-cm long tube of the gut, which is tied off at the ends after evertion on a glass rod (Kararli, 1989). The serosa becomes the inside of the sac, and the mucosa faces the outer buffer solution. As a modification of this procedure, the serosal layer and muscular layers can also be stripped off before evertion on the glass rod (Hillgren et al., 1995). The presence or absence of the serosal layer may give different transport rates of compounds, for example, salicylic acid (Hillgren et al., 1995). This has also been found for the Ussing chamber technique (see section "Ussing chamber"). An oxygenated buffer solution is injected into the sac, which is put into a flask containing the drug of interest. Samples of fluid are taken from the buffer solution in the flask. The sac is weighed before and after the experiments to compensate for fluid movement. In one modification of the method, one end of the tissue is cannulated with a polyethylene tubing (Kararli, 1989), also making it easier to withdraw samples from the serosal side of the intestine.

An advantage of this method is that it is rapid and many drugs can be tested simultaneously, especially low-permeability drugs, owing to the low volume of the serosal compartment. There is good performance as regards stirring conditions on the mucosal side, although the oxygenation of the tissue is poor, as a result of the unstirred and unoxygenated serosal layer inside the uncannulated sac. Another advantage of this method is that it needs no specialized equipment, in contrast to the Ussing chamber and cell culture models.

Disadvantages are mainly the viability issue and the diffusion through the lamina propria. Histological studies have shown that structural changes start as early as five minutes after the start of incubation, and a total disruption of the epithelial tissue can be seen after one hour (Levine et al., 1970). As for intestinal rings, there is no correction for the binding of drug substance onto the surface of the mucosa (when uncannulated sacs are used).

Ussing Chamber

The Ussing chamber technique is an old technique for studying transport across an epithelium, developed by Ussing and Zerhan in 1951. It has been used extensively in physiological studies concerning the pharmacology and physiology of ion and water fluxes across the intestinal wall. It has also recently been used for drug absorption studies using excised intestinal tissues from different animals—rabbits, dogs, rats, or monkeys (Palm et al., 1996; Ungell et al., 1997; Artursson et al., 1993; Jezyk et al., 1992; Rubas et al., 1993; Polentarutti et al., 1999)—and for human biopsies (Bijlsma et al., 1995; Söderholm et al., 1998). The method is generally based on excision of intestinal segments from the animal. These segments may be stripped of the serosa and the muscle layers and mounted between two diffusion half-cells (Grass and Sweetana, 1988) (Fig. 11). The permeability coefficients

$$P_{\text{app}} = \frac{dq}{dt} \times \frac{1}{AC_0}$$

of the compounds are calculated from the measurement of the rate of transport, dQ/dt, of molecules from one side of the segment to the other (either mucosa to serosa or serosa to mucosa), divided by the exposed area of the segment (A) and the donor concentration of the drug (C_0).

Stirring of the solutions on both sides of the membrane is very important, especially for lipophilic drugs (Karlsson and Artursson, 1991). This can be achieved either by a gas lift system, as originally proposed by Ussing and Zerhan (1951), by a more refined gas lift system, as shown by Grass and Sweetana (1988), or by stirring with rotors (Polentarutti et al., 1999). The viability of the tissues is verified with the measurement of potential difference (*PD*), short circuit current, and calculation of the transepithelial electrical resistance by Ohm's

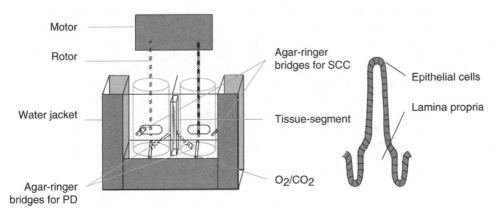

Many cell types in the epithelium and presence of a
crypt-villus axis and lamina propria

Figure 11 Schematic drawing of an Ussing chamber. Excised tissues from the animal intestine are stripped of the serosal and muscle layers and are mounted in between the two chamber halves. The experiment is run by adding the compound to one side and taking out samples from the other side for up to several hours after excision at 37°C. Oxygenation of the tissue can be performed separately from the stirring of the solutions. The viability of the tissue can be monitored simultaneously using a voltmeter and connected current generator.

law (Polentarutti et al., 1999; Söderholm et al., 1998; Ungell et al., 1992; Bijlsma et al., 1995; Sutton et al., 1992). The values that set the limits of viability should be in the range of what has been measured in vivo, for example, for rat jejunum and ileum, 5 and 6 mV, respectively. Extracellular marker molecules such as mannitol, inulin, Na-fluorescein, and PEG 4000 have been used to verify a tight epithelium (for references, see Pantzar et al., 1994) and for testing effects of enhancers and increased fluid absorption (Borchardt et al., 1996; Karlsson et al., 1994, 1999). It has also become very popular to verify a viable and intact epithelium using biochemical markers such as lactate dehydrogenase (LDH) release (Oberle et al., 1995) and morphology evaluations (Polentarutti et al., 1999; Söderholm et al., 1998). The more viable the segment, the better the interpretation of the results. Extreme values of permeability values can be discarded from the data set giving better and more reliable results and a better overall understanding of drug transport (Polentarutti et al., 1999). The model has also been used for identifying metabolites formed during transport (Ungell et al., 1992) and evaluation of carrier-mediated transport and prodrugs (Schwaan et al., 1995), although not as extensively as Caco-2.

This method has several advantages for predicting in vivo drug absorption in humans. First, there is a good correlation with the permeability coefficients of human jejunum in vivo (Lennernäs et al., 1997) for both passively transported and low- and high-permeability compounds. Second, the technique can be used for different regions of the GI tract, evaluating the regional absorption characteristics of drugs (Ungell et al., 1997; Polentarutti et al., 1999; Jezyk et al., 1992; Narawane et al., 1993; Pantzar et al., 1993). Furthermore, mucosal types (buccal, nasal, esophageal, stomach, rectal, skin) other than the intestine can be used, making it possible to evaluate other administration sites with the same model. The method using diffusion cells can also be employed for cultured monolayers using a modified insert for the monolayer membrane. The method is very useful for evaluating mechanisms of absorption. It can shed light on the importance of ionic transport processes on the transport of drug molecules because of the physiological presence of a crypt-villus axis and a heterogeneous population of cells (mature and immature as well as cells with different functions). The method also has the advantage of being available for human tissues, slices, or biopsies from surgically removed tissues (Bijlsma et al., 1995; Söderholm et al., 1998), which represents one of the most challenging developments of this method for future screening of drugs, especially for mechanistic studies and enzymatic evaluation of drugs and prodrugs for which experiments with human tissue are needed.

The major disadvantage of this absorption method is the diffusion pathways for the molecules, which are unphysiological, that is, the lack of vascular supply forces the molecules to diffuse through the lamina propria, and in the case where unstripped tissues are also used, through the serosal layer. It was recently proposed that the presence of the serosal and muscular layers might have different impacts on the transport of molecules with different physicochemical characteristics, which are both size and lipophilicity dependent (Breitholtz et al., 1999). The lamina propria, muscle layers, and serosal layer can also be different in the different animals and regional segments. Some reports have also proposed that there may be difficulties with the unstirred water layers and that there is concern regarding the stirring conditions, especially of the solution in the donor compartment. Segments from animals are often used (as for most of the absorption models), which must then be verified for human tissue. This is especially important metabolically and for carrier-mediated transport processes. The integrity and viability of the tissue must be verified simultaneously because it will strongly impair the transport of the drug molecules (see above). The model is probably not designated as an HTS tool. However, correctly used as a mechanistic secondary screening tool, data from the Ussing chamber technique are more closely related to the human situation than many of the other biological methods available.

Intestinal Perfusion Method

There are reports in the literature on the isolated perfused intestine as a technique for absorption studies and in situ perfusions (Blanchard et al., 1990; Oeschsenfahrt and Winne, 1974; Chiou, 1995; Krugliak et al., 1994; Fagerholm et al., 1996). A segment of 10 to 30 cm of the

Perfusion of intestine (gut loop)

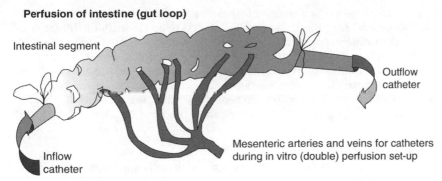

Isolated intestinal segment with intact blood flow or using artificial fluid.
With (in situ)(single perfusion) or without liver (in vitro)(double perfusion

Figure 12 Schematic drawing of the intestinal perfusion technique. The intestine of the animal is catheterized at both ends, and a flow of buffer solution of 37°C is perfused using a pump. For in vitro studies in which only the absorption over the intestine is to be measured, the vascular support can be cannulated and a separate buffer solution can be perfused through the intestine. If the influence of the liver on drug absorption is to be studied, an in situ system with an intact anesthetized animal can be used by only perfusion of the intestine, keeping the blood flow of the vascular support intact.

intestine is cannulated on both ends and perfused with a buffer solution at a flow rate of 0.2 mL/min (Fagerholm et al., 1996) (Fig. 12). The blood side can also be cannulated through the mesenteric vein and artery. The difference between in situ and in vitro is the use of the rat circulation in vivo (which is a vascular perfusion in the in vitro situation) (Windmueller et al., 1970; Fagerholm et al., 1996). This then gives the opportunity of evaluating the influence of hepatic clearance on the absorption of drugs.

Both the perfusion methods can use different evaluation systems for testing drug absorption, using the difference between "in" and "out" concentrations in the perfusion solutions and/or disappearance and appearance on both sides of the membrane and also by analyzing the drug concentration on the blood side. The permeability, usually called the P_{eff}, is calculated from the following equation:

$$P_{\text{eff}} = -Q_{\text{in}} \times \frac{\ln(C_{\text{out}}/C_{\text{in}})}{2\pi r L} \text{ (parallel tube model)} \qquad (3)$$

where Q_{in} is the flow rate, C_{in} and C_{out} are the inlet and outlet concentrations of each drug, respectively, and $2\pi r L$ is the mass transfer surface area within the intestinal segment. Different lengths are used between 10 and 30 cm, but the best flow characteristics are achieved with 10 cm (Fagerholm et al., 1996). PEG 4000 is used for corrections of fluid flow and to verify the absence of leakage in the model. In addition, as for the Ussing chamber using excised segments and Caco-2 cells, many use mannitol as a permeability marker molecule (Krugliak et al., 1994). This is more sensitive to changes in the intestinal barrier function compared with PEG 4000 alone. In situ perfusions have recently been extensively used for mechanistic studies of efflux of drugs (Lindahl et al., 1999).

The major advantage of this type of absorption method is the presence of a blood supply giving the tissue oxygen and the correct flow characteristics on the serosal side of the membrane, for example, less diffusion through the lamina propria. Second, different parts of the GI tract can be used, as in the Ussing chamber technique. Good stirring, that is, flow characteristics, of the mucosal/luminal solution has been reported (Fagerholm et al., 1996). A very good correlation with perfusions has been found to the human fraction absorbed and human permeability of different types of drugs (Fagerholm et al., 1996; Amidon et al., 1988).

The disadvantage of the method is the use of anesthesia, which has been reported to affect drug absorption (Uhing and Kimura, 1995a,b). PEG 4000 is used to verify the integrity of the barrier, which can lead to misinterpretation of the integrity of the tissue due to the high molecular weight of the marker. An additional disadvantage, although less important for mechanistic studies, is that the method is time and animal consuming, which makes it less useful for screening purposes. Some discrepancies between the disappearance rates of drugs and their appearance on the blood side have also been reported, indicating a loss of the drug in the system either by enzymatic degradation or by adhesion to the plastic catheters.

In Vivo Biological Methods

Methods primarily used are in situ perfusions of the rat gut, regionally cannulated/fistulated rats and dogs, bioavailability models in different animals, intestinal perfusions in human (Loc-i-Gut) (Lennernäs et al., 1992) (Fig. 13), and triple-lumen perfusions (Gramatté et al., 1994) and bioavailability studies in human.

For regional absorption assessments in small animals like rat, the drug substance is usually administered via a cannula situated in the region to be tested, intraduodenal, intrajejunal, intraileal, or intracolonic. Blood samples are withdrawn from an arteric/venous cannula inserted in the carotid artery/jugular vein (Borchardt et al., 1996; Sjöström et al., 1999). For regional absorption assessment in the dog, a chronic fistula is surgically inserted in the region of interest and blood samples are taken from superficial veins in the forelegs (Borchardt et al., 1996). Regional absorption differences can be seen for a compound as regards permeability coefficients (Ungell et al., 1997) and metabolism in the intestinal lumen, in the brush-border region or within the cells of the epithelium. The importance of good regional absorption performance (e.g., high and similar absorption throughout the GI tract) of a selected compound may be crucial for the development of ER formulations and should therefore be evaluated early in the screening phase for optimal drug candidate selection.

These complex studies are usually very time consuming and cost ineffective and are too complex for detailed evaluation of the mechanisms of absorption. Furthermore, only drugs that have been approved as nontoxic can be used for studies in human, and these methods are

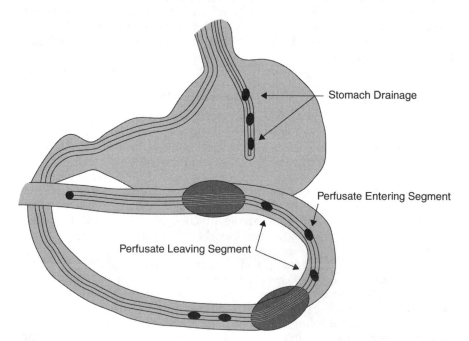

Figure 13 The multichannel tube system with double balloons allowing for segmental jejunal perfusion. The balloons are filled with air when the proximal balloon has passed the ligament of Treitz. Gastric suction is obtained by a separate tube. *Source*: From Lennernäs et al. (1992).

thus not used early in development studies. However, for the completeness of the understanding of the absorption of a certain drug, for correct information to support the pharmaceutical dosage form program, and for correlation of the performance of the more simple animal models, some experiments must be performed in vivo in animals and in humans early in the clinical phase. Such experiments include membrane permeability coefficient assessment; absorption, distribution, metabolism, and excretion (ADME) studies; dose and concentration dependency; food interactions; regional absorption performance; and evaluation of enhancer systems. All in vitro methods used, regardless of what mechanism or part of the absorption process they represent, must be correlated to the in vivo situation and, if possible, also to absorption in humans. This is not a simple evaluation since different methods represent different parts of the total process and the main barrier will affect the main part of the results. Values for in vivo absorption in human are not easy to obtain, and the values are often a result of a recalculation of data obtained for other purposes. The values of F_a for drugs in the literature are therefore most uncertain. Published, compiled data on bioavailability can be found in Benet et al. (1996).

More mechanistic studies in humans during phase I must be performed for better feedback to discovery and pharmaceutical development, and thereby for faster performance through the clinical phases. It was recently suggested that a biopharmaceutical classification of drug permeability coefficients and dissolution issues must be determined early in the development program for rational drug design (Amidon, 1996).

PERMEABILITY COEFFICIENTS VS. F_a

Using the HT-29 to 18-C1 cell line, permeabilities of various molecules have been compared with in vivo oral data (Wils et al., 1994b). This report found a threshold value of 2×10^{-6} cm/sec. Over this value, the drugs showed more than 80% absorption in vivo, and were poorly absorbed below this value. A similar threshold value can be seen for Caco-2 cells (1×10^{-6} cm/sec) (Artursson and Karlsson, 1991) and, according to a recent paper by Yazdanian et al. (1997) (0.5×10^{-6} cm/sec), for excised jejunal segments of rat in the Ussing chamber (10×10^{-6} cm/sec) (Lennernäs et al., 1997), for perfusion of the rat jejunum and for the perfused human jejunum in vivo (0.5×10^{-4} cm/sec) (Fagerholm et al., 1996). These threshold values indicate a parallel shift for different methods concerning the predictive permeability versus F_a in vivo, which was recently suggested for the methods of in situ rat perfusion, Ussing chamber with rat jejunal segments, and the perfusion of the human jejunum (Lennernäs et al., 1997) and at different laboratories using the same Caco-2 cell model (Artursson et al., 1996). The parallel shift for permeability coefficients between different methods and animals is expected since the lipid membrane composition can vary with both species and diet (Thomson et al., 1986; Ungell et al., 1997). There is no cause for concern if the ranking order is the same between the methods used.

The values of the permeability coefficients also indicate experimental windows of different sizes. The Caco-2 cells seem to operate roughly between 0.1 and 200×10^{-6} cm/sec (Artursson and Karlsson, 1991), the excised segments in the Ussing chamber between 1 and 200×10^{-6} cm/sec and the perfused rat intestine and perfused human jejunum between 0.1 and 10×10^{-4} cm/sec. A difference in the operating window can also be seen for the same model at different laboratories. Yazdanian and coworkers recently published permeability values for a vast number of compounds using the Caco-2 cell model (Yazdanian et al., 1997). In spite of the large data set in this paper, the values are difficult to interpret since they form an "all-or-none" shape of the correlation curve to F_a in humans, and the steep part of the curve shows a very narrow range in permeability values. For instance, there is a 100-fold change in F_a that shows a minor change in the permeability value, for example, 0.38×10^{-6} cm/sec for ganciclovir to 0.51×10^{-6} cm/sec for acebutalol (Yazdanian et al., 1997). The reason for this phenomenon is not known. Owing to differences in the handling of animals, age, species, food, tissues, tissue media, clones of cultured cells, or different passages, laboratories will have different prediction factors for absorption when they use the different methods available (Artursson et al., 1996; Thomson et al., 1986; Ungell et al., 1997; Ungell, 1997).

The ranking order between the different drugs might also be different between laboratories because of the different levels of viability and integrity of the biological systems used (Ungell, 1997). The integrity of the tissue change is time related, which means that there is a limit in time for use of the different systems (Levine et al., 1970; Polentarutti et al., 1999). It may also be related to buffer solutions, oxygenation of the solutions, stirring conditions, preparation of the tissues and other physical handling, and temperature (Ungell, 1997). The surface exposed to the drug is different in different models and for high- and low-permeability drugs, as suggested by Artursson et al. (1996) and Strocchi and Levitt (1993). The "true" exposed surface area is the same as the serosal surface area for cultured monolayers (Artursson et al., 1996) but is very variable for excised segments for the Ussing chamber or perfusions, depending on which region of the GI tract is used. As a result of different handling during preparation of the tissues, the effective surface area for absorption may also be different, and a time-dependent change in surface area during the course of the experiments has been reported (Polentarutti et al., 1999). The change in area by time will affect high- and low-permeability drugs differently (Strocchi and Levitt, 1993). For a full understanding of the differences in results between laboratories and between species, these parameters may perhaps be useful as a complement to other valuable information regarding the performance of the experiments and the technique used.

The variability between experiments and laboratories presents difficulties when comparing values from different laboratories. Each laboratory should therefore be careful in standardizing and correlating their own models to human absorption values before using them as predictive tools. Indeed, the guidelines from FDA regarding the use of a compound data set for classification of their candidate drugs using the BCS could be helpful in standardizing in vitro techniques (Amidon, 1996).

IN VIVO TECHNIQUES FOR STUDIES IN HUMAN

The physicochemical tests, in vitro methods, and animal experiments used in the biopharmaceutical preformulation phase can never fully reflect the conditions in human, and studies of the drug absorption prerequisites can therefore be very valuable. This is especially relevant if (1) contradictory results have been obtained in model experiments, (2) the substance has complicated absorption properties (e.g., active transport), or (3) a modified release formulation will be developed. The most important information that can be obtained in such human studies is

- intestinal drug permeability/absorption and
- bioavailability after administration at different regions in the GI tract.

This type of study is not only useful for drug substance characterization prior to formulation development but may also be performed to elucidate absorption effects of certain formulation components.

Intestinal Permeability Measurements

The extent of absorption is determined by several drug properties such as dissolution, degradation/metabolism in the GI lumen, and permeability over the GI wall. Human intestinal permeability can be quantified in vivo by the use of an intubation technique called Loc-i-Gut (Lennernäs et al., 1996) (Fig. 13). This is a multichannel tube with two balloons, which is positioned in the proximal jejunum. A closed segment is created in the jejunum by inflating the two balloons. Thereafter, an isotonic drug solution is continuously perfused through the intestine, and sampling from the segment for assessment of drug concentrations is performed in parallel. The intestinal permeability (P_{eff}) is calculated by the following equation:

$$P_{\text{eff}} = \frac{(C_{\text{in}} - C_{\text{out}})}{(C_{\text{out}})} \times \frac{Q_{\text{in}}}{2\pi rL} \tag{4}$$

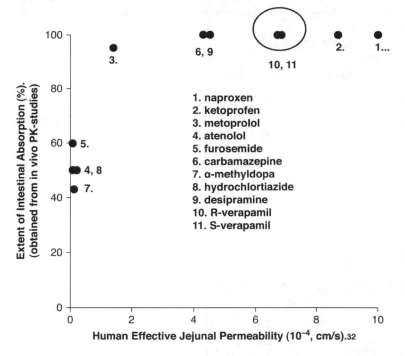

Figure 14 The relationship between fraction absorbed (F_a) drug in humans after oral administration and jejunal gut wall permeability is determined in humans for different drugs.

where C_{in} and C_{out} are the drug concentrations in the inlet solution and in the perfusate leaving the tube, respectively, and Q_{in} is the flow rate of the inlet solution. The surface of the closed segment is described by $2\pi rL$, where L is the length (10 cm) and r is the intestinal radius (1.75 cm). The recovery of a nonabsorbable marker is used to check that no fluid is leaking out of the closed segment.

The intestinal permeability has been determined by this technique for a large number of substances (Tamamatsu et al., 1997). A relationship between P_{eff} and the extent of absorption has also been established (Fig. 14), which has clearly shown that permeability can be the limiting step in the absorption process and that a certain permeability (about 4×10^{-4} cm/sec) is needed to obtain complete absorption.

It is also possible to study the influence of active carriers on the transport over the intestinal mucosa by this technique. This can be done by comparing the P_{eff} with and without an inhibitor of the carrier system in the perfusion solution or by comparing the P_{eff} for different drug concentrations in the perfusion solution. For example, the P_{eff} of verapamil was increased at higher drug concentrations in the perfusion solution (Sandström et al., 1998). An active efflux of the drug into the lumen by P-glycoprotein membrane transporters could explain this, since verapamil is known to be a substrate for this carrier.

Regional Bioavailability Assessment
The bioavailability of a drug after administration to different regions in the GI tract can be determined either by remote-control capsules or by intubation techniques. The two most frequently used remote-control devices, the "high-frequency capsule" and InteliSite, are shown in Figure 15A, B (Parr et al., 1999). The drug must be dissolved or suspended in a small volume (1 mL), which is included in a chamber or balloon in the remote-control device. The location of the device in the GI tract is determined by fluoroscopy or γ scintigraphy. When the target location has been reached, "microwaves" externally trigger a drug release mechanism and the drug appears in the intestine as a bolus dose. Markers such as radionuclides can also

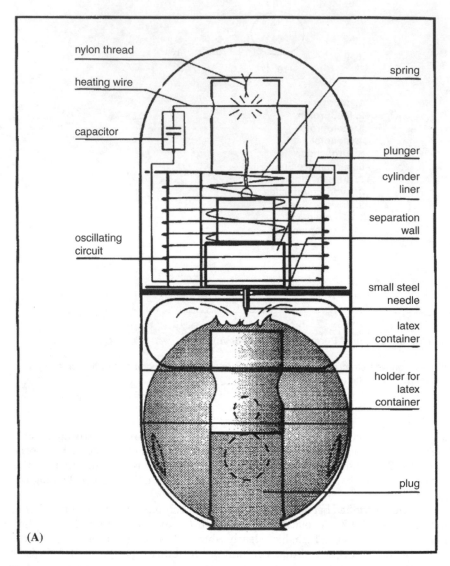

Figure 15 **(A)** The HF capsule. When the capsule has reached the intended region, it is exposed to an HF field. This induces an increased temperature in a heating wire, which leads to melting of a nylon thread and release of a steel needle. The needle perforates a latex balloon, which contains the drug solution, and the drug is released. **(B)** The InteliSite™ capsule. When the capsule has reached the desired location, it is exposed to a magnetic field, which increases the temperature in the capsule. This causes two memory alloys to straighten, which rotates the inner sleeve of the capsule. A series of slots in the sleeve surface are thereby aligned, and the drug solution is released through the openings. *Abbreviation*: HF, high frequency. (*Continued*)

be included in the device together with the drug solution to verify when drug release occurs (Bode et al., 1996).

Different intubation techniques have been used for regional absorption studies. The terminal ileum and colon can be reached either by an oral tube (Abrahamsson et al., 1997) or by colonoscopy (Gleiter et al., 1985; Parr et al., 1999). In the latter case, the tube is inserted "from the end of the colon." The position of the tube is determined by fluoroscopy before administering the drug, preferably as a solution, through the tube.

Both the types of technique have been shown to provide very valuable results, but certain pros and cons can be identified. For example, multiple doses are possible, and the rate of drug administration can be varied in the case of intubation, whereas this is presently not possible for

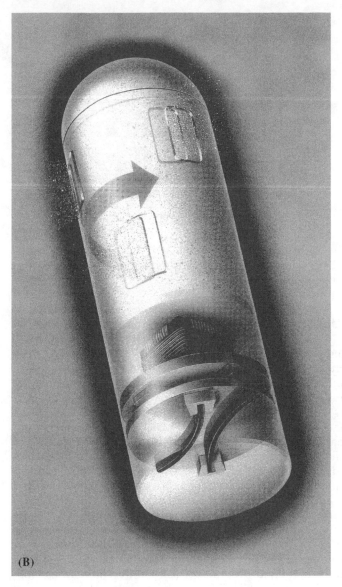

Figure 15 (*Continued*)

remote-control devices. The potential risk of not obtaining appropriate drug release at the desired site is lower for intubations, owing to its simplicity, as compared with the more highly technological remote-control devices. On the other hand, the tube or the perfusion may disturb the normal physiological flow conditions in the intestine. Furthermore, in the case of colonoscopy, the colon content must be emptied before insertion of the colonoscope, which leads to unphysiological test conditions. For both the types of technique, it is crucial to investigate drug adhesion/partitioning to the device material and drug stability for relevant time periods before starting any in vivo experiments.

In these studies, standard bioavailability variables such as the extent of bioavailability determined from area under the curve (AUC), rate of bioavailability related to peak plasma drug levels (C_{max}), and time to peak (t_{max}) are determined. A more detailed presentation of the assumptions and interpretations of bioavailability data is given in chapter 7. The bioavailability after administration in more distal parts of the intestine, such as the terminal ileum and different parts of the colon, is compared with a reference administration either as

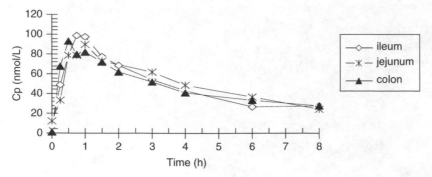

Figure 16 Mean plasma concentration of metoprolol after administration of a solution to three different regions in the GI tract by use of an intubation technique.

an oral solution or as a regional delivery to the upper small intestine. This is exemplified in Figure 16, which shows the plasma drug concentrations of metoprolol after administration to jejunum, terminal ileum, and colon ascendens or transversum.

VEHICLES FOR ABSORPTION STUDIES

Early preformulation studies are often performed to obtain initial information regarding drug absorption but may be restricted by solubility problems of the active drug. During early studies, such as in vitro methods and in vivo methods using animals, *vehicles to solubilize* the molecule are used. However, as many of these vehicles are surfactants or lipid systems, they may also act as "membrane breakers" and are therefore classified as enhancers of absorption (Oberle et al., 1995; van Hoogdalem et al., 1989; Swenson et al., 1994; Anderberg and Artursson, 1994). The absorption enhancers/vehicles may act differently on the permeability of low- and high-permeability drugs and may also affect carrier-mediated transport or metabolism, for example, chremophore and Tween 80, which are known to inhibit P-glycoprotein (Hunter and Hirst, 1997). The membrane integrity may be impaired, and whether it is the lipid fluidity or the tight junctions that are affected depends on the concentration and on the vehicle system used. The outcome of the use of the vehicle system will thereby depend on the physicochemical nature of the drug and on the metabolic pathway or transport mechanism or route it uses. There are very few reports showing the effects of vehicle systems on the integrity of the mucosal membrane. Excised intestinal segments in the Ussing chamber have been used to verify the change in permeability to mannitol and propranolol using different vehicles, both surfactant and lipid-based systems (Hanisch et al., 1998). Effects of surfactants on the viability of mucosal tissues have been reported using LDH release (Oberle et al., 1995), change in transepithelial electrical resistance (TEER) over Caco-2 cells (Anderberg and Artursson, 1994), and lipid vehicles such as monoglycerides (Borchardt et al., 1996; Yeh et al., 1994). A more comprehensive report on vehicles used can be found in Ingels et al. (2007).

At present, no inert vehicle system is available that in general will solubilize all sparingly soluble compounds during in vitro screening or that is specifically intended for in vivo administration in animals. This is, of course, impossible, since the molecules have different structural backbones and behaviors in aqueous solutions and thus have different physicochemical properties. Instead, it is advisable to use a vehicle with as few side effects as possible and, in addition, to standardize screening and to test the particular vehicle in vitro and in vivo using marker molecules (Hanisch et al., 1998, 1999; Ingels et al., 2007).

Many vehicles also give analytical problems when liquid chromatography–mass spectrometry (LC-MS) is used, for example, PEG 400, chremophoreEL, and solutol. The vehicle may, of course, impair the pharmacological effect and activity of the active drug or receptor. This must be taken into account when choosing the right vehicle for discovery screening tests and early preformulation studies.

Table 9 Most Commonly Used Classes of Enhancers to Drug Absorption from the Gastrointestinal Tract

Nonsteroidal anti-inflammatory drugs and derivatives	Mixed micelles
Sodium salicylate	Glyceryl monooleate + sodium taurocholate
Sodium 5-methoxysalicylate	Linoleic acid + HCO60
Indomethacin	Calcium-binding agents
Diclofenac	Ethylenediaminetetraacetic acid (EDTA)
Surfactants	Phenothiazines
Nonionic: polyoxyethylene ethers	Chlorpromazine
Anionic: sodium laurylsulfate	Liposomes
Cationic: quaternary ammonium compounds	Azone
Bile salts	Fatty acid derivatives of carnitine and peptides
Dihydroxy bile salts: sodium deoxycholate	Palmitoyl-DL-carnitine
Trihydroxy bile slats: sodium cholate	N-myristoyl-L-propyl-L-propyl-glycinate
Derivative: sodium tauro-24,25-dihydrofusidate	Saponins
Medium-chain fatty acids	Concanavalin A
Octanoic acid	Phosphate and phosphonate derivatives
Medium-chain glycerides	DL-α-Glycerophosphate
Glyceryl-1-monooctanoate	β-Amino-1-hydroxypropylidene-1,1-diphosphonate
Glyceryl-1-monooctanoate	Polyacrylic acid
Enamines	Diethyl maleate and diethylethoxy-
DL-Phenylalanine ethylacetoacetate enamine	Methylene malonate

Source: From van Hoogdalem et al. (1989).

Systems that *enhance drug absorption* do not always contain ingredients that act on the epithelial membrane (increased membrane permeability) but act by other mechanisms, such as by increasing the solubility, changing pH at the absorption site, or decreasing the binding to luminal material. The result of the enhancement is then an increased force in the absorption process, that is, the effective concentration at the absorption site. Some examples in the literature of enhancers can be seen in Table 9.

We must very often consider an enhancer system to be able to develop a dosage form for a drug with low bioavailability because of the difficulty in performing any more structural changes without loss of potency. The Caco-2 cells, Ussing chambers, and perfused intestinal segments methods are often used for enhancer studies or evaluation of the toxicity of the enhancers (Anderberg and Artursson, 1994; van Hoogdalem et al., 1989; LeCluyse and Sutton, 1997; Ingels et al., 2007). It has been found that the effects of enhancers on the biological system are both species and method related. For instance, it has been found that Caco-2 cell monolayers are very sensitive to surfactants, and the rat intestinal tract seems to be more sensitive than that of the rabbit (Anderberg and Artursson, 1994). Some enhancers have also been used in delivery systems for humans. Best known are the salts of the fatty acids caprate and caprylate (C8 and C10), which have been used for rectal administration of antibiotic drugs such as cefoxitin (Lindmark et al., 1997). The toxic or sensory feeling experienced with the use of the enhancers in humans has not been fully evaluated. Enhancer systems using mixtures of monoglycerides (C8 and C10), intended to increase the oral absorption in humans of a large number of different types of poorly absorbable drugs, have recently been patented, and studies on the mechanisms behind the enhancer effect have also been published (LeCluyse and Sutton, 1997; Sekine et al., 1985; van Hoogdalem et al., 1989; Constantinides, 1993; Yeh et al., 1994; Borchardt et al., 1996).

FUNCTIONAL USE OF ABSORPTION MODELS

There are different strategies for the use of these absorption models in the industry, for example, screening of structural analogues, mechanistic studies, and problem solving, as well as in early formulation perspectives and correlation to in vivo data. This means that there is no ultimate method for both the discovery and development of pharmaceutical drugs, but rather a battery of models to be used in different phases of the projects. The functional use of the different models available could be to use computational methods for the large majority of compounds, both to select drugs of interest for synthesis and to gather information on what important factors will govern the molecule through the membrane via the different transport routes (see section "Absorption/Uptake over the GI Membranes"). When analogues have been synthesized, a selected group of compounds could be run in HTS screens for solubility, permeability, and metabolic stability. The information is entered in the computational models to gather additional data and simultaneously also put into more complex prediction models of absorption and used for correlation to in vivo values found in animals. The more complex secondary screening models should also address the biopharmaceutical aspects, that is, solubility, interactions in the gut lumen, regional permeability/absorption differences, and degradation by bacteria.

HTS is mostly used in the initial phase in the discovery process, where chemical entities are tested for biological activity in specific target assays. The technology and the high-throughput standardization have also lately been discussed for the structure/absorption relationship using Caco-2 cell monolayers or other cell lines as well as intrinsic clearance determination (half-lives) for structure/stability evaluation. The overall strategy for the industry is to use this screening tool as efficiently as possible, and not necessarily for all compounds in the chemical library. The standardized systems have a high throughput where thousands of chemical compounds can be tested in a short period of time and where the time for feedback into the projects is the most important success factor. Because of the importance of the measured values resulting from such assays for a forthcoming candidate drug selection, the importance of the assay for correct prediction of the human situation becomes evident.

As concerns the absorption of drugs in the GI tract, HTS in the industry has focused on Caco-2 cell monolayer permeability assays. Other cell lines have been and are also currently being used, such as MDCK, T84 cells, CHO cells, LDCK, HT-29, and other clones of Caco-2. The purpose of using cell lines at this stage is to proceed quickly to the next step of the evaluation of a potentially available oral drug, which requires only a representative value for acceptable or nonacceptable permeability. The cell lines differ in the presence of carrier-mediated transport systems and metabolic activity, and thus the outcome differs. For the design of more specific screening tools, for example, transporters, specific cells of a certain age and differentiation are used (Döppenschmitt et al., 1998; Anderle et al., 1998; Delie and Rubas, 1997) as are cloned human transporters in cells (Artursson and Borchardt, 1997).

REFERENCES

Abdou H, ed. Theory of dissolution. In: Dissolution, Bioavailability & Bioequivalence. Easton: MACK Publishing Company, 1989:11–36.

Abrahamsson B, Lindström K, Nyberg L, et al. Regional absorption of metoprolol in humans determined by a new method suitable for studies in the whole gastro-intestinal (GI) tract. Proc Control Release Soc 1997; 24:359–360.

Altomare C, Carotti A, Trapani G, et al. Estimation of partitioning parameters of non-ionic surfactants using calculated descriptors of molecular size, polarity, and hydrogen bonding. J Pharm Sci 1997; 86:1417–1425.

Ambre JJ, Fuher LT. Effect of coadministration of aluminium and magnesium hydroxides on absorption of anticoagulants in man. Clin Pharmacokinet Ther 1973; 14:231.

Amidon GL. A biopharmaceutic classification system: update May 1996. In: Biopharmaceutics Drug Classification and International Drug Regulation. Bornem, Belgium: Capsugel Symposium Services, 1996:11–30.

Amidon GL, Sinko PJ, Fleisher D. Estimating human oral fraction dose absorbed: a correlation using rat intestinal membrane permeability for passive and carrier-mediated compounds. Pharm Res 1988; 5:651–654.

Amidon LG, Lennernäs H, Shah VP, et al. Theoretical considerations in the correlation of in vitro drug product dissolution and in vivo bioavailability: a basis for biopharmaceutical drug classification. Pharm Res 1995; 12:413–420.

Anderberg EK, Artursson P. Cell cultures to access drug absorption enhancement. In: de Boer AG, ed. Drug Absorption Enhancement. Reading: Harwood Academic Publishers, 1994:101–118.

Anderle P, Niederer E, Rubas W, et al. P-glycoprotein (P-gp) mediated efflux in Caco-2 cell monolayers: the influence of culturing conditions and drug exposure on P-gp expression levels. J Pharm Sci 1998; 87:757–762.

Arlotto MP, Trant JM, Estabrook RW. Measurement of steroid hydroxylation reactions by high performance liquid chromatography as indicator of P450 identity and function. Methods Enzymol 1991; 206:454–462.

Artursson P. Epithelial transport of drugs in cell culture I: a model for studying the passive diffusion of drugs over intestinal epithelia. J Pharm Sci 1990; 79:476–482.

Artursson P, Borchardt R. Intestinal drug absorption and metabolism in cell cultures: Caco-2 and beyond. Pharm Res 1997; 14:1655–1658.

Artursson P, Karlsson J. Correlation between oral drug absorption in humans and apparent drug permeability coefficients in human intestinal epithelial (Caco-2) cells. Biochem Biophys Res Commun 1991; 175:880–885.

Artursson P, Palm K, Luthman K. Caco-2 monolayers in experimental and theoretical predictions of drug transport. Adv Drug Deliv Rev 1996; 22:67–84.

Artursson P, Tavelin S. Studies of membrane permeability and oral absorption. Caco-2 and emerging alternatives for prediction of intestinal drug transport: a general overview. In: Van de Waterbeemd H, Lennernäs H, Artursson P, eds. Drug Bioavailability—Estimation of Solubility, Permeability and Absorption. Weinhem: Wiley-VCH, 2003: 72–89.

Artursson P, Ungell AL, Löfroth JE. Selective paracellular permeability in two models of intestinal absorption: cultured monolayers of human intestinal epithelial cells and rat intestinal segments. J Pharm Res 1993; 10:1123–1129.

Augustijns P, Annaert P, Heylen P, et al. Drug absorption studies of prodrugs esters using the Caco-2 model: evaluation of ester hydrolysis and transepithelial transport. Int J Pharm 1998; 166:45–53.

Balon K, Riebesehl BU, Müller BW. Drug liposome partitioning as a tool for the prediction of human passive intestinal absorption. Pharm Res 1999; 16:882–888.

Beigi F, Gottschalk I, Lagerqvist Hägglund C, et al. Immobilized liposome and biomembrane partitioning chromatography of drugs for prediction of drug transport. Int J Pharm 1998; 164:129–137.

Benet LZ, Oie S, Schwartz JB. Design and optimization of dosage forms regimens: pharmacokinetic data. In: Hardman JG, Limbird LE, Molinoff PB, et al., eds. Goodman and Gilman's: Pharmacological Basis of Therapy. 9th ed. New York: McGraw-Hill, 1996:1707–1792.

Bijlsma PB, Peeters RA, Groot JA, et al. Differential in vivo and in vitro intestinal permeability to lactulose and mannitol in animals and humans: a hypothesis. Gastroenterology 1995; 108:687–696.

Blanchard J, Tang LM, Earle ME. Reevaluation of the absorption of carbenoxolone using an in situ rat intestinal technique. J Pharm Sci 1990; 79:411–414.

Bode H, Brendel E, Ahr G, et al. Investigation of nifedipine absorption in different regions of the human gastrointestinal (GI) tract after simultaneous administration of ^{13}C and ^{12}C nifedipine. Eur J Clin Pharmacol 1996; 50:195–201.

Borchardt R. Rational delivery strategies to circumvent physical and metabolic barriers to the oral absorption of peptides. In: Peptides. Theoretical and Practical Approaches to Their Delivery. Bornem, Belgium: Capsugel Library, 1991:9.

Borchardt RT, Smith PL, Wilson G. Models for Assessing Drug Absorption and Metabolism. New York: Plenum Press, 1996.

Breitholtz K, Hägg U, Utter L, et al. The influence of the serosal layer on viability and permeability of rat intestinal segments in the Ussing chamber. AAPS Pharm Sci Suppl 1999; 1:S653.

Burton PS, Conradi RA, Hilgers AR, et al. The relationship between peptide structure and transport across epithelial cell monolayers. J Control Release 1992; 19:87–97.

Charman WN, Porter CJH, Mithani S, et al. Physico-chemical and physiological mechanisms for the effects of food on drug absorption: the role of lipids and pH. J Pharm Sci 1997; 86:269–282.

Chiou WL. The validation of the intestinal permeability approach to predict oral fraction of dose absorbed in humans and rats. Biopharm Drug Dispos 1995; 16:71–75.

Chong S, Dando SA, Morrison RA. Evaluation of BIOCOAT® intestinal epithelium differentiation environment (3-day cultured Caco-2 cells) as an absorption screening model with improved productivity. Pharm Res 1997; 14:1835–1837.

Coates ME, Drasar BS, Mallett AK, et al. Methodological considerations for the study of bacterial metabolism. In: Rowland IR, ed. Role of the Gut Flora in Toxicity and Cancer. London: Academic Press, 1988:1–21.

Constantinides PP. Lipid microemulsions for improving drug dissolution and oral absorption: physical and biopharmaceutical aspects. Pharm Res 1993; 12:1561–1572.

Cruciani G, Crivori P, Carrupt PA, et al. Molecular fields in quantitative structure-permeation relationships: the Volsurf approach. J Mol Struct (Theochem) 2000; 503:17–30.

Dakas CJ, Takla PG. Physicochemical interactions affecting drug in the gastrointestinal tract: a review. Epitheo Klin Farmakol Farmakokinet Int 1991; 5(3):124–142.

Delie F, Rubas W. A human colonic cell line sharing similarities with enterocytes as a model to examine oral absorption: advantages and limitations of the Caco-2 model. Crit Rev Ther Drug Carrier Syst 1997; 14:221–286.

Delie R, Rubas W. Caco-2 monolayers as a tool to examine intestinal uptake of particulates. Proc Control Release Soc 1996; 3:149–150.

Döppenschmitt S, Spahn-Langguth H, Regardh CG, et al. Radioligand binding assay employing P-glycoprotein-overexpressing cells: testing drug affinities to the secretory intestinal multidrug transporter. Pharm Res 1998; 15:1001–1006.

Dressman JB, Amidon GL, Reppas C, et al. Dissolution testing as a prognostic tool for oral drug absorption: immediate release dosage forms. Pharm Res 1998; 15:11–22.

Dressman JB, Vertzoni M, Goumas K, et al. Estimating Drug solubility in the gastrointestinal tract. Adv Drug Deliv Res 2007; 59:591–602.

Dressman JB, Yamada K. Animal models for oral drug absorption. In: Welling PG, Tse FLS, eds. Pharmaceutical Bioequivalence. New York: Dekker, 1991:235–266.

Ekins S, Durst GL, Stratford RE, et al. Three-dimensional quantitative structure-permeability relationship analysis for a series of inhibitors of rhinovirus replication. J Chem Inf Comput Sci 2001; 41: 1578–1586.

EMEA. Note for guidance on the investigation of bioavailability and bioequivalence. Geneva, Switzerland: European Agency for the Evaluation of Medicinal Products, 1998.

Eriksson L, Johansson E, Kettaneh-Wold N, et al. Multi- and Megavariate Data Analysis using Projection Methods (PCA & PLS). Umea, Sweden: Umetrics, 1999.

Fagerholm U, Johansson M, Lennernäs H. The correlation between rat and human small intestinal permeability to drugs with different physico-chemical properties. Pharm Res 1996; 13:1335.

Fallingborg J, Christensen LA, Ingelman-Nielsen M, et al. Ph-profile and regional transit times of the normal gut measured by radiotelemetry device. Aliment Pharmacol Ther 1989; 3:605–613.

FDA. Guidance for Industry—Waiver of In Vivo Bioavailability and Bioequivalence Studies for Immediate Release Solid Dosage Forms Based on a Biopharmaceutics Classification System. Rockville, MD: Food and Drug Administration, 1999.

Ganong WF. Gastrointestinal function. Digestion and Absorption. In: Ganong WF, ed. Review of Medical Physiology. 7th ed. Los Altos, CA: Lange Medical Publications, 1975.

Garberg P, Eriksson P, Schipper N, et al. Automated absorption assessment using Caco-2 cells cultivated on both sides of polycarbonate membranes. Pharm Res 1999; 16:441–445.

Gibaldi M, Feldman S. Mechanisms of surfactant effects on drug absorption. J Pharm Sci 1970; 59: 579–588.

Gleiter CH, Antonin KH, Bieck P. Colonoscopy in the investigation of drug absorption in healthy volunteers. Gastrointest Endosc 1985; 31:71–73.

Goodford PJ. A computational method procedure for determining energetically favourable binding sites on biologically important macromolecules. J Med Chem 1985; 28:849–857.

Gramattè T, Desoky EE, Klotz U. Site-dependent small intestinal absorption of ranitidin. Eur J Clin Pharmacol 1994; 46:253–259.

Grass GM, Sweetana SA. In vitro measurement of gastrointestinal tissue permeability using a new diffusion cell. Pharm Res 1988; 5:372–376.

Grosvenor MP, Löfroth JE. Interaction between bile salts and beta-adrenoceptor antagonists. Pharm Res 1995; 12:682–686.

Hanisch G, Kjerling M, Pålsson A, et al. Effects of vehicles for sparingly soluble compounds on the drug absorption in vivo. Elderly People & Medicines, Stockholm Conference Center, Alvsjo, October 11–13, 1999; (abstr).

Hanisch G, von Corswant C, Breitholtz K, et al. Can mucosal damage be minimised during permeability measurements of sparingly soluble compounds? Fourth International Conference on Drug Absorption: Towards Prediction and Enhancement of Drug Absorption, Edinburgh, 1998.

Hayeshi R, Hilgendorf C, Artursson P, et al. Comparison of drug transporter gene expression and functionality in Caco-2 cells from 10 different laboratories. Eur J Pharm Sci 2008; 35:383–396.

Hidalgo IJ, Bhatnagar P, Lee C-P, et al. Structural requirements for interaction with the oligopeptide transporter in Caco-2 cells. Pharm Res 1995; 12:317–319.

Hidalgo IJ, Raub TJ, Borchardt RT. Characterization of the human colon carcinoma cell line (Caco-2) as a model for intestinal epithelial permeability. Gastroenterology 1989; 96:736–749.

Hillgren KM, Kato A, Borchardt RT. In vitro systems for studying intestinal drug absorption. Med Res Rev 1995; 15:83–109.

Hintz RJ, Johnson KC. The effect of particle size distribution on dissolution rate and oral absorption. Int J Pharm 1989; 51:9–17.

Hjort-Krarup L, Christensen IT, Hovgaard L, et al. Predicting drug absorption from molecular surface properties based on molecular dynamics simulations. Pharm Res 1998; 15:972–978.

Hunter J, Hirst BH. Intestinal secretion of drugs: the role of P-glycoprotein and related drug efflux systems in limiting oral drug absorption. Adv Drug Deliv Rev 1997; 25:129–157.

Hörter D, Dressman JB. Influence of physicochemical properties on dissolution of drugs in the gastrointestinal tract. Adv Drug Deliv Rev 1997; 25:3–14.

Illing HPA. Techniques for microfloral and associated metabolic studies in relation to the absorption and enterohepatic circulation of drugs. Xenobiotica 1981; 11:815–830.

Imai T, Imoto M, Sakamoto H, et al. Identification of esterases expressed in Caco-2 cells and effects of their hydrolyzing activity in predicting human intestinal absorption. Drug Metab Dispos 2005; 33:1185–1190.

Ingels F, Ungell A-L, Augustijns P. Selection of solvent system for membrane, cell and tissue based permeability assessment. In: Augustijns P, Brewster M,eds. Solvent Systems and Their Selection in Pharmaceutics and Biopharmaceutics. New York: Springer, 2007: 179–221.

Ishizawa T, Sadahiro S, Hosoi K, et al. Mechanisms of intestinal absorption of the antibiotic, fosfomycin, in brush-border membrane vesicles in rabbits and humans. J Pharmacobiodyn 1992; 15: 481–489.

Jezyk N, Rubas W, Grass GM. Permeability characteristics of various intestinal regions of rabbit, dog and monkey. Pharm Res 1992; 9:1580–1586.

Kaplan SA. Biopharmaceutical considerations in drug formulation design and evaluation. Drug Metab Rev 1972; 1:15–34.

Kararli TT. Gastrointestinal absorption of drugs. Crit Rev Ther Drug Carrier Syst 1989; 6:39–86.

Kararli TT. Comparison of the gastrointestinal anatomy, physiology, and biochemistry of humans and commonly used laboratory animals. Biopharm Drug Dispos 1995; 16:351.

Karlsson J, Artursson P. A method for the determination of cellular permeability coefficients and aqueous boundary layer thickness in monolayers of intestinal epithelial (Caco-2) cells grown in permeable filter chambers. Int J Pharm 1991; 71:51–64.

Karlsson J, Ungell AL, Artursson P. Effect of an oral rehydration solution on paracellular drug transport in intestinal epithelial cells and tissues: assessment of charge and tissues selectivity. Pharm Res 1994; 11:S248.

Karlsson J, Ungell AL, Grasjo J, et al. Paracellular drug transport across intestinal epithelia: influence of charge and induced water flux. Eur J Pharm Sci 1999; 9:47–56.

Kerneis S, Bogdanova A, Kraehenbuhl JP, et al. Conversion by Peyer's patch lymphocytes of human enterocytes into M cells that transport bacteria. Science 1997; 277:949–952.

Kessler M, Acuto O, Storelli C, et al. A modified procedure for the rapid preparation of efficiently transporting vesicles from small intestinal brush border membranes. Biochim Biophys Acta 1978; 506:136–154.

Kim CD, Burton PS, Borchardt RT. A correlation between the permeability characteristics of a series of peptides using an in vitro cell culture model (Caco-2) and those using an in situ perfused rat ileum model of the intestinal mucosa. Pharm Res 1993; 10:1710–1714.

Kim JS, Oberle RL, Krummel DA, et al. Absorption of ACE inhibitors from small intestine and colon. J Pharm Sci 1994; 83:1350–1356.

Korjamo T, Honkakoski P, Toppinen MR, et al. Absorption properties and P-glycoprotein activity of modified Caco-2 cell lines. Eur J Pharm Sci 2005; 26:266–279.

Krugliak P, Hollander D, Schlaepfer CC, et al. Mechanisms and sites of mannitol permeability of small and large intestine in the rat. Dig Dis Sci 1994; 39:796–801.

Kuo S-M, Whitby B, Artursson P, et al. Carrier-mediated transport of celiprolol in rat intestine. Pharm Res 1994; 11:648–653.

Leahy DH, Lynch J, Taylor DC. Mechanisms of absorption of small molecules. In: Prescott LF, Nimmo WS, eds. Novel Drug Delivery. New York: Wiley and Sons, 1989:33–40.

LeCluyse EL, Sutton SC. In vitro models for selection of development candidates. Permeability studies to define mechanisms of absorption enhancement. Adv Drug Deliv Rev 1997; 23:163–183.

Lee C-P, de Vrueh RLA, Smith PL. Selection of development candidates based on in vitro permeability measurements. Adv Drug Deliv Rev 1997; 23:47–62.

Lennernäs H. Human jejunal effective permeability and its correlation with preclinical drug absorption models. J Pharm Pharmcol 1997; 49:627–638.

Lennernäs H, Ahrenstedt Ö,Hallgren R, et al. Regional jejunal perfusion: a new in vivo approach to study oral drug absorption in man. Pharm Res 1992; 9:1243–1251.

Lennernäs H, Nylander S, Ungell A-L. Jejunal permeability: a comparison between the Ussing chamber technique and the single-pass perfusion in humans. Pharm Res 1997; 14(5):667–671.

Lennernäs H, Palm K, Artursson P. Comparison between active and passive drug transport in human intestinal epithelial (Caco-2) cells in vitro and human jejunum in vivo. Int J Pharm 1996; 127:103–107.

Leo A, Jow PYC, Silipo C, et al. Calculation of hydrophobic constant (log P) from pi and f constants. J Med Chem 1975; 18:865–868.

Leppert PS, Fix JA. Use of everted intestinal rings for in vitro examination of oral absorption potential. J Pharm Sci 1994; 83:976–981.

Levich VG. Physicochemical Hydrodynamics. Englewood Cliffs: Prentice Hall, 1962:1–80.

Levine RR, McNary WF, Kornguth PJ, et al. Histological reevaluation of everted gut technique for studying intestinal absorption. Eur J Pharmacol 1970; 9:211–219.

Lindahl A, Persson B, Ungell A-L, et al. Surface activity and concentration dependent intestinal permeability in the rat. Pharm Res 1999; 16:97–102.

Lindahl A, Sandström R, Ungell A-L, et al. Jejunal permeability and hepatic extraction of fluvastatin in humans. Clin Pharmacol Ther 1996; 60:1.

Lindahl A, Ungell A-L, Knutson L, et al. Characterisation of fluids from the stomach and proximal jejunum in men and women. Pharm Res 1997; 14:497–502.

Lindmark T, Söderholm JD, Olaisson G, et al. Mechanism of absorption enhancement in humans after rectal administration of ampicillin in suppositories containing sodium caprate. Pharm Res 1997; 14:930–935.

Lipinski CA, Lombardo F, Dominy BW, et al. Experimental and computational approaches to estimate solubility and permeability in drug discovery and development settings. Adv Drug Deliv Rev 1996; 23:3–25.

Lundahl P, Beigi F. Immobilized liposome chromatography of drugs for model analysis of drug-membrane interactions. Adv Drug Deliv Rev 1997; 23:221–227.

Ma TY, Hollander D, Bhalla D, et al. IEC-18, a nontransformed small intestinal cell line for studying epithelial permeability. J Lab Clin Med 1992; 120:329–341.

MacAdam A. The effect of gastrointestinal mucus on drug absorption. Adv Drug Deliv Rev 1993; 11: 201–220.

Makhey VD, Guo A, Norris DA, et al. Characterization of the regional intestinal kinetics of drug efflux in rat and human intestine and in Caco-2 cells. Pharm Res 1998; 15:1160–1167.

Mannhold R, Dross KP, Rekker RF. Drug lipophilicity in QSAR practice: a comparison of experimental with calculated approaches. Quant Struct-Act Relat 1990; 9:21–28.

Matthes I, Nimmerfall F, Vonderscher J, et al. Mucus models for investigation of intestinal absorption. Part 4: comparison of the in vitro mucus model with absorption models in vivo and in situ to predict intestinal absorption. Pharmazie 1992; 47:787–791.

McEwan GTA, Lucas ML. The effect of E. coli STa enteroxine on the absorption of weakly dissociable drugs from the rat proximal jejunum in vivo. Br J Pharmacol 1990; 101:937–941.

Merino V, Freixas J, del Val Bermejo M, et al. Biophysical models as an approach to study passive absorption in drug development: 6-fluoroquinolones. J Pharm Sci 1995; 84(6):777–782.

Narawane M, Podder SK, Bundgaard H, et al. Segmental differences in drug permeability, esterase activity and ketone reductase activity in the albino rabbit intestine. J Drug Target 1993; 1:29–39.

Navia MA, Chaturvedi PR. Drug discovery today. Res Focus Rev 1996; 1:179.

Neuhoff S, Spahn-Langguth H, Regardh C-G, et al. Computational approach to predict affinity of drugs to MDR1 encoded P-glycoprotein using Mol-Surf parametrization. Arch Pharm Med Chem 1999; 331 (suppl 2):33.

Niklasson M, Brodin A, Sundelof L-O. Studies of some characteristics of molecular dissolution kinetics from rotating discs. Int J Pharm 1985; 23:97–108.

Niklasson M, Magnusson A-B. Program for evaluating drug dissolution kinetics in preformulation. Pharm Res 1985; 253–320.

Norinder U, Osterberg T, Artursson P. Theoretical calculation and prediction of Caco-2 cell permeability using MolSurf parametrization and PLS statistics. Pharm Res 1997; 14:1785–1791.

Oberle RL, Moore TJ, Krummel DAP. Evolution of mucosal damage of surfactants in rat jejunum and colon. J Pharmacol Toxicol Methods 1995; 33:75–81.

Oeschsenfahrt H, Winne D. The contribution of solvent drag to the intestinal absorption of the basic drugs amidopyridine and antipyrine from the jejunum of the rat. Naunyn Schmiedebergs Arch Pharmacol 1974; 281:175–196.

Oprea TI, Gottfries J. Toward minimalistic modeling of oral drug absorption. J Mol Graph Model 1999; 17:261–274.

Oprea TI, Gottfries J, Sherbukhin V, et al. Chemical information management in drug discovery: optimizing the computational and combinatorial chemistry interfaces. J Mol Graph Model 2000; 18:512–524.

Örnskov E, Gottfries J, Erickson M, et al. Correlation of drug absorption with migration data from capillary electrophoresis using micellar electrolytes. J Pharm Pharmacol 2005; 57:435–442.

Osiecka I, Porter PA, Borchardt RT, et al. In vitro drug absorption models. I. Brush border membrane vesicles, isolated mucosal cells and everted intestinal rings: characterization and salicylate accumulation. Pharm Res 1985; 2:284–293.

Pade V, Stavchansky S. Link between drug absorption solubility and permeability measurements in Caco-2 cells. J Pharm Sci 1998; 87:1604–1607.

Paine MR, Khalighi M, Fisher JM, et al. Characterization of interintestinal and intraintestinal variations in human CYP3A-dependent metabolism. J Pharmacol Exp Ther 1997; 288:1552–1562.

Palm K, Luthman K, Ungell AL, et al. Correlation of drug absorption with molecular surface properties. J Pharm Sci 1996; 85:32.

Palm K, Stenberg LP, Luthman K, et al. Polar molecular surface properties predict the intestinal absorption of drugs in humans. Pharm Res 1997; 14:568–571.

Pantzar N, Lundin S, Wester L, et al. Bidirectional small-intestinal permeability in the rat to common marker molecules in vitro. Scand J Gastroenterol 1994; 29:703–709.

Pantzar N, Weström BR, Luts A, et al. Regional small-intestinal permeability in vitro to different sized dextrans and proteins in the rat. Scand J Gastroenterol 1993; 28:205–211.

Parr AF, Sandefer EP, Wissel P, et al. Evaluation of the feasibility and use of a prototype remote drug delivery capsule (RDDC) for non-invasive regional drug absorption studies in the GI tract of man and beagle dog. Pharm Res 1999; 16:266–271.

Pascoe GA, Sakai-Wong J, Soliven E, et al. Regulation of intestinal cytochrome P450 and heme by dietary nutrients. Biochem Pharmacol 1983; 32:3027–3035.

Pidgeon C, Ong S, Liu H, et al. IAM chromatography: an in vitro screen for predicting drug membrane permeability. J Med Chem 1995; 38:590–594.

Pilbrant A, Cederberg C. Development of an oral formulation of omeprazol. Scand J Gastroenterol Suppl 1985; 108:113–120.

Polentarutti B, Peterson A, Sjöberg A, et al. Evaluation of viability of excised rat intestinal segments in the Ussing chamber: investigation of morphology, electrical parameters and permeability characteristics. Pharm Res 1999; 16:446–454.

Porter PA, Osiecka I, Borchardt RT, et al. In vitro drug absorption models. II: salicylate, cefoxitin, alphamethyl dopa and theophylline uptake in cells and rings: correlation with in vivo bioavailability. Pharm Res 1985; 2:293–298.

Quilianova N, Chen Y, Richard A, et al. Drug absorption screening model using rabbit intestinal brush border membrane vesicles (BBMV). AAPS Meeting in Washington on Membrane Transporters, Washington, April 1999; (abstr).

Rathbone MJ, Tucker IG. Mechanisms, barriers and pathways of oral mucosal drug permeation. Adv Drug Deliv Rev 1991; 12:41–60.

Rubas W, Jezyk N, Grass GM. Comparison of the permeability characteristics of a human colonic epithelial (Caco-2) cell line to colon of rabbit, monkey and dog intestine and human drug absorption. Pharm Res 1993; 10:113–118.

Saffran M, Kumar GS, Savariar C, et al. A new approach to the oral administration of insulin and other peptide drugs. Science 1986; 233:1081–1084.

Saitoh H, Aungst BJ. Possible involvement of multiple P-glycoprotein mediated efflux systems in the transport of verapamil and other organic cations across rat intestine. Pharm Res 1995; 12:1304–1310.

Sandström R, Karlsson A, Knutsson L, et al. Jejunal absorption and metabolism of R/S-verapamil in humans. Pharm Res 1998; 15:856–562.

Schwaan PW, Stehouwer RC, Tukker JJ. Molecular mechanism for the relative binding affinity to the intestinal peptide carrier. Comparison of three ACE inhibitors: enalapril, enalaprilat and lisinopril. Biochim Biophys Acta 1995; 1236:31–38.

Sekine M, Terashima H, Sasahara K, et al. Improvement of bioavailability of poorly absorbed II. Effect of medium-chain glyceride base on the intestinal absorption of cefmetazole sodium in rats and dogs. J Pharmacobiodyn 1985; 8:286–295.

Shamat MA. The role of the gastrointestinal microflora in the metabolism of drugs. Int J Pharm 1993; 97: 1–13.

Sjöström M, Lindfors L, Ungell A-L. Inhibition of binding of an enzymatically stable thrombin inhibitor to luminal proteases as an additional mechanism of intestinal absorption enhancement. Pharm Res 1999; 16:74–79.

Söderholm JD, Hedamn L, Artursson P, et al. Integrity and metabolism of human ileal mucosa in vitro in the Ussing chamber. Acta Physiol Scand 1998; 162:47–56.

Stewart BH, Chan OH, Jezyk N, et al. Discrimination between drug candidates using models for evaluation of intestinal absorption. Adv Drug Deliv Rev 1997; 23:27–45.

Stewart BH, Chan OH, Lu RH, et al. Comparison of intestinal permeabilities determined in multiple in vitro and in situ models: relationship to absorption in humans. Pharm Res 1995; 12(5):693–699.

Strocchi A, Levitt MD. Role of villus surface area in absorption. Dig Dis Sci 1993; 38:385.

Surendran N, Ugwu SO, Nguyen LD, et al. Absorption enhancement of melanotan-1: comparison of the Caco-2 and rat in situ models. Drug Deliv 1995; 2:49–55.

Sutton SC, Forbes AE, Cargyll R, et al. Simultaneous in vitro measurement of intestinal tissue permeability and transepithelial electrical resistance (TEER) using Sweetana-Grass diffusion cells. Pharm Res 1992; 9:316–319.

Swenson ES, Milisen WB, Curatolo W. Intestinal permeability enhancement: efficacy, acute toxicity and reversibility. Pharm Res 1994; 11:1132–1142.

Tamamatsu N, Welage LS, Idkaldek NM, et al. Human intestinal permeability of piroxicam, propranolol, phenylalanine, and PEG 400 determined by jejunal perfusion. Pharm Res 1997; 14:1127–1132.

Tanaka Y, Taki Y, Sakane T, et al. Characterization of drug transport through tight-junctional pathway in Caco-2 monolayer: comparison with isolated rat jejunum and colon. Pharm Res 1995; 12:523–528.

Thomson ABR, Keelan M, Clandinin MT, et al. Dietary fat selectively alters transport properties of rat jejunum. J Clin Invest 1986; 77:279–288.

Tsuji A, Tamai I. Carrier-mediated intestinal transport of drugs. Pharm Res 1996; 13:963–977.

Uch AS, Dressman J. Improved methodology for uptake studies in intestinal rings. Pharm Res 1997; 14 (11):S–29.

Uch AS, Hesse U, Dressman JB. Use of 1-methyl-pyrrolidone as a solubilising agent for determining the uptake of poorly soluble drugs. Pharm Res 1999; 16(6):968–971.

Uhing MR, Kimura RE. The effect of surgical bowel manipulation and anaesthesia on intestinal glucose absorption in rats. J Clin Invest 1995a; 95:2790–2798.

Uhing MR, Kimura RE. Active transport of 3-O-methyl-glucose by the small intestine in chronically catheterised rats. J Clin Invest 1995b; 95:2799–2805.

Ungell A-L. In vitro absorption studies and their relevance to absorption from the GI tract. Drug Dev Ind Pharm 1997; 23(9):879–892.

Ungell A-L, Artursson P. An overview of Caco-2 and alternatives for prediction of intestinal drug transport and absorption. In: Van de Waterbeemd H, Testa B, eds. Drug Bioavailability, Estimation of Solubility, Permeability, Absorption and Bioavailability. Weinheim: Wiley-VCH, 2009.

Ungell A-L, Karlsson J. Cell cultures in drug discovery: an industrial perspective. Van de Waterbeemd, Lennernäs, Artursson, eds. Drug Bioavailability – Estimation of Solubility, Permeability and Absorption. Wiley, 2003: 90–131.

Ungell A-L, Andreasson A, Lundin K, et al. Effects of enzymatic inhibition and increased paracellular shunting on transport of vasopressin analogues in the rat. J Pharm Sci 1992; 81:640.

Ungell A-L, Nylander S, Bergstrand S, et al. Membrane transport of drugs in different regions of the intestinal tract of the rat. J Pharm Sci 1997; 87:360–366.

Ussing HH, Zerhan K. Active transport of sodium as the source of electric current in the short-circuited isolated frog skin. Acta Physiol Scand 1951; 23:110–127.

van den Mooter G, Maris B, Samyn C, et al. Use of Azo polymers for colon-specific drug delivery. J Pharm Sci 1997; 86:1321–1327.

van der Waterbeemd H, Camenisch G, Folkers G, et al. Estimation of Caco-2 cell permeability using calculated molecular descriptors. Quant Struct-Act Relat 1996; 15:480–490.

van Hoogdalem EJ, de Boer AG, Breimer DD. Intestinal drug absorption enhancement. Pharm Ther 1989; 44:407–443.

Wacher VJ, Silvermann JA, Zhang Y, et al. Role of p-glycoprotein and cytochrome P450 3A in limiting oral absorption of peptides and peptidomimetics. J Pharm Sci 1998; 87:1322–1330.

Walter E, Kissel T, Reers M, et al. Transepithelial transport properties of peptidomimetic thrombin inhibitors in monolayers of a human intestinal cell line (Caco-2) and their correlation to in vivo data. Pharm Res 1995; 12:360.

Wenzel U, Gebert I, Weintraut H, et al. Transport characteristics of differently charged cephalosporin antibiotics in oocytes expressing the cloned intestinal peptide transporter PepT1 and in human intestinal Caco-2 cells. J Pharmacol Exp Ther 1996; 277:831–839.

Wikman A, Karlsson J, Carlstedt I, et al. A drug absorption model based on the mucus layer producing human intestinal goblet cell line HT29-H. Pharm Res 1993; 10(6):843–852.

Wils P, Warnery AA, Phung-Ba V, et al. High lipophilicity decreases drug transport across intestinal epithelial cells. J Pharmacol Exp Ther 1994a; 269:654.

Wils P, Warnery A, Phung-Ba V, et al. Differentiated intestinal epithelial cell lines as in vitro models for predicting the intestinal absorption of drugs. Cell Biol Toxicol 1994b; 10(5–6):393–397.

Windmueller HG, Spaeth AE, Ganote CE. Vascular perfusion of isolated rat gut: norepinephrine and glucocorticoid requirements. Am J Physiol 1970; 218:197–204.

Wingstrand K, Abrahamsson B, Edgar B. Bioavailability from felodipine extended-release tablets with different dissolution properties. Int J Pharm 1990; 60:151–156.

Winiwarter S, Bonham NM, Ax F, et al. Correlation of human jejunal permeability (in vivo) of drugs with experimentally and theoretically derived parameters. A multivariate data analysis approach. J Med Chem 1998; 41:4939–4949.

Yamaguchi T, Ikeda C, Sekine Y. Intestinal absorption of a beta-adrenergic blocking agent nadolol. I: comparison of absorption behaviour of nadolol with those of other beta-blocking agents in the rat. Chem Pharm Bull 1986a; 24:3362–3369.

Yamaguchi T, Ikeda C, Sekine Y. Intestinal absorption of a beta-adrenergic blocking agent nadolol. II: mechanism of the inhibitory effect on the intestinal absorption of nadolol by sodium cholate in rats. Chem Pharm Bull 1986b; 34:3836–3843.

Yamaguchi T, Oida T, Ikeda C. Intestinal absorption of a beta-adrenergic blocking agent nadolol. III: nuclear magnetic resonance spectroscopic study on nadolol-sodium cholate micellar complex and intestinal absorption of nadolol derivatives in rats. Chem Pharm Bull 1986c; 34:4259–4264.

Yang CY, Cai SJ, Liu H, et al. Immobilized artificial membranes—screens for drug membrane interactions. Adv Drug Deliv Rev 1997; 23:229–256.

Yazdanian M, Glynn SL, Wright JL, et al. Correlating partitioning and Caco-2 cell permeability of structurally diverse small molecular weight compounds. Pharm Res 1997; 15:1490–1494.

Yeh PY, Smith PL, Ellens H. Effect of medium-chain glycerides on physiological properties of rabbit intestinal epithelium in vitro. Pharm Res 1994; 11:1148–1153.

Yodoya E, Uemura K, Tenma T, et al. Enhanced permeability of tetragastrin across the rat intestinal membrane and its reduced degradation by acylation with various fatty acids. J Pharmacol Exp Ther 1994; 27:1509.

Yu LX, Lipka E, Crison JR, et al. Transport approaches to the biopharmaceutical design of oral drug delivery systems: prediction of intestinal absorption. Adv Drug Deliv Rev 1996; 19:359–376.

Yuasa H, Amidon GL, Fleischer D. Peptide carrier-mediated transport in intestinal brush border membrane vesicles of rats and rabbits: cephradine uptake and inhibition. Pharm Res 1993; 10: 400–404.

Zamora I, Oprea T, Cruciani G, et al. Surface descriptors for protein-ligand affinity prediction. J Med Chem 2003; 46:25–33.

5 | Early Drug Development: Product Design

Mark Gibson

AstraZeneca R&D Charnwood, Loughborough, Leicestershire, U.K.

THE IMPORTANCE OF PRODUCT DESIGN

It may seem obvious to state that a new product should be adequately defined before any serious product development is undertaken. In many cases, the value of the design phase is often underestimated in the rush to start development and get products to the market quickly. This can result in much wasted time and valuable resources. It can also lead to reduced staff motivation if a product is developed that is not wanted or if the product definition is constantly changing during development. The quality of the design activities can strongly influence the success of development of the right product to the market and ultimate return on investment (ROI).

Several nonpharmaceutical industries have long realized the necessity of investing time and money in an initial product design phase. The automobile, aeroplane, or shipbuilding industries, for example, would not think of gearing up for large-scale manufacture of a new model until they were satisfied with the design phase. Thorough market research will have been completed to ensure customer requirements are being met. The product definition and technical specifications will have been agreed on, and the cost of goods (CoG) estimated, so that the company is satisfied that the venture will be commercially viable! What makes it more difficult in the pharmaceutical industry are the relatively longer timelines involved and the risks and complexity associated with the development of new medicines. However, the more progressive pharmaceutical companies seem to be finally realizing the value of the product design stage to achieve successful product development and marketing of a new product.

Unfortunately, some companies still do not seem to be getting the product design process right to their cost. The following recent example of inhalable insulin has been described as "one of the drug industry's costliest failures ever," estimated to be $2.8 billion from the cost of development, closure of dedicated manufacturing plants, and unsold product (Johnson, 2007). Certain companies have invested more than 10 years and vast amounts of money on making insulin treatment more convenient for diabetes patients. The idea was that diabetics did not like to prick themselves with needles several times a day to deliver the insulin they need to balance their blood sugar. The biggest hurdle was to deliver insulin by inhaler as consistently as with a standard needle and syringe. It took a technological breakthrough to develop and launch the first inhalable insulin product in July 2006, only to abandon it in October 2007, after the product's disappointing sales performance. The company predicted that inhalable insulin would be a $2 billion-a-year product by 2010, but it only sold $12 million in the first year. There were several reasons attributed to the poor sales performance.

- The device was unwieldy and drew unfavorable reviews from doctors and investors. Some patients likened it to a bong for smoking marijuana and were embarrassed to use the device in public.
- It was taking much longer to teach patients how to use the inhaler device compared with an insulin pen, and diabetic specialists said it was hard to use.
- There were concerns about safety as only 10% of the insulin reaches the bloodstream, raising the question about the long-term effects of the other 90% remaining in the lungs.
- The inhaled treatment was approximately twice as expensive per day as the injectable insulin and some payers refused to accept the inhaled product on costs alone.

From the above, it is questionable whether there was appropriate input to the product design process. Was adequate market research really undertaken to identify what the market would accept from different customer perspectives?

Studies have shown that the initial design phase actually requires a relatively small investment, which can greatly influence the nature of the product and its ultimate commercial success (Berliner and Brimson, 1988). The ROI of the conceptual design phase was shown to be five times greater than the ROI of later development work to develop and optimize the product and manufacturing process.

A simple definition of "product design" is "the initial stage of product development, where 'global' agreement is required about the nature of the product to be developed." Figure 3 in chapter 1 illustrates where product design fits into the overall product development process. Effective product design is considered to have the following important benefits:

- To provide clear direction and objectives for the project team
- To gain buy-in and input from all the key functions at the start of development (such as pharmaceutical development, safety, clinical, manufacturing operations, quality assurance, regulatory, and commercial/marketing)
- To assess the feasibility of the project in commercial and technical terms
- To identify any risks early and hence manage them
- To avoid wasting valuable resources on developing a product that is not needed or wanted
- To provide a good reference source for the development plan

PRODUCT DESIGN CONSIDERATIONS

A useful outcome of the initial product design phase is a product design report. This should document the careful evaluation of the following key elements:

- Target product profile (TPP)/minimum product profile (MPP)
- Design specification and critical quality parameters
- Commercial and marketing considerations
- Technical issues and risk assessment
- Safety assessment considerations
- Environmental, health, and safety considerations
- Intellectual property considerations

Each of these elements is discussed in more detail below.

Target Product Profile/Minimum Product Profile

A TTP, which defines the product attributes, should be established for the intended marketed product based on all "customer" and "end-user" needs. Customers and end users include anyone in the supply chain, including both internal and external customers, such as those in manufacturing and in sales and marketing, distributors, doctors, nurses, pharmacists, and patients. Each customer wants the right product (meeting their quality expectations) at the right time and at the right price. Additionally, each customer will have his or her own specific requirements.

The TPP is often expressed primarily in clinical terms, but should also include the pharmaceutical, technical, regulatory, and commercial/marketing attributes required of the product. The TPP is based on the ideal product characteristics, which are considered to be desirable, whereas the MPP is based on the minimum product requirements, which must be met for the product to be viable and worth developing. For example, the TPP may stipulate an ideal dosing regimen of once daily. However, the MPP may state that the dosing regimen must be no more than twice daily for the product to be competitive.

The ideal attributes for a fictitious product profile example prepared for a product being developed to treat osteoarthritis is shown in Table 1.

The level of information on the dosage form and pack should provide sufficient clarity of detail to enable the pharmaceutical development group to plan their development. These

Table 1 Target Product Profile for a Fictitious Product to Treat Osteoarthritis

Key attributes	Target product profile
Disease to be treated	Osteoarthritis
Patient type (e.g., geriatric, pediatric)	Adults older than40 years, including geriatrics
Route of administration	Oral
Efficacy	Analgesic and anti-inflammatory activity better than current "criterion standard" therapy
Safety/tolerability	No GI side effects No interactions with other agents
Pharmacoeconomics	Reduced health care costs by preventing disease progression
Dosage/presentation (type/size)	Immediate release tablet No more than two strengths
Dose and dose frequency	Once daily
Pack design/type	Blister calendar pack with moisture barrier Must be able to be opened by patient Tamper evident
Process	Use standard processing equipment for tablets
Aesthetic aspects (color, flavors, taste, etc.)	Color to differentiate tablet strengths Taste masked to reduce bitterness
Territories to be marketed	United States, Europe, Japan
Cost of goods	No more than 10% of commercial price
Commercial price	Equivalent or less than current criterion standard therapy

Table 2 Example of a Pharmaceutical Product Profile for an Intravenous Solution

Key attributes	Target product profile
Dosage form presentation	Single dose, non-preserved
Primary pack	Type I clear glass vial (10 mL) rubber stopper Aluminum overseal
Secondary pack	Carton with patient instruction leaflet
Product strength range	10–50 mg in 5 mL

Excipient to be evaluated
    Tonicity adjustment
    Buffer
    Antioxidant
	
	Dextrose or saline
	Phosphate or citrate
	Sodium metabisulfite or acetylcysteine

Manufacturing process	Aseptic manufacture/sterile filtration (terminal sterilization by autoclaving not possible)

pharmaceutical attributes may be documented separately in a pharmaceutical product profile (PPP). A typical example of a PPP is shown in Table 2 for an intravenous injection product, illustrating the level of detail expected in a product design report. Similarly, a target clinical profile (TCP) can be developed by the clinical development group to document and capture the clinical characteristics required of the drug, which will meet the needs of patients, clinicians, and payers. Both the PPP and TCP can be used in conjunction with the TPP to provide a complete summary of the product design requirements.

It is clearly beneficial to conduct some early preformulation studies to characterize the candidate drug and to determine the physicochemical properties considered important in the development of the intended dosage form to support product design. Preformulation data from solubility, stressed stability, excipient compatibility, and other preformulation studies may influence the selection of the formulation dosage form and excipients. The results may also influence the choice of manufacturing process, as shown in the example in Table 2, where terminal sterilization by autoclaving has been shown not to be feasible. The preformulation data should also help to establish the critical quality parameters for the product. In chapter 6 of this book, Gerry Steele discusses in much greater detail the preformulation studies that may be undertaken to support product design.

The formulation developed for early clinical trials (phase 0 or I) is often a simple one and different from the intended commercial dosage form. A parallel development approach can significantly reduce development time by delinking early clinical supply with commercial formulation development. However, the product profile in the product design report is for the intended commercial product. This information is required at the start of development so that the final commercial product and simple clinical formulation can both be developed in parallel to avoid affecting the medical needs or timings. For example, the commercial formulation could be a film-coated tablet, but the early clinical formulation may be a simple oral solution or suspension or a hand-filled capsule. Regulatory authorities will be interested in the linkage between formulations used in early clinical studies and those used in the pivotal (phase III) studies and the final commercial product. The objective of many companies is to optimize and finalize the commercial product (formulation and process) for the start of the pivotal clinical studies to minimize any regulatory concerns.

Meeting Customer Needs

There are various methods and tools available for gathering information about customer needs to establish the product profile. It is not the intention of this book to cover this in great detail, and only an overview is given here.

A primary source of information is usually held within the pharmaceutical company, particularly if the company is already established with marketed products in a particular therapeutic area. Most companies will have a variety of information representing the voice of their customers. Much of this may be negative in the form of complaints and letters from users. These can be valuable sources of information to consider in the development of better products. It is important that all of the company's internal departments involved in product development are consulted. These internal departments include Pharmaceutical Development, Design Engineering, Manufacturing Operations, Quality Assurance, Safety/Toxicology, Medical, and Commercial/Marketing. They should be involved in the product design and product profile discussions, as they are also key internal customers. This is easier said than done because pharmaceutical organizations often lack the processes and structure to support their collaboration. The TPP should be used to facilitate joint development and "buy-in." Typically, research and development (R&D) "owns" or acts as if it owns the TPP, but ideally the process needs to be improved to incorporate real input into the TPP from all parties, or else it may become a dead document (Illert, 2007). The process needs to encourage constructive teamwork to ensure that the science, regulatory, and commercial functions' inputs are all reviewed and agreed upon. One way of doing this is to bring together all the stakeholders at one or more workshops to agree upon the development objectives and to optimize the TPP.

Once defined, the TPP provides details of the label claims that the company is seeking for the candidate drug, including the safety and efficacy requirements that should allow drug approval. Although it is not compulsory for the regulatory approval process, there are benefits of sharing the TPP with the regulators at an early stage in development as a discussion document to check with them whether the development plans are appropriate to support a marketing application.

It is important to recognize that these internal customers' perceptions and requirements may be far removed from those of external customers. If a company is venturing into a new therapeutic area, or is endeavoring to learn more about the changing needs of the market, external customers and end users in the supply chain need to be consulted for their views about current treatments and shortfalls. There are various ways of achieving this feedback. For example, surveys can be conducted by sending out questionnaires or by telephoning key customers and end users to gather perception data. Alternatively, clinics and focus groups can be set up to gain insight into customers' wants and perceptions. Clinicians, doctors, patients, or other customers may be asked to attend small focus groups, facilitated by medical, marketing, or pharmaceutical personnel, to discuss their likes and dislikes. This type of forum can be useful for demonstrating samples and prototypes of devices and drug delivery systems. Other ways of obtaining feedback include setting up individual interviews with opinion leaders in the field and generally listening to customers' comments at conferences, exhibitions, and trade shows. Consultancy organizations are often hired to gather this type of information on behalf of the pharmaceutical company developing a new product. Customer insight studies can be conducted in conjunction with the pharmaceutical company to gain a deep and clear understanding of the needs and behaviors of its customers: prescribers, patients, and all other stakeholders involved in pharmaceutical decisions. The studies try to answer the key questions such as

- What are the barriers keeping our medicines from reaching patients who would benefit from them?
- Why would physicians not prescribe our products to patients?

For example, one obstacle to the uptake of a cholesterol lowering medicine was that some physicians do not conduct frequent diagnostic tests that would lead to prescriptions. This could be overcome by providing easy-to-use blood testing equipment to the physicians so that they can diagnose more patients and prescribe the cholesterol-reducing medication.

Information gained from such customer insight studies is used by the pharmaceutical company in the design of the new medicine. The pharmaceutical development group can play a leading role in determining the pharmaceutical requirements for a new product from key customers. Customers may want more specific packs or delivery systems, and different markets still have their own preferences for different dosage forms.

Quality function deployment (QFD), also referred to as "customer-driven engineering" and "matrix product planning," is a useful quality and planning tool that uses a structured approach in defining all the customer needs or requirements and translates these into design requirements for product development. QFD seeks out both the "spoken" and "unspoken" customer requirements and maximizes "positive" quality (such as ease of use) that creates value, whereas traditional quality systems aim at minimizing negative quality (such as defects).

QFD originated in Japan in the late 1960s and was initially applied to shipbuilding, where large capital investments are made and design and planning needs to be thorough. Through the 1970s and 1980s, there was a rapid increase in the application of QFD to all industries in Japan, and in the 1980s and 1990s, it was accepted in the United States and Europe as a means of quality improvement (Akao, 1990; Day, 1993; Mizuno and Akao, 1994).

The QFD basic approach is to start with customer requirements, which are usually vague qualitative items such as easy to use, feels good, lasts a long time. These vague customer requirements are converted into internal company design requirements that are measurable and can be used objectively to evaluate the product. If the company requirements are properly introduced, the product should satisfy all the customer requirements. The company requirements must then be translated into specific parts of the product, and the characteristics of these specific parts should cause the essential functions to be performed.

Customer requirements → Company requirements (measures) → Design characteristics (specific parts)

QFD is accomplished through a series of charts, sometimes referred to as the "House of Quality" (HOQ) because the shape of the charts has a rooflike structure at the top (Fig. 1). Ideally, the chart should be developed by a cross-functional team made up of members of the core functions in product development. The first step in building the HOQ is to list the customer requirements, "the WHATs," down the left-hand side of the matrix (area 1 in Fig. 1). Each of the WHATs is translated into one or more global customer characteristics or design requirements, "the HOWs," and listed across the top of the matrix (area 2). The design requirements will usually be measurable characteristics, which can be evaluated on the completed product. The next step is to complete the relationship matrix in the center (area 3). The strength of the relationship between each customer requirement and technical requirement is depicted by using different symbols and weightings, for example, "strong" = 9, "medium" = 3, and "weak" = 1. A blank column in the relationships matrix could indicate a design requirement that is not really needed.

Next, the team completes area 4, comprising measurements for the design requirements (HOW MUCH). These objective target values should represent how good the product has to be

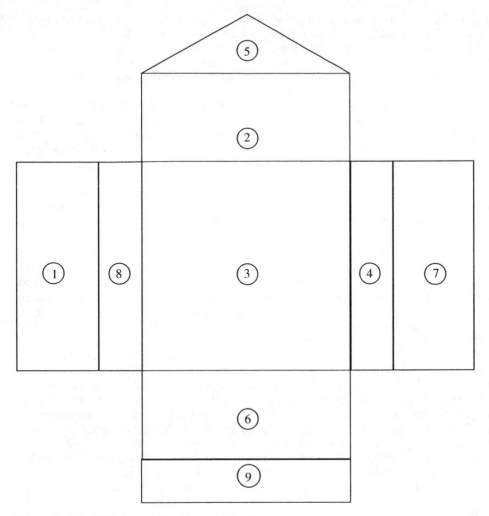

Figure 1 The QFD diagram: the House of Quality.
Key:
1. Customer requirements (WHATs)
2. Design requirements (HOWs)
3. Relationship matrix
4. Objective targets for customer's requirements (HOW MUCH)
5. Correlation matrix
6. Customer competitive assessment
7. Technical competitive assessment
8. Customer importance rating
9. Technical importance rating

to satisfy the customer and need not necessarily represent current performance levels. These values are required to provide an objective means of assuring that requirements have been met and to provide targets for further detailed development.

In area 5, the roof of the house, the correlation matrix establishes any potential synergies or conflicts between each design requirement (HOW). The purpose is to identify areas where trade-off decisions may be required. Symbols are often used to describe the strength of the relationship, for example, positive, strong positive, negative, and strong negative. From the matrix, it should be possible to identify which of the design requirements support one another and which are in conflict. Positive correlations are important because some resource efficiencies may be gained by not duplicating efforts to attain the same result. Negative correlations are also important because they indicate conditions where trade-offs are suggested. There may be ways of eliminating trade-offs by introducing some degree of innovation, which may lead to competitive advantage and patent opportunities. Trade-off resolution is achieved by adjusting the values of the targets for customer requirements (HOW MUCH).

The competitive assessment is a pair of graphs (areas 6 and 7), which depict item for item how competitive products compare with current company products. This is completed for both the customer requirements (WHATs) and the design requirements (HOWs). The customer competitive assessment is important to understand the customer's perception of the product relative to the competition, whereas the technical competitive assessment is undertaken by the company's product development experts to gain an internal view.

The final step in constructing the QFD chart is to establish the importance ratings. The customer importance rating (area 8) is based on customer assessment and is expressed as a relative scale (typically 1 to 5), with the higher numbers indicating greater importance to the customer.

It is vital that these values represent the true customer needs and not just internal company perceptions. Importance ratings for the design requirements (HOWs) are calculated by multiplying the value of the symbols in the relationship matrix for each cell (9, 3, or 1) by the corresponding customer importance rating and summing the products down the columns (area 9). The importance ratings are useful for prioritizing efforts and making trade-off decisions. The values have no direct meaning but rank in relative importance the customer and technical requirements that have to be satisfied.

Figure 2 provides a typical example of a completed top-level QFD chart for a fictitious metered dose inhaler (MDI) product to be used for the treatment of asthma.

The QFD concept can be further utilized by cascading the Voice of the Customer through a series of matrices or phases. In the product development process, this involves taking the customer requirements and defining design requirements. Some of the design requirements are translated to the next chart to establish the optimum design characteristics. This is continued to define the optimum manufacturing process requirements and production requirements. In practice, this is achieved by creating new charts in which the HOWs of the previous chart become the WHATs of the new chart, as illustrated in Figure 3.

While the QFD charts are a good planning and documentation tool, the real value is in the process of communicating and decision-making within a company because the process encourages input from multiple functional disciplines involved in product development. The active participation of the various disciplines should lead to a more balanced consideration of the customer and design requirements and, ultimately, increased customer/end-user satisfaction. Having said that, the perceived complexity of the QFD charts, and getting buy-in from across the company, can be barriers to success. However, QFD should help maintain a focus on the true requirements and requires more time to be spent at the start of development, thereby ensuring that the company determines, understands, and agrees with what needs to be done before rushing into development activities.

When appropriately applied, QFD has demonstrated that design changes are less likely later in development and has shown a corresponding reduction in development time to market (Akao, 1990).

Like any good system, QFD has evolved over the years. Modern QFD now incorporates much advancement that was not in traditional QFD. For example, traditional QFD is centered on the "4-House" approach. Some companies that do their own design work have found that this approach does not integrate well into their new product development process and is too time consuming. Modern QFD is custom tailored to identify the minimum QFD effort required with the optimum tools and sequence, making QFD more efficient and sustainable in today's lean business environment. Large, complex tools such as the HOQ are now often replaced with smaller, faster ones that provide a level of analysis that is faster and easier. In some cases, the HOQ matrix may be still useful; however, the important thing is to know when HOQ is appropriate and when it is too much team effort for the value it delivers.

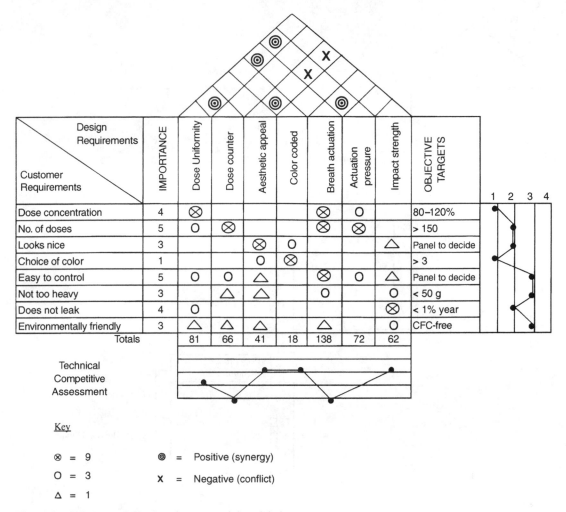

Figure 2 A fictitious QFD chart for metered dose inhaler.

Modern QFD also incorporates upgraded mathematics in the QFD matrices to meet the mathematical rigor demanded by Six Sigma precision. Traditional QFD often did not go deep enough into the Voice of the Customer to uncover unspoken needs because it began at the time when most design work was done by the customer's engineers. Modern QFD has a set of rigorous front-end tools to refine the Voice of the Customer into spoken and unspoken customer needs, leading to more innovative solutions. Additionally, Modern QFD includes psychological and lifestyle needs, not just functional needs. Today, consumers are making the purchase decision more and more on emotional needs and image issues. Lifestyle QFD (available at http://www.qfdi.org/workshop_kansei.htm) connects consumers' needs for psychological and lifestyle-enhancing solutions with product development and branding. Traditional QFD ignores bottlenecks caused by availability of certain experts. It assumed that experts were always available or would work overtime to finish the work. Modern QFD also has components for schedule deployment and project deployment based on Critical Chain Project Management to improve allocation of constrained resources and finish more projects on time. Overall, Modern QFD today provides a much better framework for integration of various innovative methods into the product development process (Mazur, 2007; Mazur, 2008).

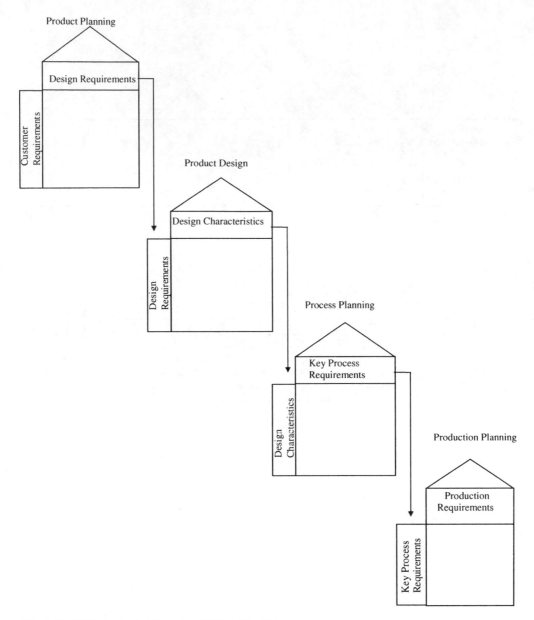

Figure 3   QFD: cascading the voice of the customer.

Design Specifications and Critical Quality Parameters
In addition to the preformulation information, there will be other considerations in the selection of the excipients and packaging components for the product. Taking the intravenous injection example in Table 2, it may be important to stipulate that any excipient used must be of parenteral grade, will comply with pharmacopoeial requirements, and be restricted to those known to be safe and acceptable to the regulatory authorities. This will reduce the risk, compared with using a novel excipient, which might be questionable to some regulatory authorities. It will also reassure the safety/toxicology department that no extra toxicological studies will be required to approve a new excipient.

Similarly, a list of requirements can be produced for the primary pack, such as the following:

- The pack will be acceptable to regulatory authorities in the countries to be marketed (other approved marketed products already use this type of pack).
- Only packs that can be multiple sourced from more than one supplier/country will be used.
- The pack must have consistency of dimensions and performance.
- The pack will meet function/user tests and specifications.

These dimensions, performance limits, and function/user test limits should be specified in the product design report.

Even though the product has not yet been developed, a high-quality product specification can be proposed with tests and limits that the product should meet at the time of manufacture and at the end of shelf life. For the intravenous product example, tests might include appearance (clear, particle free), pH, osmolality, particulate levels, sterility, and endotoxin levels. Appropriate standards or limits can also be proposed on the basis of the knowledge of similar types of products that have already been developed and from standard pharmacopoeial monographs.

Finally, in this section, it is useful to agree on what the minimum acceptable shelf life for the product should be. The product will need to be stable enough to allow time for quality control (QC) testing and quality assurance (QA) release after manufacture; distribution to wholesalers, pharmacists, and doctors; and with acceptable time for storage until prescribed and used by patients. Normally, a minimum three-year shelf life at room temperature (15–30°C) is targeted. However, if the treatment is very novel, it may be possible to justify a shorter shelf life and/or storage at lower temperatures, if stability is likely to be a problem.

Commercial and Marketing Considerations

Any pharmaceutical company's economic objective must be to maximize its ROI after launch. Therefore, the commercial viability of a new product to be developed needs to be commercially assessed at the product design stage to satisfy the company that it will achieve a satisfactory ROI. Some of the factors that should be considered in the evaluation are as follows:

- Development costs
- Timing to market
- Market size (disease prevalence, diagnosis and treatment rates, market value)
- Competition (current, developing, and impact on future market)
- Unmet medical need (effectiveness of current treatment, improvements required)
- Pricing and reimbursement (current and future)
- CoG (target)

The development costs are an estimate of the total costs of development of the product through the various stages of R&D, including preclinical, clinical, pharmaceutical (drug substance and product), and marketing costs. As a rule, the development costs will increase exponentially with development time (see Fig. 2, chap. 1), and the cost of conducting the phase III clinical studies are usually the most expensive element of the development program. Estimates of the total cost of all material, labor, and overhead costs should be included.

A major consideration for the development costs is whether to contract out some or all of the work (Spurlin et al., 1996). Contract research organizations (CROs) can offer a broad range of services covering all parts of the drug development process. In terms of product development, preformulation studies, including drug substance characterization, formulation development, stability testing, clinical trial manufacturing, and scale-up/technology transfer, are typically outsourced. In fact, most pharmaceutical companies have to contract out some aspect of R&D because of the diverse requirements and multidisciplinary nature of the work. Taken to the extreme, it is possible to create a "virtual" pharmaceutical company run by a

Table 3 Advantages and Disadvantages of Outsourcing

Advantages	Disadvantages

• More cost effective
  Reduced overhead costs
 	
  Avoid capital expenditure
  Reduced cost of good
  Reduced training costs
• Access to the best expertise, technology, and resources not available within company
• Access to patented technology
• Allows optimal use of internal resource (focus on company strengths)
• Free up resource for other purposes
 	
• Management of peaks and troughs
• Shorter time to achieve results-fast track to market
• Shared risk–joint venture
• Increased probability of success?
• Convenient and efficient
	• A big commitment and initial costs
	• Questionable quality and regulatory concerns; detailed audits required
	• Secrecy/loss of patent opportunities
	
	• Loss of technical expertise and product knowledge
	• Stagnation of in-house competence
	
	• Decreased flexibility moving resources between projects
	
	• Short-term gain—no future development of company
	• Dependability on partner

committee of project managers responsible for coordinating the outsourcing of every part of the development program (Stevenson, 1997). However, it is unlikely that major pharmaceutical companies would want to take this approach and not have any internal capability.

There are pros and cons to outsourcing, some of which are summarized in Table 3. Clearly, contracting out is not simply a commercial decision. The issues identified if outsourcing is done have to be carefully considered. One significant risk of outsourcing is if the relationship with the CRO goes sour or the CRO goes out of business. It may be difficult to find an alternative without having the detailed technical knowledge.

The outsourcing company should be aware of the potential additional costs to simply paying for a package of work. Someone from the parent company has to manage the process, and this can involve several stages such as

- selecting the CRO,
- auditing to ensure technical, commercial, and quality standards are acceptable,
- establishing a contract and agreement of the work program,
- attending reviews to discuss progress or technical issues, and
- accepting the end result.

These activities are likely to involve significant parent company investment in time, people, and costs if the outsourcing is to be successful. Some of these issues associated with using and controlling contractors are discussed further by Burton (1997).

An estimate of the timing to market is important to know to assess the positioning of the new product in relation to competitor products in development and those already marketed. The use of CROs should be able to speed up development by allowing activities to be conducted in parallel. It is also important to predict what the market size is likely to be at the time of launch on the basis of market trends. Being first to market with a new treatment can be very advantageous in determining a high commercial price. However, if other competitor products are already established, the market price may be restricted unless some significant benefit can be shown over existing treatments. For example, a novel delivery system or device that improves patient compliance might achieve a higher price than a conventional delivery system.

The potential market size can be estimated from current research data, showing the number of patients in the countries of interest and the total value of treatment. Trends in disease prevalence should be noted, whether the number of patients is increasing or decreasing. However, it should also be noted that market research can sometimes be misleading and could result in missed opportunities. A good example to illustrate this point is the introduction of a new therapeutic class of drugs where there was no existing market. Before the introduction of the H2-receptor antagonist cimetidine, there was little evidence that many people suffered from gastric ulcers. It was only after an effective treatment was available that people came forward, and an enormous market was established.

One way of assessing the commercial viability for a new product is to subtract the total development costs from the potential market share value. The potential market share value is estimated by multiplying the percentage of the potential number of patients by the potential commercial price for the new product. An alternative approach is to do the calculations based on the cost of the product or one course of treatment:

Estimated commerical return = (commercial price − cost of goods) × predicted sales volume

The commercial price that the company thinks it can obtain for the product, or for a course of treatment, will depend on some of the other factors mentioned above, such as the predicted time of market launch, the competitive positioning, and the relative cost of competitor products in the countries to be marketed. The CoG is an estimate of the sum of the cost of the drug substance, excipients, packaging materials, manufacture, labor, and overheads, among other things, that contribute to making the product.

It has been estimated that 85% of the future cost of a new product can be determined at the product design phase (Matthews, 1997). The industry average for the CoG has gradually increased over the last decade from about 10% to 20% of the commercial price. A CoG target of 5% to 10% is about the industry average, with a maximum of no more than 40%. Higher than this would be difficult to justify developing, as the margins would be too small. The choice of the commercial dosage form and manufacturing process can have a significant impact on the CoG. For example, if a product is freeze-dried, the processing costs will be extremely high because of the limited batch sizes and lengthy process involved. A less obvious example is the choice between tablets versus capsules. Cole (1998) compared the relative costs in the development and production of film-coated tablets with a dry-filled hard gelatin capsule for a new chemical entity (NCE). The relative costs in terms of development time, raw materials used, production equipment, facilities, and validation for the manufacture were considered. There is a general belief that tablets are easier and cheaper to produce than dry-fill capsules, but surprisingly, Cole found that a capsule-manufacturing facility is cheaper to build, validate, and operate than a tablet-manufacturing facility. Only when the costs of excipients are considered in isolation does the tablet process have an advantage, mainly because gelatin capsules are relatively expensive.

Technical Issues and Risk Assessment

There may be a variety of issues that should be documented in the product design report to highlight the perceived risks involved in developing the product. Some of these risks will be related to pharmaceutical development and others to clinical, safety/toxicology, or other areas.

For pharmaceutical development, risk may be associated with the technical challenges anticipated in developing a novel or complex drug delivery system or manufacturing process. Information from early preformulation and biopharmaceuticals studies should indicate the potential problems for drug delivery, formulation development, and manufacture.

There may be a lack of in-house expertise, resulting in the need to contract out the work or the need to develop an in-house capability. Alternatively, there may be a lack of in-house facilities or equipment to handle the candidate drug. These issues need to be resolved quickly or else time penalties could be incurred. Other areas of risk include the sources of excipients and packaging components. Some excipients or packaging components may only be available from one supplier, with the risk that the supplier could go out of business.

The importance of identifying these issues in a product design report is to make the company aware of the risks it is taking and to make effective plans to overcome problems and manage the risks.

Safety Assessment Considerations

In the interests of rapid product development, it is beneficial to select well-established excipients that already have regulatory approval in registered products. In the United States, specific requirements for "new" excipients are detailed in the U.S. Food and Drug Administration's *Guidance for Industry: Nonclinical Studies for the Safety Evaluation of Pharmaceutical Excipients*, published in May 2005.

According to ICH, an excipient is considered new or novel if it is used for the first time in a human drug product or by a new route of administration. In the United States, FDA maintains the Inactive Ingredient Database, which lists excipients used in approved drug products, their route of administration, and their maximum dosage. There may be situations where there are good reasons to use new excipients. There may be incompatibility problems with the candidate drug and existing excipients or there may be a need to use new excipients in a new drug delivery system. The replacement of chlorofluorocarbons (CFCs) with new hydrofluorocarbon (HFA) propellants in pressurized MDIs has been driven by environmental factors. The cost of safety testing HFA-134a and HFA-227 has been shared by a consortium of pharmaceutical companies who all had a vested interest. However, the search for novel surfactants required to suspend the drug in the new propellants has been left to individual companies, after it was discovered that none of the traditional surfactants were compatible with HFA propellants. This has resulted in many new surfactants being patented, but few have been successfully safety tested and used in marketed products.

The safety-toxicological testing of a new excipient for Europe or the United States is as extensive as that for an NCE and can take four to five years to complete. There are differences in the safety evaluation requirements for different types of formulations: oral, parenteral, and topical/transdermal. The International Pharmaceutical Excipients Council (IPEC Europe and IPEC Americas) have developed a protocol for the rational safety testing of excipients to aid the introduction of new chemical excipients (Table 4). IPEC is a federation of three independent regional industry associations based in Europe, the United States and Japan who are focused on the applicable law, regulations, and business practices of each region with respect to pharmaceutical excipients. Historically, new excipients were only reviewed by regulatory authorities in the context of new drug applications (NDAs). As a result, pharmaceutical companies were reluctant to include them in their formulations because any questions about the excipients could delay or reject their applications. To address this IPEC of the Americas has developed a New Excipient Evaluation Procedure (DeMerlis et al., 2008). The aim of this process is to provide independent evaluation of the regulatory acceptance of a new excipient before a regulatory filing of a new drug product. Although this process will not provide any type of regulatory approval, it should provide confidence to pharmaceutical companies that the excipient will be acceptable in their formulations. Supporting information for a new excipient can be provided in a drug application or in an appropriately referenced drug master file (DMF). This information includes full details of chemistry, manufacturing, and controls as well as supporting safety data. The information provided is similar in the level of detail to that provided for a drug substance. The level of information, however, may be less depending on the "newness" of the excipient.

Investment in a new excipient includes the cost of safety testing, investment in manufacturing facilities, and other development costs, including stability testing. Safety testing of a new excipient alone can be expensive. It is estimated that about $40 million to $50 million is required to allow for the cost of those materials that do not make it to the market. There is a big financial risk that the investment costs will not be recovered during the patent life of a new product. However, it may be possible to reduce these costs and timings. For example, if the new excipient is essential for the development of the new candidate drug, it may be possible to "piggyback" the safety evaluation of the new excipient onto the safety evaluation of the candidate drug itself. This approach could be particularly appropriate for parenteral products. Finally, there may be lesser considerations for excipient safety testing in novel treatments, where there is an overwhelming need to treat patients quickly and effectively, for example, for life-threatening diseases such as cancer.

Table 4 Summary of Excipient Safety Testing for Different Routes of Exposure for Humans (proposal by IPEC Europe and IPEC America)

Dermal/inhalation/tests	Oral	Mucosal	Transdermal	Topical	Parenteral	Intranasal	Ocular
Appendix 1—base set							
Acute oral toxicity	R	R	R	R	R	R	R
Acute dermal toxicity	R	R	R	R	R	R	R
Acute inhalation toxicity	C	C	C	C	C	R	C
Eye irritation	R	R	R	R	R	R	R
Skin irritation	R	R	R	R	R	R	R
Skin sensitization	R	R	R	R	R	R	R
Acute parenteral toxicity	–	–	–	–	R	–	–
Application site evaluation	–	–	R	R	R	–	–
Pulmonary sensitization	–	–	–	–	–	R	–
Phototoxicity/ photoallergy	–	–	R	R	–	–	–
Ames test	R	R	R	R	R	R	R
Micronucleus test	R	R	R	R	R	R	R
ADME-intended route	R	R	R	R	R	R	R
28-day toxicity (2 species)-intended route	R	R	R	R	R	R	R
Appendix 2							
90-day toxicity (most appropriate species)	R	R	R	R	R	R	R
Teratology (rat and rabbit)	R	R	R	R	R	R	R
Additional assays	C	C	C	C	C	C	C
Genotoxicity assays	R	R	R	R	R	R	R
Appendix 3							
Chronic toxicity (rodent, non-rodent)	C	C	C	C	C	C	C
1 Generation reproduction	R	R	R	R	R	R	R
Photocarcinogenicity	–	–	C	C	–	–	–

Abbreviations: R: required; C: conditional.

Environmental, Health, and Safety Considerations

There are increasing pressures on the pharmaceutical industry to use environmentally friendly materials in products, which are biodegradable or recyclable and do no harm to the environment. Examples are the replacement of CFCs in pressurized metered dose aerosols and the replacement of polyvinyl chloride (PVC) for alternative packaging materials in some countries. Any special restrictions on the use of materials in the product need to be identified at the product design stage. The choice of appropriate materials to suit product, customer, and environment may also have cost implications.

Another aspect is the nature of the candidate drug to be developed. Special handling requirements may be required for a very potent and potentially hazardous compound. There may be implications for the design and purchase of new facilities or equipment or the training of employees in new techniques.

Intellectual Property Considerations

Few pharmaceutical companies would venture into a long and expensive development program without a strategy for effective patent protection in place to ensure market exclusivity. Patents are legal property that prevents others using the invention (for 20 years in most countries) in exchange for a full public disclosure of information.

The pharmaceutical industry is one of the major users of the patent system, which requires that three criteria be met to grant a patent. These criteria are novelty, presence of an inventive step, and industrial applicability. Although an invention might be novel, it might not be patentable if it could have been predicted from "prior art," that is, knowledge in the public domain. Hence, there is a need for an inventive step.

At the product design stage of development, the only patent filed is likely to be for the new candidate drug. There may be a patent for a candidate drug and further patents for a new indication or a new pharmaceutical use. For example, Minoxidil, originally developed as an antihypertensive, had been discovered subsequently to be useful for the treatment of male pattern baldness. Patent protection is stronger if multiple patents can be obtained; for example, a single product could have patents covering a range of features from the candidate drug itself to the method of treatment and the delivery system. These new discoveries may only become known during development. Polymorphs (e.g., cimetidine) and hydrates (e.g., amoxycillin trihydrate) have been patented, as they have shown to have therapeutic advantages. A new formulation of the drug, delivery device, or new pharmaceutical process might allow further patent cover to be granted, to extend the exclusivity beyond that of the primary patent.

The current patent status and potential for future patents to be obtained should be highlighted in the product design report to assess the overall strength of patent protection to cover future development, and, as long as possible, market exclusivity.

CONCLUDING REMARKS

The potential benefits of conducting an initial product design stage prior to commencing product development have been emphasized in this chapter. Experience shows that the most frequent reason for terminating a project in late phase development is not because of lack of efficacy or poor safety but because the product developed does not meet the market (customer) needs. This might have been avoided if more consideration had been given to product design.

The TPP and product design report can be very useful documents to focus the company on developing the right product at the right time to the market. Of course, to be of value it is essential that the correct input has been obtained from internal and external customers. For this to happen, a pharmaceutical company's senior management has to support this approach and ensure that time and resources are allowed for the design phase activities. The most successful pharmaceutical companies are effectively using this approach.

It is important that the TPP and product design report are reviewed by the project team at milestones in the project life and updated if necessary. It is imperative that some information will change with time, for example, competitor data and information gained from conducting development studies. The introduction of a new competitor product to the market with unexpected product attributes may result in a reevaluation of the desired product profile for the new product being developed. This, in turn, can result in subsequent modifications to the preformulation and formulation development program. It is hoped that this will not be a complete change in direction, but if it is, the product design review will have alerted the company sooner rather than later to address this, and not to develop a product that is not wanted or needed.

REFERENCES

Akao Y, ed. Quality Function Deployment. Cambridge, MA: Productivity Press, 1990.
Berliner C, Brimson J, eds. Cost Management for Today's Advanced Manufacturing: The CAM-I Conceptual Design. Boston: Harvard Business School Press, 1988.
Burton W. Using and controlling subcontractors. Med Device Technol 1997; 8:14–16.
Cole G. Evaluating development and production costs: tablets versus capsules. Pharm Technol Eur 1998; (5):17–26.
Day RG. Quality Function Deployment: Linking a Company with its Customers. Milwaukee: ASQC Quality Press, 1993.
DeMerlis C, Goldring JM, Schoneker DR. Inside IPEC-Americas: New Excipient Evaluation. Pharm Technol 2008; 32(1).

Illert G. Ahead of the Game. Pharm Exec Europe 2007:32–39.

Johnson A. Insulin flop costs Pfizer $2.8 billion. The Wall Street Journal October 19, 2007.

Matthews E. Economic considerations for device design and development. Med Device Technol 1997; 8: 18–26.

Mazur G. How does Modern QFD differ from the Traditional 4-Phase QFD. QFD Institute 2007. Available at: http://www.qfdi.org/who_is_qfdi/newsletter_archive/ModernQFD_vs_Traditional_4PhaseQFD.pdf

Mazur G. QFD and Voice of the Customer in Design for Six Sigma. 2008. Available at: http://www.mazur.net/.

Mizuno S, Akao Y, eds. QFD: The Customer-Driven Approach to Quality Planning and Development, Asian Productivity Organization, Tokyo. New York: Quality Resources, 1994.

Spurlin S, Green M, Kelner L, et al. An insider's guide to outsourcing drug development—10 key steps to getting your money's worth. Pharm Technol 1996; (February): 64–76.

Stevenson R. Outsourcing and the virtual company. Chem Br 1997; (October): 29–31.

6 | Preformulation as an Aid to Product Design in Early Drug Development

Gerry Steele
AstraZeneca R&D Charnwood, Loughborough, Leicestershire, U.K.

INTRODUCTION

It is axiomatic that the physicochemical properties of candidate drugs can influence their subsequent development. The results of characterization studies carried out will influence their product design. However, in the interest of only doing necessary work, any detailed studies should only be carried out after the candidate drug has successfully overcome the safety and clinical trials performed in early development as many will fail at this stage. Since pharmaceuticals are formulated in a variety of dosage forms, the studies that should be undertaken include those of solid and solution state. In terms of solid-state evaluation, material science has assumed great importance (Cui, 2007), and this is especially true for compounds to be delivered via the inhalation route (Chow et al., 2007; Young et al., 2007). If the solid-state characteristics of the candidate drugs are less than desirable from a formulation perspective, then crystal engineering techniques can sometimes be employed to give them more amenable properties (Chow et al., 2008).

Variability of the drug candidate and excipients is the major cause of challenges in the formulation development of new compounds, and so methods for their characterization need to be available (Hagsten et al., 2008). While there are many traditional approaches to dosage form design, newer approaches based on expert systems that require knowledge of the physicochemical properties are being employed to speed up development (Rowe, 1998; Pérez et al., 2006; Branchu et al., 2007). Expert systems are discussed further in chapter 8 "Product Optimization."

SOLID DOSAGE FORMS

Since tablets and capsules account for approximately 70% of pharmaceutical preparations, an investigation into the solid-state properties of candidate drugs is an important task to be undertaken during preformulation (Wells, 1988). Generally speaking, when dealing with high-strength solid dosage forms, this formulation will be more susceptible to any drug substance variability. However, other studies are also important since, for example, the same chemical compound can have different crystal structures (polymorphs), external shapes (habits), and hence different flow and compression properties.

Carstensen et al. (1993) have usefully, although briefly, reviewed the physicochemical properties of particulate matter dealing with the topics of cohesion, powder flow, micromeritics, crystallization, yield strengths, effects of moisture, and hygroscopicity. Buckton (1995) has reviewed the surface characterization of pharmaceuticals with regard to understanding sources of variability. A general overview of the methods available for the physical characterization of pharmaceutical solids has been presented by Brittain et al. (1991). York (1994) has also dealt with these issues and produced a hierarchy of testing techniques for powdered raw material. Finally, a book dealing with the physical characterization of pharmaceutical solids by Carstensen (2001) is recommended for additional reading on this subject. The importance of powder technology in pharmaceuticals has been emphasized by Muzzio et al. (2002), who have argued that particle technology strongly affects the time to market and the length of patent protection.

Table 1 Estimated Material Demands with Respect to Development Time

Months from CD nomination	Campaign	Typical amount (kg)	Use
4	1	0.2	7-day rat and dog toxicity + pharmaceutical studies
	2	1–20	1-mo toxicity studies
			Phase I trials
10	3	30	3 and 6 month toxicity and reproductive toxicity
11			12-mo dog study
			Phase II trials
17	4	125	Oncogenicity studies
			Phase III formulation development
			Phase III trial supply
25	5	210	Phase III trial supply

There are a number of other studies that can be enacted on a candidate drug to determine other important solid-state properties, for example, particle size, powder flow, compression, and polymorphism. Therefore, when a sample undergoes initial physicochemical testing, the following parameters should be measured: particle size, true, bulk, and tapped density, surface area and properties, compression properties, and powder flow properties. Pérez et al. (2006) have devised a new expert system for the control of batch powder properties. Some of these factors will be discussed in this chapter. However, others are dealt with in more detail in chapter 11, which deals specifically with solid oral dosage forms.

The production of drug substance is usually undertaken by the process research and development department (R&D) in a typical pharmaceutical company in so-called "campaigns." The typical batch size of each campaign and its typical usage is shown in Table 1. As can be seen from this table, the output of crystallization processes employed by PR&D produces increasing quantities of drug substance material per campaign as drug development progresses (Desikan et al., 2000). It is these materials that the product development department will use for initial preformulation and continued pharmaceutical development studies. An assumption made when calculating the amount per campaign is that the maximum dose for safety assessment is 250 mg/kg. Campaign 1 material tends to be non-GMP (Good Manufacturing Practice) material and is used to support prenomination studies from a batch size of approximately 150 to 300 g.

The cost of drug substance (in raw material terms) in the early stages of development is typically in the range of US$3000 to 7000 per kg. After transferring from R&D to manufacturing operations, the cost in raw material terms for a single batch of drug substance is typically US$1 to 2 million. However, the cost per kg should be considerably reduced because of economy of scale and process optimization.

Depending on the method of crystallization (cooling crystallization, antisolvent crystallization), the subsequent isolation (filtration and drying) of the drug substance will have a specific presentation to the product development department. The crystals produced may be single crystals, but often the crystals are associated in some way with each other. Nichols et al. (2002) have defined the way crystals are associated with each other in two ways, that is, hard and soft agglomerates. They preferred this definition to aggregate and agglomerate and defined a hard agglomerate as an assemblage of crystals that is non-friable and not easily dispersed, with a soft agglomerate being the opposite.

Agglomeration, as defined by Brunsteiner et al. (2005), is the intergrowth of aggregates formed by particle collisions, through a cementation process that forms an agglomerative bond. As shown by Ålander et al. (2002), supersaturation, particle concentration, hydrodynamics, and the solvent all affect agglomeration processes. Results showed that the material crystallized from acetone showed higher levels and stronger agglomerates than samples recovered from IPA (isopropyl alcohol). This behavior was postulated to be due to IPA –OH group hydrogen bonding with H-bonding functional groups on the growing paracetamol surface; acetone being a H-bond acceptor could not partake in this process and hence agglomerated. In addition, the viscosity of acetone is approximately seven times less than that of IPA, which may also influence agglomeration. Agglomeration can be a problem since it can lead to solvent inclusions. Agglomeration involves two steps. In the first step, crystals collide and are held together by attractive forces, giving a soft agglomerate (or aggregate). In the second step, the crystals cement together to form a hard agglomerate. Agglomeration increases with supersaturation, and small particles are more likely to agglomerate than large particles. Agglomeration is also more likely between a large particle and a small particle than between two particles of similar size (Brunsteiner et al., 2005). As a test, they suggested that the powders be placed on a microscope slide and some silicone oil added. If the powders readily dispersed under gentle shearing motion of the cover slip, then the powders could be classified as a soft agglomerate. Agglomerates can be further characterized using image analysis and strength measurements (Alander et al., 2003).

Kim et al. (2005) have discussed the control of the particle properties of a drug substance by crystal engineering and its effect on drug product. This work showed how, as part of a solid supply chain, a controlled crystallization produced large crystals with a narrow distribution, which were preserved during the drying process by utilizing low shear in the filter dryer. Drug substance produced by this method was found to have reproducible formulation properties. A more general review of crystal engineering is given by Chow et al. (2008).

Drug substance quality by design (QbD) is an important new aspect in the production of pharmaceuticals. The QbD concept describes developing a design space, establishing control strategies, and defining criticality for the drug substance. As an example of the use of QbD in the manufacture of the active pharmaceutical ingredient (API) torcetapid, see Am Ende et al. (2007). In this study, they employed design of experiments (DoEs) methodologies to examine the design space of the crystallization. In addition to DoEs, process analytical technologies (PAT) are used to monitor and control crystallization processes (Yu et al., 2004; Birch et al., 2005; Byrn et al., 2006). McKenzie et al. (2006) have pointed out that adoption of these manufacturing initiatives must be accompanied by the adoption of modeling tools and efficient information management systems.

Lionberger (2007) and Yu (2008) have summarized QbD into four areas. These are

- definition of the target product quality profile that describes the performance needed to get clinical benefit and meet consumer expectation,
- product and process design,
- identifying critical parameters, and
- process monitoring and control.

Drying of drug substances after crystallization is, perhaps, a neglected area, but one that can profoundly affect their properties. This is particularly true if a hydrate is involved, which was exemplified by a paper by Cypes et al. (2004), who described the drying of a compound that existed as an anhydrate, a monohydrate, and an isopropylalcohol solvate. They pointed out that drying filtration wet cakes and fixing a set time to dry a cake was dangerous, since variability in the process may cause overdrying of the monohydrate.

Impurities
Since unwanted impurities, for example, intermediates, degradation products, and products from side reactions may have deleterious pharmacological and toxicological activities, they must be removed from the final product. The identification of impurities is thus a crucial activity in drug substance PR&D (Huang et al., 2008). Indeed, it is a regulatory requirement that the level of impurities in the drug substance be controlled (see International Committee for Harmonization (ICH) Q3a, Müller et al., 2006; Jacobson-Kram and McGovern, 2007). In addition to regulatory requirements, the incorporation of impurities in the crystal lattice can lead to crystal defects, which in turn can lead to differences in, for example, mechanical properties, dissolution behavior, and stability, which may be the basis of batch-to-batch variation (Gu and Grant, 2002). One of the main objectives of crystallization is therefore to purge the compound of these impurities to make it fit for use as the active pharmaceutical ingredient in a medicine.

ICH classifies impurities into the following categories: organic impurities (process and drug related), inorganic impurities, and residual solvents. Organic impurities include, for example, starting materials, by-products, intermediates, degradation products as well as reagents, ligands, and catalysts. Inorganic impurities can often result from the manufacturing process, and examples of these are reagents, ligands and catalysts, heavy metals, inorganic salts, and other process-related materials such as filtration aids and charcoal. Solvents are controlled though ICH guideline Q3C. In addition to these obvious impurities, polymorphs as well as enantiomeric impurities need to be considered.

Impurities can have effects on the size, shape, and polymorphic form of compounds, such that, as the synthetic chemists experiment with different synthetic routes to the drug substance, different impurities generated can alter the physical properties of the crystals generated. For example, Masui et al. (2003) found that a related substance to their drug substance, cefmatilen hydrochloride, acted as a habit modifier. During early work, it was found that the compound crystallized as fine needles. However, by controlling the reaction, the production of the impurity was reduced and the habit was modified to larger blade-like crystals. Interestingly, by crystallizing in the presence of hydroxycelluloses or polyvinyl derivatives, the habit could be modified, that is, the additives thus act as crystal engineering aids. See Hulse et al. (2008) for the effect of low levels of aluminum, at the parts per million (ppm) level, on the physical properties of paracetamol.

Impurities may also affect the polymorph that crystallizes from solution. For example, Gu et al. (2002) have reported how substances related to sulphamerazine stabilized the metastable form in a slurry experiment conducted in acetonitrile. Normally, in solution-mediated phase transformations, slurries of metastable forms will convert to the stable form. The sequence of events is dissolution of the metastable phase, nucleation of the stable phase, followed by crystal growth. The transformation of the metastable form I to form II is controlled by the crystallization of form II. However, in the presence of impurities, the nucleation and growth rates were significantly reduced in the rank order N4-acetylsulphamerazine (NSMZ) ≫ sulphadiazine > sulphamethazine (NSMZ ≫ SD > SM). Similarly, Okamoto et al. (2004) found that one of the impurities of AE1-923, a compound for pollakiuria and pain, inhibited a polymorphic transformation. The most important learning point of these studies is that the presence of impurities can affect the results of polymorph screens, since impurities can stabilize metastable forms and give a false sense of security that you are dealing with the stable form. Therefore, the use of pure material for polymorph screens is recommended, and the screen should be reconducted when route changes are made—especially if the impurity profile changes.

It should also remembered that formulations also contain excipients that have their own crystal properties, which can be altered by the incorporation of impurities with the result that batch-to-batch variation can be experienced. For example, Garnier et al. (2002) determined the effect of supersaturation and the presence of structurally related additives on the crystal growth of α-lactose monohydrate [an important excipient used in dry-powder inhalers (DPIs)]. Contrary to expectation, the crystal size of α-lactose monohydrate increased with increasing supersaturation. This was explained to be due to β-lactose strongly inhibiting crystal growth at low supersaturation. With regard to the effect of the other impurities, it was found that some impurities were able to change the habit without being incorporated into the growing crystal lattice. Indeed, α-galactose, β-cellobiose, and maltitol were found to preferentially adsorb to two specific faces of the α-lactose, leading to a flattened morphology.

Particle Size Reduction

The particle size of the drug substance is important since it can affect such things as content uniformity in tablets (Rohrs et al., 2006), bioavailability (Rasenack and Müller, 2005; Jinno et al., 2006), sedimentation, and flocculation rates in suspensions. Moreover, the inhalation therapy of pulmonary diseases demands that particles of a small particle size (2–5 μm) are delivered to the lung for the optimum therapeutic effect (Howarth, 2001; Pritchard, 2001). It is therefore important that the particle size is consistent throughout the development studies of a product to satisfy formulation and regulatory demands (Rohrs et al., 2006).

At the lead optimization stage, only small quantities (e.g., 50 mg) will be available to administer to the animal. Thus, to reduce the risk of dissolution rate limited bioavailability, the material can be ground with a mortar and pestle to reduce the particle size of the compound.

Table 2 Mill Selection Matrix

Criteria	Slurry	Fluid energy	Universal	Cone	Hammer
Particle size	Less than average	Very favorable	Very favorable	Less than average	Average
Particle distribution	Average	Very favorable	Very favorable	Favorable	Favorable
Cleaning	Less than average	Average	Average	Favorable	Less than average
Operating cost	Favorable	Unfavorable	Unfavorable	Very favorable	Favorable
Dust containment	Very favorable	Less than average	Less than average	Very favorable	Favorable
Temperature	Very favorable	Favorable	Less than average	Very favorable	Favorable
Flexibility	Average	Average	Very favorable	Favorable	Favorable

Source: From Spencer and Dalder, 1997, reproduced with permission.

However, there needs to be some caution because the process of grinding can induce a polymorphic change as shown by Lin et al. (2006). If larger quantities of drug substance are available, then ball milling or micronization can be used to reduce the particle size.

Taylor et al. (2007) have described a nanoindentation technique for predictive milling of compounds. Using a range of Pfizer compounds, they were able to calculate a fracture toughness of the material such that hardness could be calculated from the depth of the indentation. The brittleness index (BI) could then be calculated according to equation (1).

$$\mathrm{BI} = \frac{H}{K_c} \tag{1}$$

where H is the hardness and K_c is the fracture toughness. For a sildenafil citrate (Viagra®), the BI is 27.8 km$^{-\frac{1}{2}}$ (very brittle), whereas voriconazole has a BI of less than 1 (very plastic). Zügner et al. (2006) have also used nanoindentation to calculate hardness and elastic modulus of a range of compounds, which are essential when determining the conditions under which a compound is micronized. Their results showed that the elastic-plastic properties of the crystals strongly influenced their breaking behavior.

The main methods of particle size reduction have been reviewed by Spencer and Dalder (1997), who devised the mill selection matrix shown in Table 2. Chickhalia et al. (2006) have examined the effect of crystal morphology and the mill type on the disorder induced by milling. Using β-succinic acid as a model compound, which can be crystallized in plate-and-needle morphologies, size reduction was carried out in a ball-and-jet mill. They showed that the plate crystals were more susceptible to disordering in the ball mill than that in the jet mill. Interestingly, they also found that some conversion to the α-form occurred. Wilfdfong et al. (2006) have attempted to provide a theoretical framework of the disordering process induced by milling. It would appear from their investigations that disordering is a result of the crystal lattice being forced to accommodate a large number of dislocations with the net effect that, from an energetic perspective, it is effectively amorphous.

Nakach et al. (2004) have compared the various milling technologies for the particle size reduction of pharmaceutical solids. They investigated both air jet mills and impact mills. Using vitamin C (ascorbic acid) as a test substance, they concluded that the pancake mill was preferred for ultrafine grinding since it was simple to use, had a high feed rate, and was easy to clean.

Ball Milling
Ball milling is probably used most often at the preformulation stage to reduce the particle size of small amounts of a compound, especially for the preparation formulations to be administered to animals. It is also used for the preparation of co-crystals, as described in chapter 3. For a review of high-purity applications of ball milling, such as pharmaceuticals, see Vernon (1994).

Ball mills reduce the size of particles through a combined process of impact and attrition. Usually, they consist of a hollow cylinder that contains balls of various sizes, which are rotated

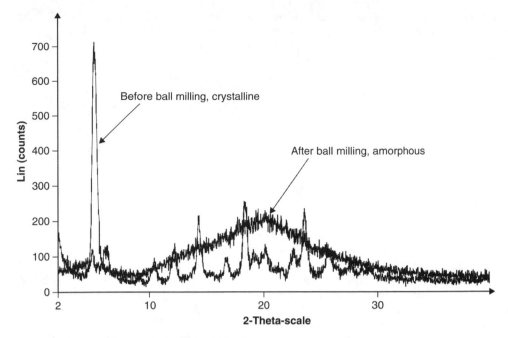

Figure 1   Effect of ball milling on a development compound.

to initiate the grinding process. There are a number of factors that affect the efficiency of the milling process, and these include rotation speed, mill size, wet or dry milling, and the amount of material to be milled.

Although ball milling can effectively reduce the particle size of compounds, prolonged milling may be detrimental in terms of its crystallinity and stability (Font et al., 1997). This was illustrated in a study that examined the effect of ball mill grinding on cefixime trihydrate (Kitamura et al., 1989). Using a variety of techniques, it was shown that the crystalline solid was rendered amorphous after four hours in a ball mill. The stability of the amorphous phase was found to be less than that of the crystalline solid, and in addition, the samples were discolored because of grinding. Thus, it is important to check this aspect of the milling process, since amorphous compounds can show increased bioavailability and possible pharmacological activity compared with the corresponding crystalline form. Ball milling may also change the polymorphic form of a compound as shown by the work conducted by Zhang et al. (2002) on the polymorphs of sulfamerazine. These workers found that when the metastable form II of this compound was milled, it resulted in a broadening and decrease in the intensities of the X-ray diffraction peaks. However, when form I (the stable form) was milled, it quickly transformed to form II. Descamps et al. (2007) have explored potential reasons why some compounds are rendered amorphous and why some may undergo a polymorphic change when milled. In particular, they pointed out that the position of the glass transition of the amorphous phase had an important bearing on the transformations that took place on milling. For example, they concluded that milling a crystalline compound well below its glass transition temperature (T_g) induced amorphization, whereas milling above the T_g caused polymorphic changes.

Figure 1 shows the X-ray Powder Diffraction (XRPD) patterns of a sample of a compound "as received" and after ball milling. After ball milling for one hour, the sample was rendered amorphous, and hence, a shorter milling period was used when preparing the sample for a suspension formulation. Polymorphic changes due to ball milling have also been followed by Raman spectroscopy (Cheng et al., 2007).

Micronization (Jet Milling)
If instrumentation and sufficient compound are available, then micronization can be undertaken. In this respect, Hosokawa has a small-scale air jet mill with a 1 in. screen, which can be used to

micronize small quantities of compound (down to ~500 mg) and is thus ideal for the preformulation stage where the amount of compound is restricted. Micronization is routinely used to reduce the particle size of active ingredients so that the maximum surface area is exposed to enhance the solubility and dissolution properties of poorly soluble compounds.

The micronization process involves feeding the drug substance into a confined circular chamber where the powder is suspended in a high-velocity stream of air. Interparticulate collisions result in a size reduction. Smaller particles are removed from the chamber by the escaping airstream toward the center of the mill where they are discharged and collected. Larger particles recirculate until their particle size is reduced. Micronized particles are typically less than 10 μm in diameter (Midoux et al., 1999). De Vegt et al. (2005a,b) have discussed some theoretical and practical aspects of the milling of organic solids in a jet mill. Zügner et al. (2006) have reported the influence of the nanomechanical crystal properties on jet milling, and the kinetics of jet milling of ethenzamide have been investigated by Fukunaka et al. (2006).

Because of the enhanced surface area, the oral bioavailability of compounds is often improved. For example, the absorption characteristics of both a micronized (8 μm) and a coarse fraction (125 μm) of felodipine were studied under two motility patterns (Scholz, 2002). The reduction in particle size led up to an approximately 22-fold increase in maximum plasma concentration and up to an approximately 14-fold increase in area under the curve, with a commensurate decrease in the time at which the maximum plasma concentration occurred. Although the absorption of felodipine from the solution and micronized suspension were not influenced by a change in the hydrodynamics, felodipine was absorbed from the coarse suspension almost twice as well in the "fed" state as under "fasted" conditions.

In addition to air jet milling, micronization by precipitation from supercritical fluids has received much attention as alternative particle size reduction method for pharmaceuticals (Martin and Cocero, 2008).

Nanoparticles
Typically, micronization can reduce the particle size of compounds to sizes in the micrometer range. However, increases in bioavailability can be obtained by further particle size reduction. To reduce the particle size into the colloidal range (10–1000 nm), other techniques such as precipitation processes, pearl milling, and high-pressure homogenization need to be employed (Gao et al., 2008). The colloidal particles produced by these processes are typically stabilized by surfactants. The precipitation technique is relatively straightforward and is usually reliant on the rapid generation of high supersaturation induced by adding an antisolvent to a solution of the compound. Pearl milling is essentially wet ball milling in the presence of a surfactant, which produces a colloidal dispersion of the compound within a few hours or days depending on the hardness of the compound and the desired particle size. High-pressure homogenization consists of passing a suspension (with a surfactant) of a compound through a narrow gap under a very high velocity. The high energy created in this region, coupled with the collisions between the particles, causes the particles to decrease in size into the colloidal region. As an alternative, Yang et al. (2008) have described the production of sumatriptan succinate nanoparticles by reactive crystallization of the two components of the salt followed by spray drying.

Effect of Milling and Micronization
Although micronization of the drug offers the advantage of a small particle size and a larger surface area, it can result in processing problems due to high dust, low density, and poor flow properties. Indeed, micronization may be counter-productive since the micronized particles may aggregate, which may decrease the surface area and compact on the surface of the equipment (Furunaka et al., 2005). In addition, changes in crystallinity of the drug can also occur, which can be detected by techniques such as microcalorimetry, dynamic vapor sorption (DVS) (Macklin et al., 2002), and inverse gas chromatography (IGC) (Buckton and Gill, 2007).

Ward and Schultz (1995) reported subtle differences in the crystallinity of salbutamol sulfate after micronization by air jet milling. They found that amorphous to crystalline conversions that were dependent on temperature and relative humidity (RH) occurred. It was suggested that particle size reduction of the powder produced defects on the surface that, if enough energy was imparted, led to amorphous regions on the surface. In turn, these regions were found to have a greater propensity to adsorb water. On exposure to moisture, these regions crystallized and expelled excess moisture. This is illustrated in Figure 2, which shows the uptake of moisture, as measured by DVS of a micronized development compound. Note how the percent mass change increases and then decreases as the RH is increased between 40% and 60% during the sorption phase. This corresponds to crystallization of the compound and subsequent ejection of the excess moisture. The compound also exhibits some hysteresis.

This effect can be important in some formulations such as DPI devices, since it can cause agglomeration of the powders and variable flow properties (Steckel et al., 2006; Young et al., 2007). In many cases, this low level of amorphous character cannot be detected by techniques such as X-ray powder diffraction. Since microcalorimetry can detect less than 10% amorphous content (the limit of detection is 1% or less), it has the advantage over other techniques such as X-ray powder diffraction or differential scanning calorimetry (DSC) (Phipps and Mackin, 2000; Mackin et al., 2002). Using the ampoule technique, with an internal hygrostat, as described by Briggner et al. (1994) (Fig. 3), the amorphous content of a micronized drug can be determined

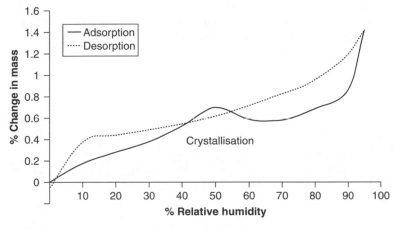

Figure 2 Dynamic vapor sorption showing crystallization effects due to moisture.

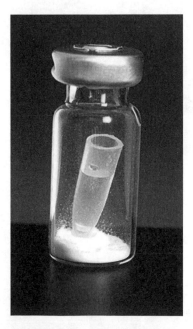

Figure 3 Internal hygrostat for microcalorimetric measurements of moisture sorption.

by measuring the heat output caused by the water vapor inducing crystallization of the amorphous regions (Fig. 4).

The crystallization of amorphous regions can cause changes to the surface of the miconized materials. For example, when Price and Young (2005) examined the effect of 70% RH on the surface of milled lactose crystals using atomic force microscopy (AFM), they found that it had undergone both morphological and physicomechanical changes. RH is not the only variable that can affect the outcome of the recrystallization process. For example, Chieng et al. (2006) have shown that the temperature of milling has an effect on the form of rantidine hydrochloride after milling. In particular, the temperature of ball milling was found to be important, for example, form I was converted to form II between 12°C and 35°C. If the milling was conducted under cold room conditions, form I was converted to the amorphous form. Another work reported by this group (Chieng et al., 2008) on the cryomilling of ranitidine polymorphs showed that both the forms were rendered amorphous by the ball mill but were found to crystallize back to the original polymorphs after two weeks.

Figure 5 shows the calibration curve of heat output versus amorphous content of a development compound. In this case, the technique is used to crystallize, or condition, these amorphous regions by exposure to elevated relative humidities. Thus, if authentic 100% amorphous and crystalline phases exist, it is possible to construct a calibration graph of heat output versus percent crystallinity so that the amount of amorphous character introduced by

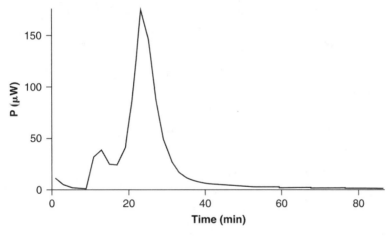

Figure 4   Crystallization peak energy versus time.

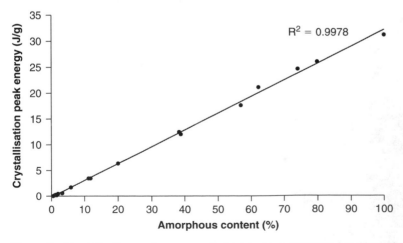

Figure 5   Crystallization peak energy versus amorphous content using microcalorimetry.

the milling process can be quantified. Ramos et al. (2005) have provided some guidance on the preparation of calibration curves when isothermal calorimetry is used in this mode.

Inverse Gas Chromatography
In addition to the DVS and microcalorimetric techniques for the characterization of surface properties of powders, another technique known as IGC can be employed (Telko and Hickey, 2007; Buckton and Gill, 2007). This technique differs from traditional gas chromatography in so far that the stationary phase is the powder under investigation. In this type of study, a range of nonpolar and polar adsorbates (probes), for example, alkanes from hexane to decane, acetone, diethyl ether, or ethyl acetate, are used. The retention volume, that is, the net volume of carrier gas (nitrogen) required to elute the probe, is then measured. The partition coefficient (K_s) of the probes between the carrier gas and surfaces of test powder particles can then be calculated. From this, a free energy can be calculated, which can show that one batch may more favorably adsorb the probes when compared with another, implying a difference in the surface energetics.

The experimental parameter measured in IGC experiments is the net retention volume, V_n. This parameter is related to the surface partition coefficient, K_s, which is the ratio between the concentration of the probe molecule in the stationary and mobile phases shown by equation (2).

$$K_s = \frac{V_n}{m} \times A_{sp} \tag{2}$$

where m is the weight of the sample in the column and A_{sp} is the specific surface of the sample in the column.

From K_s, the free energy of adsorption ($-\Delta G_A$) is defined by equation (3).

$$-\Delta G_A = RT \ln\left(K_s \times \frac{P_{sg}}{P} \right) \tag{3}$$

where P_{sg} is the standard vapor state (101 KN/m^2) and P is the standard surface pressure, which has a value of 0.338 mN/m.

IGC and molecular modeling have been used to assess the effect of micronization on dl-propranolol (York et al., 1998). The samples were jet milled (micronized) to various particle sizes, and γ_s^D was measured and plotted against their median particle size. This showed that as the particle size decreased because of the micronization process, the surface of the particles became more energetic. Interestingly, it was pointed out that the plateau region corresponded to the brittle-ductile region of this compound, as previously reported by Roberts et al. (1991). This observation implied a change in the mechanism of milling from a fragmentation to an attrition process. The data for $-\Delta G_A^{SP}$ for the tetrahydrofuran (THF) and dichloromethane probes showed that the electron donation of the surface increased as the particle size decreased. Combining these data with molecular modeling, which was used to predict which surfaces would predominate, they showed that the electron-rich naphthyl group dominated the surface of the unmilled material. This led to the conclusion that as the particle size was reduced, this surface became more exposed, leading to a greater interaction with the THF and dichloromethane probes. However, as previously noted, as milling proceeded, the mechanism of size reduction changed, which might lead to exposure of the chloride and hydroxyl moieties. More recent work on how milling affects surface properties of crystals of paracetamol has been reported by Heng et al. (2006), who found that as the crystals were reduced in size, the surfaces became more hydrophobic. This was explained by reference to the crystal structure whereby the crystals fractured along the weakest attachment energy facet, which became progressively exposed as milling progressed.

In summary, using moisture sorption, microcalorimetry, IGC, molecular modeling, and other techniques, the consequences of the particle size reduction process can be assessed. Moreover, surface energetics can be measured directly and predictions made about the nature of the surface, which could ultimately affect properties such as the flow of powders or adhesion of particles. For example, Tong et al. (2006) used IGC measurements to measure the interaction between salmeterol xinafoate powders and lactose carriers used in DPI formulations.

In addition to its use in the determination of surface properties after milling, IGC has also been used for such things as the determination of the solubility parameters of pharmaceutical excipients (Adamska et al., 2007) and determination of the of glass transitions (Surana et al., 2003; Ambarkhane et al., 2005).

Atomic Force Microscopy

AFM is a scanning probe microscopy technique that has been used in preformulation to study in great detail the surfaces of crystals (Turner et al., 2007). Imaging using AFM utilizes a sharp tip, typically made from silicon or silicon nitride (Si_3N_4), attached to a flexible cantilever that rasters across the surface using a piezoelectric scanner. This motion induced by the interaction of the tip and the surface is monitored using a laser beam that falls on photodiode detector. It can be used in a number of modes, that is, contact, "tapping," and noncontact. It has been used, for example, for characterizing polymorphs and amorphous phases and the effect of humidity on lactose (Price and Young, 2004). It has also been used to characterize crystal growth phenomena (Thomson et al. (2004).

Time-of-Flight Secondary Ion Mass Spectroscopy

Time-of-flight secondary ion mass spectroscopy (Tof SIMS) is a surface characterization technique. Surface mass spectrometry techniques measure the masses of fragment ions that are ejected from the surface of a sample to identify the elements and molecules present. Tof SIMS instruments with mass resolution of 10^{-3} to 10^{-4} amu are achievable. This enables Tof SIMS to be sensitive to ppm/ppb. Tof SIMS has been used in the pharmaceutical arena (Muster and Prestidge, 2002). In this study, face-specific surface chemistries of polymorphs I and III were characterized.

Particle Size Distribution Measurement

It is known that the particle size distribution of a pharmaceutical powder can affect the manufacturability, stability, and bioavailability of immediate-release tablets (Tinke et al., 2005). The Food and Drugs Administration (FDA) recommends that a suitable test method and acceptance criteria be established for the particle size distribution of a drug substance.

Snorek et al. (2007) has discussed the concepts and techniques of particle size analysis and its role in pharmaceutical sciences and gives the range of size measurement methods commonly used and the corresponding approximate useful size range (Snorek et al., 2007). The most readily available laboratory techniques include sieving (Brittain and Amidon, 2003), optical microscopy in conjunction with image analysis, electron microscopy, the Coulter counter, and laser diffraction (Xu et al., 2003). It is usual that a powder shows a distribution of particle sizes often represented as a Gaussian distribution (log normal).

Sieve Analysis

Sieving is a simple, well-established technique to determine the particle size distribution of powders whereby the particles pass through a set of screens of decreasing size due to agitation or sonication. The sample is introduced on the top sieve, and the agitation causes the powder to move through the rest of the sieves, and the particle size distribution is determined from the weight of compound remaining on each sieve. The particle size distribution data is then presented as a percentage of the material retained on each sieve. Like all techniques for particle size analysis, it has its strengths and weaknesses. The major strength of sieve analysis is its relative simplicity. However, the nature of the sieves is such that, for example, acicular crystals may pass through the sieve via their short axis.

Laser Diffraction and Scattering

Laser diffraction has become the most popular method of particle size analysis because of its ease of use, fast analysis times, and high reproducibility (Xu, 2000). The use of this technique is based on light scattered through various angles, which is directly related to the diameter of the particle. Thus, by measuring the angles and intensity of scattered light from the particles, a particle size distribution can be deduced. It should be noted that the particle diameters reported are the same as those that spherical particles would produce under similar conditions.

Two theories dominate the theory of light scattering; the Fraunhofer and Mie theories. In the former, each particle is treated as spherical and essentially opaque to the impinging laser light. Mie theory, on the other hand, takes into account the differences in refractive indices between the particles and the suspending medium. If the diameter of the particles is above 10 μm, then the size produced by utilizing each theory is essentially the same. However, discrepancies may occur when the diameter of the particles approaches that of the wavelength of the laser source.

The following are the values reported from diffraction experiments:

$D[v,0.1]$ is the size of particles for which 10% of the sample is below this size.
$D[v,0.5]$ is the volume (v) median diameter for which 50% of the sample is below and above this size.
$D[v,0.9]$ gives a size of particle for which 90% of the sample is below this size.
$D[4,3]$ is the equivalent volume mean diameter calculated from equation (4), which is as follows:

$$D[4, 3] = \frac{\sum d^4}{\sum d^3} \tag{4}$$

where d is the diameter of each unit.
$D[3,2]$ is the surface area mean diameter; also known as the Sauter mean.

Log difference represents the difference between the observed light energy data and the calculated light energy data for the derived distribution.

Span is the measurement of the width of the distribution and is calculated from equation (5).

$$\text{Span} = \frac{D[v, 0.9] - D[v, 0.1]}{D[v, 0.5]} \tag{5}$$

The dispersion of the powder is important in achieving reproducible results. Ideally, the dispersion medium should have the following characteristics:

- Should have a suitable absorbency
- Should not swell the particles
- Should disperse a wide range of particles
- Should slow sedimentation of particles
- Should allow homogeneous dispersion of the particles
- Should be safe and easy to use

In terms of sample preparation, it is necessary to deaggregate the samples so that the primary particles are measured. To achieve this, the sample may be sonicated, although there is a potential problem of the sample being disrupted by the ultrasonic vibration. To check for this, it is recommended that the particle dispersion be examined by optical microscopy standards for laser diffraction given in the standard.

The Malvern Mastersizer (Malvern Instruments, Malvern, U.K.) is an example of an instrument that measures particle size by laser diffraction on the basis of the Mie theory, and the Helos laser diffraction instrument (Sympatec GmbH, Clausthal-Zellerfeld, Germany) represents a Fraunhofer-based system.

Although laser light diffraction is a rapid and highly repeatable method in determining the particle size distributions of pharmaceutical powders, the results obtained can be affected by particle shape. For example, Xu et al. (2003) compared the particle size distributions

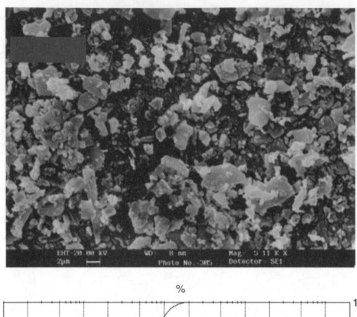

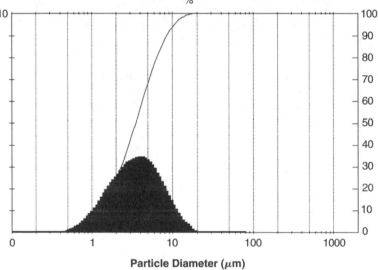

Figure 6   Scanning electron microscopy of a micronized powder and particle size measured by laser diffraction.

obtained from laser diffraction experiments, electrical zone sensing, and dynamic image analysis (DIA). They found that for spherical particles or particles with small aspect ratio, all instruments returned similar results. However, as the shape of the particle size distribution became more extreme, the laser diffraction instrument tended to overestimate the breadth of the size distribution. Thus, when dealing with anisotropic particle shape, caution should be exercised on the quotation of a particle size.

Figure 6 shows the particle size distribution of a micronized powder determined by scanning electron microscopy (SEM) and laser light scattering. Table 3 shows the data obtained from the laser diffraction analysis shown in Figure 6.

Another laser-based instrument, relying on light scattering, is the aerosizer. This is a particle-sizing method based on a time-of-flight principle as described by Niven (1993). The aerosizer with aero-disperser is specifically designed to carry deaggregated particles in an airstream for particle sizing. Mendes et al. (2004) have used this instrument to evaluate the Ventilan Rotocaps™ and Bricanyl Tubohaler™ DPIs.

Table 3 Particle Size Distribution of a Micronized Powder Measured by Using Laser Diffraction

Size (µm)	Volume under %	Size (µm)	Volume under %	Size (µm)	Volume under %	Size (µm)	Volume under %
0.05	0.00	0.65	1.09	4.30	60.67	28.15	100.00
0.12	0.00	0.81	2.58	5.29	71.18	34.69	100.00
0.15	0.00	1.00	5.08	6.52	80.61	42.75	100.00
0.19	0.00	1.23	8.90	8.04	88.21	52.68	100.00
0.23	0.00	1.51	14.24	9.91	93.69	64.92	100.00
0.28	0.00	1.86	21.22	12.21	97.18	80.00	100.00
0.35	0.00	2.30	29.72	15.04	99.08		
0.43	0.03	2.83	39.38	18.54	99.87		
0.53	0.34	3.49	49.86	22.84	100.00		
Range: 45 mm	Beam: 2.40 mm		Sampler: MS1				Obs': 15.8%

Presentation: 2$$D	Analysis: polydisperse	Residual: 0.117%
Modifications: none		
Concentration = 0.0062% volume	Density = 1.427 g/cm^3	SSA = 1.6133 m^2/g
Distribution: volume	D[4,3] = 4.34 µm	D[3,2] = 2.61 µm
D[v,0.1] = 1.29 µm	D[v,0.5] = 3.50 µm	D[v,0.9] = 8.54 µm
Span = 2.071E + 00	Uniformity = 6.515E − 01	

Photon Correlation Spectroscopy or Quasi-Elastic Elastic Light Scattering

For submicron materials, particularly colloidal particles, photon correlation spectroscopy (PCS) [quasi-elastic elastic light scattering (QELS)] is the preferred technique. This technique has been usefully reviewed by Phillies (1990). Often this technique is coupled with zeta potential measurements so that the dispersion stability can be assessed. Examples of the use of PCS in the literature include the characterization of nebulized buparvaquone nanosuspensions (Hernandez-Trejo et al., 2005) and the characterization of liposomes (Ruozi et al., 2005). PCS relies on the Doppler shift in the wavelength of the scattered laser light, and from the autocorrelation function, a z-average particle size is derived and can be used to measure particles in the size range 3 nm to 3 µm. In addition to the size of the particles, a polydispersity index (a measure of the width of the distribution) is also derived. An example of a commercial PCS is the Malvern Zetasizer manufactured by Malvern Instruments (U.K.) (Grau et al., 2000).

Image Analysis

Optical microscopy is a simple but powerful technique for the examination of crystal size and shape (Lerke and Adams, 2003). It can give a quick estimation of the average size of crystals, but for a more quantitative measure, the microscopic images need to be coupled with image analysis software to increase the accuracy, decrease the tediousness of manual counting, and minimize operator bias. Recent advances in high-speed camera and more powerful computers have been combined to such an extent that it is now possible to perform DIA. An example of DIA is Sympatec's QicPic, which can capture images of particles in an airstream (see Yu and Hancock, 2008 for details of this technique). In essence, the QicPic uses rear illumination with a visible pulsed (1–500 Hz) light source synchronized with a high-speed camera running at 500 frames per second. The sample is delivered to this detection system via a dry-powder feeder where air is flowing at 100 m/s. During the course of an experiment, approximately 10^5 particle images are counted. Yu and Hancock compared the data obtained from samples that were spherical or rod-shaped and their mixtures with the measurements obtained from a laser diffraction instrument. The initial analysis indicated that the QicPic overestimated the amount of rod-shaped particles in the mixture, but when other data with respect to apparent density were taken into account, good agreement between the computed and experimental data was obtained.

In an interesting extension to image analysis is its use in following the recrystallization of, for example, amorphous cefadroxil (Parkkali et al., 2000).

Surface Area Measurements

The surface area of a solid pharmaceutical is an important parameter since such secondary properties such as dissolution and bioavailability (as predicted by the Noyes–Whitney equation) can be affected. Surface areas are usually determined by gas adsorption (nitrogen or krypton), and although there are a number of theories describing this phenomenon, the most widely used is the Bruner, Emmet, and Teller (BET) method. Adsorption methods for surface area determination have been reviewed in detail by Sing (1992). Two methods are used, that is, multipoint and single-point.

Without going into too much theoretical detail, the BET isotherm for type II (typical for pharmaceutical powders) adsorption processes is given by equation (6).

$$\left\{ \frac{\dot{z}}{(1-z)} V \right\} = \frac{1}{cV_{mon}} + \frac{(c-1)z}{cV_{mon}} \tag{6}$$

where $z = P/P_o$, V the volume of gas adsorbed, V_{mon} the volume of gas at monolayer coverage, and c is related to the intercept. It can be seen that equation (6) is of the form of a straight line. Thus, by plotting $\{z/(1-z)V\}$ versus z, a straight line of slope $(c-1)/cV_{mon}$ and intercept $1/cV_{mon}$ will be obtained. According to the U.S. Pharmacopoeia (USP), the data are considered to be acceptable if, on linear regression, the correlation coefficient is not less than 0.9975, that is, r^2 is not less than 0.995.

Figure 7 shows the full adsorption isotherm of two batches of the micronized powder shown earlier in Figure 6.

It should be noted that, experimentally, it is necessary to remove gases and vapors that may be present on the surface of the powder. This is usually achieved by drawing a vacuum or purging the sample in a flowing stream of nitrogen. Raising the temperature may not always be advantageous. For example, Phadke and Collier (1994) examined the effect of degassing temperature on the surface area of magnesium stearate obtained from two manufacturers. In this study, helium at a range of temperatures between 23°C and 60°C was used in single and

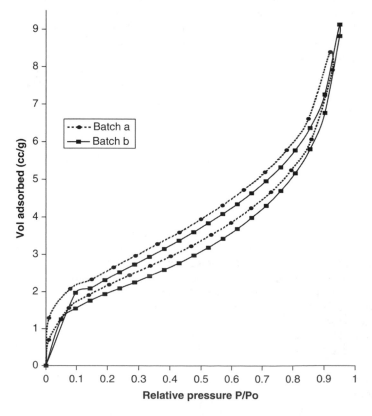

Figure 7 Full type IIb adsorption isotherm for two batches of a micronized powder.

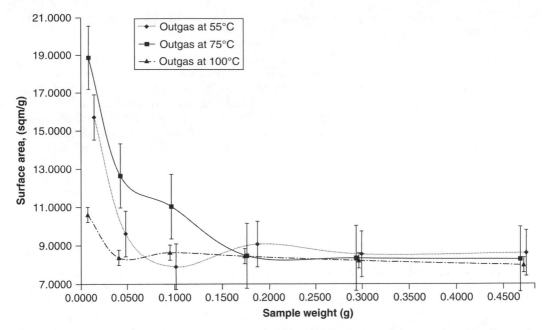

Figure 8 Effect of sample weight and degassing temperature on the surface area of micronized powder.

multipoint determinations. It was found that the specific surface area of the samples decreased with an increase in temperature. From other measurements using DSC and thermogravimetric analysis (TGA), it was found that raising the temperature changed the nature of the samples. Hence, it was recommended that magnesium stearate should not be degassed at elevated temperatures. Further work on the difficulty in measuring the surface area of magnesium stearate has been reported by Andrès et al. (2001).

Figure 8 shows the effect of sample weight and temperature of degassing on a sample of a micronized powder using a Micromeritics Gemini BET analyzer. From this plot, it can be seen that the weight of the sample can have a marked effect on the measured surface area of the compound under investigation. Therefore, to avoid reporting erroneous surface areas, the sample weight should not be too low and in this case be greater than 300 mg.

In an interesting paper by Joshi et al. (2002a), they reported that after micronization, the specific surface area increased after storage at 25°C. This was attributed to postmicronization stress relief via intraparticle crack formation.

True Density

Density can be defined as the ratio of the mass of an object to its volume. Therefore, the density of a solid is a reflection of the arrangement of molecules in a solid. In pharmaceutical development terms, knowledge of the true density of powders has been used for the determination of the consolidation behavior. For example, the well-known Heckel relation [equation (7)] requires knowledge of the true density of the compound.

$$\ln\left[\frac{1}{(1-D)}\right] = KP + A \qquad (7)$$

where D is the relative density, which is the ratio of the apparent density to the true density, K is determined from the linear portion of the Heckel plot, and P is the pressure. Sun (2005) has pointed out that an inaccurate true density value can affect powder compaction data. Using a novel mathematical model (Sun, 2004), it was shown that to achieve 4% accuracy, a true density with less than 0.28% error was required. The densities of molecular crystals can be increased by compression. For example, while investigating the compression properties of acetylsalicylic acid using a compaction simulator, increases in the true density were found (Pedersen and Kristensen, 1994).

- Information about the true density of a powder can be used to predict whether a compound will cream or sediment in a metered-dose inhaler (MDI) formulation. The densities of the hydrofluoroalkane (HFA) propellants, 227 and 134a, which have replaced chlorofluorocarbons (CFCs) in MDI formulations, are 1.415 and 1.217 g/cm^3, respectively. Traini et al. (2007) have reported the true densities of the inhalation drugs budesonide and formoterol fumarate dihydrate as 1.306 and 1.240 g/cm^3, respectively. Suspensions of compounds that have a true density less than these figures will cream (rise to the surface) and those that are denser will sediment. Those that match the density of the propellant will stay in suspension for a longer period (Williams et al., 1998). It should be noted, however, that the physical stability of a suspension is not merely a function of the true density of the material.

The true density is thus a property of the material and is independent of the method of determination. In this respect, the true density can be determined using three methods: displacement of a liquid, displacement of a gas (pycnometry), or floatation in a liquid. These methods of measuring true density have been evaluated by Duncan-Hewitt and Grant (1986). They concluded that whereas liquid displacement was tedious and tended to underestimate the true density, displacement of a gas was accurate but needed relatively expensive instrumentation. As an alternative, the floatation method was found to be simple to use, inexpensive, and, although more time consuming than gas pycnometry, accurate.

Gas pycnometry is probably the most commonly used method in the pharmaceutical industry for measuring true density. For details of the measurement of density by gas pycnometry, the reader should, for example, refer to Pharm Forum 20, 7222 (1994). All gas pycnometers rely on the measurement of pressure changes as a reference volume of gas, typically helium, is added to or deleted from the test cell. Experimentally, measurements should be carried out in accordance with the manufacturers' instructions. However, it is worth noting that artifacts may occur. For example, Figure 9 shows the measured true density of a number of tableting excipients as a function of sample weight. As can be seen, at low sample

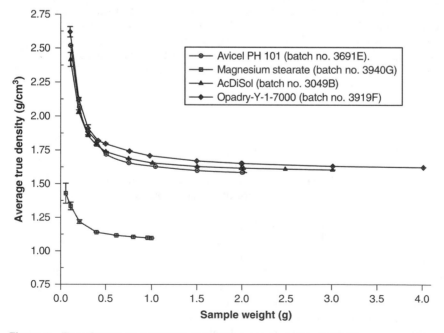

Figure 9   True density as a function of sample mass for some excipients.

weights, the measured true density was seen to increase, making the measurements less accurate. Viana et al. (2002) have systematically investigated pycnometry and showed that accuracies of the technique to the nearest 0.001% g/cm^3 could not be guaranteed.

The true density of organic crystals can also be calculated from the crystal structure of the compound and can be accessed via the Mercury program supplied by the Cambridge Crystallographic Data Centre (CCDC). As a further sophistication, Sun (2007) has examined the variability of this value and found that, on average, a relative standard deviation (RSD) of $\sim 0.4\%$ is typical for a calculated crystal structure. He also found that the true density increased as the temperature decreased. The experiments carried out by Viana et al. (2002) pointed out that true densities determined by pycnometry appeared to be less than those calculated from the crystal structure.

Coa et al. (2008) have used two empirically derived predictive methodologies to estimate the true densities of some drug substances. Both the methods showed good agreement with measured values and thus may be valuable when very limited amounts of compound are available for experimental measurements.

Flow and Compaction of Powders

Although at the preformulation stage, only limited quantities of candidate drug are available, any data generated on flow and compaction properties can be of great use to the formulation scientist. The data provided can give guidance on the selection of the excipients to use, the formulation type, and the manufacturing process to use, for example, direct compression or granulation. It is important that once the habit and size distribution of the test compound have been determined, the flow and compaction properties are evaluated, if the intended dosage form is a solid dosage form. York (1992) has reviewed the crystal engineering and particle design for the powder compaction process, and Thalberg et al. (2004) has compared the flowability tests for inhalation powders (ordered mixtures). The techniques investigated include the poured bulk density, compressed bulk density, an instrument known as the AeroFlow, and a uniaxial tester. Other shear testing includes ring shear testers (Hou and Sun, 2008), the angle of repose, Carr's index, Hausner ratio, etc. (see Hickey et al., 2007a, b for a good review of the various methods available).

The European Pharmacopoeia (Ph Eur) contains a test on flowability of powders based on how a powder flows vertically out of a funnel. Using data from a range of excipients, Schüssele and Bauer-Brandl (2003) have argued that the powder flow using this technique should be expressed as volume per unit time rather than mass per unit time as recommended by the Ph Eur Soh et al. (2006) have proposed some new indices of powder flow based on their avalanching behavior, that is, avalanche flow index (AFI) and cohesive interaction index (CoI), using the commercially available AeroFlow^{TM} instrument.

The compaction properties of the API are critical in their formulation, and such parameters such as yield stress and strain rate sensitivity (SRS) and their measurement are important.

The compression of flow powders is dealt with in more detail in chapter 11 "Oral Solid Dosage Forms. With respect to the preformulation screening of candidate drugs for solid dosage forms, a protocol to examine their compression properties devised by Aulton and Wells (1988) can be carried out. Their scheme is shown in Table 4. Essentially, the compound is compressed using an IR and die set under 10 tons of pressure, and the resulting tablets are tested with regard to their crushing strength.

The interpretation of crushing strengths is as follows. If the crushing strengths are of the order B > A > C, the material probably has plastic tendencies. Materials that are brittle are usually independent of the scheme, while elastic material can behave in a variety of ways, for example,

1. A will cap or laminate,
2. B will probably maintain integrity but will be very weak, and
3. C will cap or laminate.

Figure 10 shows a scanning electron micrograph of a compound (remacemide HCl) that had poor compression properties. Notice how the top of the compact has partially detached

Table 4 Compression Protocol

| | 500 mg drug + 1% magnesium stearate | | |
	A	B	C
Blend in a tumbler mixer for	5 min	5 min	30 min
Compress in 13 mm die set	75 MPa	75 MPa	75 MPa
Compacts in a hydraulic press at dwell time of	2 sec	30 sec	2 sec
Store tablets in sealed container at room temperature to allow equilibration	24 hr	24 hr	24 hr
Perform crushing strength			

Source: From Aulton and Wells (1988).

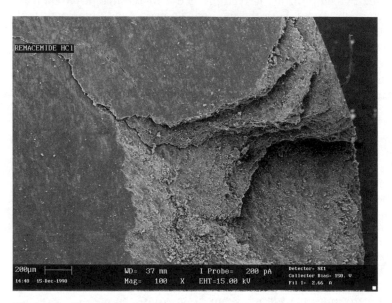

Figure 10 Scanning electron microscopy of a compound that undergoes capping and lamination.

(capping) and how the compact has separated into layers (lamination) (Yu et al., 2008). For further details on remacemide HCl, an *N*-methyl-D-aspartate (NMDA) antagonist that was investigated as a potential treatment of epilepsy, Parkinson's and Huntingdon's diseases (Schachter and Tarsy, 2000).

As shown by Otsuka et al. (1993), it is always worth checking the effect of compression on a powder if the compound is known to be polymorphic. Using the XRPD patterns of chlorpropamide forms A and C, they examined the effect of temperature and compression force on the deagglomerated powders and found that both the forms were mutually transformed.

Computational methods of predicting the mechanical properties of a powder from the crystal structure are now being explored. There appears to be a relationship between the indentation hardness and the molecular structure of organic materials. However, a prerequisite for predicting indentation hardness is knowledge of the crystal structure (Roberts et al., 1994). Payne et al. (1996) have used molecular modeling to predict the mechanical properties of aspirin and forms A and B of primodone. The predicted results of the Young's modulus were found to be in good agreement with those determined experimentally, and thus, compaction measurements might not always be necessary if they are difficult to perform.

Color

Color is a useful observation when describing different batches of drug substance since it can sometimes be used as an indicator of solvent presence, or, more importantly, an indication of degradation. In addition, subtle differences in color may be due to variations in the particle size distribution. Usually, color is subjective and is based on individual perception. However, more quantitative measurements can be obtained by using, for example, reflectance spectroscopy (Berberich et al., 2002, Rhee et al., 2008). The method is based on the CIELAB color system, which gives a precise representation of the color perception of humans. For full details of the CIELAB system, the reader is referred to the paper by Rhee et al. (2008) or the USP. Rhee et al.'s conclusions were that spectrocolorimetry was a useful drug-excipient screening tool, particularly because it was cheaper and faster than other methods. However, they added a note of caution by stating that the values obtained were only comparable when the measurements were carried out on comparable instruments.

Stark et al. (1996) have observed color changes during accelerated stability testing of captopril tablets, flucloxacillin sodium capsules, cefoxitin sodium powder for injection, and theophylline CR (controlled release) tablets. Under ambient conditions, only the flucloxacillin sodium and cefoxitin were observed to show any significant coloring. However, under stress conditions of accelerated stability testing, a linear relationship between color formation and the drug content of the formulations was found except for the theophylline tablets, where discoloration occurred in the absence of any significant degradation. Interestingly, the rate of coloring was found to obey the Arrhenius equation. The authors proposed that the shelf life of the formulations could be specified using the Commission Internationale d'Eclairage or International Commission on Illumination (CIE) system for color.

Electrostaticity

Powders can acquire an electrostatic charge during processing, the extent of which is related to the aggressiveness of the process and the physicochemical properties (Lachiver et al., 2006). It is important since it has been shown that, for example, electrostatic deposition is among the most important factors in deposition of drug substances in the lung (Hinds, 1999). Table 5, from BS5958, gives the range of values that arise because of various processes. Static electrification of two dissimilar materials occurs by the making and breaking of surface contacts (tribo-electrification) (Watanabe et al., 2007). Simply put, charge accumulation is due to electron transfer and depends on a number of factors such as surface resistivity of the materials in contact, the roughness of the surface, and contaminations (Elajnaf et al., 2007). Thus, the extent of the electrostatic charge accumulation will increase as the surfaces collide and contact, for example, by increasing the agitation time and intensity of a powder in a mixer. The net results will therefore increase the spot charge over the particle surfaces and adhesive characteristics. This technique has been used to prepare drug-carrier systems known as an interactive mixture.

The net charge on a powder may be either electropositive or electronegative. Although the process is not fully understood, it is generally accepted that charging occurs as a result of electron transfer between materials of different electrical properties. It has been shown that increased RH of the atmosphere has the effect of decreasing the electrostaticity of powders (Rowley and Macklin, 2007). The electrostatic charge of bulk solids can be measured using a Faraday pail (Carter et al., 1992).

The electrostatic charges on the surface of a powder can affect the flow properties of powders. An electric detector can determine the electric field generated by the electrostatic charges on the surface of the powder. This acts as a voltmeter and allows the direct determination of both polarity and absolute value of the electrostatic field. Rowley (2001) has reviewed the ways in which the electrostatic interactions in pharmaceutical powders can be quantified.

Table 5 Mass Charge Density Arising from Various Operations (BS5958)

Operation	Mass charge density (μC/kg)
Sieving	10^{-3} to 10^{-5}
Pouring	10^{-1} to 10^{-3}
Scroll feed transfer	1 to 10^{-2}
Grinding	1 to 10^{-1}
Micronizing	10^{2} to 10^{-1}

Source: Reproduced from BS5958 with permission of BSI under licence number 2001SK/0091. Complete standards can be obtained from BSI Customer Services, 389 Chiswick High Road, London, W4 4AL.

Kwok et al. (2008) have investigated the electrostatic properties of DPI aerosols of Pulmicort® and Bricanyl® Turbuhalers®. In this study, they investigated the effect of RH on the performance of these inhalers and found that although both generated significant charge, different RHs did not affect their mass output. Bricanyl appeared to be more affected by the RH of the atmosphere, whereby the charge decreased with increasing RH. Pulmicort, on the other hand, showed a decrease in particle charge at 40% RH and then increased with increasing RHs. Young et al. (2007) also showed that the electrostaticity of micronized sulbutamol sulfate was reduced at RHs greater than 60%. In an interesting application of AFM, Bunker et al. (2007) observed the charging of a single particle of lactose as it was either dragged or tapped on a glass slide. They also showed that as the RH increased, the charge was dissipated.

Caking

Caking can occur after storage and involves the formation of lumps or the complete agglomeration of the powder. A number of factors have been identified that predispose a powder to exhibit caking tendencies. These include static electricity, hygroscopicity, particle size, and impurities of the powder, and, in terms of the storage conditions, stress temperature, RH, and storage time can also be important. The caking of 11-amino undeconoic acid has been investigated, and it was concluded that the most important cause of the observed caking with this compound was its particle size (Provent et al., 1993). The mechanisms involved in caking are based on the formation of five types of interparticle bonds. These are

- bonding resulting from mechanical tangling,
- bonding resulting from steric effects,
- bonds via static electricity,
- bonds due to free liquid, and
- bonds due to solid bridges.

The caking tendency of a development compound was investigated when it was discovered to be lumpy after storage. An experiment was performed on the compound whereby it was stored at different RHs (from saturated salt solutions) for four weeks in a dessicator. Results revealed that caking was evident at 75% RH, with the compound forming loosely massed porous cakes (Table 6). Thermogravimetric analysis of the samples showed that caked samples lost only a small amount of weight on heating (0.62% w/w), which indicated that only low levels of moisture were required to produce caking for this compound.

It is known that micronization of compounds can lead to the formation of regions with a large degree of disorder, which, because of their amorphous character, are more reactive compared with the pure crystalline substance. This is particularly true on exposure to moisture and can lead to problems with caking, which is detrimental to the performance of the product. It has been argued that these amorphous regions transform during moisture sorption because of surface sintering and recrystallization at relative humidities well below the critical RH. Fitzpatrick et al. (2007) have shown that when amorphous lactose is raised above its T_g, it becomes sticky, cohesive, and eventually cakes (Listiohadi et al., 2008).

Table 6 Effect of moisture on the caking of a development compound

% Relative humidity	Moisture content (%)	Appearance and flow properties
0	0.31	Free-flowing powder; passed easily through sieve
11.3	0.24	Ditto
22.5	0.27	Less-flowing powder
38.2	0.32	Base of powder bed adhered to petri dish, however, material above this flowed
57.6	0.34	Less free flowing
75.3	0.62	Material caked
Ambient	0.25	Base of powder adhered to petri dish

Polymorphism Issues

Because polymorphism can have an effect on so many aspects of drug development, it is important to fix the polymorph (usually the stable form) as early as possible in the development cycle and probably before campaign 3. The FDA has produced guidance for industry: ANDAs: Pharmaceutical Solid Polymorphism Chemistry, Manufacturing, and Controls Information (http://www.fda.gov/cder/guidance/7590fnl.htm). Raw et al. (2004) have reported this in the literature, but the reader should consult the FDA Web site for the most up-to-date guidance.

While it is hoped that the issue polymorphism is resolved during prenomination and early development, it can remain a concern when the synthesis of the drug is scaled up into a larger reactor or transferred to another production site. In extreme cases and despite intensive research, work may have only produced a metastable form and the first production batch produces the stable form. Dunitz and Bernstein (1995) have reviewed the appearance of and subsequent disappearance of polymorphs. Essentially, this describes the scenario whereby, after nucleation of a more stable form, the previously prepared metastable form could no longer be made.

The role of related substances in the case of the disappearing polymorphs of sulphathiazole has been explored (Blagden et al., 1998). These studies showed that a reaction by-product from the final hydrolysis stage could stabilize different polymorphic forms of the compound depending on the concentration of the by-product. Using molecular modeling techniques, they were able to show that ethamidosulphthiazole, the by-product, influenced the hydrogen bond network and hence form and crystal morphology.

In the development of a reliable commercial recrystallization process for dirithromycin, Wirth and Stephenson (1997) proposed that the following scheme should be followed in the production of Candidate Drugs

.

1. Selection of the solvent system
2. Characterization of the polymorphic forms
3. Optimization of process times, temperature, solvent compositions, etc.
4. Examination of the chemical stability of the drug during processing
5. Manipulation of the polymorphic form, if necessary

While examples of disappearing polymorphs exist, perhaps more common is the crystallization of mixtures of polymorphs. Many analytical techniques have been used to quantitate mixtures of polymorphs, for example, XRPD has been used to quantitate the amount of cefepime: 2HCl dihydrate in cefepime, 2HCl monohydrate (Bugay et al., 1996). As noted by these workers, a crucial factor in developing an assay based on a solid-state technique is the production of pure calibration and validation samples. Moreover, while the production of the forms may be straightforward, production of homogeneously mixed samples for calibration purposes may not be so. To overcome this problem, a slurry technique was employed, which satisfied the NDA requirements, to determine the amount of one form in the other. The criteria employed are as follows:

1. A polymorphic transformation did not occur during preparation or analysis.
2. A limit of detection of 5% (w/w) of the dihydrate in monohydrate.
3. Ease of sample preparation, data acquisition, and analysis.
4. Ease of transfer to a quality control (QC) environment.

Calibration samples were limited to a working range of 1% to 15% w/w, and to prepare the mixes, samples of each form were slurried in acetone to produce a homogeneous mixture of the two.

With respect to solid dosage forms, there have been a few reports on how processing affects the polymorphic behavior of compounds (Morris et al., 2001). For example, the effect of polymorphic transformations that occurred during the extrusion-granulation process of carbamazepine granules has been studied by Otsuka et al. (1997). Results showed that granulation using 50% ethanol transformed form I into the dihydrate during the process. Wet granulation (using an ethanol-water solution) of chlorpromazine hydrochloride was found to produce a phase change (Wong and Mitchell, 1992). This was found to have some advantage since form II (the initial metastable form) was found to show more severe capping and lamination compared with form I, the (stable) form produced on granulation. Using a range of compounds, Wikström et al. (2008) have studied factors that influence the anhydrate-to-hydrate conversion during wet granulation and concluded that the transformation was a function of such things as the compound's solubility, surface properties, seeds, and the shear forces involved in wet granulation. However, even this paper noted that better models were needed to understand the complexities of the transformations. Solvate formation may have some advantages. For example, Di Martino et al. (2007) showed that the desolvated dioxane solvate of nimesulide had better tableting properties than the known polymorphs of the compound, which appears to represent a viable method of improving the compression properties of drug substances.

Polymorphism is not only an issue with the compound under investigation, that is, excipients also show variability in this respect. For example, it is well known that the tablet lubricant magnesium stearate can vary depending on the supplier. In one study, Wada and Matsubara (1992) examined the polymorphism with respect to 23 batches of magnesium stearate obtained from a variety of suppliers. Using DSC they classified the batches into six groups—interestingly, the polymorphism was not apparent by XRPD, IR, or SEM observations. In another report, Barra and Somma (1996) examined 13 samples of magnesium stearate from three suppliers. They found that there was variation not only between the suppliers but also in the lots supplied by the same manufacturer.

It is well known that polymorphism is a function of temperature and pressure, thus under the compressive forces that compounds experience under tableting conditions phase transformations may be possible. However, Német et al. (2005) have sounded a note of caution when conducting analysis of compressed samples. They reported that DSC measurements tended to amplify the transformation of form B to form A of famotidine.

SOLUTION FORMULATIONS

Development of a solution formulation requires a number of key pieces of preformulation information. Of these, solubility (and any pH dependence) and stability are probably the most important. As noted by Meyer et al. (2007), with over 350 parenteral products marketed worldwide, these probably represent the most common solution formulation type. The principles and practices governing the formulation development of parenteral products have been reviewed by Sweetana and Akers (1996). Strickley (1999, 2000, 2001) has produced a useful series of papers detailing the formulation of a large number of compounds delivered by the parenteral route. A further review by Strickley (2004) has detailed solubilizing excipients for both oral and injectable formulations. Rowe et al. (1995) have described an expert system for the development of parenteral products (see also chapter 9).

Solubility Considerations

One of the main problems associated with developing a parenteral or any other solution formulation of a compound is its aqueous solubility. For a poorly soluble drug candidate, there are several strategies for enhancing its solubility. These include pH manipulation, cosolvents, surfactants, emulsion formation, and complexing agents; combinations of these methods can also be used (Ran et al., 2005). More sophisticated delivery systems, for example, liposomes, can also be considered.

pH Manipulation

Since many compounds are weak acids or bases, their solubility will be function of pH. Figure 11 shows the pH-solubility curve for sibenadit HCl salt with pK_as at 6.58 and 8.16. When the acid-base titration method (Serrajudden and Mufson, 1985) was used, the solubility curve showed a minimum pH between 6 and 8. Below this pH region, the solubility increased

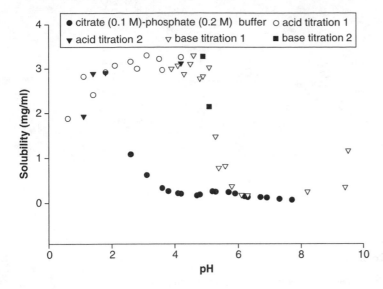

Figure 11 pH-solubility curve of sebenidet hydrochloride.

as the pK_a was passed to reach a maximum between pH 2 and 4 and then decreased because of the common ion effect. As the second pK_a was passed in the alkaline region, the solubility again increased. However, when the solubility experiments were performed in 0.2 M citrate-phosphate buffer, the solubility of the compound decreased, and this illustrates the effect that ionic strength can have on drug solubility. Clearly, the region between pH 2 and 5 represents the best area to achieve the highest solubility. However, caution should be exercised if the solution needs to be buffered, since this can decrease the solubility, as in this case. Myrdal et al. (1995) found that a buffered formulation of a compound did not precipitate on dilution and did not cause phlebitis. In contrast, the unbuffered drug formulation showed the opposite effects. These results reinforce the importance of buffering parenteral formulations instead of simply adjusting the pH.

Cosolvents

The use of cosolvents has been utilized quite effectively for some poorly soluble drug substances. It is probable that the mechanism of enhanced solubility is the result of the polarity of the cosolvent mixture being closer to the drug than in water. This was illustrated in a series of papers by Rubino and Yalkowsky (1984, 1985, 1987), who found that the solubilities of phenytoin, benzocaine, and diazepam in cosolvent and water mixtures were approximated by the log-linear equation (8).

$$\log S_m = f \log S_c + (1 - f) \log S_w \tag{8}$$

where S_m is the solubility of the compound in the solvent mix, S_w the solubility in water, S_c the solubility of the compound in pure cosolvent, f the volume fraction of cosolvent, and σ the slope of the plot of $\log \left(\dfrac{S_m}{S_w} \right)$ versus f. Furthermore, they related σ to indexes of cosolvent polarity such as the dielectric constant, solubility parameter, surface tension, interfacial tension, and octanol-water partition coefficient.

It was found that the aprotic cosolvents gave a much higher degree of solubility than the amphiprotic cosolvents. This means that if a cosolvent can donate a hydrogen bond, it may be an important factor in determining whether it is a good cosolvent. Deviations from log-linear solubility were dealt with in a subsequent paper (Rubino and Yalkowsky, 1987).

Figure 12 shows how the solubility of a development drug increases in a number of water-solvent systems.

Care must be taken when attempting to increase the solubility of a compound, that is, a polar drug might actually show a decrease in solubility with increasing cosolvent composition (Gould et al., 1984).

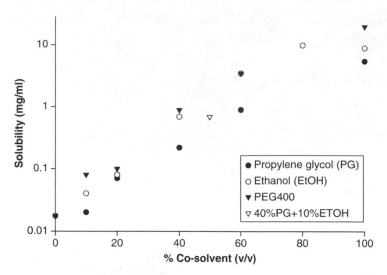

Figure 12   Solubility as a function of cosolvent volume for a development compound.

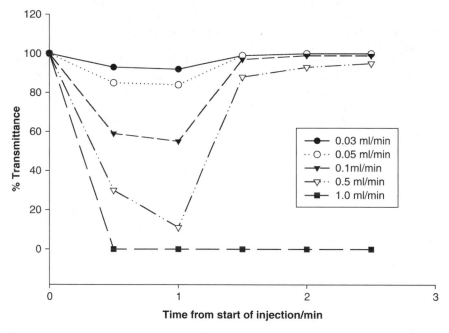

Figure 13   Effect of flow rate on the precipitation of a polyethylene glycol 400 solution of a drug.

It is often necessary to administer a drug parenterally at a concentration that exceeds its aqueous solubility. Cosolvents offer one way of increasing drug solubility, but the amount of cosolvent that can be used in a parenteral intravenous (IV) formulation is often constrained by toxicity considerations. It may cause hemolysis (Amin, 2006), or the drug may precipitate when diluted or injected, causing phlebitis (Johnson et al., 2003). Prototype formulations are often tested on animals, which is undesirable if a reliable in vitro technique can be employed.

Yalkowsky and coworkers (1983) have developed a useful in vitro technique based on UV spectrophotometry for predicting the precipitation of a parenteral formulations in vivo following injection. Figure 13 shows the effect of injection rate on the transmittance at 600 nm of a polyethylene glycol (PEG) 400 formulation of a compound being introduced into flowing saline. As shown, the faster the injection rate, the more precipitation was detected by the spectrophotometer. This simple technique can be used to assess whether precipitation of a compound might occur on dilution or injection. Johnson et al. (2003) have now validated this approach for screening formulations.

Narazaki et al. (2007a,b) have developed equations for estimating the precipitation of pH-cosolvent solubilized formulations. The equation takes account of the effect of the cosolvent on the pK_a of the compound and any buffering components, which have determining effects on its solubility. In the case of the model compound used, phenytoin, more precipitation occurred on dilution when compared with a pH-controlled formulation.

While cosolvents can increase the solubility of compounds, on occasion, they can have a detrimental effect on their stability. For example, a parenteral formulation of the novel antitumor agent carzelsin (U80,244) using a PEG 400/absolute ethanol/polysorbate 80 (PET) formulation in the ratio 6:3:1 v/v/v has been reported (Jonkman-De Vries et al., 1995). While this formulation effectively increased the solubility of the compound, this work showed that interbatch variation of PEG 400 could affect the stability of the drug because of pH effects.

One point that is often overlooked when considering cosolvents is their influence on buffers or salts. Since these are conjugate acid-base systems, it is not surprising that introducing solvents into the solution can result in a shift in the pK_a of the buffer or salt. These effects are important in formulation terms, since many injectable formulations that contain cosolvents also contain a buffer to control the pH (Rubino, 1987).

Emulsion Formulations
Oil-in-water (o/w) emulsions have been successfully employed to deliver drugs with poor water solubility (Date and Nagarsenker, 2008). In preformulation terms, the solubility of the compound in the oil phase (often soybean oil) is the main consideration while using this approach. However, the particle size of the emulsion and its stability (physical and chemical) also need to be assessed (Tian et al., 2007). Ideally, the particle size of the emulsion droplets should be in the colloidal range to avoid problems with phlebitis. For example, Intralipid 10% (a soybean o/w emulsion) was found to consist of "artificial chylomicrons" (oil droplets) with a mean diameter of 260 nm and liposomes with a diameter of 43 nm (Férézou et al., 2001). To achieve this size, a microfluidizer should be used, since other techniques may produce droplets of a larger size, as shown in Table 7 (Lidgate, 1990). Emulsions are prepared by homogenizing the oil in water in the presence of emulsifiers, for example, phospholipids, which stabilize the emulsion via a surface charge and also a mechanical barrier. Intravenous emulsions can be sterilized by autoclaving, which gives a high level of assurance of sterility. However, careless aseptic techniques can compromise the patient. In this situation, the inclusion of antimicrobial additives could be considered. To this end, Han and Washington (2005) have investigated the effect of antimicrobial additives on the stability of Diprivan®, an intravenous anesthetic emulsion.

The particle size and zeta potential of emulsions can be measured using instruments that combine PCS and surface charge measurements (Tian et al., 2007). Driscoll et al. (2001) have compared a light obscuration (LO) and laser diffraction to examine the stability of parenteral nutrition mixtures–based intravenous emulsions. From this study, they concluded that LO was a better technique for detecting globules greater than 5 μm in diameter. They recommended two key measurements, that is, the mean droplet size and the large droplet size, since without these it is impossible to guarantee the safety of the emulsion (large droplets can cause thrombophlebitis).

Table 7 Size of Emulsion Droplets Produced by Various Methods

Method of manufacture	Particle size (μm)
Vortex	0.03–24
Blade mixer	0.01–8
Homogenizer	0.02–2
Microfluidizer	0.07–0.2

Source: From Lidgate (1990), reproduced with permission.

Physical instability of emulsions can take a number of forms, for example, creaming, flocculation, coalescence, or breaking, while chemical instability can be due to hydrolysis of the stabilizing moieties. To assess the stability of the emulsion, heating and freezing cycles as well as centrifugation can be employed (Yalabik-Kas, 1985b). Chansiri et al. (1999) have investigated the effect of steam sterilization (121°C for 15 minutes) on the stability of o/w emulsions. They found that emulsions with a high negative zeta potential did not show any change in their particle size distribution after autoclaving. Emulsions with a lower negative value, on the other hand, were found to separate into two phases during autoclaving. Because the stability of phospholipids-stabilized emulsion is dependent on the surface charge, they are normally autoclaved at pH 8 to 9. Similarly, Han et al. (2001) found that when two formulations of propofol were shaken and subjected to a freeze-thaw cycle, the formulation that had a more negative zeta potential (−50 vs. −40 mV) was more stable. There was also a difference in pH of the formulations, with the less stable formulation having a pH between 4 and 5 compared with pH 8 for the more stable formulation (AstraZeneca's Diprivan).

An interesting extension of this approach of solubilizing a poorly soluble compound is the SolEmuls® technology described by Junghanns et al. (2007). In this technique, a nanosuspension of amphotericin was generated, mixed with a Lipofundin®, a conventional lipidic emulsion, and then subjected to high-pressure homogenization. Results indicted that this formulation approach produced better antifungal effects when compared with the commercially available Fungizone®.

In recent years, microemulsions have been investigated as a way of solubilizing drugs for intravenous delivery (Date and Nagarsenker, 2008). In contrast to the conventional emulsions described above, microemulsions are thermodynamically stable, complex dispersions consisting of micro domains of oil and water, which are stabilized by alternating films of surfactants and co-surfactants. The droplet size of microemulsions is generally less than 150 nm. One feature of microemulsions is that they are clear in contrast to the milk-like appearance of the conventional emulsions.

Stability Considerations

The second major consideration with respect to solution formulations is stability. The stability of pharmaceuticals, from a regulatory point of view, is usually determined by forced degradation studies. These studies provide data on the identity of degradants, degradation pathways, and the fundamental stability of the molecule. Guidance for the industry on how to conduct stability testing of new drug substances and products is given in the ICH guideline Q1A (R2). See Reynolds et al. (2002) and Alsante et al. (2007) for a detailed account on the regulatory requirements of forced degradation studies and recommended degradation conditions.

Notari (1996) has presented some arguments regarding the merits of a complete kinetic stability study. He calculated that with reliable data and no buffer catalysis, sixteen experiments were required to provide a complete kinetic stability study. If buffer ions contribute to the hydrolysis, then each species contributes to the pH-rate expression. Thus, for a single buffer, for example, phosphate, a minimum of six experiments were required. A stock solution of the compound should be prepared in an appropriate solvent and a small aliquot (e.g., 50 µL) added to, for example, a buffer solution at a set pH. This solution should be maintained at a constant temperature, and the ionic strength may be controlled by the addition of KCl (e.g., $I = 0.5$). After thorough mixing, the solution is sampled at various time points and assayed for the compound of interest. If the reaction is very fast, it is recommended that the samples be diluted into a medium that will stop or substantially slow the reaction, for example, a compound that is unstable in acid may be stable in an alkaline medium. Cooling the solution may also be useful. Slow reactions, on the other hand, may require longer-term storage at elevated temperature. In this situation, solutions should be sealed in an ampoule to prevent loss of moisture. If sufficient compound is available, the effect of, for example, buffer concentration should be investigated. Of course, such studies can be automated, for example, Symyx Technologies (Santa Clara, California, U.S.) offer their Automated Forced Degradation System for high-throughput forced degradation studies. This platform produces degradation libraries of stressed samples of liquid formulations, which are then heated and sampled over

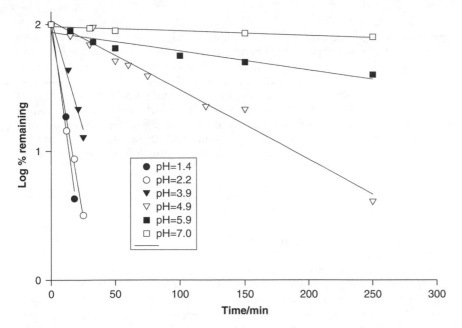

Figure 14   First-order hydrolysis decomposition of a compound (25°C).

time at 55°C, 70°C, and 85°C, and the compound degradation is followed with time. From these measurements, library arrays of first-order kinetic plots are generated, and predictions of room temperature stability of the compound are produced (Carlson et al., 2005).

The first-order decomposition plot of an acid-labile compound with respect to pH is shown in Figure 14. Clearly, this compound is very acid labile, and even at pH 7, some decomposition is observed. A stable solution formulation would, therefore, be difficult to achieve in this pH range. However, a solution formulation at lower pHs might be possible, depending on how long it needed to be stored. To get an estimate of how long this might be, Arrhenius experiments should be undertaken. As an example of this methodology, Jansen et al. (2000) followed the decomposition of gemcitabine, formulated as a lyophilized powder, at pH 3.2 at four different temperatures from which an Arrhenius plot was used to calculate the decomposition rates at lower temperatures. From the data generated, they concluded that a solution formulation of gemcitabine was feasible if the solution was stored in a refrigerator.

A detailed paper on the mechanistic interpretation of pH-rate profiles is that by Loudon (1991). Van der Houwen et al. (1997) have reviewed the systematic interpretation of pH degradation profiles. The rate profiles obtained when the pH is varied can take a number of forms. However, Loudon (1991) makes the point that they "usually consist of linear regions of integral slope connected by short curved segments." Indeed, the linear regions generally have slopes of −1, 0, or +1, and "any pH-rate profile can be regarded as a composite of fundamental curves."

It is also possible that compounds may be formulated in cosolvent systems for geriatric or pediatric use where administration of a tablet would be difficult (Chang and Whitworth 1984). In addition, cosolvents are routinely employed in parenteral formulations to enhance the solubility of poorly soluble drugs. For example, Tu et al. (1989) have investigated the stability of a nonaqueous formulation for injection based on 52% *N,N*-dimethylacetamide and 48% propylene glycol. By stressing the preparation with regard to temperature, they found that by using Arrhenius kinetics, the time for 10% degradation at 25°C would be 885 days. The solution also discolored when stressed. Furthermore, it is also sometimes useful to assess the effect of ethanol/acid on the stability of compounds that can be taken concurrently, for example, temazepam (Yang, 1994).

Stability to Autoclaving

For parenteral formulations, a sterile solution of the compound is required. According to Meyer et al. (2007), one-third of the 350 parenteral products on sale worldwide are multi-dose formulations, which require the inclusion of an antimicrobial preservative. The most commonly used preservatives are benzyl alcohol, chlorobutanol, m-cresol, phenol, phenoxyethanol, propylparaben, and thiomersal. Of these, benzyl alcohol and combinations of methyl and propylparaben are the most popular. See Meyer et al. (2007) for further details of the use of preservatives in parenteral formulations. Of course, one of the limiting factors of the use of a preservative is its compatibility with the active ingredient, and these studies should be undertaken during the preformulation stage of development. In addition, other formulation ingredients may affect the effectiveness of the antimicrobial agent (Meyer et al., 2007).

A terminal sterilization method is preferred, rather than aseptic filtration, because there is a greater assurance of achieving sterility. As noted by Moldenhauer (1998), the regulatory authorities will require a written justification to explain why a product is not terminally sterilized. Therefore, for a sterile formulation product, it is mandatory to assess whether it is stable to autoclaving as part of any preformulation selection process. Autoclaving (usually 15 minutes at 121°C) at various pHs is undertaken after which the drug solutions should be evaluated for impurities, color, pH, and degradation products. Clearly, if one compound shows superior stability after autoclaving, then this will be the one to take forward.

The effect of the autoclave cycle, that is, fill, heat-up, peak dwell, and cool-down on the theoretical chemical stability of compounds intended for intravenous injection, has been investigated by Parasrampuria et al. (1993). Assuming first-order degradation kinetics, that is, hydrolysis, the amount of degradation was calculated for any point during the above process. Although the results were calculated for the first-order kinetics, the authors estimated that the calculations were applicable to other reaction orders, that is, zero and second.

Acceptable reasons for not proceeding with a terminally sterilized product are

- pH changes,
- color changes,
- carbonate buffering loss,
- container closure problems, and
- drug or excipient degradation.

Effect of Metal Ions and Oxygen on Stability

After hydrolysis, oxidation is the next most important way by which a drug can decompose in both the solid and liquid states. It is a complex process that can take place by way of such mechanisms as autoxidation, nucleophilic or electrophilic additions, and electron transfer reactions (Hovorka and Schneich, 2001). In addition, some excipients have been shown to contain impurities (such as peroxides and metal ions), which can promote oxidative degradation. Therefore, in formulation terms, the removal of oxygen and trace metal ions and the exclusion of light may be necessary to improve the stability of oxygen-sensitive compounds (Waterman et al., 2002). Formulation aids to this end include antioxidants and chelating agents and, of course, the exclusion of light where necessary. As an example, Li et al. (1998) showed that a formulation of AG2034 could be stabilized through using nitrogen in the ampoule headspace and the inclusion of an antioxidant. Antioxidants are substances that should preferentially react with oxygen and hence protect the compound of interest toward oxidation. A list of water- and oil-soluble antioxidants is given in Table 8 (Akers, 1982).

Reformulation screening of the antioxidant efficiency in parenteral solutions containing epinephrine has been reported by Akers (1979), who concluded that screening was difficult on the basis of the redo potential, and complicated by a complex formulation of many components. To assess the stability of compounds toward oxidation, a number of accelerated (forced) degradation studies need to be undertaken Alsante et al. (2007). As an example, Freed et al. (2008) examined the forced degradation of a number of compounds.

Caution should be exercised when including antioxidants, since a number of reports have pointed out that some antioxidants, for example, sulfites, can have a detrimental effect on

Table 8 List of Water- and Oil-Soluble Antioxidants

Water soluble	Oil soluble
Sodium bisulfite	Propyl gallate
Sodium sulfite	Butylated hydroxyanisole
Sodium metabisulfite	Butylated hydroxytoluene
Sodium thiosulfate	Ascorbyl palmitate
Sodium formaldehyde sulfoxylate	Nordihydroguaiaretic acid
L- and d-ascorbic acid	Alpha-tocopherol
Acetylcysteine	
Cysteine	
Thioglycerol	
Thioglycollic acid	
Thiolactic acid	
Thiourea	
Dithithreitol	
Glutathione	

Source: From Akers (1982), reproduced with permission.

the stability of certain compounds (Asahara et al., 1990). Thus, oxygen-sensitive substances should be screened for their compatibility with a range of antioxidants. It should also be noted that bisulphite has also been known to catalyze hydrolysis reactions (Munson et al., 1977).

Trace metal ions can affect stability and can arise from the bulk drug, formulation excipients, or glass containers (Allain and Wang, 2007). The effect of metal ions on the solution stability of fosinopril sodium has been reported (Thakur et al., 1993). In this case, the metal ions were able to provide, through complexation, a favorable reaction pathway. Metal ions can also act as degradation catalysts by being involved in the production of highly reactive free radicals, especially in the presence of oxygen. The formation of these radicals can be initiated by the action of light or heat, and propagate the reaction until they are destroyed by inhibitors or by side reactions that break the chain (Hovorka and Schöneich, 2001).

Ethlenediaminetetraacetic Acid and Chelating Agents
Because of the involvement of metal ions in degradation reactions, the inclusion of a chelating agent is often advocated (Pinsuwan et al., 1999). The most commonly used chelating agents are the various salts of ethylenediaminetetraacetic acid (EDTA). In addition, the use of hydroxyethylenediaminetriacetic acid (HEDTA), diethylenetriaminepentacetic acid (DPTA), and nitrilotriacetate (NTA) has been assessed for their efficiency in stabilizing, for example, isoniazid solutions (Ammar et al., 1982).

EDTA has pK_a values of $pK_1 = 2.0$, $pK_2 = 2.7$, $pK_3 = 6.2$, and $pK_4 = 10.4$ at 20°C. Generally, the reaction of EDTA with metal ions can be described by equation (9).

$$M^{n+} + Y^{4-} \rightarrow MY^{(4-n)+} \tag{9}$$

In practice, however, the disodium salt is used because of its greater solubility. Hence,

$$M^{n+} + H_2Y \rightarrow MY^{(n-4)+} + 2H^+ \tag{10}$$

From equation (10), it is apparent that the dissociation (or equilibrium) will be sensitive to the pH of the solution. Therefore, this will have implications for the formulation.

The stability of the complex formed by EDTA–metal ions is characterized by the stability or formation constant, K. This is derived from the reaction equation and is given by equation (11).

$$K = \frac{[(MY)^{(n-4)^+}]}{[M^{n^+}][Y^{4-}]} \tag{11}$$

Stability constants (expressed as log K) of some metal ion–EDTA complexes are shown in Table 9.

Table 9 Metal Ion–Ethylenediaminetetraacetic Acid Stability Constants

Ion	log K	Ion	log K	Ion	log K
Ag^+	7.3	Co^{2+}	16.3	Fe^{3+}	25.1
Li^+	2.8	Ni^{2+}	18.6	Y^{3+}	18.2
Na^+	1.7	Cu^{2+}	18.8	Cr^{3+}	24.0
Mg^{2+}	8.7	Zn^{2+}	16.7	Ce^{3+}	15.9
Ca^{2+}	10.6	Cd^{2+}	16.6	La^{3+}	15.7
Sr^{2+}	8.6	Hg^{2+}	21.9	Sc^{3+}	23.1
Ba^{2+}	7.8	Pb^{2+}	18.0	Ga^{3+}	20.5
Mn^{2+}	13.8	Al^{3+}	16.3	In^{3+}	24.9
Fe^{2+}	14.3	Bi^{3+}	27.0	Th^{4+}	23.2

Equation (11) assumes that the fully ionized form of $EDTA^{4-}$ is present in solution. However, at low pH, other species will be present, that is, $HEDTA^{3-}$, H_2EDTA^{2-}, and H_3EDTA^-, as well as the undissociated H_4EDTA. Thus, the stability constants become conditional on pH.

The ratio can be calculated for the total uncombined EDTA (in all forms) to the form $EDTA^{4-}$. Thus, the apparent stability constant becomes K/α_L, and hence,

$$\alpha_L = \frac{[EDTA]_{\text{all forms}}}{[EDTA^{4-}]} \tag{12}$$

Thus,

$$K_H = \frac{K}{\alpha_L} \text{ Or } \log K_H = \log K - \alpha_L \tag{13}$$

where $\log K_H$ is known as the conditional stability constant.

Fortunately, α_L can be calculated from the known dissociation constants of EDTA, and its value can be calculated from equation (14).

$$\alpha_L = \left\{1 + \frac{[H^+]}{K_4} + \frac{[H^+]}{K_4 K_3} + \ldots\right\} = 1 + 10^{(pK_4 - pH)} + 10^{(pK_4 + pK_3 pH)} + \ldots \tag{14}$$

Thus, at pH 4, the conditional stability constants of some metal-EDTA complexes are calculated as follows:

$$\log K_H \text{ EDTABa}^{2+} = 0.6$$
$$\log K_H \text{ EDTAMg}^{2+} = 1.5$$
$$\log K_H \text{ EDTACa}^{2+} = 3.4$$
$$\log K_H \text{ EDTAZn}^{2+} = 9.5$$
$$\log K_H \text{ EDTAFe}^{3+} = 17.9$$

Thus, at pH 4, the zinc and ferric complexes will exist. However, calcium, magnesium, and barium will only be weakly complexed, if at all.

The inclusion of EDTA is occasionally not advantageous since there are a number of reports of the EDTA catalyzing the decomposition of drugs (Medenhall, 1984; Nayak et al., 1986). Citric acid, tartaric acid, glycerin, sorbitol, etc., can also be considered as complexing agents. However, these are often ineffective. Interestingly, some formulators resort to amino acids or tryptophan because of a ban on EDTA in some countries (Wang and Kowal, 1980).

Surface Activity

Many drugs show surface-active behavior because they have the correct mix of chemical groups that are typical of surfactants. The surface activity of drugs can be important since they show a greater tendency to adhere to surfaces or solutions may foam. The surface activity of compounds can be determined using a variety of techniques, for example, surface tension

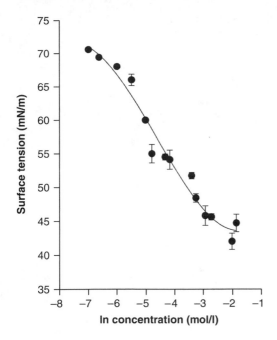

Figure 15 Plot of surface tension versus the natural log of the concentration for a primary amine hydrochloride.

measurements using a Du Nouy tensiometer, a Whilhelmy plate or conductance measurements. Figure 15 shows the surface tension as a function of concentration (using a Du Nouy tensiometer) of remacemide hydrochloride solutions in water. The surface tension of water decreased because of the presence of the compound. However, there was no break, which would have been indicative of micelle formation. Even when the pH of the solution was adjusted to 7, where a solubility "spike" had been observed, the surface tension was not significantly different to that observed for water alone. Thus, although the compound was surface active, it did not appear to form micelles, probably because of steric effects.

The surface-active properties of MDL 201346, a hydrochloride salt, have been investigated by a number of techniques including conductivity measurements (Streng et al., 1996). It was found that it underwent significant aggregation in water at temperatures greater than 10°C. Moreover, a break in the molar conductivity versus square root of concentration was noted, which corresponded to the critical micelle concentration (cmc) of the compound and aggregation of 10 to 11 molecules. In addition to surface-active behavior, some drugs are known to form liquid crystalline phases with water, for example, diclofenac diethylamine (Kriwet and Muller, 1993). Self-association in water (vertical stacking) of the novel anticancer agent brequiner sodium (King et al., 1989) has been reported.

Osmolality

Body fluids, such as blood, normally have an osmotic pressure, which is often described as corresponding to that of a 0.9% w/v solution of sodium chloride, and, indeed, a 0.9% w/v NaCl solution is said to be iso-osmotic with blood. Solutions with an osmotic pressure lower than 0.9% w/v NaCl are known as hypotonic, and those with osmotic pressure greater than this value are said to be hypertonic. The commonly used unit to express osmolality is osmol, and this is defined as the weight in grams per solute, existing in a solution as molecules, ions, macromolecules, etc., that is osmotically equivalent to the gram molecular weight of an ideally behaving nonelectrolyte.

Pharmaceutically, osmotic effects are important in the parenterals and ophthalmic field, and work is usually directed at formulating to avoid the side effects or finding methods of administration to minimize them. The ophthalmic response to various concentrations of sodium chloride is shown in Table 10 (Flynn, 1979).

Osmolality determinations are usually carried out using a cryoscopic osmometer, which is calibrated with deionized water and solutions of sodium chloride of known concentration.

Table 10   Ophthalmic Response to Various Concentrations of Sodium Chloride

% NaCl	Opthalmic response
0.0	Very disagreeable
0.6	Perceptibly disagreeable after 1 min
0.8	Completely indifferent after long exposure
1.2	Completely indifferent after long exposure
1.3	Perceptibly disagreeable after 1 min
1.5	Somewhat disagreeable after 1 min
2.0	Disagreeable after 0.5 min

Source: From Flynn (1979), reproduced with permission.

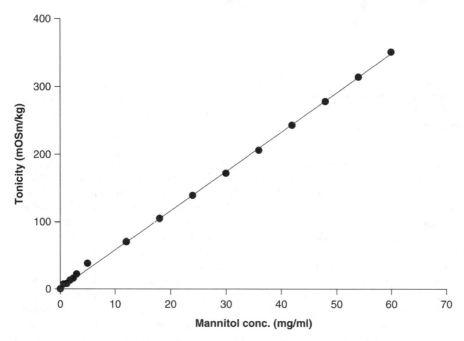

Figure 16   Plot of tonicity versus concentration for mannitol in water.

Using this technique, the sodium chloride equivalents and freezing point depressions for more than 500 substances have been determined and reported in a series of papers by Hammarlund and coworkers (Hammerlund, 1981). Figure 16 shows the osmolality of mannitol-water solutions.

Cyclodextrins are used for the solubility enhancement of poorly soluble drugs, and Zannou et al. (2001) have determined the osmotic properties of the sulfobutyl and hydroxypropyl derivatives. In an interesting set of measurements to accompany the osmometry measurements, they conducted osmolality measurements on frozen solutions using DSC. Sodium chloride solutions of known osmolality were used as calibrants.

FREEZE-DRIED FORMULATIONS

If a drug in solution proves to be unstable, then an alternative formulation approach will be required, and freeze-drying is often used to produce the requisite stability. A common prerequisite for this method of production of a freeze-dried formulation is restricted to those that have enough aqueous solubility and stability over the time course of the process.

However, if the compound is unstable in water, then an alternative solvent such as *t*-butanol may be employed (Ni et al., 2001). Preformulation studies can be performed to evaluate this approach and to aid the development of the freeze-drying cycle. Briefly, freeze-drying consists of three main stages: (*i*) freezing of the solution, (*ii*) primary drying, and (*iii*) secondary drying (Tang and Pikal, 2004). In many cases, the inclusion of excipients is necessary, which act as bulking agents and/or stabilizing agents. Thus, production conditions should be evaluated to ensure that the process is efficient and that it produces a stable product (Schwegman et al., 2005). The first stage, therefore, is to characterize the freezing and heating behavior of solutions containing the candidate drug, and in this respect, DSC and freeze-drying microscopy can be used as described by Thomas and Cannon (2004). Schwegman et al. (2005) have produced some good advice with regard to the formulation and process development of freeze-dried formulations. Since mannitol is a common excipient used in the formulated product, the sub-ambient behavior of its solutions is of importance (Kett et al., 2003).

To understand the processes taking place during freezing a solution containing a solute, it is worth referring to the phase diagram described by Her and Nail (1994). This shows that as a solution of a compound is cooled, the freezing point is depressed because of the presence of an increasing concentration of the dissolved solute. If the solute crystallizes during freezing, a eutectic point is observed. If crystallization does not take place, the solution becomes super-cooled and thus becomes more concentrated and viscous. Eventually, the viscosity is increased to such an extent that a glass is formed. This point is known as the T_g.

Measurement of the glass transition of frozen solution formulation of the candidate drug is an important preformulation determination since freeze-drying an amorphous system above this temperature can lead to a decrease in viscous flow of the solute (due to a decrease in viscosity) after the removal of the ice. This leads to what is commonly known as "collapse," and for successful freeze-drying, it should be performed below the T_g. Consequences of collapse include high residual water content in the product and prolonged reconstitution times. In addition, the increase in the mobility of molecules above the T_g may lead to in-process degradation (Pikal and Shah, 1990).

Figure 17 shows the glass transition, as determined by DSC, of a trial formulation of a candidate drug. The glass transition was measured by freezing a solution of the compound in a DSC pan and then heating the frozen solution. It should be noted that T_g is usually a subtler event compared with the ice-melt endotherm, and so the thermogram should be examined

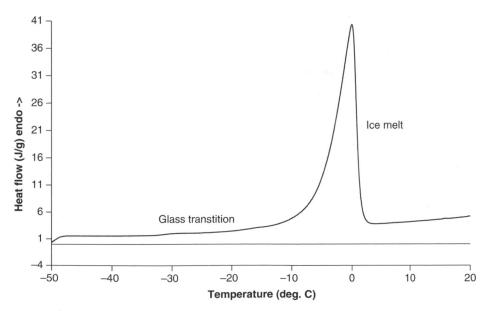

Figure 17 DSC thermogram showing a glass transition of heated frozen drug solution.

very carefully (Fig. 17). In some cases, an endotherm due to stress relaxation may be superimposed on the glass transition. It is possible to resolve these events by using the related technique, modulated DSC (MDSC) or dynamic DSC (DDSC) (Kett, 2001).

If during freezing the solutes crystallize, the first thermal event detected using DSC will be the endotherm that corresponds to melting of the eutectic formed between ice and the solute. This is usually followed by an endothermic event corresponding to the melting of ice. Figure 18 shows this behavior for a saline solution. Normally, freeze-drying of these systems are carried out below the eutectic melting temperature (Williams and Schwinke, 1994). Another way of detecting whether a solute or formulation crystallizes on freezing is to conduct sub-ambient X-ray diffractometry (Cavatur and Suryanarayanan, 1998).

If a lyophilized drug is amorphous, then knowledge of the glass transition temperature is important for stability reasons. Chemically, amorphous compounds are usually less stable than their crystalline counterparts. This is illustrated in Table 11, which shows some stability data for an amorphous compound (produced by lyophilization) and the crystalline hydrate form of the compound.

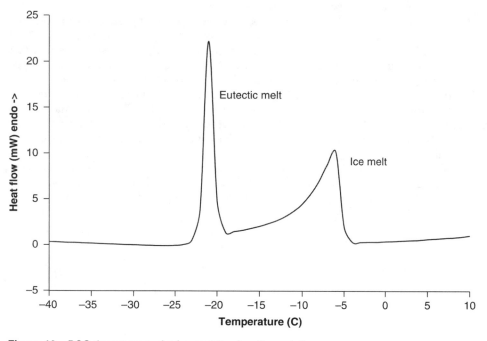

Figure 18   DSC thermogram of a frozen 9% w/v saline solution.

Table 11   Stability Data for an Amorphous (Lyophilized) and Crystalline Hydrate Form of a Compound

	Storage conditions	Time (mo)	Moisture content (% w/w)	Total impurities (% w/w)
Crystalline		Initial	15.98	0.53
	25°C/16% RH	1	15.78	0.54
	25°C/60% RH	1	15.50	0.56
	40°C/75% RH	1	15.76	0.59
Amorphous		Initial	4.83	0.47
	25°C/16% RH	1	8.31	0.57
	25°C/60% RH	1	12.55	0.69
	40°C/75% RH	1	12.72	1.44

Abbreviation: RH, relative humidity.

Although the moisture content of the amorphous form was increased, it did not crystallize. Other work showed that at relative humidities greater than 70%, the sample crystallized (O'Sullivan et al., 2002). It is important to note that moisture has the effect of lowering the glass temperature, which in turn increases the propensity of instability. This appears to be due to water acting as a plasticizer such that molecular mobility is increased, thus facilitating reactivity (Shalaev and Zografi, 1996).

Duddu and Weller (1996) have studied the importance of the glass transition temperature of an amorphous lyophilized aspirin-cyclodextrin complex. Using DSC, the glass transition was found to be 36°C followed by an exothermic peak, believed to be due to aspirin crystallization. The glass transition at this temperature was also observed by using dielectric relaxation spectroscopy. When the aspirin/hydroxypropylcyclodextrin (HPCD) loophole was exposed to higher humidities, the T_g was reduced to a temperature below room temperature and the product became a viscous gel. Craig et al. (1999) have reviewed the physicochemical properties of the amorphous state with respect to drugs and freeze-dried formulations, and Nail and Seales (2007) have discussed QdD (Quality by Design) aspects of their development and scale-up of freeze-dried formulations.

SUSPENSIONS

If the drug substance is not soluble, then the compound may be administered as a suspension. This might be the formulation approach used for oral administration of drugs to animals for safety studies, for early-phase clinical studies in humans, or for the intended commercial dosage form, for example, ophthalmic, nasal, oral, etc. Data considered to be important for suspensions at the preformulation stage include solubility, particle size, and propensity for crystal growth and chemical stability. Furthermore, during development, it will be important to have knowledge of the viscosity of the vehicle to obtain information with respect to settling of the suspended particles, syringibility, and physical stability (Akers, 1987). In a report on the preformulation information required for suspensions, Morefield et al. (1987) investigated the relationship between the critical volume fraction as a function of pH. They noted that "it is usually desirable to maximize the volume fraction of solids to minimize the volume of the dose."

It should be obvious that for a successful suspension, insolubility of the candidate drug is required. While for large hydrophobic drugs like steroids, this may not be a problem, weak acids or bases may show appreciable solubility. In this instance, reducing the solubility by salt formation is a relatively common way to achieve this end. For example, a calcium salt of a weak acid may be sufficiently insoluble for a suspension formulation. However, difficulties may arise because of hydrate formation, for example, with concomitant crystal growth. Hoelgaard and Møller (1983) found that metronidazole formed a monohydrate on suspension in water. Zietsman et al. (2007) have shown that this conversion can be prevented by using Avicel RC-591 as a suspending agent.

Another way crystals can grow in suspension that is not attributable to a phase change is by Otswald ripening. This is the result of the difference in solubility between small and large crystals, as predicted by equation (15).

$$\frac{RT}{M} \ln\left(\frac{S_2}{S_1}\right) = \frac{2\sigma}{\rho}\left(\frac{1}{r_1} - \frac{1}{r_2}\right) \qquad (15)$$

where R is the gas constant, T the absolute, S_1 and S_2 the solubilities of crystals of radii r_1 and r_2, respectively, σ the specific surface energy, ρ the density, and M the molecular weight of the solute molecules. Otswald ripening is promoted by temperature changes during storage, particularly if there is a strong temperature-solubility relationship. Therefore, as the temperature is increased, the small particles of the drug will dissolve, which is followed by crystal growth as the temperature is decreased. Ziller and Rupprecht (1988a) have reported the design of a control unit to monitor crystal growth. However, simple microscopic observation may be all that is necessary to monitor the growth of crystals. If a phase change occurs, then the usual techniques may be used to assess the solid-state form of the compound produced on storage such as DSC, HSM (hot stage microscopy), or XRPD. Various polymeric additives may be employed to inhibit drug crystallization. Ziller and Rupprecht (1988b) found that polyvinylpyrollidone (PVP) and bovine serum albumin inhibit crystal growth using a variety of compounds. Similarly, Douroumis and Fahr (2007) found that PVP and hydroxypropylmethylcellulose (HPMC) were effective in preventing the growth of carbamazepine nanosuspension.

It is a pharmacopoeial requirement that suspensions should be redispersible if they settle on storage. However, the pharmacopoeias do not offer a suitable test that can be used to characterize this aspect of the formulation. In an attempt to remedy this situation, Deicke and Süverkrüp (1999) have devised a mechanical redispersibility tester, which closely simulates the action of human shaking. The crystal habit may also affect the physical stability of the formulation. For example, Tiwary and Panpalia (1999) showed that trimethoprim crystals with the largest aspect ratio showed the best sedimentation volume and redispersibility.

If the suspension is for parenteral administration, it will need to be sterilized. However, terminal heat sterilization can affect both its chemical and physical stabilities, the latter usually observed as crystal growth or aggregation of the particles (Na et al., 1999). Another measure of suspension stability is the zeta potential, which is a measure of the surface charge. However, various studies have shown that it is only useful in some cases. For example, Biro and Racz (1998) found that the zeta potential of albendazole suspensions was a good indicator of stability, whereas Duro et al. (1998) showed that the electrical charge of pyrantel pamoate suspensions was not important for its stabilization.

As noted above, the particle size of suspensions is another important parameter in suspension formulations. The particle size distribution can be measured using a variety of techniques including laser diffraction. A point to note in laser diffraction is the careful selection of the suspending agent. This was illustrated by Akinson and White (1992), who used a Malvern Mastersizer to determine the particle size of a 1% methylcellulose in the presence of seven surface-active agents (Tween 80, Tween 20, Span 20, Pluronic L62, Pluronic F88, Cetomacogol 100, and sodium lauryl sulfate). The particle size of the suspensions was measured as a function of time, and surprisingly, Tween 80, which is widely used in this respect, was found to be unsuitable for the hydrophobic drug under investigation. Other surfactants also gave poor particle size data, for example, Tween 20, Cetomacrogol 1000, Pluronic F88, and sodium lauryl sulfate. This arose from aggregation of the particles, and additionally, these suspensions showed slower drug dissolution into water. Span 20 and Pluronic L62 showed the best results, and the authors cautioned the use of a standard surface-active agent in preclinical studies.

Usually, suspensions are flocculated so that the particles form large aggregates that are easy to disperse—normally, this is achieved using potassium or sodium chloride (Akers et al., 1987). However, for controlled flocculation suspensions, sonication may be required to determine the size of the primary particles (Bommireddi et al., 1998).

Although high performance liquid chromatography (HPLC) is the preferred technique for assessing the stability of formulations, spectrophotometry can also be used. Girona et al. (1988) used this technique for assessing the stability of an ampicillin-dicloxacillin suspension. Rohn (2004) has reported that rheology could be used as a rapid screening technique for testing the stability of drug suspensions. He claims that by monitoring the tan delta parameter, the stability of the suspension could be predicted. Furthermore, the oscillation frequency sweep test gave information on the viscoelastic properties of the suspension, which could be used to screen potential suspending agents.

TOPICAL/TRANSDERMAL FORMULATIONS

Samir (1997) has reviewed preformulation aspects of transdermal drug delivery. This route of delivery offers several potential advantages compared with the oral route such as avoidance of fluctuating blood levels, no first-pass metabolism, and no degradation attributable to stomach acid. However, the transdermal route is limited because of the very effective barrier function of the skin. Large, polar molecules do not penetrate the stratum corneum well. The physicochemical properties of candidate drugs that are important in transdermal drug delivery include molecular weight and volume, aqueous solubility, melting point, and log *P*. Clearly, these are intrinsic properties of the molecule and as such will determine whether or not the compounds will penetrate the skin. Furthermore, since many compounds are weak acids or bases, pH will have an influence on their permeation.

One way in which the transport of zwitterionic drugs though skin has been enhanced was to form a salt. This was demonstrated by Mazzenga et al. (1992), who showed that the rank order of epidermal flux of the salts of phenylalanine across the epidermis was hydrobromide > hydrochloride > hydrofluoride > phenylalanine. Thus, like most other delivery routes, it is worth considering salt selection issues at the preformulation stage to optimize the delivery of the compound via the skin.

The formulation in which the candidate drug is applied to the skin is another important factor that can affect its bioavailability. In transdermal drug delivery, a number of vehicles may be used, such as creams, ointments, lotions, and gels. The solubility of the compound in the vehicle needs to be determined. Problems can arise from crystal growth if the system is supersaturated; for example, phenylbutazone creams were observed to have a gritty appearance attributable to crystal growth (Sallam et al., 1986). Indeed, in matrix patches, crystals of estradiol hemihydrate or gestodene of up to 800 μm grew during three months of storage at room temperature (Lipp and Müller, 1999). Needle-like crystals of the hydrate of betamethasone-17 valerate were found by Folger and Muller-Goymann (1994) when creams were placed on storage.

Chemical and physical stability also needs to be considered. For example, Thoma and Holzmann (1998) showed that dithranol showed a distinct instability in the paraffin base due to light, but was stable when protected from light. In terms of kinetics, Kenley et al. (1987) found that the degradation in a topical cream and that in ethanol-water solutions were very similar in the pH range 2 to 6. This suggested that the degradation of this compound occurred in an aqueous phase or compartment that was undisturbed by the oily cream excipients. If the compound decomposes because of oxidation, then an antioxidant may have to be incorporated. In an attempt to reduce the photodegradation of a development compound, Merrifield et al. (1996) compared the free acid of compound with a number of its salts, each of which they incorporated into a white soft paraffin base. Their results (Table 12) showed that after a one-hour exposure in a SOL2 light-simulation cabinet, the disodium salt showed significant degradation.

Martens-Lobenhoffer et al. (1999) have studied the stability of 8-methoxypsoralen (8-MOP) in various ointments. They found that after 12 weeks of storage, the drug was stable in Unguentum Cordes and Cold Cream Naturel. However, the Unguentum Cordes emulsion began to crack after eight weeks. When formulated in a carbopol gel, 8-MOP was unstable.

The physical structure of creams has been investigated by a variety of techniques, for example, DSC, TGA, microscopy, reflectance measure, rheology, Raman spectroscopy, and dielectric analysis (Peramal et al., 1997). Focusing on TGA and rheology, Peramal et al. (1997) found that when aqueous BP creams were analyzed by TGA, there were two peaks in the derivative curve. It was concluded that these were attributable to the loss of free and lamellar water from the cream, and therefore TGA could be used as a quality-control tool. The lamellar structure of creams can also be confirmed using small-angle X-ray measurements (Niemi and

Table 12 Light Stability of the Salts of a Candidate Drug in a White Soft Parrafin Base

| | % Initial compound after 1-hr exposure in SOL2 | | |
Salt/form	0.1% concentration	0.5% concentration	2.0% concentration
Free acid (micronized)	51.0	80.0	85.9
Free acid (unmicronized)	69.4	nd	nd
Disodium (unmicronized)	9.9	3.6	nd
Ethylenediamine (unmicronized)	51.9	65.1	nd
Piperazine (unmicronized)	79.9	88.2	nd

Abbreviation: nd, not detected.
Source: From Merrifield et al. (1996).

Laine, 1991). For example, the lamellar spacings of a sodium lauryl sulfate, cetostearyl alcohol and liquid paraffin cream were found to increase in size as the water content of the cream increased until, at greater than 60% water, the lamellar structure broke down. This was correlated with earlier work that showed that at this point, the release of hydrocortisone was increased (Niemi et al., 1989).

Atkinson et al. (1992) have reported the use of a laser diffraction method to measure the particle size of drugs dispersed in ointments. In this study, they stressed the fact that a very small particle size was required to ensure efficacy of the drug. In addition, the size of the particles was especially important if the ointment was for ophthalmic use where particles must be less than 25 μm. While the particle size of the suspended particles can be assessed microscopically, laser diffraction offers a more rapid analysis.

INHALATION DOSAGE FORMS

As noted by Sanjar and Matthews (2001), delivering drugs via the lung is not new since the absorption of nicotine by smoking of tobacco has been known for centuries, and before inhalation drug delivery devices, some asthma medications were administered in cigarettes. In addition, anesthetic gases are routinely administered by inhalation. For many years now, however, respiratory diseases such as asthma and chronic obstructive pulmonary disease (COPD) have been treated by inhaling the drug from a pressurized metered-dose inhaler (pMDI), DPI, or a nebulizer solution. Although pMDIs remain the most popular devices for the delivery of drugs to the lungs, DPIs have gained in popularity over the years (Gonda, 2000). For example, Taylor and Gustafsson (2005) stated that in 2004, 292 million pMDIs and 113 million DPIs were sold worldwide: In another article, Colthorpe (2003) has estimated that, on a daily basis, 500 million people carry a pMDI. Smyth and Hickey (2005) have estimated that there are greater than 11 DPIs in use and a similar number under development. See this publication for a list of devices and compounds. Islam and Gladki (2008) have reviewed DPI device reliability.

Because of the large surface area available, drug delivery via the lung has a number of advantages over the oral route since the rate of absorption of small molecules from the lung is only bettered by the intravenous route, and thus the bioavailability is usually higher than that obtained from drug delivery by the oral route. This is particularly true for hydrophobic compounds, which can show extremely rapid absorption (Cryan et al., 2007). However, drug deposition in the lung can be problematic and requires the drug to be reduced in size to between 2 and 6 μm for optimal effect (Pritchard, 2001; Howarth, 2001). If the particle size is greater than 6 μm, the compound is deposited in the mouth and esophageal region, and there is no clinical effect apart from the part that is swallowed. Particles of size 2 μm, on the other hand, are deposited in the peripheral airways/alveoli.

Metered-Dose Inhalers

In pMDI technology, CFC propellants are being replaced with the ozone-friendly HFAs 134a and 227 (McDonald and Martin (2000). For an overview of the environmental hazards and exposure risk of hydrofluorocarbons (HFCs), see Tsai (2005). In pMDI drug delivery systems,

$$F_3C \longrightarrow CF_2H \qquad\qquad F_3C \overset{H}{\underset{F}{\rule{0pt}{1.6em}|}} CF_3$$

134a   227

the drugs are formulated as a suspension or as a solution depending on the solubility of the drug in the propellant (or the addition of a cosolvent). Hoye et al. (2008) have investigated the solubility of 36 organic solutes in HFA 134a, and it was found that calculations of solubility from an ideal solubility viewpoint did not agree well with experimental values. However, addition of other terms such as log P, molar volume, molecular weight, etc., showed a better correlation and could provide an initial estimate of the solubility of a compound in HFA 134a. Traini et al. (2006) have described a novel apparatus for the determination of the solubility of salbutamol sulfate, budesonide, and formoterol fumarate dihydrate in propellant 134a. Their device allows the pMDI to be actuated into a collection vessel from which the amount that has been dissolved is assessed (using HPLC) after the propellant has evaporated. Another technique, based on direct injection from a pMDI into the injector port of an HPLC, for determining compound solubility in pMDIs has been described by Gupta and Myrdal (2004, 2005). An earlier method for determining the solubility of drugs in aerosol propellants has been described by Dalby et al. (1991). At room temperature, the propellants are gases, therefore, special procedures are required in separating the excess solid from the solution in the aerosol can; in this case, it is a simple filtration from one can to another. The propellent from the can containing the filtrate is then allowed to evaporate, and the residue is assayed for the drug using, for example, HPLC. Appreciable drug solubility may lead to particle growth, however, this may be overcome by the appropriate choice of salt if the compound is a weak acid or base. Thus, although suspensions offer the advantage of superior chemical stability (Tiwari et al. (1998), they may have problematic physical stability in terms of crystal growth or poor dispersion properties. In this respect, Tzou et al. (1997) examined whether the free base or the sulfate salt of albuterol (salbutamol) had the best chemical and physical stability for a pMDI formulation. Results showed that all of the sulfate formulations were chemically stable for up to 12 months, however, the base was less stable. In terms of physical stability, the base formulations showed crystal growth and agglomeration, illustrating the need for a salt selection process to be undertaken.

One significant challenge in the transition from the CFCs to HFAs is that the surfactants and polymers used as suspension stabilizers in CFC formulations are not soluble enough in the HFAs to be effective. For example, sorbitan monoleate (Span 85), commonly used in CFC formulations, is not soluble in HFA 134a or 227, however, other surfactants and polymers have been screened for their effectiveness in stabilizing propellant suspensions with some success. Some solubility of the surfactant in the propellant is a prerequisite, and while some suitable agents have been identified, they have not been progressed because of their potential toxicity in the lung. Some apparent solubilities of surfactants in HFAs 134a and 227 are shown in Table 13 (Vervaet and Byron, 1999).

It would of value to know if and how much surfactant or polymer was adsorbed by the particles. In an attempt to understand this process, Blackett and Buckton (1995) used

Table 13 Apparent Solubilities of Some Surfactants in HFA 134a and HFA 227

Surfactant	hydrophile-lipophile balance (HLB)	Apparent solubility (% w/w)	
		HFA 134a	HFA 227
Oleic acid	1.0	<0.02	<0.02
Sorbitan trioleate	1.8	<0.02	<0.01
Propoxylated PEG	4.0	≈3.6	1.5−15.3
			32.0−60.3
Sorbitan monooleate	4.3	<0.01	<0.01
Lecithin	7.0	<0.01	<0.01
Brij 30	9.7	≈1.8	0.8−1.2
Tween 80	15.0	<0.03	0−10.0
			25.0−89.8
Tween 20	16.7	≈0.1	1.4−3.5
PEG 300	20	≈4.0	1.5−4.3
			16.1−100
Polyvinylpyrollidone, PVA		>0.1	
Oligolactic acids		≈2.7	

Abbreviations: HFA, hydrofluoroalkane; PEG, polyethylene glycol.
Source: From Vervaet and Byron (1999), with permission from Elsevier.

isothermal microcalorimetry. The system investigated was the model CFC Arcton 113, salbutamol sulfate (crystalline and partially crystalline), and oleic acid or Span 85 as stabilizers. Using a perfusion-titration setup, they titrated suspensions of the drug with solutions of the surfactant and followed heat output as a function of time. It was shown that the heat output and adsorption were different depending on the crystallinity of the sample; that is, there was less heat output for the more energetic, partially crystalline sample. From these data, it was hypothesized that the orientation of the surfactant molecule during adsorption was different depending on the surface energy of the particles in suspension.

Drug substances for inhalation therapy via a pMDI (and DPIs) are reduced in size by micronization to particles of approximately 1 to 6 μm, which are capable of penetrating the deep airways and impact at the site of action. As noted earlier, micronization can cause problems because of the reduction in crystallinity and poor flow properties as a result of the milling process (Buckton, 1997). The effect of micronization on samples can be assessed by a variety of techniques, for example, DVS, microcalorimetry, and IGC. For example, IGC has been used to determine the surface properties of two batches of salbutamol sulfate (Ticehurst et al., 1994). This group also investigated the surface properties of α-lactose monohydrate (an excipient used in DPIs, see next section) using this technique to detect batch variation (Ticehurst et al., 1996). It was hypothesized that these differences in surface energetics between the nominally equivalent batches were due to small variations in surface crystallinity or purity. One common way of removing the high-energy portions from the surface is to condition the powder with moist air, which crystallizes the amorphous regions (Ahmed et al., 1996).

Williams et al. (1999) have reported the influence of ball milling and micronization on the formulation of triamcinolone acetonide (TAA) for MDIs. Both methods reduced the particle size of the powder, however, ball milling produced material with a greater amorphous content. This was shown by solution calorimetry measurements. Although the ball-milled material was less crystalline, it was found to have the smallest particles and the highest respirable fraction.

It is possible that a number of physical changes can occur because of suspension in the propellant. The first is due to Ostwald ripening, a phenomenon described earlier in this chapter. This arises when the compound shows some solubility in the propellant resulting in particle growth and caking. In this process, the smallest micronized particles dissolve and then recrystallize on the larger particles. As shown by Phillips et al. (1993), optical microscopy can be used to assess the crystal growth of micronized salicylic acid in CFC pMDIs. In this study, the increase in the axial ratio (length/breadth) of the crystals was measured as a function of time. Although the crystals continued to grow after an initial increase in the axial ratio, after some time, it did not change. It was therefore concluded that axial ratios of crystals should always be determined by microscopy to detect any physical instability in the early stages of MDI formulation development. In another paper by this group, Phillips et al. (1994) have investigated the surfactant-promoted crystal growth of micronized methylprednisolone in trichloromono-fluoromethane (CFC-11). The effect of drug concentration, surfactant type, and composition on the solubility of methylprednisolone was determined and related to the observed crystal growth in suspension. In particular, high concentrations of Span 85 (sorbitan trioleate) were found to increase the solubility of the compound, with the consequence of crystal growth. Oleic acid and lower concentrations of Span 85, on the other hand, showed little particle size change. In addition to an increase in particle size, the crystals may also solvate the propellants, and this may also lead to crystal growth. Apart from the obvious increase in particle size of the suspension, there are a number of techniques that can be used to confirm the existence of the solvate. These include DSC, TGA, hot-stage microscopy, XRPD, and infrared spectroscopy.

An example of this phenomenon is a development compound that was found to have changed from a micronized powder to much larger particles after storage in propellant. When the recovered crystals were analyzed using TGA, a mass loss of 25.5% was detected in the range of 40°C to 100°C. This thermal event was also evident in the DSC, which showed an endotherm corresponding to solvent loss followed by an exotherm probably due to crystallization. Hot-stage microscopy showed that, when heated in silicone oil, a gas was evolved as the temperature was raised. This is illustrated in Figure 19. Notice how the crystals broke apart as the gas was released as the temperature was raised.

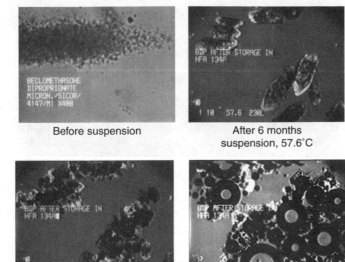

Before suspension

After 6 months
suspension, 57.6°C

65.5°C

73.9°C

Figure 19 HSM photographs of an inhalation drug before and after suspension in gHFA 134a.

To confirm that the crystals had solvated the propellant, infrared spectroscopy provided a useful test, whereby the main difference was the appearance of a medium-strong peak at 1289/cm. By reference to standard tables of infrared stretching frequencies, this new peak was assigned as a C-F stretch that, with the other information, lead to the conclusion that the compound had solvated the propellant gas (134a).

For pMDIs, the compatibility of the propellants with the valve elastomers also needs to be evaluated. For example, Tiwari et al. (1998) investigated the effect of 134a on a number of valve elastomers and found that it adversely affected the performance of the valve. Inhalation dosage forms are discussed in more detail in chapter 10.

Dry-Powder Inhalers

DPIs do not rely on the CFC or HFA propellant gases and are hence more "environmentally friendly" than MDIs. There are a number of devices that can deliver drugs to the lung as dry powders, for example, Turbuhaler™ and Diskhaler™. DPIs rely on a larger carrier particle such as α-lactose monohydrate to which the drug is attached. (The lactose is usually fractionated such that it lies in the size range 63–90 μm.) On delivery, the drug detaches from the lactose, and because the drug is micronized, it is delivered to the lung, whereas the lactose is swallowed. The use of alternative carriers, such as erythitol, mannitol, and trehalose, has been investigated by Jones et al. (2008). As noted elsewhere, micronization is a somewhat aggressive method of particle size reduction commonly used for inhalation compounds. A common way of restoring the crystallinity after this process is to condition the surface of the micronized drug by exposing it to elevated relative humidities or organic vapors. The net effect of this procedure is to crystallize the amorphous regions, making the powder better suited for formulation in a DPI. Brodka-Pfeiffer et al. (2003) have described work on the conditioning of salbutamol sulfate. As noted elsewhere, crystallization from supercritical fluids has been investigated as a method for producing micronized particles for inhalation (Martin and Cocero, 2008). Young and Price (2004) have examined the effect of humidity on the aerosolization of micronized salbutamol sulfate. Using DVS, AFM, and twin-stage impinger data, they showed that at increased humidities, the fine-particle fraction for both samples decreased because of the amorphous character induced by the micronization process: the crystallization of the amorphous regions due to the elevated humidity causes the particles to fuse to the lactose carrier.

The performance of DPIs is governed by a number of factors such as van der Waals, electrostatic, and capillary forces (Young et al., 2003a, b; Jones and Price, 2006; Jones et al., 2008). When formulating a DPI, considerable attention needs to be paid to the physical form of the drug substance. For example, it needs to have a reasonably high melting point (>80°C), not show significant moisture uptake (probably less than 2% w/w), not taste significantly, and not be significantly colored. Of these, moisture sorption is arguably the most important since moisture can affect the deagglomeration of the compound from the lactose carrier (Maggi et al., 1999; Young et al., 2003). The use of hydrates in DPI formulations can be problematic, particularly those that sorb moisture to form non-stoichiometric hydrate (see chapter 10). It is recommended that these physical forms be avoided because of potential difficulties with deagglomeration. For example, Young et al. (2003, 2006) examined the effect of storing disodium cromoglycate (a channel hydrate that takes up moisture from the atmosphere nonstoichiometrically for 12 hours at 15%, 30%, 45%, 60%, and 75% RH). Not unsurprisingly, the delivered dose and the fine-particle dose were decreased with increasing RH. Clarke et al. (2000), on the other hand, found that the stoichiometric channel hydrate, nedocromil sodium trihydrate, when stored between 12% and 76% RH, did not have a perceptible effect on its performance. However, storage of the micronized powder above 86%RH, where the trihydrate converts to the heptahemihydrate, caused a significant reduction of the deaggregation performance. The effect of storing two DPI devices under hot and humid conditions showed that the performance of one DPI was affected in vitro (Borgström et al., 2005).

As noted by Jashnani and Byron (1996), in formulation terms, it is always worth optimizing the salt form of a compound. In this study, the performance of dry-powder aerosol generation in different environments for the sulfate, adipate (diethanolate), and stearate salts of albuterol were determined. Overall, the stearate emptied and aerosolized best from the inhaler and showed the least sensitivity to environmental factors such as temperature and humidity. Another use of low-solubility salts is to mask the taste of compounds that is unpleasant when delivered by DPI (or pMDI for that matter). By lowering the solubility and hence dissolution rate, the taste can often be effectively eliminated.

It has also shown that the polymorphic form of the lactose used can affect the aerosolization properties of the formulation. The results showed that, as function of flow rate, the β-form was easily entrained but held on to the drug particles most strongly. The anhydrous α-form showed the opposite behavior, and the α-form (the monohydrate) showed intermediate behavior. Processing of lactose was the subject of a paper by Young et al. (2007).

Micronized particles form strong agglomerates, and the size of these agglomerates, among other things, depends on the surface free energy of the powder. Since micronization can change the surface free energy of a material, the adherence properties of the compound will also be changed. For example, Podczeck et al. (1994, 1995a,b) have performed adhesion and autoadhesion measurements of salmeterol xinafoate particles of various sizes to compacted lactose monohydrate surfaces using a centrifuge technique. This work was followed up by work investigating the adhesion force of micronized salmeterol xinafoate particles to pharmaceutically relevant surface materials (Podeczeck et al., 1996). Results showed that long contact times with PVC, polyethylene, or aluminum should be avoided because the adhesion force between the drug and these surfaces was much higher than that between it and the lactose carrier. Thus, detachment and loss of drug in the formulation could occur. In another study, Podczeck et al. (1996a, b) investigated the adhesion strength of some salts of salmeterol to lactose and other substrates with varying surface roughness, surface free energy, and Young's modulus. It was concluded that many of these factors play a part, as well as chemical forces, and that only experimental assessment could indicate whether the material was suitable.

Using AFM, Bérard et al. (2002) showed that an increased RH increased the adhesion between their probe molecule, zanamivir, and lactose. As has been noted earlier, micronized particles can contain amorphous regions, which can be crystallized at elevated levels of RH. However, the recrystallization process can lead to particle growth, with bridges being formed between the micronized particles (Brodka-Pfeiffer et al., 2003).

Because lactose is the most commonly used carrier excipient in DPIs, its compatibility with the drug substance should be assessed, particularly if it is a primary amine (see the section on compatibility). The physicochemical characteristics of some alternative carrier particles have been described by Byron et al. (1996). The effect of the surface morphology of lactose carriers on the inhalation properties of pranlukast hydrate has been reported

Table 14 Solubility of an Sibenadit HCl in Water and Isotonic Saline as a Function of Temperature

Solvent	Solubility (μg/mL)		
	4°C	25°C	40°C
Water	1789	2397	6837
Saline	<30	61	157

(Kawashima et al., 1998). The lactose carriers investigated were pharmatose 325M, pharmatose 200M (sieved to ~60 μm), and fluidized-bed granulated lactose. Results showed that with increasing specific surface area and roughness, the effective index of inhalation decreased because of the drug being held more tightly in the inhaled airstream. Therefore, character-ization of the carrier particles by, for example, surface area measurements, SEM, as well as other solid-state techniques is recommended in preformulation activities for DPIs. Jones and Price (2006) have shown that inclusion of fine lactose particles improved the performance of a DPI formulation.

Nebulizer Solutions

Nebulizer formulations are normally solutions, however, suspensions are also used, for example, the insoluble steroid budesonide has been successfully formulated for delivery by nebulization (Dahlback, 1994). Some important preformulation considerations for nebulizers are stability, solubility, viscosity, and surface tension (McCallion et al., 1996; Nikander, 1997). In terms of solubility, the common ion effect may be important where, for example, a hydrochloride salt is to be dissolved in saline. In addition, the temperature dependence of the solubility of the drug may be important, for example, Taylor et al. (1992) found that the temperature of a solution of a pentamidine isethionate decreased by up to 13°C, causing the drug to crystallize from solution. The osmolality of solutions has been found to increase during nebulization, although the pH does not appear to do so (Schoeni and Kraemer, 1989).

Table 14 shows solubility data for the potential inhalation drug sebenadit hydrochloride, which was to have been delivered by a pMDI and as a nebulizer solution (Cosgrove et al., 2005).

These data show the increase in solubility of the compound with respect to temperature and how the presence of the chloride ion depressed its solubility. Wong-Beringer et al. (2008) have performed in more depth investigation into the optimal physicochemical properties for the delivery of the antibiotic caspofungin by nebulizer solution. They found that caspofungin required dilution with a 0.9% w/v sodium chloride adjusted to between pH 6.17 and 6.26 with sodium hydroxide to give a solution that had an osmolality that was optimal for delivery to the lung.

If the drug is insoluble, it is important that for a suspension formulation, the drug is micronized to a size of less than 2 μm (Dahlback, 1994). The particle size distribution of nebulized droplets can be measured using, for example, laser diffraction (Clark et al., 1995). Validation experiments showed that laser diffraction was robust and reliable and that the diffraction data was a good measure of the particle size of the aerosolized droplets.

Nebulized inhalation drugs are often admixed with others, however, their physical and chemical compatibility should be to assess before proceeding. For a discussion of this aspect of nebulizer therapy, see Kamin et al. (2007).

COMPATIBILITY

Compatibility studies are conducted to accelerate the development of formulations by allowing formulators to eliminate those excipients that cause API degradation. Factors that affect the compatibility between drugs and potential formulation aids include local pH and water content, which affect the chemical stability of the API. Typically, incompatibilities can arise because of either intrinsic degradation of the API and is facilitated by the excipients or a

Table 15 Known Reactivities of Some Functional Groups

Functional group	Incompatibilities	Type of reaction
Primary amine	Mono- and disaccharides	Amine-aldehyde and amine-acetal
Ester, cyclic, lactone	Basic components	Ring-opening ester-base hydrolysis
Carbonyl, hydroxyl	Silanol	Hydrogen bonding
Aldehyde	Amine carbohydrates	Aldehyde-amine Schiff base or glycosylamine
Carboxyl	Bases	Salt formation
Alcohol	Oxygen	Oxidation to aldehydes and ketones
Sulfhydryl	Oxygen	Dimerization
Phenol	Metals	Complexation
Gelatin capsule shell	Cationic surfactant	Denaturation

Source: From Monkhouse (1993), reproduced with permission.

covalent chemical reaction between the API and the excipients (Damien, 2004). Of course, it is worth checking whether there are any known incompatibilities, as shown in Table 15 (Monkhouse, 1993). After checking for any known incompatibilities, experimental investigations of compatibility should be undertaken. Akers (2002) has reviewed drug-excipient interactions with respect to parenteral formulations.

While the Maillard reaction between lactose and primary amines is well known, the same reaction between the secondary amine fluoxetine hydrochloride (Prozac) and lactose has recently been reported (Wirth et al., 1998). In the solid-state water content, lubricant concentration and temperature were also found to influence the degradation. In addition to the chemical reactions noted above, the drug may interact to form a molecular compound. For example, solid-state interactions between trimethoprim and antimicrobial paraben esters to form a 1:1 molecular compound have been reported (Pedersen et al., 1994).

When conducting compatibility studies, there are four steps to be considered, which are as follows:

1. Sample preparation
2. Statistical design
3. Storage conditions
4. Method of analysis

Traditionally, a binary mixture of drug and the excipient being investigated is intimately mixed, the ratio of drug to excipient being often 1:1; however, other mixtures may also be investigated. These powder samples, one set of which is moistened, are then sealed into ampoules to prevent moisture loss. These are then stored at a suitable temperature and analyzed at various time points using HPLC, DSC, FTIR (Fourier transform infra-red), or TGA as appropriate (Stulzer et al., 2008). Using DSC alone is not recommended since it can throw up false negatives and positives and should be used as guide only. Indeed, Larkshama et al. (2008) have concluded that DSC experiments need to be supported by other techniques such as FTIR and HPLC. The use of microthermal analytical technologies such as localized thermomechanical analysis (L-TMA), localized differential thermal analysis (L-DTA), nanosampling, thermally assisted particle manipulation (TAPM), and photothermal microspectrometry (PTMS) has been described by Harding et al. (2008). It is fair to say, however, that these are quite specialized techniques not widely available in industry at this point in time. Alternatively, the drug in suspension with excipients may be investigated (Waltersson, 1986). Table 16 shows data for 250 mg of remacemide hydrochloride mixed with 250 mg of spray-dried lactose and dispensed into clear, neutral glass ampoules. Half of the ampoules were sealed without further treatment, and to the others, 25 µl of distilled water was added prior to sealing. The ampoules were then stored at 25°C for 1, 4, and 12 weeks.

As expected, there is clear evidence of incompatibility between the amine hydrochloride and the spray-dried lactose. However, the results also showed that moisture was the catalyst for decomposition as no degradation was observed in the dry state even after 12 weeks' storage at 90°C.

Table 16　Compatibility Study Between Remacemide HCl and Spray-Dried Lactose

Water added (µl)	Storage temperature (°C)	Storage time (wk)	Color	Moisture by TGA	% Drug recovered
0	25	1	White	2.6	101.2
		4	White	2.6	99.4
		12	White	2.6	102.8
	70	1	White	2.6	105.0
		4	White	2.6	101.8
		12	Off-white	2.5	100.3
	90	1	White	2.6	102.5
		4	White	2.6	98.5
		12	Off-white	2.2	100.2
25	25	1	White	2.6	93.6
		4	White	6.8	102.6
		12	White	5.0	88.4
	70	1	Brown	3.2	91.4
		4	Brown/black	N/I[a]	99.7
		12	Brown/black	N/I	74.4
	90	1	Brown	4.0	98.5
		4	Brown/black	N/I	90.0
		12	Black	N/I	51.4

[a]Thermogram not interpretable because of extensive sample degradation.

Ahlneck and Lundgren (1985) have described methods for the evaluation of solid-state stability and compatibility between drugs and excipients. Three methods were studied and compared isothermally and non-isothermally, viz. suspension, storage of powders, and compacts at specified humidities and elevated temperatures. It was concluded that the suspension technique was good for fast screening of chemical instability. The other solid-state procedures were found to be better predictors of the solid dosage form.

The storage conditions used to examine compatibility can vary widely in terms of temperature and humidity, but a temperature of 50°C for storage of compatibility samples is considered appropriate. Some compounds may require higher temperatures to make reactions proceed at a rate that can be measured over a convenient time period. Methods of analysis also vary widely, ranging from thermal methods, for example, DSC, microcalorimetry or chromatographic techniques like TLC and HPLC.

DSC has been used extensively for compatibility studies (Holgado et al., 1995). Although only milligram quantities of drug are needed for a DSC experiment, the interpretation of the thermograms may be difficult and conclusions may be misleading on the basis of DSC experiments alone (van Dooren, 1983; Joshi et al., 2002b), Nonetheless, the technique remains in use, for example, Verma and Garg (2005) and Araujo et al. (2005). The original protocol for DSC compatibility testing was proposed by van Dooren (1983), who suggested the following scheme:

1. Run the drug candidate and excipients individually
2. Run mixtures of the drug candidate and excipients immediately after mixing
3. Run the drug candidate and excipients individually after three weeks at 55°C
4. Run the drug candidate–excipient mix after three weeks at 55°C
5. Run the single components and mixtures after three weeks at 55°C only if the curves of the mixtures before and after storage at this temperature differ from each other

An excipient that is particularly desired may be investigated further by examining different weight ratios with the drug. This method of compatibility testing has been criticized by Chrzanowski et al. (1986), who found that the DSC compatibility method was an unreliable compatibility predictor for fenretinide and three mefenidil salts with various direct compression excipients. They concluded that an isothermal stress (IS) method (which requires a specific, quantitative assay method, for example, HPLC, for either test substance or its degradation products) was preferred for its accuracy over DSC in compatibility testing. In addition, the IS method gave quantitative information. Disadvantages of the IS system compared with DSC are that the tests tend to consume more compound than the DSC test and are conducted over longer storage times, one to two months at 60°C to 80°C. However, the whole point of DSC is speed of prediction, so DSC may be of use if the amount of drug available is small and an idea of compatibility is required (Venkataram et al. 1995). On the other hand, although DSC may be used to predict that interactions may occur, it provides little insight into the nature of the interaction (Hartauer and Guillory, 1991). Although most investigators use only binary mixtures of drug and excipient, Damien (2004) notes that the interactions are often complex and active substance-excipient compatibility studies must not be limited to simple binary mixtures.

Microcalorimetry has also been used in excipient compatibility studies (Phipps et al., 1998). In this study, 1:1 mixtures were prepared using a ball mill and examined for incompatibility by sealing samples in glass crimped vials using a microcalorimeter at 50°C at a set RH. After an equilibration period of between one to four days, thermal data were collected over 15 hours. Generally, the data from the thermal activity monitor (TAM) was comparable to the corresponding HPLC analysis. However, it was less successful in prediction when mixtures containing a hygroscopic component was present. Another work by Selzer et al. (1998) has shown that microcalorimetry can be used to detect incompatibility. However, since microcalorimetry only detects heat flow, they made the point that physical events such as crystallinity changes would be superimposed on the heat output signal. They also found that experimental temperatures close to the ambient could not be employed because the enthalpy change was not large enough.

In solid dose form technology, Monkhouse (1993) has argued that it may be a better idea to make tablets with proven excipient blends in a compaction simulator using representative compression forces. This, it was claimed, would use a small amount of the candidate drug and also take into account factors such as mixing, granulation, and compression. Then only if the tablet is proven to be unstable, should retrospective examination of the incompatibility be undertaken to identify the excipients that are incompatible. Indeed, according to this author, any formulations that do not contain lactose and magnesium stearate should be successful! Other investigators may have different experiences and may not have access to a compaction simulator. It is also worth being aware of processing-induced incompatibilities such as that reported by Wardrop et al. (2006), who found that even after conventional compatibility testing, degradation of their compound in a trial formulation was observed. The incompatibility was traced to an unusual anhydrate-to-amorphous transition that occurred because of granulation. A new dry process was developed, and polarized light microscopy was used to confirm the presence of the crystalline anhydrate after formulation.

Like other aspects of the work in the modern pharmaceutical industry, automation and high-throughput techniques are being employed to speed up the process. For example, Wyttenbach et al. (2005) have described a miniaturized high-throughput compound-excipient compatibility protocol, which included statistical experimental design techniques. In essence, they used 96-well technology, whereby the compound was mixed with the excipients in a ~1:100 ratio and stored under accelerated conditions of elevated temperature and humidity. At various time points, the mixtures were analyzed using fast gradient HPLC. Combined with the statistical experimental design factor interaction plots can be generated, and all this can be achieved using 0.1 mg of compound per data point. Workers from Pfizer (Thomas and Naath, 2008) have also reported an automated 96-well plate compatibility system, which can weigh and blend mixtures, conduct accelerated stress stability, extract the sample, and perform HPLC analysis. They have termed this system as drug-excipient compatibility automated system (DECCAS). Wakasawa et al. (2008) have conducted drug-excipient compatibility studies using a robotic system, which automatically dispenses, weighs, and stores powder samples, and then analyzes the drug substance using ultra-performance liquid chromatography (UPLC). After storage at 70°C for nine days, the samples are examined for degradation.

REFERENCES

Adamska K, Voelkel A, Héberger K. Selection of solubility parameters for characterization of pharmaceutical excipients. J Chromatogr A 2007; 1171:90–97.

Ahlneck C, Lundgren P. Methods for the evaluation of solid-state stability and compatibility between drug and excipient. Acta Pharm Suec 1985; 22:305–314.

Ahmed H, Buckton G, Rawlins DA. Use of isothermal microcalorimetry in the study of small degrees of amorphous content of a hydrophobic powder. Int J Pharm 1996; 130:195–201.

Akers MJ. Preformulation screening of antioxidant efficiency in parenteral solutions. J Parenter Drug Assoc 1979; 33:346–356.

Akers MJ. Antioxidants in pharmaceutical products. J Parenter Sci Technol 1982; 36:222–228.

Akers MJ. Excipient-drug interactions in parenteral formulations. J Pharm Sci 2002; 91:2283–2300.

Akers MJ, Fites AL, Robinson RL. Formulation design and development of parenteral suspensions. J Parenter Sci Technol 1987; 41:88–96.

Alander EM, Uusi-Pentilla MS, Rasmsuon AC. Characterization of paracetamol agglomerates by image analysis and strength measurements. Powder Tech 2002; 130:298–306.

Alsante KM, Ando A, Bronw R, et al. The role degradant profiling in active pharmaceutical ingredients and drug products. Adv Drug Deliv Rev 2007; 59:29–37.

Am Ende D, Bronk KS, Mustakis J, et al. API quality by design example from the torcetrapib manufacturing process. J Pharm Innov 2007; 2:71–86.

Ambarkhane AV, Pincott K, Buckton G. The use of inverse gas chromatography and gravimetric vapour sorption to study transitions in amorphous lactose. Int J Pharm 2005; 294:129–135.

Amin K, Dannenfelser R-S. In vitro hemolysis: guidance for the pharmaceutical scientist. J Pharm Sci 2006; 95:1173–1176.

Ammar HO, Ibrahim SA, El-Mohsen A. Effect of chelating agents on the stability of injectable isoniazid solutions. Pharmazie 1982; 37:270–271.

Andrès C, Bracconi P, Pourcelot Y. On the difficulty of assessing the specific surface area of magnesium stearate. Int J Pharm 2001; 218:153–163.

Araujo AAS, Storpirtis S, Mercuri LP, et al. Thermal analysis of the antiretroviral zidovudine (AZT) and evaluation of the compatibility with excipients used in solid dosage forms. Int J Pharm 2005; 260:303–314.

Asahara K, Yamada H, Yoshida S, et al. Stability prediction of nafamostat mesylate in an intravenous admixture containing sodium bisulfite. Chem Pharm Bull 1990; 38:492–497.

Atkins TW, White S. Hydrophobic drug substances: the use of laser diffraction particle size analysis and dissolution to characterize surfactant stabilized suspensions. Spec Publ R Soc Chem 1992; 102:133–142.

Atkinson TW, Greenway MJ, Holland SJ, et al. The use of laser diffraction particle size analysis to predict the dispersibility of a medicament in a paraffin based ointment. Spec Publ R Soc Chem 1992; 102:139–152.

Aulton M, Wells JA. Pharmaceutics. The science of dosage form design. In: Aulton ME, ed. Preformulation. Edinburgh: Churchill Livingstone, 1988.

Barra J, Somma R. Influence of the physicochemical variability of magnesium stearate on its lubricant properties: possible solutions. Drug Dev Ind Pharm 1996; 22:1105–1120.

Bérard V, Lesniewska E, Andrès C, et al. Dry powder inhaler: influence of humidity on topology and adhesion studied by AFM. Int J Pharm 2002; 232:213–224.

Bererich J, Dee KH, Hayauchi Y, et al. A new method to determine discoloration kinetics of uncoated white tablets occurring during stability testing an application of instrumental colour measurement in the development pharmaceutics. Int J Pharm 2002; 234:55–66.

Birch M, Fussel SJ, Higginson PD, et al. Towards a PAT-based strategy for crystallization development. Org Proc Res Dev 2005; 9:360–364.

Biro EJ, Racz I. The role of zeta potential in the stability of albendazole suspensions. STP Pharma Sci 1998; 8:311–315.

Blackett PM, Buckton G. A microcalorimetric investigation of the interaction of surfactants with crystalline and partially crystalline salbutamol sulphate in a model inhalation aerosol system. Pharm Res 1995; 12:1689–1693.

Blagden N, Davey RJ, Rowe R, et al. Disappearing polymorphs and the role of reaction byproducts: the case of sulphathiazole. Int J Pharm 1998; 172:169–177.

Bommireddi A, Li L, Stephens D, et al. Particle size determination of a flocculated suspension using a light scattering particle analyzer. Drug Dev Ind Pharm 1998; 24:1089–1093.

Branchu S, Rogueda PG, Plumb AP, et al. A decision-support tool for the formulation of orally active, poorly soluble compounds. Eur J Pharm Sci 2007; 32:128–139.

Briggner L-E, Buckton G, Bystrom K, et al. The use of microcalorimetry in the study of changes in crystallinity induced during the processing of powders. Int J Pharm 1994; 105:125–135.

Brittain HG, Amidon G. Critical overview of the proposed particle size analysis tests. Am Pharm Rev 2003; 68–72.

Brittain HG, Bogdanowich SJ, Bugey DE, et al. Physical characterization of pharmaceutical solids. Pharm Res 1991; 8:963–973.

Brodka-Pfeiffer K, Häusler H, Grass P, et al. Conditioning following powder micronization: influence on particle growth of salbutamol sulfate. Drug Dev Ind Pharm 2003; 29:1077–1084.

Brunsteiner M, Jones AG, Pratola F, et al. Towards a molecular understanding of crystal agglomeration. Crystal Growth Des 2005; 5:3–16.

Buckton G. Surface characterization: understanding sources of variability in the production and use of pharmaceuticals. J Pharm Pharmcol 1995; 47:265–275.

Buckton G. Characterisation of small changes in the physical properties of powders of significance for dry powder inhaler formulations. Adv Drug Deliv Rev 1997; 26:17–27.

Buckton G, Gill H. The importance of surface energetics of powders for drug delivery and the establishment of inverse gas chromatography. Adv Drug Deliv Rev 2007; 59:1474–1479.

Bugay DE, Newman AW, Findlay WP. Quantitation of cefepime-2HCl dihydrate in cefepime-2HCl monohydrate by diffuse reflectance IR and powder X-ray diffraction techniques. J Pharm Biomed Anal 1996; 15:49–61.

Bunker MJ, Davies MC, James MB, et al. Direct observation of single particle electrostatic charging by atomic force microscopy. Pharm Res 2007; 24:1165–1169.

Byron PR, Naini V, Phillips EM. Drug carrier selection—important physicochemical characteristics. Respir Drug Deliv 1996; 5:103–113.

Byrn SR, Liang JK, Bates S, et al. PAT—process understanding and control of active pharmaceutical ingredients. PAT J Proc Anal Technol 2006; 3:14–19.

Cao X, Leyva N, Anderson SR, et al. Use of prediction methods to estimate true density of active pharmaceutical ingredients. Int J Pharm 2008; 355:231–237.

Carlson E, Chandler W, Galdo I, et al. Automated integrated forced degradation and drug-excipient compatibility studies. J Assoc Lab Automat 2005; 10:374–380.

Carstensen JT. Advanced Pharmaceutical Solids, Vol 110, Drugs and the Pharmaceutical Sciences. New York: Marcel Dekker Inc., 2001.

Carstensen JT, Ertell C, Geoffroy J-E. Physico-chemical properties of particulate matter. Drug Dev Ind Pharm 1993; 19:195–219.

Carter PA, Rowley G, Fletcher EJ, et al. An experimental investigation of triboelectrification in cohesive and non-cohesive pharmaceutical powders. Drug Dev Ind Pharm 1992; 18:1505–1526.

Cavatur RK, Suryanarayanan R. Characterization of frozen aqueous solutions by low temperature X-ray powder diffractometry. Pharm Res 1998; 15:194–199.

Chang H-K, Whitworth CW. Aspirin degradation in mixed polar solvents. Drug Dev Ind Pharm 1984; 10:515–526.

Chansiri G, Lyons RT, Patel MV. Effect of surface charge on the stability of oil/water emulsions during steam sterilization. J Pharm Sci 1999; 88:454–458.

Cheng W-T, Lin SH, Li M-J. Raman micro spectroscopic mapping or thermal or thermal system used to investigate milling-induced solid-state conversion of famotidine. J Raman Spectrosc 2007; 38: 1595–1601.

Chieng N, Rades T, Saville D. Formation and physical stability of the amorphous phase of ranitidine hydrochloride polymorphs prepared by cryo-milling. Eur J Pharm Biopharm 2008; 68:771–780.

Chieng N, Zujovic Z, Bowmaker G, et al. Effect of milling conditions on the solid-state conversion of ranitidine hydrochloride form I. Int J Pharm 2006; 327:36–44.

Chikhalia V, Forbes RT, Storey RA, et al. The effect of crystal morphology and mill type on milling induced crystal disorder. Eur J Pharm 2006; 27:19–26.

Chow AHL, Tong HHY, Chattopadhyay P, et al. Particle engineering for pulmonary drug delivery. Pharm Res 2007; 24:411–437.

Chow K, Tong HHY, Lum S, et al. Engineering of pharmaceutical materials: an industrial perspective. J Pharm Sci 2008; 97:2855–2877.

Chrzanowski FA, Ulissi BJ, Fegely BJ, et al. Preformulation excipient compatibility testing. Application of a differential scanning calorimetry method versus a wet granulation simulating isothermal stress method. Drug Dev Ind Pharm 1986; 12:783–800.

Clark AR. The use of laser diffraction for the evaluation of the aerosol clouds generated by medical nebulizers. Int J Pharm 1995; 115:69–78.

Clarke MJ, Tobyn MJ, Staniforth JN. Physicochemical factors governing the performance of nedocromil sodium as a dry powder aerosol. J Pharm Sci 2000; 89:1160–1169.

Colthorpe P. Industry experiences of the HFA transitions. Drug Deliv Syst Sci 2003; 3:41–43.

Cosgrove SD, Steele G, Plumb AP, et al. Understanding the polymorphic behaviour of sibenadit hydrochloride through detailed studies integrating structural and dynamical assessment. J Pharm Sci 2005; 94:2403–2415.

Craig DQM, Royall PG, Kett VL, et al. The relevance of the amorphous state to pharmaceutical dosage forms: glassy drugs and freeze dried systems. Int J Pharm 1999; 179:179–207.

Cryan A-A, Sivadas N, Garci-Contreras L. In vivo animal models for drug delivery across the lung mucosal barrier. Adv Drug Deliv Rev 2007; 59:1133–1151.

Cui Y. A materials science perspective of pharmaceutical solids. Int J Pharm 2007; 339:3–18.

Cypes SH, Wenslow RM, Thomas SM, et al. Drying an organic monohydrate: crystal form instabilities and a factory–scale drying scheme to ensure monohydrate preservation. Org Proc Res Dev 2004; 8: 576–582.

Dahlback M. Behaviour of nebulizing solutions and suspensions. J Aerosol Med 1994; 7(suppl):S13–S18.

Dalby RN, Phillips EM, Byron PR. Determination of drug solubility in aerosol propellants. Pharm Res 1991; 8:1206–1209.

Damien G. Development of a solid dosage form compatibility studies on the active substance-excipients. STP Pharma Prat 2004; 14:303–310.

Date AA, Nagarsenker MS. Parenteral microemulsions: an overview. Int J Pharm 2008; 55:19–30.

De Vegt O, Vromans H, Faassen F, et al. Milling of organic solids in a jet mill. Part 1: determination of the selection function and related mechanical material properties. Part Part Syst Charact 2005a; 133–140.

De Vegt O, Vromans H, Faassen F, et al. Milling of organic solids in a jet mill. Part 2: checking the validity of the predicted rate of breakage function. Part Part Syst Charact 2005b; 22:261–267.

Deicke A, Süverkrüp R. Dose uniformity and redispersibility of pharmaceutical suspensions I: quantification and mechanical modelling of human shaking behaviour. Eur J Pharm Biopharm 1999; 48:225–232.

Descamps M, Willart JF, Dudognon E, et al. Transformation of pharmaceutical compounds upon millling and co-milling. The role of T_g. J Pharm Sci 2007; 96:1398–1407.

Desikan S, Anderson SR, Meenan PA, et al. Crystallization challenges in drug development: scale-up from laboratory to pilot plant and beyond. Curr Opin Drug Discov Devel 2000; 3:723–733.

Di Martino P, Censi R, Barthélémy C, et al. Characterization and compaction behaviour of nimesulide crystal forms. Int J Pharm 2007; 342:137–144.

Douroumis D, Fahr A. Stable carbamazepine colloidal systems using the cosolvent technique. Eur J Pharm Sci 2007; 30:367–374.

Driscoll DF, Etzler F, Barber TA, et al. Physicochemical assessment of parenteral lipid emulsions: light obscuration versus laser diffraction. Int J Pharm 2001; 219:21–37.

Duddu SP, Weller K. Importance of glass transition temperature in accelerated stability testing of amorphous solids: case study using a lyophilized aspirin formulation. J Pharm Sci 1996; 85:345–347.

Duncan-Hewitt WC, Grant DJW. True density and thermal expansivity of pharmaceutical solids: comparison of methods and assessment of crystallinity. Int J Pharm 1986; 28:75–84.

Dunitz JD, Bernstein J. Disappearing polymorphs. Acc Chem Res 1995; 28:193–200.

Duro R, Alverez C, Martinez-Pachecon R, et al. The adsorption of cellulose ethers in aqueous suspensions of pyrantel pamoate: effects of zeta potential and stability. Eur J Pharm Biopharm 1998; 45:181–188.

Elajnaf A, Carter P, Rowley G. The effect of relative humidity on electrostatic charge decay of drugs and excipients used in dry powder inhaler formulation. Drug Dev Ind Pharm 2007; 33:967–974.

Férézou J, Gulik A, Domingo N, et al. Intralipid 10%: physicochemical characterization. Nutrition 2001; 17:930–933.

Fitzpatrick JJ, Hodnett M, Twomney M, et al. Glass transition and the flowability and caking of powders containing amorphous lactose. Powder Technol 2007; 178:119–128.

Flynn GL. Isotonicity-colligative properties and dosage form behaviour. J Parenteral Drug Assoc 1979; 33: 292–315.

Folger M, Möller-Goymann CC. Investigations on the long-term stability of an O/W cream containing either bufexamac or betamethasone-17-valerate. Eur J Pharm Biopharm 1994; 40:58–63.

Font J, Muntasell J, Cesari E. Amorphization of organic compounds by ball milling. Mat Res Bull 1997; 32: 1691–1696.

Freed AL, Strhmeyer HE, Mahjour M, et al. pH Control of nucleophilic/electrophilic oxidation. Int J Pharm 2008; 357:180–188.

Fununaka T, Golman B, Shinohara K. Batch grinding kinetics of ethenzamide particles by fluidized-bed jet-milling. Int J Pharm 2006; 311:89–96.

Garnier S, Petit S, Coquerel G. Influence of supersaturation and structurally related additives on the crystal growth of α-lactose monohydrate. J Cryst Growth 2002; 234:207–219.

Girona V, Pacareu C, Riera A, et al. Spectrophotometric determination of the stability of an ampicillin – dicloxacillin suspension. J Pharm Biomed Anal 1988; 6:23–28.

Goa L, Zhang D, Chen M. Drug nanocrystals for the formulation of poorly soluble drugs and its application as a potential drug delivery system. J Nanopart Res 2008; 10:845–862.

Gonda I. The ascent of pulmonary drug delivery. J Pharm Sci 2000; 89:940–945.

Gould PL, Goodman M, Hanson PA. Investigation of the solubility relationship of polar, semi-polar and non-polar drugs in mixed co-solvent systems. Int J Pharm 1984; 19:149–159.

Grau MJ, Kayer O, Müller RH. Nanosuspensions of poorly soluble drugs – reproducibility of small-scale production. Int J Pharm 2000; 196:155–157.

Gu C-H, Chaterjee K, Young V Jr., et al. Stabilization of a metastable polymorph of sulfamerazine by structurally related additives. J Cryst Growth 2002; 235:471–481.

Gu C-H, Grant DJW. Relationship between particle and impurity incorporation during crystallization of (+)-pseudoephdrine hydrochloride, acetaminophen and adipic acid from aqueous solution. Pharm Res 2002; 19:1068–1070.

Gupta A, Myrdal PB. On-line high-performance liquid chromatography method for analyte quantification from pressurized metered dose inhalers. J Chromatogr A 2004; 1033:101–106.

Gupta A, Myrdal PB. A comparison of two methods to determine the solubility in aerosol propellants. Int J Pharm 2005; 292:201–209.

Hagsten A, Larsen CC, Sonnergaard JM, et al. Identifying sources of batch-to-batch variation in processability. Powder Technol 2008; 183:213–219.

Hammerlund ER. Sodium chloride equivalents, cryoscopic properties, and hemolytic effects of certain medicinals in aqueous solution iv: supplemental values. J Pharm Sci 1981; 70:1161–1163.

Han J, Davis SS, Washington C. Physical properties and stability of two emulsion formulations of propofol. Int J Pharm 2001; 215:207–220.

Han J, Washington C. Partition of antimicrobial additives in an intravenous emulsion and their effect on emulsion physical stability. Int J Pharm 2005; 288:263–271.

Harding L, Qi S, Hill G, et al. The development of microthermal analysis and photothermal microspectroscopy as novel approaches to drug-excipient compatibility studies. Int J Pharm 2008; 354: 149–157.

Hartauer KJ, Guillory JK. A comparison of diffuse reflectance FT-IR spectroscopy and DSC in the characterization of a drug excipient interaction. Drug Dev Ind Pharm 1991; 17:617–630.

Heng JYY, Bismark A, Lee AF, et al. Anisotropic surface energetics and wettability of macroscopic form I paracetamol crystals. Langmuir 2006; 22:2760–2769.

Her L-H, Nail SL. Measurement of the glass transition temperatures of freeze concentrated solutes by differential scanning calorimetry. Pharm Res 1994; 11:54–59.

Hernandez-Trejo N, Kayser O, Steckel H, et al. Characterization of nebulized buparvaquone nano-suspensions-effect of nebulization technology. J Drug Target 2005; 13:499–507.

Hickey AJ, Mansour HM, Telko MJ, et al. Physical characterization of component particles included in dry powder inhalers. I. Strategy review and static characteristics. J Pharm Sci 2007a; 96:1282–1301.

Hickey AJ, Mansour HM, Telko MJ, et al. Physical characterization of component particles included in dry powder inhalers II. Dynamic characteristics. J Pharm Sci 2007b; 96:1302–1319.

Hinds WC. Aerosol Technology: Properties, Behaviour and Measurement of Airborne Particles. New York: Wiley, 1999:191–192.

Hoelgaard A, Møller N. Hydrate formation of metronidazole benzoate in aqueous suspensions. Int J Pharm 1983; 15:213–221.

Holgado MA, Fernandez-Arevalo M, Gines JM, et al. Compatibility study between carteolol hydro-chloride and tablet excipients using differential scanning calorimetry and hot stage microscopy. Pharmazie 1995; 50:195–198.

Hou H, Sun CC. Quantifying effects of particulate properties on powder flow properties using a ring shear tester. J Pharm Sci 2008; 97:4030–4039.

Hovorka SW, Schneich C. Oxidative degradation of pharmaceuticals: theory, mechanisms and inhibition. J Pharm Sci 2001; 90:253–269.

Howarth PH. Why particle size should affect clinical response to inhaled therapy. J Aerosol Med 2001; 14(suppl 1):S27–S34.

Hoye JA, Gupta A, Myrdal PB. Solubility of solid solutes in HFA-134a with a correlation to physico-chemical properties. J Pharm Sci 2008; 97:198–208.

Huang Y, Ye Q, Guo Z, et al. Identification of critical process impurities and their impact on process research and development. Org Proc Res Dev 2008; 12:632–636.

Hulse WL, Grimsey IA, de Matas M. The impact of low-level inorganic impurities on key physicochemical properties of paracetamol. Int J Pharm 2008; 349:61–65.

Islam N, Gladki E. Dry powder inhalers (DPIs)-a review of device reliability and innovation. Int J Pharm 2008; 360:1–11.

Jacobson-Kram D, McGovern T. Toxicological overview of impurities in pharmaceutical products. Adv Drug Deliv Rev 2007; 59:38–42.

Jansen PJ, Akers MJ, Amos RM, et al. The degradation of the antitumor agent gemcitabine hydrochloride in an acidic aqueous solution at ph 3.2 and identification of degradation products. J Pharm Sci 2000; 89:885–891.

Jashnani RN, Byron PR. Dry powder aerosol generation in different environments: performance comparisons of albuterol, albuterol sulfate, albuterol adipate and albuterol stearate. Int J Pharm 1996; 130:13–24.

Jinno J-I, Kamada N, Miyake M, et al. Effect of particle size reduction on dissolution and oral absorption of a poorly water-soluble drug, cilostazol, in beagle dogs. J Control Release 2006; 111:56–64.

Johnson JLH, He Y, Yalkowsky SH. Prediction of precipitation-induced phlebitis: a statistical validation of an in vitro model. J Pharm Sci 2003; 92:1574–1581.

Jones MD, Harris H, Hooton JC, et al. An investigation into the relationship between carrier-based dry powder inhalation performance and formulation cohesive-adhesive force balances. Eur J Pharm Biopharm 2008; 69:496–507.

Jones MD, Price R. The influence of fine excipient particles on the performance of carrier-based dry powder inhalation formulations. Pharm Res 2006; 23:1665–1674.

Jonkman-De Vries JD, Rosing H, Henrar REC, et al. The influence of formulation excipients on the stability of the novel antitumor agent carzelesin (U-80,244) PDA. J Pharm Sci Technol 1995; 49:283–288.

Joshi BV, Patil VB, Pokharkar VB. Compatibility studies between carbamazepine and tablet excipients using thermal and non-thermal methods. Drug Dev Ind Pharm 2002; 28:687–694.

Joshi V, Dwivedi S, Ward GH. Increase in specific surface area of budesonide during storage postmicronization. Pharm Res 2002; 19:7–12.

Junghanns J-U, Buttle I, Müller RH, et al. SolEmuls®: a way to overcome the drawback of parenteral administration of insoluble drugs. Pharm Dev Techol 2007; 12:437–445.

Kamin W, Scwabe A, Krämer I. Physicochemical compatibility of fluticasone-17-propionate nebulizer suspension with ipratropium and albuterol nebulizer solutions. Int J COPD 2007; 2:599–607.

Kawashima Y, Sergano T, Hino T, et al. Effect of surface morphology of carrier lactose on dry powder inhalation property of pranlukast. Int J Pharm 1998; 172:179–188.

Kenley RA, Lee MO, Sakumar L, et al. Temperature and pH dependence of fluocinolone acetonide degradation in a topical cream formulation. Pharm Res 1987; 4:342–347.

Kett V. Modulated temperature differential scanning calorimetry and its application to freeze drying. Eur J Parenteral Sci 2001; 6:95–99.

Kett VL, Fitzpatrick S, Cooper B, et al. An investigation into the subambient behaviour of aqueous mannitol using differential scanning calorimetry, cold stage microscopy, and X-ray diffractometry. J Pharm Sci 2003; 92:1919–1929.

Kim S, Lotz B, Lindrud M, et al. Control of the particle properties of a drug substance by crystallization engineering and the effect on drug product formulation. Org Proc Res Dev 2005; 9:894–901.

King S, Ying O, Basita AM, et al. Self-association and solubility behavior of a novel anticancer agent, brequinar sodium. J Pharm Sci 1989; 78:95–100.

Kitamura S, Miyamae A, Koda S, et al. Effect of grinding on the solid-state stability of cefixime trihydrate. Int J Pharm 1989; 56:125–134.

Kriwet K, Muller-Goymann CC. Binary diclofenac diethylamine-water systems: micelles, vesicles, and lyotropic liquid crystals. Eur J Pharm Biopharm 1993; 39:234–238.

Kwok PCL, Chan HK. Effect of relative humidity on the electrostatic charge properties of dry powder inhaler aerosols. Pharm Res 2008; 25:277–288.

Lachiver ED, Abatzoglou N, Cartilier L, et al. Insights into the role electrostatic forces on the behaviour of dry pharmaceutical systems. Pharm Res 2006; 23:997–1007.

Lerke SA, Adams SA. Development and validation of a particle size distribution method for analysis of drug substance. Am Pharm Rev 2003; 66:88–91.

Li S, Wang W, Chu J, et al. Degradation mechanism and kinetic studies of a novel anticancer agent, AG2034. Int J Pharm 1998; 167:49–56.

Lidgate DM, Fu RC, Fleitman JS. Using a microfludizer to manufacture parenteral emulsions. Pharm Tech Int 1990; 30–33.

Lin S-Y, Cheng W-T, Wang S-L. Thermodynamic and kinetic characterization of polymorphic transformation of famotidine during grinding. Int J Pharm 2006; 318:86–91.

Lionberger RA. Regulatory aspects of the use of new particle engineering technologies. Am Pharm Rev 2007; 80–84.

Lipp R, Müller-Fahrnow A. Use of X-ray crystallography for the characterization of single crystals grown in steroid containing transdermal drug delivery systems. Eur J Pharm Biopharm 1999; 47:133–138.

Listiohadi Y, Hourigan JA, Sleigh RW, et al. Moisture sorption, compressibility and caking of lactose polymorphs. Int J Pharm 2008; 359:123–134.

Loudon GM. Mechanistic interpretation of pH-rate profiles. J Chem Ed 1991; 68:973–984.

Mackin L, Zanon R, Min Park J, et al. Quantification of low levels (<10%) of amorphous content in micronised active batches using dynamic vapour sorption and isothermal microcalorimetry. Int J Pharm 2002; 231:227–236.

Maggi L, Bruni R, Conte U. Influence of the moisture on the performance of a new dry powder inhaler. Int J Pharm 1999; 177:83–91.

Martens-Lobenhoffer J, Jens RM, Losche D, et al. Long term stability of 8-methoxypsoralen in ointments for topical PUVA therapy ("Cream-PUVA"). Skin Pharmacol Appl Skin Physiol 1999; 12:266–270.

Martin A, Cocero MJ. Micronization processes with supercritical fluids: fundamentals and mechanisms. Adv Drug Deliv Rev 2008; 60:339–350.

Masui Y, Kitaura Y, Kobayashi T, et al. Control of crystal habit and size of cefmatilen hydrochloride with a habit modifier. Org Proc Res Dev 2003; 7:334–338.

Mazzenga GC, Berner B, Jordan F. The transdermal delivery of zwitterionic drugs II: the flux of zwitterion salt. J Control Release 1992; 20:163–170.

McCallion ONM, Taylor KMG, Bridges PA, et al. Jet nebulisers for pulmonary drug delivery. Int J Pharm 1996; 130:1–11.

McDonald KJ, Martin GP. Transition to CFC-free metered dose inhalers-into the new millennium. Int J Pharm 2000; 201:89–107.

McKenzie P, Kiang S, Tom J, et al. Can pharmaceutical process development become high tech? AIChE J 2006; 52:3990–3994.

Mendes PJ, Raposo A, Sousa JMM, et al. Sizing of powders in inhalers with an aerosizer® according to a mixed experimental factorial design. Aerosol Sci 2004; 35:509–527.

Merrifield DR, Carter PL, Clapham D, et al. Addressing the problem of light instability during formulation development. In: Tønnesen HH, ed. Photostability of Drugs and Drug Formulations. London: Taylor & Francis, 1996:141–154.

Meyer BK, Ni A, Hu B, et al. Antimicrobial preservative use in parenteral products: past and present. J Pharm Sci 2007; 96:3155–3167.

Midoux N, Hosek P, Pailleres L, et al. Micronization of pharmaceutical substances in a spiral jet mill. Powder Technol 1999; 104:113–120.

Moldenhauer JE. Determining whether a product is steam sterilizable. PDA J Pharm Sci Technol 1998; 52:28–32.

Monkhouse DC. Excipient compatibility possibilities and limitations in stability prediction. In: Crim W, Krummen K, eds. Stability Testing in the EC, Japan and the USA. Scientific and Regulatory Requirements. Paperback APV. 32. Stuttgart: Wissenschaftlidie Verlassgellscaft mbH, 1993:67–74.

Morefield EM, Feldkamp JR, Peck GE, et al. Preformulation information for suspensions. Int J Pharm 1987; 34:263–265.

Morris KR, Griesser UJ, Eckhardt CJ, et al. Theoretical approaches to physical transformations of active pharmaceutical ingredients during manufacturing processes. Adv Drug Deliv Rev 2001; 48:91–114.

Müller L, Mauthe RJ, Riley CM, et al. A rationale for determining, testing, and controlling specific impurities in pharmaceuticals that possess potential for genotoxicity. Regul Toxicol Pharmacol 2006; 44:198–211.

Munson JW, Hussain A, Bilous R. Precautionary note for use of bisulphite in pharmaceutical formulations. J Pharm Sci 1977; 66:1775–1776.

Muster TH, Prestidge CA. Face specific surface properties of pharmaceutical crystals. J Pharm Sci 2002; 91:1432–1444.

Muzzio F, Shinbrot T, Glasser BJ. Powder technology in the pharmaceutical industry: the need to catch up fast. Powder Technol 2002; 124:1–7.

Myer BK, Binghua AN, Shi L. Antimicrobial preservative use in parenteral products: past and present. J Pharm Sci 2007; 96:3155–3167.

Myrdal PB, Simamora P, Surakitbanharn Y, et al. Studies in phlebitis. VII: in vitro and in vivo evaluation of pH-solubilized levemopamil. J Pharm Sci 1995; 84:849–852.

Na GC, Stevens HS Jr., Yuan BO, et al. Physical stability of ethyl diatrizoate nanocrystalline suspension in steam sterilization. Pharm Res 1999; 16:569–574.

Nail SL, Searles JA. Elements of quality by design in development and scale-up of freeze-dried parenterals. Biopharm Int 2008; 21:44–52.

Nakach M, Authelin J-R, Chamayou A, et al. Comparison of various milling technologies for grinding pharmaceutical powders. Int J Miner Process 2004; 74S:S173–S181.

Narazaki R, Sanghvi R, Yalkowsky SH. Estimation of drug precipitation upon dilution of pH-controlled formulations. Mol Pharm 2007a; 4:550–555.

Narazaki R, Sanghvi R, Yalkowsky SH. Estimation of drug precipitation upon dilution of pH-cosolvent solubilized formulations. Chem Pharm Bull 2007b; 55:1203–1206.

Nayak AS, Cutie AJ, Jochsberger T, et al. The effect of various additives on the stability of isoproternol hydrochloride solutions. Drug Dev Ind Pharm 1986; 12:589–601.

Német Z, Hegedüs B, Szántay C Jr., et al. Pressurization effects on the polymorphic forms of famotidine. Thermochim Acta 2005; 430:35–41.

Ni N, Tesconi M, Tababi E, et al. Use of pure *t*-butanol as a solvent for freeze-drying: a case study. Int J Pharm 2001; 226:39–46.

Nichols G, Bryard S, Bloxham MJ, et al. A review of the terms agglomerate and aggregate with a recommendation for nomenclature used powder and particle characterization. J Pharm Sci 2002; 91:2103–2109.

Niemi L, Laine E. Effect of water content on the microstructure of an o/w cream. Int J Pharm 1991; 68: 205–214.

Niemi L, Turakka L, Kahela P. Effect of water content and type of emulgator on the release of hydrocortisone from o/w creams. Acta Pharm Nord 1989; 1:23–30.

Nikander K. Some technical, physicochemical and physiological aspects of nebulization of drugs. Eur Respir Rev 1997; 7:168–172.

Niven RW. Aerodynamic particle-size testing using a time-of-flight aerosol beam spectrometer. Pharm Technol 1993; 17:64–78.

Notari RE. On the merits of a complete kinetic stability study. Drug Stab 1996; 1:1–2.

O'Sullivan D, Steele G, Austin TK. Investigations into the amorphous and crystalline forms of a development compound. In: Levine H, ed. Amorphous Food and Pharmaceutical Systems. Cambridge: Royal Society of Chemistry, Special Publication No. 281, 2002:220–230.

Okamoto M, Hamano M, Igraashi K, et al. The effects of impurities on crystallization of polymorphs of a drug substance of AE1-923. J Chem Eng Jpn 2004; 37:1224–1231.

Otsuka M, Hasegawa H, Matsuda Y. Effect of polymorphic transformation during the extrusion-granulation process on the pharmaceutical properties of carbmazepine granules. Chem Pharm Bull 1997; 45:894–898.

Otsuka M, Matsuda Y. Physicochemical characterization of phenobarbital polymorphs and their pharmaceutical properties. Drug Dev Ind Pharm 1993; 19:2241–2269.

Parasrampuria J, Li LC, Dudleston A, et al. The impact of an autoclave cycle on the chemical stability of parenteral products. J Parenter Sci Technol 1993; 47:177–179.

Parkkali S, Lehto V-P, Laine E. Applying image analysis in the observation of recrystallization of amorphous cefadroxil. Drug Dev Ind Pharm 2000; 5:433–438.

Payne RS, Roberts RJ, Rowe RC, et al. The mechanical properties of two forms of primidone predicted from their crystal structures. Int J Pharm 1996; 145:165–173.

Pedersen S, Kristensen HG. Change in crystal density of acetylsalicylic acid during compaction. STP Pharma Sci 1994; 4:201–206.

Pedersen S, Kristensen HG, Cornett C. Solid-state interactions between trimethoprim and parabens. STP Pharma Sci 1994; 4:292–297.

Peramal VL, Tamburie S, Craig DQM. Characterisation of the variation in the physical properties of commercial creams using thermogravimetric analysis and rheology. Int J Pharm 1997; 155:91–98.

Pérez P, Suñé-Negre JP, Miñarro M, et al. A new expert systems (SeDeDM Diagram) for control batch powder formulation and preformulation drug products. Eur J Pharm Biopharm 2006; 64:351–359.

Phadke DS, Collier JL. Effect of degassing temperature on the specific surface area and other physical properties of magnesium stearate. Drug Dev Ind Pharm 1994; 20:853–858.

Pharm Forum 20, 7222, 1994.

Phillies GDJ. Quasielastic light scattering. Anal Chem 1990; 62:1049A–1057A.

Phillips EM, Byron PR. Surfactant promoted crystal growth of micronized methylprednisolone in trichloromonofluoromethane. Int J Pharm 1994; 110:9–19.

Phillips EM, Byron PR, Dalby RN. Axial ratio measurements for early detection of crystal growth in suspension-type metered dose inhalers. Pharm Res 1993; 10:454–456.

Phipps MA, Mackin LA. Application of isothermal microcalorimetry in solid-state drug development. Pharm Sci Technol. Today 2000; 3:9–17.

Phipps MA, Winnike RA, Long ST, et al. Excipient compatibility as assessed by isothermal microcalorimetry. J Pharm Pharmacol 1998; 50(suppl):9.

Pikal MJ, Shah S. The collapse temperature in freeze-drying: dependence on measurement methodology and rate of water removal from the glassy phase. Int J Pharm 1990; 62:165–186.

Pinsuwan S, Alverez-Núñez, Tabibi ES, et al. Degradation kinetics of 4-dedimethylamino sancycline, a new anti-tumor agent, in aqueous solutions. Int J Pharm 1999; 181:31–40.

Podczeck F, Newton JM, James MB. Assessment of adhesion and autoadhesion forces between particles and surfaces: I. The investigation of autoadhesion phenomena of salmeterol xinafoate and lactose monohydrate particles using compacted powder surfaces. J Adhes Sci Technol 1994; 8:1459–1472.

Podczeck F, Newton JM, James MB. Assessment of adhesion and autoadhesion forces between particles and surfaces. Part II. The investigation of adhesion phenomena of salmeterol xinafoate and lactose monohydrate particles in particle-on particle and particle-on-surface contact. J Adhes Sci Technol 1995a; 9:475–486.

Podczeck F, Newton JM, James MB. Adhesion and autoadhesion measurements of micronized particles of pharmaceutical powders to compacted powder surfaces. Chem Pharm Bull 1995b; 43:1953–1957.

Podczeck F, Newton JM, James MB. The adhesion force of micronized salmeterol xinafoate to pharmaceutically relevant surface materials. J Phys D Appl Phys 1996a; 29:1878–1884.

Podczeck F, Newton JM, James MB. The influence of physical properties of the materials in contact on the adhesion strength of particles of salmeterol base and salmeterol salts to various substrate materials. J Adhes Sci Technol 1996b; 10:257–268.

Price R, Young PM. Visualization of the crystallization of lactose from the amorphous state. J Pharm Sci 2004; 93:155–164.

Price R, Young PM. On the physical transformations of processed pharmaceutical solids. Micron 2005; 36:519–524.

Pritchard JN. The influence of lung deposition on clinical response. J Aersol Med 2001; 14(suppl 1):S19–S26.

Provent B, Chulia D, Carey J. Particle size and caking tendency of a powder. Eur J Pharm Biopharm 1993; 39:202–207.

Ramos R, Gaisford S, ad Buckton G. Calorimetric determination of amorphous content in lactose: a note on the preparation of calibration. Int J Pharm 2005; 300:13–21.

Ran Y, Jain A, Yalkowsky SH. Solubilization and preformulation studies on PG-300995 (an anti-HIV drug). J Pharm Sci 2005; 94:297–303.

Rasenack N, Müller BW. Poorly water-soluble drugs for oral delivery—a challenge for pharmaceutical development. Pharm Ind 2005; 67:447–451.

Raw AS, Furness MS, Gill DS, et al. Regulatory considerations of pharmaceutical solid polymorphism in abbreviated new drug applications (ANDAs). Adv Drug Deliv Rev 2004; 56:397–414.

Reynolds DW, Facchine JF, Mullaney JF, et al. Available guidance and best practices for conducting forced degradation studies. Pharm Technol 2002; 26:48–54.

Rhee Y-S, Park C-W, Shin Y-S, et al. Application of instrumental evaluation of color for the pre-formulation and formulation of rabeprazole. Int J Pharm 2008; 350:122–129.

Roberts RJ, Rowe RC, York P. The relationship between Young's modulus of elasticity of organic solids and their molecular structure. Powder Tech 1991; 65(3):139–146.

Roberts RJ, Rowe RC, York P. The relationship between indentation hardness of organic solids and their molecular structure. J Mater Sci 1994; 29:2289–2296.

Rohn CL. Rheology: a rapid screening method for testing the stability of drug suspensions. Am Lab 2004; 36: 20–21.

Rohrs BR, Amidon GE, Meury RH, et al. Particle size limits to meet USP content uniformity criteria for tablets and capsules. J Pharm Sci 2006; 95:1049–1059.

Rowe RC, Wakerly MJ, Roberts RJ, et al. Expert systems for parenteral development. PDA J Pharm Sci Technol 1995; 49:257–261.

Rowe RC, Roberts RJ. Artificial intelligence in pharmaceutical product formulation: knowledge-based and expert systems. Pharm Sci Tech Today 1998; 1:153–159.

Rowley G. Quantifying electrostatic interactions in pharmaceutical solid systems. Int J Pharm 2001; 227: 47–55.

Rowley G, Macklin LA. The effect of moisture sorption on electrostatic charging of selected pharmaceutical excipient powders. Powder Technol 2003; 135–136:50–58.

Rubino JT. The effects of cosolvents on the action of pharmaceutical buffers. J Parenter Sci Technol 1987; 41: 45–49.

Rubino JT, Yalkowsky SH. Cosolvency and deviations from log-linear solubilization. Pharm Res 1987; 4: 231–235.

Ruozi B, Tosi G, Forni F, et al. Atomic force microscopy and photon correlation spectroscopy: two techniques for rapid characterization of liposomes. Eur J Pharm Sci 2005; 25:81–89.

Sallam E, Saleem H, Zaru R. Polymorphism and crystal growth of phenylbutazone in semisolid preparations. Part one: characterisation of isolated crystals from commercial creams of phenyl-butazone. Drug Dev Ind Pharm 1986; 12:1967–1994.

Samir RD. Preformulation aspects of transdermal drug delivery systems. In: Ghosh TK, Pfister WR, eds. Transdermal Topical Drug Delivery Systems. Buffalo Grove: Interpharm Press, 1997:139–166.

Sanjar S, Matthews J. Treating systemic diseases via the lung. J Aerosol Med 2001; 14(suppl 1):S51–S58.

Schachter SC, Tarsy D. Remacemide: current status and clinical applications. Exp Opin Invest Drugs 2000; 9: 871–833.

Schoeni MH, Kraemer R. Osmolality changes in nebulizer solutions. Agents Actions 1989; 31:225–228.

Scholz A, Abrahamsson B, Diebold SM, et al. Influence of hydrodynamics and particle size on the absorption of felodipine in labradors. Pharm Res 2002; 19:42–46.

Schüssele A, Bauer-Brandl A. On the measurement of flowability according to the European pharmacopoeia. Int J Pharm 2003; 257:301–304.

Schwegmann JJ, Hardwick LM, Akers MJ. Practical formulation and process development of freeze-dried products. Pharm Dev Technol 2005; 10:151–173.

Selzer T, Radau M, Kreuter J. Use of isothermal heat conduction microcalorimetry to evaluate stability and excipient compatibility of a solid drug. Int J Pharm 1998; 171:227–241.

Serrajudin ATM, Mufson D. pH-solubility profiles of organic bases and their hydrochloride salts. Pharm Res 1985; 2:65–68.

Shalaev EY, Zografi G. How does residual water affect the solid-state degradation of drugs in the amorphous state? J Pharm Sci 1996; 85:1137–1141.

Sing KSW. Adsorption methods for surface area determination. In: Stanley-Wood NG, Lines RW, eds. Particle Size Analysis. Proc. 25th Anniv. Confr., 1991. Cambridge: The Royal Society of Chemistry, 1992:13–32.

Smyth HDC, Hickey AJ. Carriers in dry powder delivery. Implications for inhalation system design. Am J Drug Deliv 2005; 3:117–132.

Snorek SM, Bauer JF, Chidambaram N, et al. PQRI recommendations on particle-size analysis of drug substances used in oral dosage forms. J Pharm Sci 2007; 96:1451–1467.

Soh JLP, Liew CV, Heng P. New indices to characterize powder flow based on their avalanching behaviour. Pharm Dev Technol 2006; 11:93–102.

Spencer R, Dalder B. Sizing up grinding mills. Chem Eng 1997; 84–87.

Stark G, Fawcett JP, Tucker IG, et al. Instrumental evaluation of color of solid dosage forms during stability testing. Int J Pharm 1996; 143:93–100.

Steckel H, Mrakefka P, te Wierik H, et al. Effect of milling and sieving on functionality of dry powder inhalation products. Int J Pharm 2006; 309:51–59.

Streng WH, Yu DH-S, Zhu C. Determination of solution aggregation using solubility, conductivity, calorimetry, and pH measurements. Int J Pharm 1996; 135:43–52.

Strickley RG. Parenteral formulations of small molecules therapeutics marketed in the United States part I. PDA J Parent Sci Technol 1999; 53:324–349.

Strickley RG. Parenteral formulations of small molecules therapeutics marketed in the United States part II. PDA J Parent Sci Technol 2000; 54:69–96.

Strickley RG. Parenteral formulations of small molecules therapeutics marketed in the united states part III. PDA J. Parent Sci Technol 2001; 54:152–169.

Strickley RG. Solubilizing excipients in oral and injectable formulations. Pharm Res 2004; 21:201–230.

Stulzer HK, Tagliari MP, Cruz AP, et al. Compatibility studies between piroxicam and pharmaceutical excipients used in solid dosage forms. Pharm Chem J 2008; 42:215–219.

Sun CC. Development of a novel method for deriving true density of pharmaceutical solids including hydrates and water-containing formulated powders. J Pharm Sci 2004; 93:646–653.

Sun CC. Quantifying errors in tableting data analysis using the Ryshkewitch equation due to inaccurate true density. J Pharm Sci 2005; 94:2061–2063.

Sun CH. Thermal expansion of organic crystals and precision of calculated crystal density: a survey of Cambridge Crystal Database. J Pharm Sci 2007; 96:1043–1052.

Surana R, Randall L, Pyne A, et al. Determination of glass transition temperature and in situ study of the plasticizing effect of water by inverse gas chromatography. Pharm Res 2003; 20:1647–1654.

Sweetana S, Akers MJ. Solubility principles and practices for parenteral drug dosage form development. PDA J Parenter Sci Technol 1996; 50:330–342.

Tang X, Pikal MJ. Design of freeze-drying processes for pharmaceuticals: practical advice. Pharm Res 2004; 21:191–200.

Taylor A, Gustafsson P. Do all dry powder inhalers show the same pharmaceutical performance? Int J Clin Pract 2005; 59(suppl 149):7–12.

Taylor KMG, Venthoye G, Chawla A. Pentamidine isethionate delivery from jet nebulisers. Int J Pharm 1992; 85:203–208.

Taylor LJ, Papadopoulos DG, Dunn PJ, et al. Predictive milling of pharmaceutical materials using nanoindentation of single crystals. Org Proc Res Dev 2004; 8:674–679.

Telko MJ, Hickey AJ. Critical assessment of inverse gas chromatography as a means of assessing surface free energy and acid-base interaction of pharmaceutical powders. J Pharm Sci 2007; 96:2647–2654.

Thakur AJ, Morris K, Grosso JA, et al. Mechanism and kinetics of metal ion mediated degradation of fosinopril sodium. Pharm Res 1993; 10:800–809.

Thalberg K, Lindholm D, Axelsson A. Comparison of different flowability tests for powders for inhalation. Powder Technol 2004; 146:206–213.

Thoma K, Holzmann C. Photostability of dithranol. Eur J Pharm Biopharm 1998; 46:201–208.

Thomas M, Cannon AJ. Low temperature thermal analyses are key to formulation design. Pharm Technol 2004; (suppl):20–27.

Thomas VH, Naath M. Design and utilization of the drug-excipient chemical compatibility automated system. Int J Pharm 2008; 359:150–157.

Thompson C, Davies MC, Roberts CJ, et al. The effects of additives on the crystal growth of paracetamol (acetaminophen) crystals. Int J Pharm 2004; 280:137–150.

Tian L, He H, Tang X. Stability and degradation kinetics of an etoposide-loaded parenteral lipid emulsion. J Pharm Sci 2007; 96:1719–1728.

Ticehurst MD, Rowe RC, York P. Determination of the surface properties of two batches of salbutamol sulphate by inverse gas chromatography. Int J Pharm 1994; 111:241–249.

Ticehurst MD, York P, Rowe RC, et al. Characterisation of the surface properties of α-lactose monohydrate with inverse gas chromatography used to detect batch variation. Int J Pharm 1996; 141:93–99.

Tinke AP, Vanhoutte K, Vanhoutte M, et al. Laser diffraction and image analysis as a supportive analytical tool in the pharmaceutical development of immediate release direct compression formulations. Int J Pharm 2005; 297:80–88.

Tiwari D, Goldman D, Dixit S, et al. Compatibility evaluation of metered dose inhaler elastomers with tetrafluoroethane (P134a), a non-CFC propellant. Drug Dev Ind Pharm 1998; 24:345–352.

Tiwari D, Goldman D, Malick WA, et al. Formulation and evaluation of albuterol metered dose inhalers containing tetrafluoroethane (P134a), a non-CFC propellant. Pharm Dev Technol 1998; 3:163–174.

Tiwary AK, Panpalia GM. Influence of crystal habit on trimethoprim suspension formulation. Pharm Res 1999; 16:261–265.

Tong HH, Shekunov BY, York P, et al. Predicting the aerosol performance of dry powder inhalation formulations b) interparticulate interaction analysis using inverse gas chromatography. J Pharm Sci 2006; 95:228–233.

Traini D, Young PM, Price R, et al. A novel apparatus for the determination of solubility in pressurized metered dose inhalers. Drug Dev Ind Pharm 2006; 32:1159–1163.

Traini D, Young PM, Rogueda P, et al. In vitro investigation of drug particulates interactions and aerosol performance of pressurized metered dose inhalers. Pharm Res 2007; 24:125–135.

Tsai W-T. An overview of environmental hazards and exposure risk of hydrofluorocarbons. Chemosphere 2005; 61:1539–1547.

Tu Y-H, Wang D-P, Allen LV. Stability of a nonaqueous trimethoprim preparation. Am J Hosp Pharm 1989; 46:301–304.

Turner YTA, Roberts CJ, Davies MC. Scanning probe microscopy in the field of drug delivery. Adv Drug Deliv Rev 2007; 59:1453–1473.

Tzou T-S, Pachta RR, Coy RB, et al. Drug form selection in albuterol-containing metered-dose inhaler formulations and its impact on chemical and physical. J Pharm Sci 1997; 86:1352–1357.

Van der Houwen OAGJ, de Loos MR, Beijnen JH, et al. Systematic interpretation of pH-degradation profiles. A critical review. Int J Pharm 1997; 155:137–152.

Van Dooren AA. Design for drug-excipient interaction studies. Drug Dev Ind Pharm 1983; 9:43–55.

Verma RK, Garg S. Selection of excipients for extended release formulations of glipizide through drug-excipient compatibility testing. J Pharm Biomed Anal 2005; 38:633–644.

Vernon B. Using a ball mill for high-purity milling applications. Powder Bulk Eng 1994; 8:53–62.

Vervaet C, Byron PR. Drug-surfactant-propellant interactions in HFA-formulations. Int J Pharm 1999; 186:13–30.

Viana M, Jouannin P, Pontier C, et al. About pycnometric density measurements. Talanta 2002; 57: 583–593.

Wada Y, Matsubara T. Pseudo-polymorphism and crystalline transition of magnesium stearate. Thermochim Acta 1992; 196:63–84.

Wakasawa T, Sano K, Hirakura Y, et al. Solid-state compatibility studies using a high-throughput and automated forced degradation system. Int J Pharm 2008; 355:164–173.

Waltersson JO. Factorial designs in pharmaceutical preformulation studies. Part 1. Evaluation of the application of factorial designs to a stability study of drugs in suspension form. Acta Pharm Suec 1986; 23:129–138.

Wang Y-CJ, Kowal RR. Review of excipients and pHs for parenteral products used in the United States. J Parenter Drug Assoc 1980; 34:452–462.

Ward GH, Schultz RK. Process-induced crystallinity changes in albuterol sulfate and its effect on powder physical stability. Pharm Res 1995; 12:773–779.

Wardrop J, Law D, Qiu Y, et al. Influence of solid phase and formulation processing on stability of abbott-232 tablet formulations. J Pharm Sci 2006; 95:2380–2392.

Watanabe H, Ghadiri M, Matsuyama T, et al. Triboelectrification of pharmaceutical powders by particle impact. Int J Pharm 2007; 334:149–155.

Waterman KC, Adami RC, Alsante KM, et al. Stabilization of pharmaceuticals to oxidative degradation. Pharm Dev Technol 2002; 7:1–32.

Wells JI. Pharmaceutical Preformulation. The Physicochemical Properties of Drug Substances. Chichester: Ellis Horwood Ltd., 1988.

Wikström H, Rantanen J, Gift AD, et al. Toward to understanding of the factors influencing anhydrate-to-hydrate transformation kinetics in aqueous environments. Cryst Growth Des 2008; 8:2684–2693.

Wilfdong PLD, Hancock BC, Moore MD, et al. Towards an understanding of the structurally based potential for mechanically activated disordering of small molecule organic crystals. J Pharm Sci 2006; 95:2645–2656.

Williams NA, Shwinke DL. Low temperature properties of lyophilized solutions and their influence on lyophilization cycle design: pentamidine isothionate. J Pharm Sci Technol 1994; 48:135–139.

Williams RO III, Brown J, Liu J. Influence of micronization methodon the performance of a suspension triamcinolone acetonide pressurized metered-dose inhaler formulation. Pharm Dev Technol 1999; 4:167–179.

Williams RO III, Repka M, Liu J. Influence of propellant composition on drug delivery from a pressurized metered dose inhaler. Drug Dev Ind Pharm 1998; 24:763–770.

Williams RO III, Rodgers TL, Liu J. Study of solubility of steroids in hydrofluoroalkane propellants. Drug Dev Ind Pharm 1999; 25:1227–1234.

Wirth DD, Baertschi SW, Johnson RA, et al. Maillard reaction of lactose and fluoxetine hydrochloride, a secondary amine. J Pharm Sci 1998; 87:31–39.

Wirth DD, Stephenson GA. Purification of dirithromycin. Impurity reduction and polymorph manipulation. Org Proc Res Dev 1997; 1:55–60.

Wong MWY, Mitchell AG. Physicochemical characterization of a phase change produced during the wet granulation of chlorpromazine hydrochloride and its effects on tableting. Int J Pharm 1992; 88: 261–273.

Wong-Beringer A, Lambros MP, Beringer PM, et al. Suitability of casofungin for aerosol delivery. Physicochemical profiling and nebulizer choice. Chest 2008; 128:3711–3716.

Wyttenbach N, Birringer C, Alsenz J, et al. Drug-excipient compatibility testing using a high-throughput approach and statistical design. Pharm Dev Technol 2005; 10:499–505.

Xu R. Particle Characterization: Light Scattering Methods. Dordrecht, The Netherlands: Kluwer Academic Publishing, 2000.

Xu R, Andreina Di Guida OA. Comparison of sizing small particles using different technologies. Powder Technol 2003; 132:145–153.

Yalabik-Kas HS. Stability assessment of emulsion systems. STP Pharma 1985; 1:978–984.

Yalkowsky SH, Valvani SC, Johnson BW. In vitro method for detecting precipitation of parenteral formulations after injection. J Pharm Sci 1983; 72:1014–1017.

Yang SK. Acid catalyzed ethanolysis of temazepam in anhydrous and aqueous ethanol solution. J Pharm Sci 1994; 83:898–902.

Yang Z-Y, Le Y, Hu TT, et al. Production of ultrafine sumatriptan succinate particles for pulmonary delivery. Pharm Res 2008; 25:2012–2018.

York P. Crystal engineering and particle design for the powder compaction process. Drug Dev Ind Pharm 1992; 18:677–721.

York P. Powdered raw materials: characterizing batch uniformity. Respir Drug Deliv IV, 1994:83–91.

York P, Ticehurst MD, Osborn JC, et al. Characterisation of the surface energetics of milled dl-propranolol hydrochloride using inverse gas chromatography and molecular modelling. Int J Pharm 1998; 174:179–186.

Young PM, Chan H-K, Chiou H, et al. The influence of mechanical processing of dry powder inhaler carriers on drug aerosolization performance. J Pharm Sci 2007; 96:1331–1341.

Young PM, Price R. The influence of humidity on the aerosolization of micronized and SEDS produced salbutamol sulphate. Eur J Pharm Sci 2004; 22:235–240.

Young PM, Price R, Tobyn MJ, et al. Investigations into the effect of humidity on drug-drug interactions using the atomic force microscope. J Pharm Sci 2003a; 92:815–822.

Young PM, Price R, Tobyn MJ, et al. Effect of humidity on aerosolization of micronized drugs. Drug Dev Ind Pharm 2003b; 29:959–966.

Young PM, Sung A, Traini D, et al. Influence of humidity on the electrostatic charge and aerosol performance of dry powder inhaler carrier based systems. Pharm Res 2007; 24:963–970.

Young PM, Tobyn MJ, Price MJ, et al. The use of colloid probe microscopy to predict aerosolization performance in dry powder inhalers: AFM and in vitro correlation. J Pharm Sci 2006; 95:1800–1809.

Yu C-Y, Hancock BC, Mills A, et al. Numerical and experimental investigation of capping mechanisms during pharmaceutical tablet compaction. Powder Technol 2008; 181:121–129.

Yu LX. Pharmaceutical quality by design product and process development, understanding, and control. Pharm Res 2008; 25:781–791.

Yu W, Hancock BC. Evaluation of dynamic image analysis for characterizing pharmaceutical excipient particles. Int J Pharm 2008; 361:150–157.

Zannou EA, Streng WH. Osmotic properties of sulfobutylether and hydroxypropyl cyclodextrins. Pharm Res 2001; 18:1226–1231.

Zhang GG, Gu C, Zell MT, et al. Crystallization and transactions of sulfamerazine polymorphs. J Pharm Sci 2002; 91:1089–1100.

Zietsman S, Killian G, Worthington M, et al. Formulation development and stability studies of aqueous metronidazole benzoate suspensions containing various suspending agents. Drug Dev Ind Pharm 2007; 33:191–197.

Ziller KH, Rupprecht H. Control of crystal growth in drug suspensions. 1) Design of a control unit and application to acetaminophen suspensions. Drug Dev Ind Pharm 1988a; 14:2341–2370.

Ziller KH, Rupprecht HH. Control of crystal growth in drug suspensions. Part 2. Influence of polymers on dissolution and crystallization during temperature cycling. Pharm Ind 1988b; 52:1017–1022.

Zügner S, Marquardt K, Zimmermann I. Influence of nanomechanical crystal properties on the communication process of particulate solids in spiral jet mills. Eur J Pharm Biopharm 2006; 62:194–201.

7 | Biopharmaceutical Support in Formulation Development

Bertil Abrahamsson and Anna-Lena Ungell
AstraZeneca, Mölndal, Sweden

INTRODUCTION

The pharmaceutical formulation plays an important role in the delivery of a drug to the body. The clinical benefit of a drug molecule can thereby be optimized by delivering the right amount at the right rate to the right site at the right time. For example, extended-release (ER) formulations have been used for a long time to control the rate of absorption and thereby keep drug levels within the therapeutic interval during an entire dosage interval. More examples of biopharmaceutical properties that can be provided by oral formulations are given in Table 1. In the future, the pharmaceutical possibilities for improving clinical utility may be extended to include site-specific drug delivery systems that reach systemic targets, such as cancer cells and the central nervous system (CNS), or gene delivery to cell nuclei. Such areas of drug delivery are, however, outside the scope of the present chapter.

To achieve the potential clinical benefits that can be provided by a formulation, as exemplified in Table 1, biopharmaceutical input is needed from the start of preformulation, through formulation development, to documentation for regulatory applications. The main objective is to obtain and verify desirable drug-delivery properties for a pharmaceutical formulation. The key activities are as follows:

- Characterization of relevant physicochemical, pharmacokinetic/dynamic prerequisites provided by the drug molecule
- Identification of the relevant biopharmaceutical targets and hurdles in formulation development
- Definition of test methods/study designs needed to obtain the biopharmaceutical targets in the formulation development and correct interpretation of the study results obtained
- Choice of suitable drug form, formulation principles, and excipients

In addition, understanding of the physiological processes that may interact with the biopharmaceutical function of the dosage form is crucial.

Successful biopharmaceutical input during development can make a significant contribution to clinical efficiency and tolerability of a drug product. In certain cases, such as poorly absorbable drugs or drugs that are degraded in the gut, the biopharmaceutical aspects can make the difference between a new useful product or an aborted development program of a potentially very useful drug compound. Additionally, appropriate use of biopharmaceuticals will also contribute to a time and cost-efficient development process.

The present chapter is limited to presentations and uses of different biopharmaceutical test methods in formulation development, such as

- in vitro dissolution testing,
- bioavailability studies,
- in vitro/in vivo correlation (IVIVC) of drug dissolution,
- use of animal models in in vivo studies of formulations, and
- in vivo imaging of formulations by γ-scintigraphy.

Table 1 Examples of Biopharmaceutical Properties of Oral Dosage Forms

Biopharmaceutical target	Formulation function
Increase amount absorbed/reduced variability of amount absorbed	Dissolution or permeability enhancement Protection from degradation in GI tract
Control rate of absorption	Extended release Pulsed release
Control site of delivery	Gastric retention Colon release Mucoadhesive

This chapter is strongly focused on oral drug delivery. The relevant principles and methods involved in biopharmaceutical characterization of a drug molecule, mainly applied in the preformulation phase, are described in chapter 4, "Biopharmaceutical Support in Candidate Drug Selection."

IN VITRO DISSOLUTION

In vitro dissolution testing of solid dosage forms is the most frequently used biopharmaceutical test method in formulation development. It is used from the start of dosage form development and in all subsequent phases. Examples of different purposes of dissolution testing in research and development are as follows:

- Investigation of drug release mechanisms, especially for ER formulations
- Obtaining a predefined target release profile and robust formulation properties regarding influences of physiological factors (e.g., pH and food) on the drug release
- Generation of supportive data to bioavailability studies as an aid in interpretation of in vivo results
- Validation of manufacturing processes
- Investigation of effects of different storage conditions
- Batch quality control (QC)
- A surrogate for bioequivalence studies

An in vitro dissolution method for batch QC is always defined for a new solid dosage form product. However, this method may not be sufficient for all the different aims of dissolution testing that might arise. The choice of dissolution method and test conditions should therefore be adapted to best serve their purpose. For example, simplicity and robustness are crucial properties of a QC method; whereas physiological relevance may overrule these factors when a method is used for in vivo predictions.

Standard in vitro dissolution testing models two processes: the release of drug substance from the solid dosage form and drug dissolution. Drug release is determined by formulation factors such as disintegration/dissolution of formulation excipients or drug diffusion through the formulation. Drug dissolution is affected by the physicochemical substance properties (e.g., solubility, diffusivity), solid-state properties of the substance (e.g., particle surface area, polymorphism), and formulation properties (e.g., wetting, solubilization). In vitro dissolution testing should thus provide predictions of both the drug release and the dissolution processes in vivo. Therefore, in most situations, the use of in vitro dissolution will be meaningless if the method used does not provide some correlation with in vivo data or resemblance with the physiological conditions in the gastrointestinal (GI) tract. To reach this goal, the choice of dissolution apparatus and test medium should be carefully considered. Another important aspect in the development and definition of a new method is that it must be designed and operated in such a way that drug release and dissolution are not sensitive to minor variations in the operating conditions.

This chapter will provide some practical considerations for developing and using in vitro dissolution methods. Aspects of study design and evaluation of in vitro dissolution data will also be discussed. For additional information on in vitro dissolution testing, *Pharmaceutical Dissolution Testing* (Dressman and Krämer, 2005), the *FIP Guidelines for Dissolution Testing of Solid Oral Products* (1997), *Handbook of Dissolution Testing* (Hansson, 2007), pharmacopoeias, and regulatory guidelines are recommended.

Dissolution Apparatus

The most well established apparatuses are those described in the pharmacopoeias. Four methods, mainly intended for oral solid dosage forms, are described in the U.S. Pharmacopoeia (USP) XXIV (1) the rotating basket method (USP I), (2) the rotating paddle method (USP II), (3) the reciprocating cylinder (USP III), and (4) the flow-through method (USP IV). All of these methods, except for the reciprocating cylinder, are also described in the European Pharmacopoeia (EP), although the equipment specifications are not identical to those in the USP. These methods are schematically presented in Figure 1.

- USP I: The dosage form is placed in a cylindrical basket that is covered by a mesh. The basket is immersed in the dissolution medium and rotated at a speed of between 25 and 150 rpm. The standard beaker has a volume of 1 L, but smaller and larger volume vessels, for example, 0.25 and 4 L, are also available. The mesh size in the basket wall can also be varied.
- USP II: The dosage form moves freely in the same type of glass beaker as used for USP I. A paddle is rotated at a speed of 25 to 150 rpm. The dosage form may be placed in a steel helix, a "sinker," to avoid floating.
- USP III: The formulation is placed in a cylindrical glass tube with steel screens in the bottom and at the top. The mesh size of the tube may vary. This tube is moved up and down in a larger tube that contains the dissolution fluid. The amplitude of the inner tube movements is 5–40 dips/min, and the volume of the outer tube is 300 mL. Tubes containing 100 mL and 1 L are also available. The inner tube can be moved during the dissolution process between different outer tubes, which may hold different dissolution fluids.
- USP IV: The formulation is placed in a thermostated flow cell. The dissolution fluid is pumped through the cell in a pulsating manner at a constant rate, typically between 4 and 16 mL/min. Before the inlet flow reaches the formulation, it is passed through a bed of glass pellets to create a laminar flow. A filter is placed in the cell at the outlet side of the formulation. The cell is available in different sizes/designs, and tablet holders are available as an option.

USP and the EP describe four additional apparatuses mainly intended for transdermal or dermal delivery: the paddle over disc (USP V, EP), the extraction cell method (EP), the cylinder method (USP VI, EP), and the reciprocating holder method (USP VII). A large number of other noncompendial methods have been described. Most of them could be categorized as

- modified USP methods,
- rotating flask methods (Koch, 1980), and
- dialysis methods (El-Arini et al., 1990).

An example of a commercially available (VanKel, Cary, North Carolina, U.S.) alternative to the standard USP II method is one that consists of a glass vessel that has been modified by introducing a peak in the bottom (Fig. 2). This modification has been introduced to create appropriate stirring in all parts of the vessel and thereby avoid formation of poorly agitated heaps of undissolved material. Another more recent development of nonstandard USP methods is the TIM machine (Blanquet, 2004). This method, originally developed for absorption studies of nutritionals but now applied for dissolution testing of pharmaceuticals, represents a more complex approach aiming to better mimic the fluid dynamics and hydrodynamics of the GI tract. This kind of approach has low throughput, is labor-intensive, and variability sources are difficult to control. Therefore, presently they have the potential to replace in vivo studies rather than simpler in vitro dissolution tests.

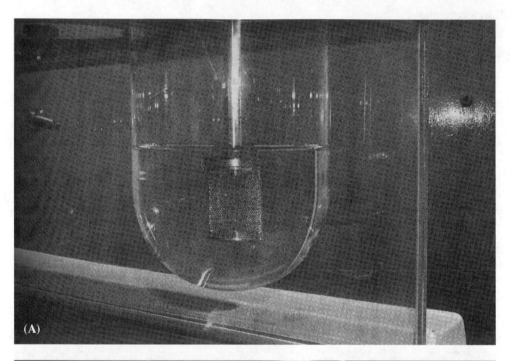

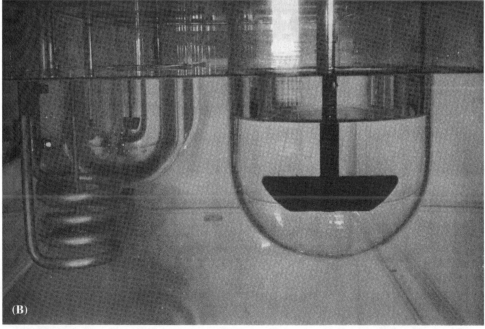

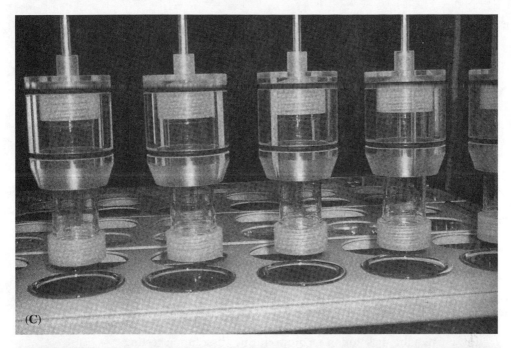

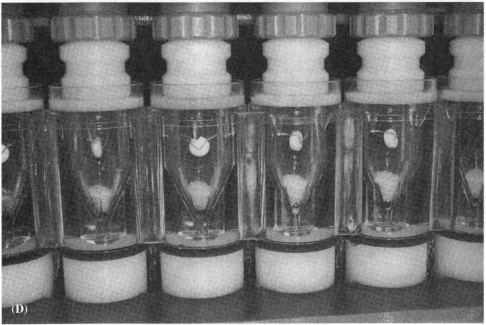

Figure 1 Different dissolution apparatuses: (**A**) the rotating basket (USP I) dissolution apparatus, (**B**) the rotating paddle (USP II), (**C**) the reciprocating cylinder (USP III) dissolution apparatus, (**D**) flow-through cell (USP IV). *Abbreviation*: USP, U.S. Pharmacopoeia.

The choice of dissolution apparatus will be specific for each formulation, and the following factors should be considered:

- Correlation to in vivo data
- Risk for hydrodynamic artifacts
- Regulatory guidelines
- Drug solubility

Standard USP vessel   Peak vessel

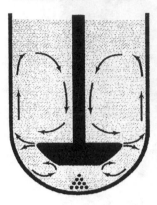
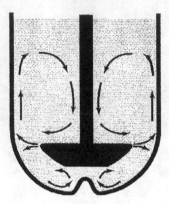

Conventional   **Peak Vessel**

Figure 2 Standard and modified (peak vessel) USP II dissolution apparatuses including illustrations of the different flow patterns within the beakers and photographs taken at a paddle stirring rate of 100 rpm showing a heap of pellets beneath the paddle in the standard method compared to the desirable dispersion of pellets in the modified method.

- Need to change the dissolution medium during dissolution testing
- Ease of operation, in-house know-how, and suitability for automation

As a general guideline in the choice of dissolution test apparatus, the simplest and most well established method should be chosen, with respect to both in-house know-how and regulatory aspects. In most cases, this is the USP II paddle method or the USP I rotating basket method. However, if satisfactory performance cannot be obtained by these methods, other methods should be considered. Primarily, the USP III and USP IV methods, and noncompendial methods could also provide relevant advantages.

Correlation of the in vitro dissolution to the in vivo dissolution is a crucial property of a dissolution test. The major difference in this respect between different apparatus is the hydrodynamic conditions. It has been argued for some of the methods, such as the USP IV flow-through cell or a rotating flask with baffles, that an in vivo–like situation is created in the in vitro test. However, this hypothesis has not been verified by any experimental means for any method, and it is clear that no apparatus mimics the full complexity of the motility patterns in the GI tract. A recommended approach is therefore to evaluate different apparatuses on a case-by-case basis using IVIVC studies (see sect. "Bioavailability Studies") to reveal which method provides the most desirable results.

The potential for hydrodynamic artifacts (e.g., floating, clogging of material to screens, coning below paddle, adhesion to equipment of the formulation, or variable flow conditions in the vicinity of the formulation because of other reasons) is strongly formulation dependent and thus has to be evaluated for each type of formulation. To detect artifacts, careful visual inspection of the dissolution test equipment is crucial. Video recordings can be used to aid such investigations.

The present regulatory guidelines in the United States and Europe propose the use of USP I and USP II as the methods of choice. Other methods, both compendial and noncompendial, could be acceptable, but the rationale for not using USP I and USP II must be clearly stated and supported by experimental data. In generic product development, complete dissolution methods, including the apparatus, are provided for many products in the USP and should thus be the first choice in a regulatory context. It should be noted, however, that this is not applicable in all cases. A dissolution method that is well functioning for a certain formulation type may provide high variability, artifacts, or poor IVIVC for other dosage forms. Thus, in particular, for ER formulations or dosage forms containing dissolution-enhancing principles, different dissolution tests may be needed for different formulations, although the drug substance is the same.

For sparingly soluble substances, the volume in standard vessel methods may not be sufficient to dissolve the dose. In this case, the USP IV flow-through method is beneficial, since it provides a continuous renewal of the dissolution fluid. However, the maximum flow rate limits the amount of drug that could be dissolved in this method. Sufficient solubility cannot be obtained for a rapidly releasing formulation of a drug with very low solubility in relation to the dose.

In certain cases, it is desirable to change the dissolution medium during the dissolution test. For example, a more physiologically relevant medium is desired with changes of the conditions (e.g., pH) corresponding to the differences along the GI tract. Both USP III and USP IV permit such changes without significant interruptions of the dissolution process.

Irrespective of the chosen apparatus, the equipment must be set up and handled in a way that both minimizes the variability of the dissolution and avoids artifacts. The most common source to such variability or artifacts is hydrodynamic factors, but unwanted chemical reactions or temperature shifts could also occur. Alterations of hydrodynamics, as well as changes of temperature, can both affect the dissolution of a drug substance and the release of a substance from the dosage form. Chemical reactions in the test medium may cause degradation of the drug substance or some formulation excipient, which may affect the dissolution or may lead to misinterpretation of the results. Examples of different sources to variability for the USP apparatuses are summarized below.

- USP I: Clogging of basket screen, positioning of basket
- USP II: Adherence of formulation to the beaker wall, floating, "entrapment" of solid material in the stagnant area beneath the paddle, positioning of the paddle
- USP III: Floating, adherence to tube wall or bottom screen, clogging of screens, disappearance of undissolved material through the screens
- USP IV: Clogging of filter, variations in flow rate

Some other factors that could potentially cause problems are not specific for a certain apparatus. These general factors include vibrations, variations in agitation rate, impurities due to poor cleaning or to trace amounts of metals from dissolution equipment, variations in dissolution fluid components, and poor quality of dissolution media components. Another factor relevant for lipophilic compounds is migration of the drug substance into fillers and plastic material.

Choice of Agitation Intensity

All compendial dissolution apparatuses can be operated at different agitation intensities. The three most outstanding aspects to consider when deciding at which level the tests should be performed are

1. correlation to in vivo data,
2. variability of dissolution results, and
3. regulatory guidelines and pharmacopoeial recommendations.

The U.S. regulatory agency recommends a stirring rate of 50 to 100 rpm for USP I and 50 to 75 rpm for USP II.

The above-proposed agitation intensities should be used if IVIVCs cannot be improved or the variability in dissolution data can be improved by other settings. The major problem associated with a too low agitation is that solid material is not sufficiently well dispersed, which delays the dissolution. On the other hand, the possibility to discriminate between different formulations/batches with different dissolution properties might be lost at a too intensive agitation.

Sometimes a dissolution test is performed with the aim to investigate the robustness of the release properties toward potential changes of the physiological conditions in vivo. In this case, tests at different agitation intensities should be considered to model different intestinal motilities. The use of more than one apparatus may also be considered.

Choice of Dissolution Test Media

The choice of dissolution medium is highly dependent on the purpose of the dissolution study, but the following aspects should always be considered:

- Correlation to in vivo data
- Resemblance of physiological conditions in the GI tract
- Regulatory and pharmacopoeial recommendations
- Drug solubility and stability properties at different pH values
- Known sensitivity of the formulation function for different medium factors

Attainment of IVIVC is a key aspect in the choice of dissolution test medium. However, it is not recommended to choose a test medium only on the basis of correlation to in vivo data. The dissolution test medium should also be relevant for the physiological conditions in the GI tract. Components and physicochemical characteristics of the GI fluids that might be considered in the choice of dissolution medium were discussed in chapter 4. The in vivo conditions are not static, but the fluids are constantly changing along the GI tract because of absorption of water and nutrients; secretions of enzymes, carbonate, salts and bile; and digestive processes. It is therefore clear that it is not realistic to reconstitute the full complexity of the in vivo conditions in an in vitro test. An approach has to be taken where the most relevant factors are included, on the basis of the knowledge of the solubility of the drug substance and the release mechanism of the dosage form. Examples of some dissolution test media that have been proposed to be physiologically relevant are given in Table 2 (USP, 2008; Dressman et al., 1998). An update of the physiologically more relevant simulated gastric and intestinal media developed by Dressman et al. has now been revised to even better reflect the GI fluids on the basis of more recent characterizations of real human GI fluids (Jantratid, 2008).

Another important aspect in the selection of a dissolution test medium is the need to consider the saturation solubility of drug in the test medium in relation to the drug dose tested. Drug dissolution will depend on the amount of drug in the solution if the dissolved amount of drug in the test medium approaches the saturation solubility. This can be understood from the Noyes-Whitney equation (see equation 1 in chapter 4, "Biopharmaceutical Support in Candidate Drug Selection"); the dissolution rate will be affected by the drug concentration in the dissolution medium (C_t) if C_t is not much less than the saturation solubility (C_s). This is not a desirable situation since, if C_t controls the rate of dissolution, the test may not be discriminative for factors related to the formulation performance. Another disadvantage, if C_t is significant in relation to C_s, is that the dissolution rate will be dose dependent, and different results will be obtained for different strengths of the same formulation. Finally, it can be assumed, in most cases, that C_t does not affect the in vivo dissolution rate due to the continuous removal of drug from the GI lumen by the drug absorption process that keeps

Table 2 Examples of Dissolution Test Media Including Physiological Components

USP-simulated gastric fluid	2 g/L NaCl 3.2 g/L pepsin 0.06 M HCl
USP-simulated intestinal fluid	0.05 M KH$_2$PO$_4$ 0.015 M NaOH 10.0 g/L pancreatin pH adjusted to 6.8 by HCl or NaOH
Simulated gastric fluid–fasted state (Dressman et al., 1998)	0.01–0.05 M HCl 2.5 g/L Na lauryl sulfate 2 g/L NaCl
Simulated intestinal fluid–fasted state (Dressman et al., 1998)	0.029 M KH$_2$PO$_4$ 5 mM sodium taurocholate 1.5 mM lecithin 0.22 M KCl pH adjusted to 6.8 by NaOH

the drug concentrations in the GI tract at a level far below C_s. Consequently, it is desirable to choose a dissolution test method that provides a high enough saturation solubility to avoid dependence on C_t. C_s should be at least three to five times higher than C_t when the total dose has been dissolved. Such conditions have been termed "sink conditions." In the first instance, maximum volume or flow of test medium should be used to obtain sink conditions. Adjustment of the pH to a level that provides optimal solubility should be considered for proteolytic drugs without neglecting the aspects of physiological relevance. For drugs with a very low solubility in relation to the administered dose, the above-described approaches will not provide sufficient drug solubility in the test media. In those cases, a surfactant should be added to the test medium in amounts above its critical micelle concentration (CMC) to solubilize the drug. The solubility can thereby be increased several hundred orders of magnitude. This approach is also favored due to the occurrence in vivo of drug solubilizing micelles formed in the presence of bile acids. However, the use in vitro of bile acids in standard methods is not recommended due to variations in quality and high costs, and it will still be almost impossible to simulate the in vivo complexity. Therefore, synthetic surfactants are the first choice, and sodium lauryl sulfate (SLS) has been especially recommended (Shah et al., 1989). Due to the risk of specific interactions between the formulation and SLS (of no in vivo relevance) or poor solubilization capacity for certain drugs, other synthetic surfactants may be considered on a case-by-case basis. An example of the first case is illustrated in Figure 3, where the in vitro dissolution-time profiles of a poorly soluble compound, felodipine, are shown for three different hydrophilic matrix ER tablets (Fig. 3) when three different surfactants [SLS, CTAB (cetyltrimethylammonium bromide), and Tween] were used to obtain sink conditions (Abrahamsson et al., 1994). SLS interacted with the gel-forming excipient, which led to much less of a difference in drug dissolution rate between the three different tablets, compared with the use of the other surfactants. It is also important to realize that attainment of sink conditions does not guarantee that the in vitro results correlate to the in vivo performance, because of other effects. The discriminating power of a dissolution test may be lost if the solubility of the drug is too favorable in the dissolution medium. For example, an in vitro dissolution method including SLS in amounts providing sink conditions was used to test three other felodipine ER tablets. No difference was obtained in vitro for the three tablets, which contained different forms of the drug substance, whereas one of the tablets provided almost no bioavailability in vivo due to poor dissolution (Johansson and Abrahamsson, 1997). Thus, general recommendations of the amount and type of solubilizer to be used in an in vitro test medium may be misleading, and the test medium should preferably be based on correlation to relevant in vivo data for poorly soluble substances.

On the basis of the knowledge of the substance solubility, release mechanisms from the dosage forms, and known interactions with key excipients, certain components may be of special importance to include or exclude in the dissolution test medium. This has to be considered on a case-by-case basis. Two examples are given below.

Example 1
Hard gelatine capsules have the potential to be cross-linked during storage, which leads to formation of non–water soluble capsules. However, this does not affect the in vivo dissolution due to the presence of enzymes that digest the gelatine. Thus, the presence of pepsin and pancreatin in simulated gastric and intestinal fluids, respectively, may be especially important in the dissolution testing of hard gelatine capsules (Digenis et al., 1994).

Example 2
The ionic concentration in the test medium can affect both the drug solubility and the release mechanism for modified-release formulations. One example of the latter case is hydrophilic gel matrix tablets, a type of ER tablet that forms a gel layer in contact with the GI fluids. Solutes will affect the hydration of the gel matrix and, thereby, affect the drug release rate.

It has been shown for such tablets that the correlation to in vivo data can be completely lost by use of inappropriate ionic compositions in the test medium (Abrahamsson et al., 1998a). For ER formulations with osmotically driven drug release, a decreased drug release rate

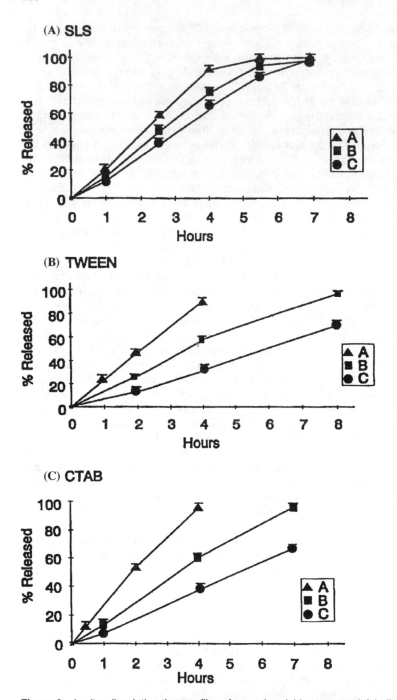

Figure 3 In vitro dissolution-time profiles of a poorly soluble compound, felodipine, for three different hydrophilic matrix ER tablets (**A–C**) when three different surfactants (SLS, CTAB, and Tween) were used in the dissolution test medium at levels providing "sink conditions." *Abbreviations*: ER, extended-release; SLS, sodium lauryl sulfate; CTAB, cetyltrimethylammonium.

approaching no release will occur for high ionic concentrations in the test medium, and misleading in vitro results may be obtained if a relevant ionic composition is not used (Lindstedt et al., 1989).

The concern for variability in dissolution results is of special significance when setting up a specification test method to be used for batch release but may also be considered for other

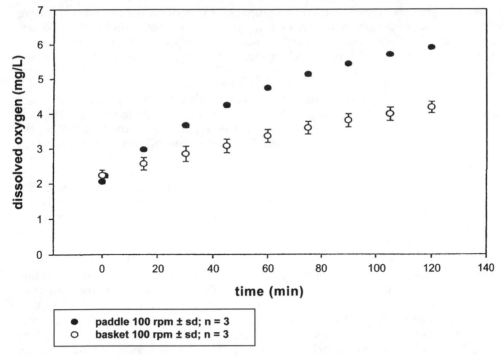

Figure 4 Oxygen concentration in deaerated dissolution test medium at different times in the USP I and USP II apparatuses at an agitation speed of 100 rpm.

tests. To reduce variability in dissolution results due to the test medium, the quality aspects of the dissolution media components that could affect the drug dissolution and release must be identified, and appropriate qualities of the components should be defined. This is especially important for the use of surfactants to provide micellar solubilization in the test medium (Crison et al., 1997). Another potential source of variability is impurities in the components that may alter the solubility or catalyze degradation of labile drugs. It is also important to see that the dissolution test medium is stable, that is, the components are not degraded or precipitated during the dissolution test period. This is of no concern for plain buffer systems but is more relevant for complex media including physiological components.

Dissolved air in the dissolution medium could, under certain circumstances, be located as air bubbles on the surface of the dosage form or released solid material. This will clearly affect the dissolution process by reducing wetting and the available surface area for dissolution in an uncontrolled way. To avoid this problem, the dissolution media has to be deaerated. A method for deaeration on the basis of heating and filtration can be found in USP XXIV. Other methods have also been described (Diebold and Dressman, 1998). It is, however, important to realize that the reaeration of deaerated water is a rapid process. The oxygen content increases significantly during filling of the in vitro dissolution test vessel as well as during the dissolution experiment (Diebold and Dressman, 1998) (Fig. 4).

Other Study Design Aspects
The design aspects of dissolution testing include, primarily, the choice of sampling intervals and number of tablets to be tested. Batch control often includes the testing of 6 individual units, whereas testing for regulatory purposes most often requires the testing of 12 individual units. In batch control of immediate-release (IR) formulations, one test point is most commonly used to assure complete dissolution (e.g., 80% or 85% of the total dose) at a specified time point (e.g., after 30–60 minutes), whereas three time points are required for ER formulations. For more slowly dissolving IR formulations, or poorly soluble drugs, a two-point dissolution test, that is, sampling at two different times, has been proposed (FDA, 1997b). For regulatory

purposes, when in vitro dissolution is used as a surrogate for bioequivalence studies, multiple time point determinations may also be required for IR formulations; if not, complete dissolution is not obtained within 15 minutes. For ER formulations, a more frequent sampling schedule than three time points is recommended during development, or as surrogate for in vivo bioequivalence studies, to reveal the full character of the dissolution profile. For example, the biphasic release pattern or a significant lag phase may not be detected if too few samples are collected.

Another design aspect of dissolution tests occurs when several parameters in the dissolution test method are varied. This could be the situation when looking for the best correlation to in vivo data, testing the robustness of the dissolution method, or testing the robustness of the dissolution properties of a certain formulation toward different physiological factors. The traditional approach has been to vary one factor at a time, while keeping the others at a constant level. The main disadvantages of this design approach are the numerous experiments needed when many factors have to be investigated, and the risk of suboptimization when there are interactions between different study variables. Statistical experimental design has been applied to dissolution testing during recent years as a method of reducing these problems. For full information regarding design and evaluation of such experiments, statistical textbooks such as *Statistics for Experimenters* (Box et al., 1978) are recommended, since the aim of the present chapter is only to provide a short introduction to this topic.

The basic principle of experimental design is to vary all factors concomitantly according to a randomized and balanced design, and to evaluate the results by multivariate analysis techniques, such as multiple linear regression or partial least squares. It is essential to check by diagnostic methods that the applied statistical model appropriately describes the experimental data. Unacceptably poor fit indicates experimental errors or that another model should be applied. If a more complicated model is needed, it is often necessary to add further experimental runs to correctly resolve such a model.

An example of a design aimed at validation of a dissolution method is given below (Gottfries et al., 1994). Seven factors were included, and each one was tested at two different levels plus one center point (i.e., all factors are set at a level in the middle between the high and low levels). In this case, there were $2^7 - 128$ number of unique experiments that could be performed, excluding the center point, to cover all possible combinations of the low and high-level settings of the seven different factors. Such a large number of experiments are seldom practically and economically justified. However, in statistical design, it is possible to do fractional designs; that is, a limited number of all possible experiments is chosen according to balanced design. In the present case, only 16 experiments, excluding the center point, were performed, and the settings in all experimental runs are presented in Table 3. The center point was replicated four times to assess experimental variability. The most common ways to present the results are shown in Figures 5 and 6. In Figure 4, the bars represent the effect on the amount of drug dissolved after four hours of each variable when varying the setting from the center to the upper level. The most predominant effects were provided by the stirring rate (St), temperature (T), ionic strength (Ion), the square of T, interaction between St and buffer volume (Buf) and interaction between T and Ion. Figure 6 is a surface response plot that displays the dissolution response at different levels of two selected variables while others are held constant at the mid-level. It is also possible to use an obtained model to predict dissolution results for any experimental setting within the tested domain. In this case, dissolution profiles were simulated for all possible combinations of settings within a series of predetermined limits to determine acceptable limits for methodological variation.

Examples of applications of statistical designs for optimizing correlations with in vivo data and for the testing of a formulation under different experimental conditions to elucidate the sensitivity of the drug release toward different physiological factors have also been published (Abrahamsson et al., 1998a; Abuzarur-Aloul et al., 1997).

Assessment of Dissolution Profiles

It is often desirable to present the dissolution results by some response variable. The most common descriptor is the amount dissolved at a certain time point. For rapidly dissolving dosage forms, it may be sufficient to provide the amount dissolved, for example, at 15 or

Table 3 Worksheet Illustrating a Statistical Experimental Design for Evaluating the Effect on the Dissolution of Variations of the Test Conditions in an In Vitro Dissolution Method

Experiment no.	Stirring speed (rpm)	pH	Concentration of CTAB (%)	Temperature (°C)	Basket position (cm)	Ionic strength of buffer (M)	Buffer volume (mL)
1	110.0	6.0	0.50	34.0	2.0	0.05	510.0
2	110.0	6.0	0.30	34.0	2.0	0.15	490.0
3	110.0	7.0	0.50	34.0	0.0	0.15	490.0
4	110.0	7.0	0.30	34.0	0.0	0.05	510.0
5	110.0	7.0	0.50	40.0	2.0	0.15	510.0
6	110.0	6.0	0.50	40.0	0.0	0.05	490.0
7	110.0	7.0	0.30	40.0	2.0	0.05	490.0
8	110.0	6.0	0.30	40.0	0.0	0.15	510.0
9	100.0	6.5	0.40	37.0	1.0	0.10	500.0
10	100.0	6.5	0.40	37.0	1.0	0.10	500.0
11	100.0	6.5	0.40	7.0	1.0	0.10	500.0
12	100.0	6.5	0.40	37.0	1.0	0.10	500.0
13	100.0	6.5	0.40	37.0	1.0	0.10	500.0
14	90.0	7.0	0.50	34.0	2.0	0.05	490.0
15	90.0	6.0	0.50	34.0	0.0	0.15	510.0
16	90.0	6.0	0.30	34.0	0.0	0.05	490.0
17	90.0	7.0	0.30	34.0	2.0	0.15	510.0
18	90.0	6.0	0.30	40.0	2.0	0.05	510.0
19	90.0	7.0	0.30	40.0	0.0	0.15	490.0
20	90.0	7.0	0.50	40.0	0.0	0.05	510.0
21	90.0	6.0	0.50	40.0	2.0	0.15	490.0
A1	110.0	7.0	0.50	40.0	0.0	0.15	490.0
A2	90.0	6.0	0.30	40.0	0.0	0.05	490.0
A3	110.0	7.0	0.50	40.0	0.0	0.05	510.0
A4	90.0	6.0	0.50	34.0	0.0	0.05	510.0
A5	90.0	7.0	0.50	34.0	2.0	0.15	490.0
A6	100.0	6.5	0.40	34.0	1.0	0.10	500.0
A7	100.0	6.5	0.40	40.0	1.0	0.10	500.0
A8	100.0	6.5	0.40	37.0	1.0	0.10	490.0
A9	100.0	6.5	0.40	37.0	1.0	0.10	510.0

Source: From Gottfries et al. (1994).

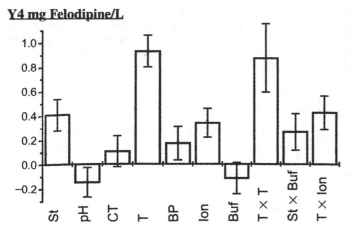

Y4 mg Felodipine/L

Figure 5 Scaled and centered coefficients for felodipine in vitro dissolution after four hours (Y4). The height of the bars illustrates the change in response estimated for a relative increase of each factor from the mid-point level to the high level in the factorial design. The different factors were stirring speed (St), pH, concentration cetyltrimethylammonium bromide (CT), temperature (T), basket position (BP), ionic strength (Ion), buffer volume (Buf), square of T (T × T), interaction terms between St and Buf (St × Buf) and between T and Ion (T × Ion). *Source*: From Gottfries et al. (1994).

30 minutes. For dosage forms where it is relevant to study the whole profile, more sophisticated methods are needed, since the use of a single point neglects all other data points.

Any model can be applied to in vitro dissolution data and fitted by linear or nonlinear regression, as appropriate. Sometimes a first-order model $[A(t) = A - Ae^{-kt}]$, where $A(t)$ is the

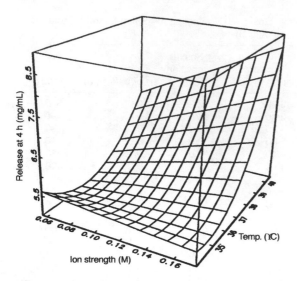

Figure 6 Response surface of felodipine dissolved in vitro after four hours expressed as drug concentration at different ionic strengths and temperatures. *Source*: From Gottfries et al. (1994).

amount dissolved after time t, A is the initial amount, and k is the first-order dissolution rate constant, or even a zero-order model [$A(t) = A - Akt$] is sufficiently sophisticated to determine a dissolution rate that is representative for the whole process. However, a more general equation that is commonly applied to dissolution data is the Weibull equation (Langenbucher, 1976)

$$A(t) = A_\infty \times \left[1 - e^{-\left[(t-t_{\text{lag}})/\tau_{\text{d}}\right]^\beta}\right] \qquad (1)$$

where $A(t)$ is the amount dissolved at time t, A_∞ is the final plateau level of amount dissolved in the dissolution-time curve, and t_{lag} is the duration of an initial period of no dissolution. τ_{d} is a rate parameter, more specifically it is a scale factor of the time axis. Two curves differing only in τ_{d} appear as being stretched or compressed along the time axis. Finally, β is a parameter that characterizes the shape of the curve. At β values of 0 and 1, the dissolution-time curve follows zero- and first-order kinetics, respectively.

Another approach to obtain a parameter that describes the dissolution rate is to use statistical moments to determine the mean dissolution time (MDT) (von Hattingberg, 1984). This method has the advantage of being applicable to all types of dissolution profiles, and it does not require fitting to any model. The only prerequisite is that data points are available close to the final plateau level. The MDT can be interpreted as the most likely time for a molecule to be dissolved from a solid dosage form. In the case of zero- and first-order dissolution processes, the MDT corresponds to the time when 50% and 63.2% have been released, respectively. The MDT is determined from

$$\text{MDT} = \frac{i \sum t_i \times \Delta M_i}{M_0} \qquad (2)$$

where t_i is the midpoint of the ith time period during which the fraction ΔM_i has been released and M_0 is the final amount released. The length of each time period is given by the sampling intervals.

A special case occurs when two dissolution profiles are compared. This is often the case when a change has been introduced in the composition, manufacturing process, or manufacturing site. The aim is then to maintain the same dissolution properties as for the original version. Such comparisons of dissolution profiles are performed by calculating a similarity factor, f_2, which is calculated as follows from cumulative mean data (Shah et al., 1998):

$$f_2 = 50 \times \log\left\{\left[1 + \left(\frac{1}{n}\right)\sum_{t=1}^{n}(R_t - T_t)^2\right]^{-0.5} \times 100\right\} \qquad (3)$$

where n is the number of time points in the dissolution-time curve and R_t and T_t are the cumulative amount dissolved at time t for the reference and test formulation, respectively. The number of time points, n, should be at least 3, but only including one value close to the final plateau level ($\geq 85\%$). From a regulatory perspective, f_2-values greater than 50 ensure that the profiles are similar enough (FDA, 1997b) and if $f_2 = 100$, the test and reference products have identical dissolution-time curves. An f_2-value of 50 corresponds to an average difference between the test and reference curves of 10%. This test is not relevant for very rapidly dissolving formulations (i.e., complete release within 15 minutes), since differences in the dissolution profiles between formulations that are so rapid is of no in vivo relevance.

Validation of In Vitro Dissolution Methods

High quality and valuable in vitro dissolution tests are obtained by a rational design of test method as described above. However, there are different means to validate the method, that is, to verify that the method functions as intended. These include

- dissolution tests with USP calibrator tablets,
- robustness testing, and
- comparison with in vivo results.

Disintegrating as well as nondisintegrating USP calibrator tablets are available with a specified dissolution profile for each apparatus. These tablets are used to control the dissolution apparatus and to allow it to operate as intended, so that the hydrodynamic conditions are satisfactory. However, it should be noted that certain formulations might be more sensitive to such factors than are the calibrator tablets.

Another important aspect in validation of a new dissolution method is to investigate how sensitive the dissolution results of the product, for which the method has been developed, are for minute variations in operating conditions. Examples of factors to consider in such a test are temperature of test medium, rotational speed, volume, sampling procedure, medium compositions, and testing performed by different operators. On the basis of such robustness tests of the method, limits can be defined for acceptable variations of test conditions. Statistical design may be useful to apply in situations such as those demonstrated earlier in this chapter.

Comparison of in vitro dissolution results with corresponding in vivo data for different formulations to verify that the in vitro methods predict the in vivo dissolution properties (see sect. "In Vitro/In Vivo Correlations") is already preferably used in the design of the test method. However, if not so, the in vivo validity of the method should be investigated at a later stage, especially for modified release formulations and poorly soluble drugs.

BIOAVAILABILITY STUDIES

In bioavailability studies, the drug plasma concentrations, and potentially the amount of drug/ metabolites in urine, are followed over an appropriate time interval after administration to derive drug absorption parameters. There are basically two different aspects of the function of the formulation that can be evaluated: (1) rate of drug dissolution and/or release and (2) extent of drug that is made available for absorption.

The drug dissolution or release rate will directly determine the absorption rate in cases where this is the rate-limiting step in the absorption process. The formulation may also affect the extent of absorption, for example, when

- dissolution enhancers are used for poorly soluble compounds,
- absorption enhancers are used for poorly permeable drugs,
- the drug release is incomplete from the formulation, and
- the formulation provides a means of avoiding degradation in the GI tract.

The importance and the need to study these factors increase if the substance has problematic absorption properties, or if the aim is to develop an advanced formulation, such as a modified release product, or if a dosage form affects the biopharmaceutical properties in any other way.

Bioavailability studies are performed during formulation development at different stages and for several reasons to

- obtain and verify the desirable dissolution and release properties,
- study the influence of physiological factors such as food,
- establish bioquivalence between clinical trial and commercial formulations after changes of a formulation,
- develop and validate IVIVCs for in vitro dissolution test methods.

Although all these different types of studies aim to investigate the influence of the dosage form on the rate and extent of absorption, different designs and means to evaluate the data are applied. This chapter describes different ways to assess the formulation function from plasma concentration data obtained in bioavailability studies. Certain study design aspects will also be pointed out. For a more basic understanding of pharmacokinetics, specialized textbooks should be consulted, such as *Clinical Pharmacokinetics—Concepts and Applications* (Rowland and Tozer, 1995).

Aspects of Study Design

Single-Dose Studies

Single-dose studies are most sensitive for evaluation of absorption properties and should generally be used for evaluation of formulations. The main exception is if the regulatory guidelines require repeated dosing studies. The drug should be administered under fasting conditions (overnight) together with 200 mL of water. No food should generally be allowed for four hours after intake, and the subjects should thereafter follow a standardized meal schedule during the study day.

Crossover Designs

In crossover designs, the same subjects receive test and reference formulations to avoid the influence of any interindividual differences that could affect the plasma concentration–time profile. For drugs with a very long half-life (several weeks), a parallel group design (i.e., each formulation is studied in different groups of subjects) may be applied for practical reasons to shorten the duration of the study. A parallel group design could also be used if the interindividual (between subjects) variability of the bioavailability variables is of the same magnitude as the intraindividual (within-subject) variability. Additionally, other standard design principles such as randomization should be used, as described in more detail in statistical textbooks.

Washout Period

A washout period, that is, a minimum number of days between administration of each formulation, is needed to avoid influence of the previous administration on the plasma concentration profile of the following formulation. As a rule of thumb, the washout period should be at least five times the elimination half-life of the drug under investigation.

Reference Formulation

In almost all studies, a reference formulation is needed, either as a comparator for assessment of relative performance compared to the test formulation, or as a simple vehicle, to characterize the drug substance pharmacokinetics. If the aim is to investigate the influence of certain formulations on the rate and extent of absorption, which is the case in early development or IVIVC studies, an oral solution of the drug is the first choice as a reference formulation. Stability of the solution, regarding drug compound degradation and precipitation, is an important factor to verify before study start. Inclusion of a parenteral reference formulation, if feasible, provides additional information, as will be further discussed below.

Number of Subjects

The number of subjects to be included in the study will be determined by the inherent variability in drug substance pharmacokinetics, the magnitude of effects that are of interest, the desired confidence in conclusions, costs, time, ethical aspects and where relevant, and regulatory guideline recommendations. Three different situations may be identified that require different algorithms to determine the sample size:

1. The aim is to determine the absorption characteristics for a certain formulation, for example, in an IVIVC study. In this case, the question for the pharmaceutical scientist is how precise the mean estimates of primary variables must be, that is, how wide confidence intervals around the mean are acceptable.
2. The aim is to investigate the difference between two or more formulations. In this case, the question is how large a difference between the formulations can be of interest to detect at a certain statistical significance level.
3. The aim is to establish bioequivalence between two formulations by obtaining a confidence interval for the difference within specified limits. In this case, the main question is how large a risk the investigator is willing to take to obtain nonconclusive results. Inclusion of more subjects will decrease the width of the confidence interval and thereby reduce the risk of not meeting the acceptance criteria.

Statisticians often make calculations of a suitable number of subjects. However, for an understanding of these calculations, any basic statistical textbook is recommended for the first two cases, and in the case of bioequivalence studies, another reference (Hauschke et al., 1999) is suggested.

Plasma Sampling

The plasma-sampling schedule has to be designed so that the desired accuracy of the primary bioavailability variables can be obtained. In cases of evaluation of formulation performance, it is crucial to have frequent sampling during the absorption phase. In addition, at least three samples should be obtained during the major terminal elimination phase to obtain a relevant measure of the rate constant for this phase, which is needed for a correct estimate of the extent of absorption. Numerous late plasma samples, when the drug concentration is below the limit of quantification of the bioanalytical assay, should be avoided.

Food

Food may not only affect drug substance pharmacokinetics, such as first-pass metabolism or drug clearance; it may also influence drug dissolution, or by other means, the function of the dosage form. For example, with food, drug residence time in the stomach will be increased, the pH will be changed, motility will be altered, and bile and pancreatic secretions will increase. All these factors could potentially affect drug release and dissolution from a solid formulation. It is therefore relevant to study the influence of food on rate and extent of drug dissolution/release during development. Such a study should include an oral solution, to allow for a distinction between the effects of food on formulation and drug substance. The dosage forms are typically administered immediately after intake of the food. Since almost all medications are administered in the morning, studies are usually performed together with a breakfast. The composition of the meal has to be well defined, since variations can introduce unwanted variability.

Generally, a heavy breakfast (approximately 1000 calories and 50% of the energy content from fat) should be used, since this is supposed to stress potential food effects. A proposal for a standardized composition of a heavy breakfast is displayed in Table 4 (FDA, 1997c).

Table 4 Example of a Standardized Breakfast to Be Used in Food Interaction Studies

2 Eggs fried in butter	4 ounces of hash brown potatoes
2 Strips of bacon	8 ounces of whole milk
2 Slices of toast with butter	

Assessments

Evaluation of drug plasma concentrations is an indirect way of estimating the rate and amount of drug dissolution and/or absorption. Several assumptions are therefore needed, irrespective of which of the metrics described below are applied

- In crossover studies, drug substance pharmacokinetics, including first-pass metabolism, distribution and clearance, should be identical within the same subject, between administrations of different formulations.
- Linear pharmacokinetics within the investigated rate of delivery (dose/time units) of the drug to the body, that is, the plasma concentration–time profile, should be identical for different doses after correction for dose. The most common reason for nonlinear pharmacokinetics is dose-dependent first-pass metabolism. This phenomenon does not just occur at high doses, but has also been shown for the slow delivery rates obtained by ER formulations.

In cases where the in vivo dissolution/release rate is going to be quantified in some way from plasma concentrations, it is important to emphasize that this is only relevant if this is the rate-limiting step in the absorption process. If other factors are affecting the absorption rate, estimations of the in vivo dissolution will be confounded. Examples of such confounding factors in determination of the in vivo dissolution rate are

- gastric emptying (assuming negligible absorption over the gastric mucosa),
- low drug permeability over the gastric wall,
- degradation in the GI tract,
- complex-binding of the drug to any component in the GI tract, and
- enterohepatic circulation, that is, intact drugs are excreted by the bile into the intestine.

In vivo evaluation of formulations thus requires a high level of knowledge regarding the drug substance absorption properties obtained both by in vitro and in vivo methods described in this chapter and in chapter 4, and also by basic pharmacokinetic studies, a review of which is outside the scope of the present chapter.

Standard Bioavailability Variables

The standard bioavailability variables after a single-dose administration are the maximum plasma concentration (C_{max}), the time to reach C_{max} (t_{max}), and the area under the plasma concentration–time curve from time zero to infinity (AUC).

C_{max} and t_{max} are used as characteristics of the absorption rate and may thereby be affected by the drug dissolution and release, as discussed above. However, both variables are affected by several pharmacokinetic properties other than the absorption rate (K_a) as shown in equations (4) and (5), which describe C_{max} and t_{max}, respectively, for a first-order absorption process

$$C_{max} = \frac{F \times D(K_a/K_e)^{-K_e(K_a - K_e)}}{V_d} \tag{4}$$

$$t_{max} = \frac{2.303 \times \log(K_a/K_e)}{K_a - K_e} \tag{5}$$

where F is the extent of oral drug bioavailability expressed as a fraction, D is the administered dose, K_e is the first-order elimination rate constant, according to one compartment model, and V_d is the volume of distribution.

Thus, C_{max} and t_{max} are not useful as pure measures of the absorption rate but can be used in comparisons between different formulations. Another disadvantage is that they are single-point estimates, which does not take into account all data sampled during the absorption process. In the case of rapid dissolution processes, it is difficult to accurately localize the true maximum, and frequent plasma sampling during the absorption phase is especially crucial in getting reasonably good estimates. The main merit of C_{max}, besides simplicity, is its potential clinical relevance, that is, when the peak plasma concentration is related to maximal pharmacological effects or adverse effects.

AUC is used to evaluate the extent of absorption, which may be affected by the formulation, as discussed above. AUC is a composite variable determined not only by the extent of bioavailability (F) but also by the systemic drug clearance (Cl) and the dose (D) as described by

$$AUC = \frac{D \times F}{Cl} \qquad (6)$$

Thus, AUC is only of interest as a relative variable, where the AUC for a test formulation is related to a reference. If the AUC-ratio is determined for a formulation in relation to an oral solution, the influence of the dosage form on the extent of absorption can be determined, that is, if $AUC_{solid}/AUC_{solution} \neq 1$, the deviation from 1 can be attributed to the formulation, provided that the above-stated assumptions hold. AUC is also a primary variable in bioequivalence studies.

The calculation of AUC is commonly determined by the linear trapezoidal rule. In this procedure, the sum of the areas of a series of trapezoids, which are formed between the data points for two adjacent times, is calculated (Fig. 7). This approximate method requires that blood sampling be frequent enough so that the curvature of the plasma concentrations between two data points is negligible. For example, in the ascending part, the plasma concentration curve has a convex profile, and a straight line will provide an overestimation of the AUC. Applying a modified version, the log trapezoidal rule, can reduce this problem. The area under each segment between two data points for the linear trapezoidal (equation 7) and logarithmic trapezoidal (equation 8) methods are determined by

$$AUC(t_n, t_{n+1}) = \left(\frac{C_n + C_{n+1}}{2}\right) \times (t_{n+1} - t_n) \qquad (7)$$

$$AUC(t_n, t_{n+1}) = \left(\frac{C_n - C_{n+1}}{\ln\frac{C_n}{C_{n+1}}}\right) \times (t_{n+1} - t_n) \qquad (8)$$

where C_n is the drug concentration for the nth plasma sample obtained at time t_n. It is imperative in single-dose studies, which are generally most suitable for evaluation of dosage form performance, to determine the AUC from time zero to infinity. This requires that the

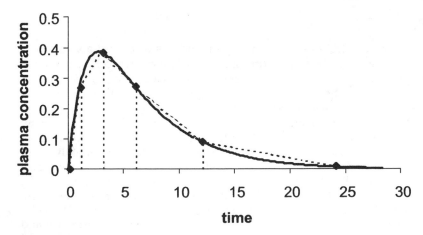

Figure 7 Drug plasma concentration–time curve illustrating formation of trapezoids, in calculation of the area under the curve.

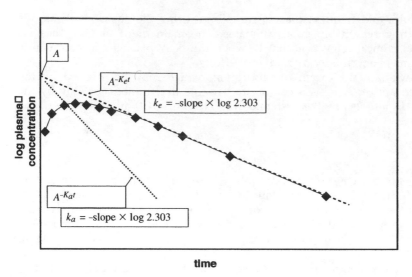

time

Figure 8 Logarithmic drug plasma concentration–time curve for an oral administration illustrating the K_e and first-order K_a. *Abbreviations*: K_a, absorption rate constant; K_e, elimination rate constant.

remaining area from the last measured data point ($C_{t_{last}}$) to infinity be extrapolated, and is made from the following equation:

$$\text{AUC}_{t_{last}-\infty} = \frac{C_{t_{last}}}{K_e} \tag{9}$$

where K_e is the elimination rate constant that is determined from the slope of the terminal log-linear plasma concentration–time profile (Fig. 8) by linear regression. To obtain a reliable estimate of AUC, the extrapolated area ($\text{AUC}_{t_{last}-\infty}$) should not exceed 10% of the total AUC.

C_{max} and AUC are also used as primary variables in bioequivalence studies, that is, studies aiming to establish that a test and a reference product provide similar enough plasma concentration–time profiles to be exchanged without altering the clinical effects. Such studies are, for example, performed in NDA programs to compare the clinical trial formulations with the "to-be-marketed" product, at post-approval changes of composition, manufacturing process or site of a product, and to document a generic versus the original product. More details regarding performance and evaluation of such studies can be found in appropriate guidelines (FDA, 2000; EMEA, 1998).

Model-Dependent Analysis
An absorption rate, which could reflect dosage form performance, as discussed above, could be determined from plasma concentration data by fitting the data to a pharmacokinetic model. The absorption rate could be a zero-order or first-order rate constant, that is, the amount absorbed is constant over time or the absorption rate decreases exponentially over time, respectively. The choice of model also depends on how many phases in the log-plasma concentration–time profiles are identified after the peak concentration, that is, how many compartments are needed to describe the plasma concentration–time profile. The model may also include a lag time (t_{lag}) before absorption starts. A comprehensive description of different models can be found in Gabrielsson and Weiner (1997). Model dependent analysis could also be used to determine the standard bioavailability variables such as C_{max}, t_{max}, and AUC. Fitting the plasma concentration data to the suitable model is done by nonlinear regression. Computer programs designed for pharmacokinetic modeling are available, such as NONLIN (Pharsight Corp., Mountain View, California, U.S.). More details regarding performance and evaluation of nonlinear regressions for this purpose can be found elsewhere (Gabrielsson and Weiner, 1997).

In the case of one-compartment disposition pharmacokinetics, that is, when the declining part of the plasma concentration–time curve can be approximated by a one log-linear phase, a first-order rate constant (K_a) can be determined according to

$$Ae^{-K_a t} = Ae^{-K_e t} - C_t \tag{10}$$

where A is determined from the intercept with the y-axis of the extrapolated log-linear elimination phase (Fig. 8), K_e is the first-order rate constant that describes the elimination phase, and C is the plasma concentration at time t. The difference between the extrapolated elimination phase and the actual plasma concentration ($Ae^{-K_e t} - C_t$) is plotted versus time, which thus equals $Ae^{-K_a t}$ and describes the absorption phase. The K_a can then be determined from the slope of the line in a log-linear plot as shown in Figure 8.

Moment Analysis

Moment analysis provides the means to determine a model independent characteristic of the absorption rate or dissolution rate (Riegelman and Collier, 1980). A single value characterizing the rate of the entire dissolution or absorption process is obtained, which is called the mean absorption or dissolution time (MAT and MDT, respectively). These parameters can be determined without any assumptions regarding absorption or disposition pharmacokinetics, apart from the general prerequisites of linear pharmacokinetics and absence of intraindividual variability described above. MAT/MDT can be interpreted as the most probable time for a molecule to become absorbed/dissolved, on the basis of a normal Gaussian distribution.

If these processes follow zero- or first-order kinetics, MAT/MDT corresponds to 50% and 63% absorbed/dissolved, respectively. MDT is especially useful for correlations with in vitro data since this in vivo variable corresponds to the MDT determined from in vitro dissolution data, as described in the section "In Vitro Dissolution".

MAT and MDT for a test formulation are determined from drug plasma concentrations–time data obtained in a single-dose study according to the following equations:

$$\text{MRT} = \frac{\text{AUMC}_{0-\infty}}{\text{AUC}_{0-\infty}} \tag{11}$$

$$\text{MAT} = \text{MRT}_{\text{test}} - \text{MRT}_{\text{IV}} \tag{12}$$

$$\text{MDT} = \text{MRT}_{\text{test}} - \text{MRT}_{\text{oral solution}} \tag{13}$$

where MRT is the mean residence time, which includes the complete time from intake to elimination of the drug. $\text{AUMC}_{0-\infty}$ is the area under the curve of the product of time t and the plasma concentration versus time from zero to infinity, and $\text{AUC}_{0-\infty}$ is the area under the plasma concentration–time curve, as defined above. Thus, administration of an oral or intravenous (IV) reference administration is needed to calculate MAT and MDT, respectively, except when the drug substance follows one-compartment pharmacokinetics. In this case, the MAT can be determined without a reference according to the following formula:

$$\text{MAT}_{\text{test}} = \text{MRT}_{\text{test}} - \left(\frac{1}{K_e}\right) \tag{14}$$

that is, MRT and K_e are determined from the plasma concentration–time profile for the test formulation according to the procedures described above.

In Vivo Dissolution/Absorption-Time Profiles

A full-time course in vivo dissolution- or absorption-time profile is generally the most informative way of evaluating formulation performance from the plasma concentration–time data. The methods described in the present chapter all have the advantage over the modeling of zero- or first-order rate constants, in that no assumptions have to be made regarding the kinetics of the absorption phase. Some of the methods provide an estimate of the

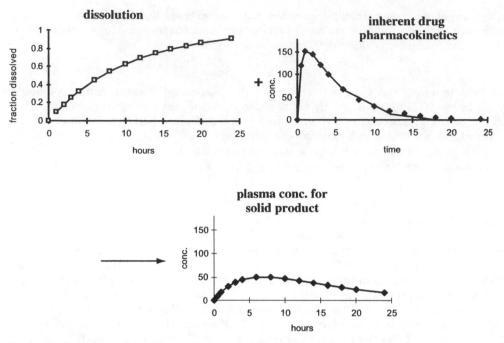

Figure 9   Illustrations of the different functions included in deconvolution/convolution.

absorption-time profile, rather than the in vivo dissolution-time profile. However, in the context of evaluating formulation performance, the former measure is fully valid, provided that the drug dissolution/release is the rate-determining step in the absorption process.

The method of choice for determination of in vivo dissolution- or absorption-time profiles is *deconvolution*. In deconvolution, three components are defined: input, weighting, and response functions, as exemplified in Figure 9. The input function corresponds to the entry of drug into the body, that is, the in vivo dissolution- or absorption-time profiles for the oral test formulation. The weighting function corresponds to the time course of the drug within the body, as described by the plasma concentration–time profile after administration of an oral or IV reference solution, and the response function is described by the plasma concentration–time curve for the test formulation. In deconvolution, the input function is determined from data that describe the weighting and response functions, that is, the in vivo dissolution- or absorption-time profile is calculated from the plasma concentration–time data of the test formulation and a reference solution. It is also possible to calculate the response function from available data of the input and weighting functions, that is, the plasma concentration–time profile for a solid oral dosage form is simulated from in vitro dissolution data and plasma concentration–time data for a solution. This latter procedure is called *convolution*. The three most common definitions of the input, weighting, and response functions in deconvolution/ convolution are presented in Table 5.

Different deconvolution algorithms have been described (Tucker, 1983). However, further descriptions in the present chapter will be limited to numerical deconvolution (Langenbucher, 1982). The merits of this equation compared to others are the relative

Table 5   Definitions of the Different Functions in Deconvolution/Convolution

Input (I)	Weighting (W)	Response (R)
	Plasma concentration–time profile for	Plasma concentration–time profile for
Dissolution-time profile or solid formulation	Oral solution	Solid formulation
Absorption-time profile or solid formulation	IV solution	Solid formulation
Absorption-time profile for oral solution	IV solution	Oral solution

simplicity of the algorithm and the lack of any modeling of the plasma concentration–time data to be used in the assessment of the input profile. The fractional amount dissolved or absorbed (I) is calculated by the following deconvolution algorithm:

$$I_1 = \frac{R_1 T}{W_1}$$

$$I_2 = \frac{R_2/(T - I_1)W_2}{W_1}$$

$$I_3 = \frac{R_3/(T - I_1)(W_3 - I_2)W_2}{W_1} \tag{15}$$

$$I_n = \frac{R_n/(T - I_1)(W_n - I_2)(W_{n-1} - \cdots - I_{n-1})W_2}{W_1}$$

where W_i and R_i are the plasma concentrations for the ith time representing the weighting and response functions, respectively. These plasma concentration–time profiles are divided into finite intervals of equal time T before the plasma concentrations can be entered into the equation described above. Interpolations are generally needed between the measured data points to obtain such data. A common method for performing such interpolations is the point-area method (Vaughan and Dennis, 1978).

A drawback of deconvolution algorithms is that they are not stable. Small inconsistencies or noise in the data could, in some cases, lead to input time profiles that oscillate by increasing amplitude, that is, no meaningful interpretation of such results can be made. Such problems could be overcome by changing the time interval T, by suitable interpolation or by smoothing/modeling of the plasma concentration data used as weighting and response functions.

The plasma concentration for a solid product can be estimated from in vitro dissolution data and plasma concentration–time data for a reference formulation by rearranging equation (15) to a convolution algorithm

$$R_1 = I_1 W_1 T$$

$$R_2 = (I_1 W_2 + I_2 W_1)T$$

$$R_3 = (I_1 W_3 + I_2 W_2 + I_3 W_1)T \tag{16}$$

$$R_n = (I_1 W_n + I_2 W_{n-1} + \cdots + I_n W_1)T$$

The convolution algorithm (equation 16) is stable, in contrast to deconvolution procedures.

Two other methods have been described that require modeling of the disposition pharmacokinetics but not of the absorption phase. For drugs with disposition pharmacokinetics that can be approximated by a one-compartment model, that is, the declining part of the plasma concentration–time curve can be approximated by a one log-linear phase, the following equation can be applied to determine the fractional amount absorbed (A) at different times t after administration (Wagner and Nelson, 1963):

$$A(t) = \frac{C_t + (K_e \times \text{AUC}_{0-t})}{(K_e \times \text{AUC}_{0-\infty})} \tag{17}$$

where K_e and AUC have been defined previously in this chapter. This equation is known as the *Wagner–Nelson method*. The main advantage of this method is that the absorption-time profile can be determined without administration of any reference formulation, provided that the elimination rate constant can be accurately determined from the post-absorption phase of the plasma concentration–time curve of the test formulation. Another merit of the Wagner–Nelson method is the simple calculation procedure compared to other methods. An important limitation of the Wagner–Nelson method is that the amount absorbed is expressed as the fraction of the total amount absorbed, that is, the asymptotic plateau level of the absorption-time profile will always be 1.0. Thus, no conclusions can be drawn from such data regarding completeness of drug release or dissolution.

For drugs that are best described by a two-compartment pharmacokinetic model, the absorption-time profile can be determined by the *Loo–Riegelman method* (Loo and Riegelman, 1968). However, this method requires administration of an IV bolus dose to determine the disposition pharmacokinetics. Therefore, this method does not provide any clear advantages compared to deconvolution.

Fractional Amount Absorbed

The fractional *amount of drug absorption* (F_a) can be defined as the amount of intact drug that permeates the gastric wall. It is related to the absolute bioavailability (F), that is, the fraction of the administered drug that reaches the systemic circulation, according to the following equation:

$$F = F_a \times F_h \times F_g \tag{18}$$

where F_h and F_g are the fractions of the administered drug that escape first-pass metabolism in the liver and the gut wall, respectively, before entering the systemic circulation. F_a is of special relevance for elucidation of formulation performance, because it is affected by the completeness of dissolution/release, the success in avoiding degradation in GI tract and/or potential effects of the formulation on drug permeability.

F_a can be estimated from plasma concentration–time data and urine data. In the former case, administration of a reference IV solution is needed, in addition to administration of the test formulation. F_a can be approximately determined from the following series of algorithms:

$$F_a = \frac{F}{1 - E_h} \tag{19}$$

$$F = \left(\frac{AUC_{oral}}{AUC_{IV}}\right) \times \left(\frac{dose_{IV}}{dose_{oral}}\right) \tag{20}$$

$$E_h = \frac{Cl_{h_{blood}}}{Q_h} \tag{21}$$

$$Cl_{h_{blood}} = Cl_{h_{plasma}} \times blood : plasma\ concentration\ rate \tag{22}$$

$$Cl_{h_{plasma}} = Cl_{tot} - CLr \tag{23}$$

$$Cl_{tot} = \frac{dose_{IV}}{AUC_{IV}} \tag{24}$$

$$CLr = f_e \times Cl_{tot} \tag{25}$$

$$f_e = \frac{A_u}{F \times dose} \tag{26}$$

where E_h is the hepatic elimination ratio, $Cl_{h_{blood}}$ is the hepatic blood clearance and Q_h is the hepatic blood flow, which is assumed to be 1.5 L/min in man. The partition of drug between blood and plasma has to be experimentally determined. Cl_{tot} is the total systemic plasma clearance, CLr is the renal plasma clearance, f_e is the fraction of drug excreted unchanged in urine, and A_u is the total amount of drug excreted unchanged in urine. It should be realized that this is only an approximate method since neither the blood flow nor the blood/plasma drug ratio is measured during the absorption process. In addition, it has to be assumed that all first-pass metabolism is performed by the liver. Systemic clearance is only provided by the liver and kidneys, and hepatic metabolism is linear within the concentration range encompassed by high levels during the first-pass through the liver and lower levels returned from the systemic circulation.

If a radioactively labeled drug is administered intravenously and orally, the F_a can be more simply estimated from the oral/intravenous ratio, corrected for dose, of total radioactivity in the urine. This requires that urine collection continue over a time period long enough to provide almost complete emptying of the radioactivity. Furthermore, to get reasonable precision, a significant amount of metabolites and/or unchanged drug has to be excreted by the kidneys. Finally, it has to be assumed that the parent drug molecule is not degraded in the GI tract and is subsequently absorbed as the metabolite.

IN VITRO/IN VIVO CORRELATIONS

The correlation between in vitro and in vivo dissolution, or other in vivo characteristics, is useful during several stages of formulation development. For example, in early formulation development, it may be desirable to establish the in vivo relevance of the dissolution method used for screening of different candidate formulations. During later development phases, IVIVCs can be used to validate the batch control dissolution test method, or as a guide when setting the dissolution specification limits. IVIVC may also form a basis for replacing bioequivalence studies with simpler in vitro dissolution studies for modified release formulations, both during development and in connection with later post-approval changes (EMEA, 1999; FDA, 1997a).

It should be possible to establish IVIVCs provided that the following prerequisites are fulfilled.

- Drug release or dissolution is the rate-limiting step in the absorption process.
- The in vitro dissolution method provides in vivo relevant results.
- Unbiased estimates of the in vivo dissolution-time profiles are obtained from plasma concentration–time data (see sect. "Bioavailability Studies").

The drug release or dissolution can only be expected to fulfill the first prerequisite given above in cases of modified release formulations and poorly soluble drugs. In other cases, such as rapidly dissolving formulations of highly soluble drugs, or drugs with low permeability over the GI wall, gastric emptying and transport over the gastric mucosa, respectively, will determine the absorption kinetics. Thus, IVIVCs are not possible to obtain in those cases, since permeability and gastric emptying are not at all modeled by an in vitro dissolution test method.

It is important to realize that an established IVIVC is not a general characteristic of a drug compound that can freely be applied to all kinds of oral formulations. An IVIVC is, rather, specific for a certain type of formulation. The main limitation of IVIVCs is the problem of defining how large the changes made to a specific formulation can be without affecting the applicability of an established correlation.

Reports have been published in the case of ER tablets, showing that the relationship between in vitro and in vivo data could be altered by changing the quality of a critical excipient (Abrahamsson et al., 1994). The most conservative approach is to apply IVIVC only to formulation changes that are covered by the formulations included in the establishment of a correlation. However, provided that good knowledge exists regarding drug absorption properties, function of the dosage form and role of critical excipients, as well as the in vitro dissolution under various physiologically relevant conditions, somewhat wider applications are possible with reasonable confidence.

Three different types of correlation have been defined, levels A, B, and C, as described in Table 6. The following part of this chapter will describe how these levels are established and their respective roles, merits, and disadvantages.

Valuable additional information on IVIVCs can be found in Brockmeier (1986) and in Young et al. (1997).

Table 6 Different Types of In Vitro/In Vivo Correlations of Drug Dissolution

Type	Description	Example
Level A	In vitro and in vivo dissolution-time profiles are superimposable	
Level B	Relationship established between MDTvitro and MDTvivo determined by statistical moment analysis	
Level C	Relationship established between single-point in vitro dissolution rate characteristic and bioavailability variables	

Level A

Level A correlation is generally the most desirable form, since the in vitro method completely mimics the in vivo results, and a direct correspondence exists at each time point. The achievement of an in vitro method that models the entire in vivo process confers confidence in the method's capability as a surrogate for in vivo studies. This allows for predictions from in vitro data of complete absorption-time and plasma concentration–time profiles in early formulation development as well as in later phases, when relevant in vitro specification limits are settled. In addition, it is only level A correlations that are accepted by regulatory agencies as a basis for replacing in vivo bioequivalence studies with in vitro dissolution tests.

The development and evaluation of a level A correlation consists of the following steps:

1. Design and assessment of in vitro dissolution studies and human bioavailability studies
   - Choice/development of formulations
   - Study design aspects
   - Assessment of in vivo absorption/dissolution-time data
2. Establishment of an IVIVC
   - Relationship between in vitro and in vivo data
3. Evaluation of predictability
   - Prediction of drug plasma concentrations from in vitro model
   - Comparisons of predicted and measured bioavailability variables by calculation of the prediction error

Design and Assessment of In Vitro Dissolution Studies and Human Bioavailability Studies

It is possible to establish a level A correlation on the basis of data from only one formulation. However, this will not be sufficient for regulatory purposes in most cases, and an established correlation should preferably be validated by additional data. The most common approach is therefore to include several formulations with different in vitro release rates. Formulations with different release rates for IVIVC studies may be obtained by (1) choosing batches with different rates due to batch-to-batch variation, (2) altering the manufacturing process in a way that affects dissolution rate, (3) altering the amount or quality of critical excipients, or (4) altering the particle size or crystal form of the active drug substance. The ideal formulations for an IVIVC study should provide differences in the release rate of a magnitude that could be detected in vivo on top of the inherent pharmacokinetic variation. Furthermore, the mechanism of the variation of release rate should be known, and the modifications performed to obtain the different batches should be relevant for variations that may occur in normal production.

The in vivo bioavailability studies should generally be single dose, crossover studies with administration under fasting conditions, of formulations with different release rates, and a reference solution. The primary response variable in bioavailability studies aimed at establishing IVIVCs is the assessment of an in vivo dissolution-time or an absorption-time profile. Further details regarding assessment of such data are given in the section "Bioavailability Studies." The number of subjects to be included should be on the basis of the desired precision in the mean estimate of the dissolution-time profile.

The in vitro dissolution program may comprise tests under several conditions to find the optimal method (see sect. "In Vitro Dissolution") or may only include testing by use of a tentative production control method. It is crucial that frequent sampling be applied to appropriately characterize the entire dissolution-time curve, since tentative test points in a product specification are generally not sufficient. An adequate number of individual tablets should be tested. For regulatory purposes, 12 individual dosage units from each batch are usually required.

Establishing an IVIVC

When the obtained in vitro and in vivo dissolution-time curves for all included formulations are superimposable without further mathematical modeling, no additional steps are needed to establish an IVIVC. However, at times, some scaling of the in vitro data must be done to obtain superimposable curves. The same scaling factor should be used for all formulations. Linear scaling is recommended, especially in cases where few formulations (<3) are included in the IVIVC, although the use of nonlinear scaling functions has also been proposed. The scaling may be performed in two dimensions, either as a time scaling or as a scaling of the amount dissolved, at a certain time point. In the first case, the in vitro and in vivo time curves are made superimposable by the scaling of the time axis (Fig. 10A). The rationale for this approach is that the drug release/dissolution follows the same type of kinetics in vitro and in vivo, but the differences between the in vitro milieu and physiological conditions affect the rates. Another reason for time scaling may be lag times in vivo due to gastric emptying, which cannot be reflected by an in vitro test. An easy way to obtain a scaling function is to plot the time points from the in vitro and in vivo dissolution-time curves when equal amounts of drug have been dissolved, and subsequently fit a linear function to the data by linear regression. This function should then be used to transform the in vitro dissolution-time points to obtain an in vivo relevant dissolution-time curve. Another principle for scaling between in vitro and in vivo dissolution data is to adjust the y-axis, that is, the in vitro dissolution data, by the linear scaling factor ($y = kx$) to reach the same level when the dissolution process has been completed (Fig. 10B). Thus, the scaling factor k is determined from the ratio of the asymptotic plateau levels obtained in the in vitro and in vivo dissolution-time curves. The rationale for using this approach is that there may be differences in the extent of bioavailability between test and reference formulations that cannot be attributed directly to the formulation performance, but more to indirect effects (e.g., first-pass metabolism) due to the differences in the rate of administration or site of absorption.

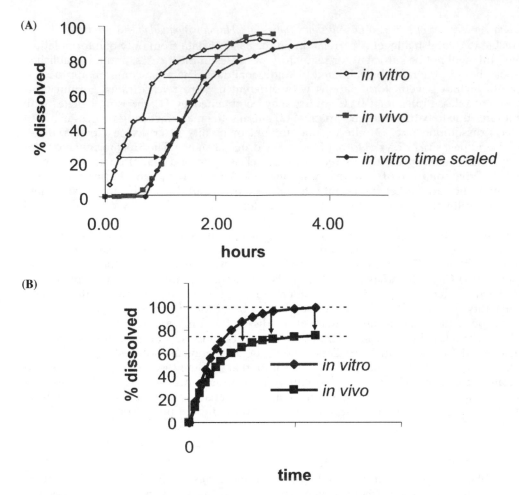

Figure 10 (**A**) Cumulative in vitro and in vivo dissolution-time curves, illustrating the time-scaling procedure of an in vitro dissolution-time curve to obtain an in vivo predictive in vitro model. (**B**) Cumulative in vitro and in vivo dissolution-time curves, illustrating a case where an in vivo predictive in vitro model can be obtained by scaling of the amount dissolved based on the ratio between the asymptotic plateau levels (*dashed lines*).

Evaluation of IVIVCs

The in vivo predictability of an in vitro model with or without a scaling function should be evaluated. A subjective assessment can be made by comparing the modeled in vitro dissolution data and the corresponding in vivo dissolution-time curves in a graph. However, a more stringent approach, applied in regulatory contexts, is to predict the plasma concentration–time profiles from the in vitro model and compare them to measured in vivo data. The latter step is performed by comparing the estimated and measured primary bioavailability variables, C_{max} and AUC.

　　　The plasma concentration–time data of a test formulation can be predicted from a dissolution-time profile, obtained from the in vitro model, and measured plasma concentrations for a reference formulation in the IVIVC bioavailability study (e.g., an oral solution), by use of convolution (see previous section). The difference in C_{max} and AUC based on predicted and measured plasma concentrations can be numerically assessed for each formulation by a simple estimation of the relative difference, denoted prediction error (PE), as follows:

$$\%PE = \left(\frac{\text{observed value} - \text{predicted value}}{\text{observed value}}\right) \times 100 \qquad (27)$$

This evaluation may be performed either by use of the same data, as included in the establishment of an IVIVC (internal predictability), or by use of other data sets (external predictability). The criteria for concluding a level A IVIVC in a regulatory context requires, in the case of internal predictability, an average percentage PE of $\leq 10\%$ for C_{max} and AUC, respectively, and the percentage PE for each formulation regarding these two bioavailability variables should not exceed 15% (FDA, 1997a).

Level B

A level B correlation is based on comparisons between MDT in vitro and MDT in vivo, or MAT. MDT and MAT are average rate characteristics, which take into account all data points. They are determined by statistical moment analysis, as described in the sections "In Vitro Dissolution" and "Bioavailability Studies" for in vitro and in vivo data, respectively.

To establish a level B correlation, in vitro and in vivo data for at least three formulations with different release properties are required. Each formulation provides one pair of in vitro and in vivo MDT values. A level B correlation can be concluded if a linear relationship is obtained between the in vitro and in vivo MDT values by use of linear regression.

Level B correlations can be used when level A correlations are not possible, due to different dissolution profiles in vitro and in vivo. The establishment of a level B correlation implies that the dissolution method can discriminate between formulations that are different in vivo. This provides an increased confidence in the suitability of a product control method or a method to be used for optimization during development. It is also possible to use a level B correlation for the scaling of the in vitro dissolution rate to obtain a more in vivo relevant estimate of the dissolution process. For example, if MDTvivo ∞ 2MDTvitro, the dissolution process is on average twice as fast in vivo compared to in vitro. The main disadvantage of level B correlations compared to level A correlations is lack of the possibility to predict the entire in vivo dissolution- and plasma concentration–time profiles from in vitro data. Therefore, level B correlations have very limited use in regulatory contexts.

Level C

A level C correlation establishes a single-point relationship between a measure of the in vitro dissolution rate, for example, the time when 50% of the dose has been dissolved ($t_{50\%}$), and a bioavailability variable, for example, C_{max} or AUC. Thus, a corresponding approach is applied as for level B correlations. An advantage of level C correlations, compared to level A and B correlations, is that no reference formulation is needed in the in vivo studies. Another advantage of a level C correlation is that the in vitro dissolution data are directly related to a bioavailability variable that can be more easily interpreted in a clinical context, compared to dissolution-time profiles and MDT. Level C correlations could also be useful for rapidly releasing formulations to assess at which level a formulation variable, such as tablet disintegration time or drug particle size, becomes a rate-limiting step in the absorption process and starts to affect the bioavailability variables. An example of such usage of a level C correlation is given in Figure 11. In this case, an initial phase is found where the in vivo variable is independent of the in vitro dissolution rate, followed by a linear relationship at slower dissolution rates. This could be useful in establishing the discriminating power of the

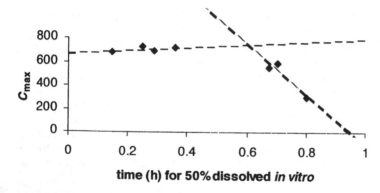

time (h) for 50% dissolved *in vitro*

Figure 11   Mean maximal plasma concentrations (C_{max}) versus time when 50% has been dissolved in vitro for seven different immediate release formulations. Two linear relationships have been identified, and the cross-section between the two lines indicates the critical dissolution rate at which the dissolution becomes the rate-limiting step in the absorption process.

dissolution test, optimizing the formulation during development and establishing biopharma-ceutically relevant specifications for drug particle size or other critical manufacturing variables.

The disadvantages of single-point level C correlations are that

- it is not possible to predict entire plasma concentration–time profiles from in vitro data,
- the single-point estimates, such as $t_{50\%}$ and C_{max}, do not take into account the majority of data points obtained in the in vitro and in vivo studies, and
- the bioavailability variable is influenced by several other pharmacokinetic drug properties that are not intended to be modeled by the dissolution test.

Single-point level C correlations, therefore, also have a limited use for regulatory purposes.

ANIMAL MODELS

Man is the ultimate model for in vivo evaluations, such as bioavailability studies or other investigations of new formulations. However, the use of animal models can provide some important advantages.

- The possibility to perform early in vivo studies during preclinical drug development before studies in man are possible.
- The use of advanced sampling techniques and other manipulations of experimental conditions are not possible in man.
- These studies are cheaper and faster than studies in man.

Animal models may thus not only be used as a screening tool before studies are performed in humans, but also for later mechanistic evaluations of findings obtained in human studies.

The main limitation of the usage of animal models is that no single species resembles all physiological properties of man. This introduces a risk that the results obtained in the animal model are not relevant for the situation in man. In the evaluation of oral dosage forms, the main aspects to consider are physiological features of the GI tract, such as dimensions, residence times in different segments, motility patterns, secretions, physical and physico-chemical characteristics of GI fluids, the presence of enzymes that could metabolize drugs, and critical excipients, since these factors could directly affect the formulation performance. In cases where the main study variable is the drug plasma concentration, other factors such as the presence of active drug transporters over the GI wall or species differences in first-pass metabolism may also confound the extrapolation of animal data to man. These problems can be handled by choosing the best possible animal model and an appropriate study design and by integrating knowledge of differences between animal and man in the interpretation of obtained results.

Choice of Animal Model

The great majority of studies are performed in dogs. They are, together with other animals such as pigs and monkeys, generally the most suitable species due to many anatomical and physiological similarities with man. Pigs and monkeys, however, have some practical disadvantages compared to dogs, such as being more difficult to train, the need for larger space, ethical concerns, and high costs. Rabbits are also used to some extent, despite some fundamental physiological differences to humans. Smaller animals such as rodents, common in other preclinical experiments, are often too small to allow administration of solid formulations.

The initial approach should be to first identify which formulation properties are critical for its in vivo function. Thereafter, all potential physiological factors that may influence this function should be identified and the correlation between the animal and man regarding those factors should be considered. For example, in the case of a pH-dependent enteric-coat

Table 7 Comparison of Anatomical and Physiological Data for the Cecum and Colon of Humans, Dogs, Swine, and Rhesus Monkeys

Parameter	Human	Dog	Swine	Monkey
Length (autopsy) (m)	7	4	15–20	5 cm
(in vivo) (m)	3	1.5		(duodenum)
Duodenal diameter (cm)	3–4	2–2.5	2.5–3.5	1.5–2
Villi				
Length	0.5–1.5		0.5–1	
Shape	Filamentous	Long, slender		Ridges, leaflike
Peyer's patches: location	Ileum	Duodenum, Jejunum, ileum	Jejunum, ileum, colon	Ileum
Secretions				
Bile				
Major acid	Cholic	Cholic	Hyocholic	
Concentration by gallbladder	×5	×8–10	×2	
Flow rate (L/day)	0.8–1	0.1–0.4		
Pancreatic juice flow rate (mL/min)	1	2–3	1	
Intestinal pH				
Fasted	6.1 (5.6–6.4)[a]	6.5–7.5	7.2 (duodenum)	7–9; 5.5–6.0
Fed	5.4 (5.0–5.8)[a]	6.5–6.9		
Cecum				
Length (cm)	7	12–15	20–30	5–6
Diameter (cm)	6		8–10	
Volume (L)	About 1	0.25	1.5–2.2	
Colon				
Length, overall (m)	0.9–1.5	0.6–0.75	4–4.5	0.4–0–5
Length, ascending colon (cm)	20		Long, coiled	10
Diameter (cm)	6	Similar to SI	8–10	
Haustrae	Present	Absent	Present	Present
Microbial metabolism, colon	Volatile fatty acids Vitamins	Very minor Vitamins	Volatile fatty acids	
pH, colon	6 (upper) 7.5 (lower)			

[a]Lower duodenum.
Source: From Dressman and Yamada (1991).

formulation, the dissolution of the coating layer will clearly be a critical formulation variable. The pH in the stomach and small intestine, as well as gastric emptying, will all be critical variables. If the correlation of such parameters with man is poor for all available animal models, there is no rationale for performing such studies if the deviations cannot be accounted for when interpreting the results.

Physiological and anatomical characteristics for different species are summarized in Table 7 (Dressman and Yamada, 1991). Some additional information of relevance for the use of animal models in formulation studies can be found in other review articles (Kararli, 1995; Ritschel, 1987; Martinez, 2002).

The most frequently used animal is the dog, which can in many cases be an acceptable model due to its similarity to man regarding anatomy, motility pattern, GI residence times, and many secretory components. However, cases exist where favorable results in dogs have not been verified in subsequent human studies. Examples of differences that could lead to pitfalls in formulation development studies are the following:

- No basal acid secretion in the stomach during fasted state, and thereby often close to neutral pH in contrast to the acidic human pH. However, an acidic pH may be induced in some individuals without intake of food. This has to be specially considered, for

example, when drug solubility is pH dependent and for enteric-coated formulations, for which drug release is dependent on the pH in the GI tract.
- The dog has a higher bile salt concentration than man, which could potentially lead to too favorable conditions for dissolution of very low water soluble drugs.
- Higher passive intestinal permeability than in man of low permeability compounds.
- Fed state could be introduced by coprophagy, which may lead to the tablets and capsules being retained in the stomach for a long time.
- The residence time in the colon is much shorter than in man, making the dog a poor model for long-acting ER formulations, due to the risk of incomplete drug release before the formulation is expelled from the body.
- The microbiological activity in the distal parts of the intestine is much less than in man, which has implications for drugs or excipients that are metabolized by gut flora enzymes, or drug release principles, on the basis of this process.

Study Design Aspects in Bioavailability Studies

Most investigations in animals aimed at evaluating new formulations are bioavailability studies, that is, the rate and extent of dissolution/release is determined from plasma concentration–time data. There may be differences in drug absorption, first-pass metabolism, distribution, and elimination between animals and man, which will lead to different plasma concentration–time profiles. However, this is a minor problem in the evaluation of dosage forms, provided that an oral drug solution is included in the study as a reference. Thereby, it is possible to eliminate the influence of pharmacokinetic factors other than those purely related to the formulation function. The same methods and assumptions should be applied as described in the section "Bioavailability Studies."

In most animal studies, the dose is given as the amount of drug in relation to body weight. In an evaluation of dosage form, it is preferable to administer the doses intended for humans to avoid development of specific low-dose formulations for animal studies. Two prerequisites of specific significance for the usefulness of this approach are (1) no toxicological effects at the given dose and (2) no saturation of any process involved in the drug absorption.

In the *administration of* solid *dosage forms* to dogs, the formulation is placed into the posterior pharynx followed by closing the dog's mouth. A feeding tube is subsequently inserted into the trachea, and 50 to 75 mL of water is administered. Liquid formulations are administered directly through a feeding tube. For administration to pigs or monkeys, applicators are often used to insert the dosage form. Small solid formulations (<5 mm) may also be administered to rats in this manner.

Many animals, including dogs, rats, rabbits, and monkeys eat excrement, which is called *coprophagy*. This could alter the physiological conditions in the GI tract, such as fasting/fed motility, secretions, and microflora, and thereby lead to an uncontrolled study situation. Furthermore, drug or metabolites that have been excreted by feces could be reabsorbed, which will obscure interpretation of bioavailability data. Thus, coprophagy has to be prevented by using cages with bottom screens and by placing plastic collars around the animal's neck, preventing the animal from reaching its anus.

Additional information on design of bioavailability studies in animals can be found in Ritschel (1987).

IMAGING STUDIES

Noninvasive imaging can be used to study the dosage form after administration in man or animals. The amount of radioactivity administered in such studies is at such a low level that no known hazards exist for study subjects. Several factors of relevance for the function of the formulation can thus be monitored directly in vivo. Potential study variables are given below:

- Residence time in different parts of the GI tract
- Location of a formulation within the GI tract at a certain time point

- Transit/emptying times in the GI tract
- Distribution of multiple units or liquid vehicles in the GI tract
- "Pharmacoscintigraphy"—relation of drug plasma concentrations to location of dosage form
- Disintegration/erosion of solid formulations
- Release of a marker substance from the formulation

More detailed overviews of different applications of imaging in in vivo studies of formulations can be found in Wilding et al. (1991) and Digenis et al. (1998a, b).

The imaging data can be used either as the main study variable, for example, in case of regional GI treatments, or to provide complementary information to bioavailability data. In the latter case, the obtained information regarding the location and performance of the formulation could often be crucial for correct interpretation of the bioavailability data, especially in the case of modified release formulations. Data obtained from imaging studies are generally not required by regulatory agencies, but they may well be used as supportive information in an NDA file.

Gamma scintigraphy has been established as the method of choice for in vivo imaging studies of formulations. Other methods such as positron emission tomography (PET), magnetic resonance imaging (MRI), ultrasound, and X ray have a much more limited applicability. Recently, the use of detecting low magnitude magnetic signals (magnetic marker monitoring) has emerged as an interesting alternative to γ-scintigraphy for studies of single units. In this technique, the dosage unit is labeled with a few milligrams of magnetized ferric oxide and monitored by a magnetometer previously used in studies of biomagnetism (Weitsches, 2005). This method has advantages by means of data quality, for example, temporal and spatial resolution, as well as practical aspects such as avoidance of radionuclides.

In γ-scintigraphy, the formulation is visualized by γ-radiation emitted from trace amounts of one or two radionuclides that have to be included in the dosage form. These types of studies in humans or animals are often performed at specialized Contract Research Organizations or at university hospitals. They involve several disciplines, besides traditional biopharmaceutical and pharmaceutical competence, such as radiochemical, nuclear medicinal, or other imaging expertise. However, it is crucial that the pharmaceutical/biopharmaceutical scientist, who understands the critical manufacturing variables and the biopharmaceutical function of a dosage form, cooperates with the radiation and imaging expertise in the design and evaluation of such studies. Furthermore, manufacturing and in vitro testing of labeled formulations may often be an in-house activity at the company developing the formulation of interest. The present chapter will include an introduction of the basic principles of γ-scintigraphy, different aspects of labeling of formulations, and performance of in vivo studies.

Basic Principles of γ-Scintigraphy

The physical principles of γ-scintigraphy are based on the fact that a radionuclide emits electromagnetic γ-rays at decay to stable isotopes. The decay of a radionuclide is logarithmic, and the half-life $(t_{1/2})$ is a key characteristic determined by the following equation:

$$A_t = A_0 e^{-kt} \tag{28}$$

where A_t and A_o are the radioactivity at time t and zero, respectively; k is a first-order decay constant, expressed in the same time unit as t. The decay half-life equals $\ln 2/k$. The amount of radioactivity is expressed in Bequerel (Bq), which corresponds to decay/sec or Curie (Ci), where 1 Ci = 3.7×10^{10} Bq. The γ-rays travel at the speed of light and permeate effectively through the formulation, body tissue, and air, although some energy is lost when the photon hits atoms. Such attenuation of the γ-radiation follows the following equation:

$$I_l = I_0 \times e^{-\mu l} \tag{29}$$

where I_l is the intensity of the radiation after traveling the length l through a material with an attenuation coefficient μ and I_0 is the intensity of the radiation before it hits the material.

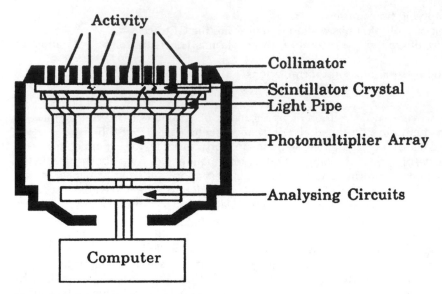

Figure 12   Schematic drawing of a γ-camera.

Typical lengths (l) in water and lead, which reduce the intensity to half of its initial value ($I_0/2$) for radionuclides used in formulation studies, are about 0.5 m and 1 mm, respectively.

    A schematic picture of a γ-camera is shown in Figure 12. The radiation enters the γ-camera through a collimator, which is a lead shield with many small holes. The purpose of the collimator is to limit the field of view and thereby prevent radiation from nontarget areas, such as naturally existing background radiation, from reaching the detectors. When the γ-ray has passed the collimator, it hits an NaI(Tl) crystal and a light impulse is created. An array of photomultipliers is used to determine the position of the light. The signal is then digitalized, and a picture can be produced, or other quantifications can be performed with computer programs. Two radionuclides can be monitored simultaneously if they produce different peak photon energies. This makes it possible to concomitantly administer two formulations with different labeling for head-to-head comparisons under identical conditions. Primarily, an image is obtained, which consists of a two-dimensional matrix of, for example, 64 × 64 units called pixels. The radioactivity gathered during the sampling period within each pixel will provide different colors on an image where most often black-blue-red-yellow-white corresponds to different intensities from very low to maximum. Examples of γ-camera images of a labeled multiple unit formulation at different times after intake are given in Figure 13. The data behind the construction of the γ-camera image may be further analyzed to obtain various quantifications, as described further below. The spatial resolution, that is, the minimum

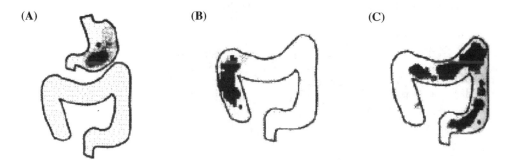

Figure 13   Example of a series of γ-camera images of pellet formulation obtained at 0.5 hour (**A**), 10 hours (**B**), and 24 hours (**C**).

distance between two labeled objects that can be distinguished by the camera, is dependent on the radionuclide, collimator, and distance from the object to the detector. A normal value of the spatial resolution obtained in phantom studies to mimic the in vivo situation is about 0.5 cm.

Labeling of Formulations

Labeling Principles

Radionuclides are generally introduced in the formulation by physical mixture rather than chemical bonding. The simplest procedure is to mix a radionuclide solution with other excipients, that is, in a normal granulation step, thereby getting an even distribution of the marker in the formulation. A formulation, or one of its intermediate states, could also be soaked in a solution of the radionuclide. Other methods are inclusion of the radiomarker as discrete particles formed by binding to a resin, precipitation as a poorly soluble salt or oxide, coating with nondissolving material or polymeric material, or by combinations thereof. Such particulate marker material could be included at well-defined positions within the formulation, or by random distribution of a multitude of particles. A formulation may include two radionuclides with different energies to follow more than one process at the same time.

The two main aspects in the radiolabeling of a formulation that will guide the choice of labeling principle are (1) that the labeling should provide an unbiased estimate of the decided imaging study variables and (2) that the function of the dosage form is unaltered. For example, if the purpose is to study the location of a solid dosage form at various times in the GI tract, it is critical that the marker is not released from the formulation. In addition, if the formulation is of a disintegrating type, it should be possible to conclude when this has happened to avoid the location of a free marker being interpreted as the position of the formulation. If the aim is to study drug release from the formulation, the radionuclide should be released from the formulation at a rate that corresponds to the drug of interest. The greatest risk for altered formulation performance by the labeling is if "microscale" manufacturing equipment has to be used or if other nonstandard manufacturing conditions exist to minimize radioactive exposure to laboratory personnel.

In Vitro Evaluation

Before performing an in vivo study, in vitro testing must be used to see if the intended function of the radiolabeling has been met and that the properties of the formulation are unaffected by the labeling. In these tests, the amount of radionuclide released from the formulation should be determined at physiologically relevant conditions. The amount of released radionuclide could be determined by liquid scintigraphy for assessment of radionuclide in solution and/or by assessing the remaining radioactivity in the solid dosage form by an ionic chamber detector.

Choice of Type and Amount of Radionuclide

Several radionuclides are suitable for use in imaging studies of formulations as outlined in Table 8. In the choice of radionuclide, the following aspects should be considered:

- Half-life of radionuclide
  - Duration of γ-measurements
  - Time needed for manufacturing and QC in advance of study start

Table 8 Radionuclides Suitable for Labeling of Formulations, Including Decay Half-Life $t_{1/2}$ and Peak Photon Energy

Radionuclide	$t_{1/2}$	Energy (keV)	Comments
Technetium (^{99m}Tc)	6.0 hr	140	
Indium (^{111}In)	2.8 days	173–247	
Iodine (^{131}I)	8 days	364	
Chromium (^{51}Cr)	28 days	320	
Samarium (^{153}Sm)	46.7 hr	69–103	Obtained by neutron activation
Erbium (^{170}Er)	7.5 hr	112–308	Obtained by neutron activation
Ytterbium (^{175}Yb)	4.2 days	114–396	Obtained by neutron activation
Barium (^{138}Ba)	84 min	166	Obtained by neutron activation

- Energy of radionuclide
  - Sensitivity of γ-camera crystal to detect radiation
  - Combination of two radionuclides with different energies for simultaneous measurements
- Suitability of physicochemical properties of available chemical forms of the radionuclide
  - Provide unbiased estimates of desired imaging variables
  - No systemic absorption

Most radionuclides are available as complexes [e.g., ^{99m}Tc-diethylenetriaminepentaacetic acid (DTPA)], or as oxides. The chemical and physicochemical state of the radionuclide should not be altered by either the formulation excipients and/or the physiological conditions in the GI tract. Such effects could lead to the radionuclide disappearing from the formulation in an unintended manner, thereby obscuring data evaluation. The amount of radioactivity included in a formulation is determined by the precision and variability that is required in the γ-scintigraphic measurements and by the acceptable level of radiation exposure to study subjects.

Safety Aspects in Manufacturing and Analysis of Radiolabeled Formulations
Radiation exposure is one of the most well-studied hazards to human health, but it has not been possible to link any increased incidence of impaired health at the levels of exposure that are allowed for laboratory personnel. However, higher radiation exposure is harmful, which has several important implications. First, key prerequisites are that personnel involved in the handling of radioactive material are properly educated in how to avoid unnecessary exposure to people and the environment, appropriate protective and dosimetry devices are used, and a plan is implemented for the handling and disposal of material. Second, it is usually not possible to use normal laboratory or pilot plant-scale equipment, since such batch sizes will require the handling of excessive amounts of radioactivity. Therefore, "microscale" equipment may be developed for certain processes.

Neutron Activation
Neutron activation is an elegant way to avoid restrictions and hurdles introduced by the handling of radioactive material in the manufacturing of formulations. Especially favorable is the possibility of using standard equipment and operation conditions. In this procedure, small amounts of a stable isotope, typically a few milligrams, are included in the formulation. The labeled formulation is subsequently exposed to a neutron flux, and the stable isotope is thereby transformed to a radioactive isotope upon capture of a neutron. The most commonly used isotopes for this purpose are listed in Table 8. Several of the listed radionuclides are available in both enriched and natural forms; the use of the former, however, requires a less stable isotope to be included and/or less neutron radiation, at the disadvantage of higher costs. The main potential problem connected with neutron activation of dosage forms is the risk of affecting tablet function or causing degradation of the active compound as well as of excipients. Therefore, this has to be checked on a case-by-case basis before the start of in an in vivo study. Another potential problem is the creation of radionuclides, other than the intended one, which will obscure data interpretation and increase radiation exposure. If the undesirable isotopes have a significantly shorter half-life than the labeling isotope, this problem can be handled by waiting for a suitable time period such that the activity of the unintended isotope has declined, whereas significant activity remains for the desired radionuclide. One example of a common stable isotope that unintentionally can form radionuclides by neutron flux is sodium (^{24}Na, $t_{1/2} = 15$ hours).

Reviews of different applications of neutron activation in studies of dosage forms can be found in Digenis and Sandefer (1991).

Conduct of In Vivo Studies

Practical Procedures
The subject is positioned in front of a γ-camera, or between two cameras, one in front of the subject and one behind (Fig. 14). The latter principle is needed when making quantifications of

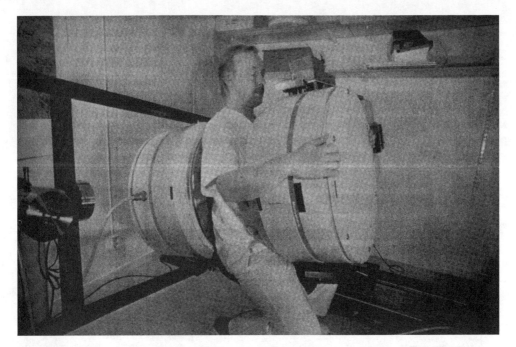

Figure 14 A γ-camera investigation with two opposite cameras.

radioactivity at different positions in the GI tract to avoid influence of the position-dependent attenuation of γ-radiation, whereas one camera system is generally sufficient for locating single units. Systems with cameras that circulate around the subject for creation of three-dimensional images are also available, but their use in formulation studies in man are restricted by the higher amounts of radioactivity needed in the formulation to obtain reliable data. The field of vision usually covers the entire GI tract in most subjects, but sometimes the position of the camera has to be adjusted to cover the lower parts of the abdomen.

The data collection can be dynamic, that is, the subject is constantly located in front of the γ-camera system, and signals are constantly gathered into images within very short time frames (often < 1 minute). This procedure may be advantageous to follow very rapid processes. In most cases, radiation is gathered over a finite time period to generate pictures. The time period for collecting radiation to one picture, typically 30 seconds to 1 minute, is mainly determined by quality requirements on picture/variability in quantitative data and the risk of moving artifacts.

Data Evaluation
It is almost always of interest to determine the localization, emptying times from one segment to another or transit times through a segment of the formulation in the GI tract. An example of the gastric emptying and colon transit time of a nondisintegrating tablet and small pellets after administration with a breakfast are given in Figure 15. Normally, it is possible to identify the stomach, terminal ileum, cecum, ascending/transversal/descending/sigmoidal colon, or rectum. In contrast to other parts of the GI tract, it is more difficult to obtain a precise position in the small intestine because of the anatomy.

The location of a single unit in the GI tract is determined from the position of the γ-camera image. Since no image of the GI anatomy is obtainable, an external radioactive marker may be positioned at a well-defined anatomical position as a reference point in the determination of the radiolabeled formulation. Another approach for facilitating determination of position is to administer a radiolabeled reference solution, which will provide images of certain intestinal parts, such as the stomach. In the case of solid multiple particles, or liquid

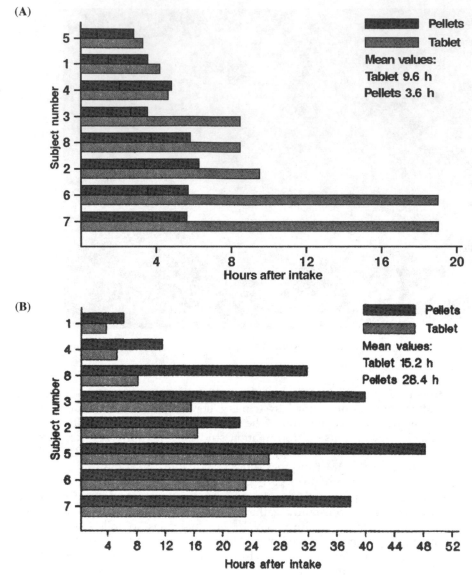

Figure 15 Gastric emptying time after administration with breakfast (**A**) and colon residence time (**B**) for a nondisintegrating tablet and pellet formulation in eight individual subjects. *Source*: From Abrahamsson et al. (1996).

formulations, the emptying, transit or arrival time is a continuous process over a certain time interval. This is exemplified in Figure 16, which shows the amount of food and a floating antacid remaining in the stomach at different times. The emptying or arrival processes from, or to, a certain region are determined by defining a region encompassing the area of interest. The number of counts obtained within this region is determined at several time points after correction for background radiation. The number of counts is often expressed as a percentage, defining the value obtained in the stomach immediately after administration as 100%. A rate constant, for example, the gastric emptying time, can then be determined from the emptying-time profile by applying moment analysis (see sect. "In Vitro Dissolution"), a model containing a rate constant or by just determining the time point when 50% has been emptied, based on the type of data presented in Figure 16. The gastric emptying of solids and liquids is often

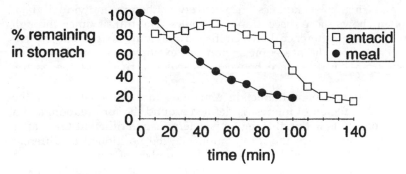

Figure 16 The gastric emptying of a meal and a floating antacid formulation after concomitant administration.

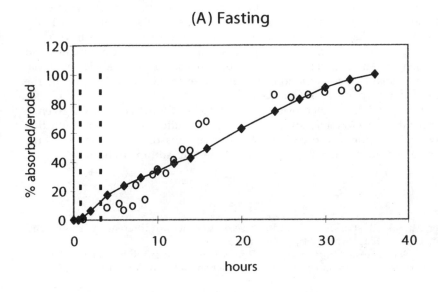

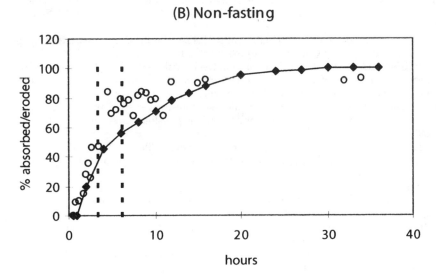

Figure 17 Tablet erosion (*circles*) and cumulative drug absorption (*diamonds*) for a hydrophilic matrix ER tablet after administration under (**A**) fasting and (**B**) nonfasting conditions in one subject. The two dashed vertical lines represent gastric emptying and colon arrival, respectively. The figures illustrate the correspondence between tablet erosion and drug absorption. In addition, the figures also show that the more rapid absorption after intake with food is caused by an increased erosion rate *Abbreviation*: ER, extended release. *Source*: From Abrahamsson (1998b).

approximated by zero- and first-order kinetics, respectively, although individual data, especially for particles, often shows more discontinuous profiles. The transit times through a segment are determined as the difference between the arrival time to the subsequent compartment and the emptying from the preceding region. For example, the small intestinal transit time is determined from the difference between the colon arrival and the gastric emptying times.

In quantification of the amount of radionuclide remaining in a formulation, for the monitoring of a release process, a region of interest is defined around the formulation, and a quantification of the number of counts within this region is determined at different times after correction for background radiation. Since the formulation may be positioned at different depths in the body at different times, which will affect the number of counts, obtaining simultaneous measurements by a posterior and anterior camera is necessary to avoid artifacts. The geometric mean of the number of counts obtained by the two cameras is used as the characteristic of the release process. The data may be expressed in a percentage, where the number of counts obtained within the formulation immediately after intake is defined as 100%. It is important to have frequent data sampling, since a certain number of images have to be discarded because of formulation movements during data collection or other anomalies and artifacts. A special problem in data evaluation could occur if release of radiolabeled material gather together with the remaining formulation, which, for example, may happen in the terminal ileum due to normal physiological function.

An example of determination of tablet erosion of a hydrophilic ER matrix tablet is given in Figure 17 where determinations were made after administration under fasting and nonfasting conditions. The scintigraphic erosion data revealed the underlying reason for an increase of the drug absorption rate obtained after nonfasting compared to fasting administration.

REFERENCES

Abrahamsson B, Alpsten M, Bake B, et al. *In vitro* and *in vivo* erosion of two different hydrophilic gel matrix tablets. Eur J Pharm Biopharm 1998a; 46:69–75.

Abrahamsson B, Alpsten M, Bake B, et al. Drug absorption from nifedipine hydrophilic matrix extended-release (ER) tablet–Comparison with an osmotic pump tablet and effect of food. J Control Release 1998b; 52:301–310.

Abrahamsson B, Alpsten M, Jonsson UE, et al. Gastro-intestinal transit of a multiple-unit formulation (metoprolol CR/ZOK) and a non-disintegrating tablet with the emphasis on colon. Int J Pharm 1996; 140:229–235.

Abrahamsson B, Johanson D, Torstensson A, et al. Evaluation of solubilizers in the drug release testing of hydrophilic matrix extended-release tablets of felodipine. Pharm Res 1994; 11:1093–1097.

Abuzarur-Aloul K, Gjellan K, Sjölund M, et al. Critical dissolution test of oral system based on statistically designed experiments. I. Screening of critical fluids and *in vitro/in vivo* modelling of extended release coated spheres. Drug Dev Ind Pharm 1997; 23:749–760.

Blanquet S, Zeijdner E, Beyssac E, et al. A dynamic artificial gastrointestinal system for studying the behavior of orally administered drug dosage forms under various physiological conditions. Pharm Res 2004; 21:585–591.

Box G E P, Hunter WG, Hunter JS. Statistics for Experimenters. New York: Wiley, 1978:291–432.

Brockmeier D. *In vitro/in vivo* correlation of dissolution using moments of dissolution and transit times. Acta Pharm Technol 1986; 32:164–174.

Crison J R, Weiner ND, Amidon GL. Dissolution media for *in vitro* testing of water-insoluble drugs: effect of surfactant purity and electrolyte on *in vitro* dissolution of carbamazepine in aqueous solutions of sodium lauryl sulfate. J Pharm Sci 1997; 86:384–388.

Diebold SM, Dressman JB. Dissolved oxygen as a measure for de- and re-aeration of aqueous media for dissolution testing. Dissolution Technol 1998; 5:13–16.

Digenis GA, Gold TB, Shah VP. Cross-linking of gelatin capsules and its relevance to their *in vitro-in vivo* performance. J Pharm Sci 1994; 83:915–921.

Digenis GA, Sandefer E. Gamma scintigraphy and neutron activation techniques in the *in vivo* assessment of orally administered dosage forms. Crit Rev Ther Drug Carrier Syst 1991; 7:309–345.

Digenis GA, Sandefer EP, Page RC, et al. Gamma scintigraphy: an evolving technology in pharmaceutical formulations development—Part 1. Pharm Sci Technol Today 1998a; 1:100–107.

Digenis GA, Sandefer EP, Page RC, et al. Gamma scintigraphy: an evolving technology in pharmaceutical formulations development—Part 2. Pharm Sci Technol Today 1998b; 1:160–165.

Dressman JB, Amidon GL, Reppas C, et al. Dissoluting testing as a prognostic tool for oral drug absorption: immediate release dosage forms. Pharm Res 1998; 15:11–22.

Dressman JB, Krämer J. Pharmaceutical Dissolution Testing. Boca Raton, FL: Taylor & Francis Group LLC, 2005.

Dressman JB, Yamada K. Animal models for oral drug absorption. In: Welling PG, Tse FLS, Dighe SV, ed. Pharmaceutical Bioequivalence. New York: Marcel Dekker, 1991:235–266.

El-Arini SK, Shiu GK, Skelly JP. Theophylline-controlled release preparations and fatty food: an *in vitro* study using the rotating dialysis cell method. Pharm Res 1990; 7:1134–1140.

EMEA. Note for Guidance on the Investigation of Bioavailability and Bioequivalence. London: European Agency for the Evaluation of Medicinal Products, 1998.

EMEA. Note for Guidance on Quality of Modified Release Products A: Oral Dosage Forms. B: Transdermal Dosage Forms Section 1 (Quality). London: European Agency for the Evaluation of Medicinal Products, 1999.

FDA. Guidance for Industry—Extended Release Oral Dosage Forms: Development, Evaluation, and Application of In vitro/In vivo Correlations. Rockville, MD: Food and Drug Administration, 1997a.

FDA. Guidance for Industry—Dissolution Testing of Immediate Solid Oral Release Dosage Forms. Rockville, MD: Food and Drug Administration, 1997b.

FDA. Guidance for Industry—Food-Effect Bioavailability and Bioequivalence Studies. Rockville, MD: Food and Drug Administration, 1997c.

FDA. Guidance for Industry—BA and BE Studies of Orally Administered Drug Products—General Considerations. Rockville, MD: Food and Drug Administration, 2000.

FIP. Guidelines for dissolution testing of solid oral products. Dissolution Technol 1997; 4:5–14.

Gabrielsson J, Weiner D. Pharmacokinetic/Pharmacodynamic Data Analysis: Concepts and Applications. Stockholm, Sweden: Swedish Pharmaceutical Press, 1997.

Gottfries J, Ahlbom J, Harang V, et al. Validation of an extended release tablet dissolution testing system using design and multivariate analysis. Int J Pharm 1994; 106:141–148.

Hansson R, Gray V. Handbook of Dissolution Testing. 3rd ed. Springfield, OR: Aster Publishing Corp., 2007.

Hauschke D, Kieser M, Diletti E, et al. Sample size determination for proving equivalence based on the ratio of two means for normally distributed data. Stat Med 1999; 18:93–105.

Jantratid E, Janssen N, Reppas C, et al. Dissolution media simulating conditions in the proximal human gastro-intestinal tract: an update. Pharm Res 2008; 25:1663–1676.

Johansson D, Abrahamsson B. *In vivo* evaluation of two different dissolution enhancement principles for a sparingly soluble drug administered as extended release (ER) tablet. Proceedings of the International Symposium on Controlled Release of Bioactive Materials. Control Release Soc 1997; 24:363–364.

Kararli TT. Comparison of the gastrointestinal anatomy, physiology, and biochemistry of humans and commonly used laboratory animals. Biopharm Drug Dispos 1995; 16:351–380.

Koch HP. The Resotest apparatus. A universally applicable biopharmaceutical experimental tool. Methods Find Exp Clin Pharmacol 1980; 2:97–102.

Langenbucher F. Parametric representation of dissolution-rate curves by the RRSBW distribution. Pharm Ind 1976; 38:472–477.

Langenbucher F. Numerical convolution/deconvolution as a tool for correlating *in vitro* with *in vivo* drug availability. Pharm Ind 1982; 44:1166–1172.

Lindstedt B, Ragnarsson G, Hjartstam J. Osmotic pumping as a release mechanism for membrane-coated drug formulations. Int J Pharm 1989; 56:261–268.

Loo JC, Riegelman S. New method for calculating the intrinsic absorption rate of drugs. J Pharm Sci 1968; 57:918–928.

Martinez M, Amidon G, Clarke L, et al. Applying the biopharmaceutics classification system to veterinary pharmaceutical products. Part II: Physiological considerations. Adv Drug Deliv Rev 2002; 54:825–850.

Riegelman S, Collier P. The application of statistical moment theory to the evaluation of *in vivo* dissolution time and absorption time. J Pharmacokinet Biopharm 1980; 8:509–530.

Ritschel WA. *In vivo* animal models for bioavailability assessment. STP Pharma 1987; 3:125–141.

Rowland M, Tozer TN. Clinical Pharmacokinetics—Concepts and Applications. Philadelphia: Williams & Wilkins, 1995.

Shah VP, Konecny JJ, Everett RL, et al. *In vitro* dissolution profile of water insoluble drug dosage forms in the presence of solubilizers. Pharm Res 1989; 6:162–168.

Shah VP, Tsong Y, Sathe P, et al. *In vitro* dissolution profile comparison—statistics and analysis of the similarity factor, f_2. Pharm Res 1998; 15:889–896.

Tucker GT. The determination of *in vivo* drug absorption rate. Acta Pharm Technol 1983; 29:159–164.

USP. U.S. Pharmacopoeia XXXI. Rockville, MD: United States Pharmacopoeial Convention, Inc., 2008.

Vaughan P, Dennis M. Mathematical basis of point-area deconvolution method for determining *in vivo* input function. J Pharm Sci 1978; 67:663–665.

von Hattingberg HM. Moment analysis *in vitro* and *in vivo*. Methods Find Exp Clin Pharmacol 1984; 6:589–595.

Wagner JG, Nelson E. Per cent absorbed time plots derived from blood level and/or urinary excretion data. J Pharm Sci 1963; 52:610–611.

Weitsches W, Kosch O, Mönnikes H, et al. Magnetic marker monitoring: an application of biomagnetic measurement instrumentation and principles for the determination of the gastrointestinal behaviour of magnetically marked solid dosage forms. Adv Drug Deliv Rev 2005; 57:1210–1222.

Wilding IR, Coupe AJ, Davis SS. The role of gamma-scintigraphy in oral drug delivery. Adv Drug Deliv Rev 1991; 7:87–117.

Young D, Devane JG, Butler J. In Vitro–in Vivo Correlations. New York, London: Plenum Press, 1997.

8 | Product Optimization

Mark Gibson
AstraZeneca R&D Charnwood, Loughborough, Leicestershire, U.K.

PURPOSE AND SCOPE

The major objective of product optimization is to ensure that the product selected for further development (the intended commercial product) is fully optimized and complies with the design specification and critical quality attributes (CQAs) described in the Target Product Profile and Product Design Report (refer to chap. 5). The traditional approach to product development described in the original version of this book emphasized that the following key outputs should be obtained from this stage of development:

- A quantitative formula defining the grades and quantities of each excipient and the quantity of candidate drug
- Defined pack
- Defined drug, excipient, and component specifications
- Defined product specifications

Although these are all still important, a paradigm shift led by the regulators in how products should be developed has added another dimension to the key outputs from product optimization. A series of quality-by-design (QbD) regulatory initiatives, including process analytical technology (PAT) and the ICH guidances [ICH Q8, pharmaceutical development; ICH Q9, quality risk management (QRM); ICH Q10, pharmaceutical quality systems (PQSs)], have been introduced to change the outputs from product optimization. The emphasis has changed from the need to demonstrate that the product will consistently meet relatively tight specifications to a new situation of being able to demonstrate that the product is controlled within a broader "design space." Product optimization studies are conducted to determine the critical formulation attributes and critical process parameters and to assess the extent of their variation on quality attributes of the drug product, and hence to define the design space. Once this is defined, then changes within that design space should not require further regulatory approval. This QbD approach encourages the need for a greater scientific understanding of the product/process and to firmly link product development with manufacturing design. As continuous quality verification is built-in with PAT-based manufacturing and process control strategies, traditional end-product testing and tight product specifications should become less significant and the desired state of "real-time release" should be possible.

The Food and Drug Administration (FDA) (Nasr et al., 2008; Wechsler, 2007) has led the way in encouraging drug developers to adopt this new quality-based approach to achieve a shared vision to reach the "desired state" of drug manufacturing in the 21st century, whereby

- product quality and performance should be achieved and assured by design of effective and efficient manufacturing processes and
- product specifications should be based on mechanistic understanding of how formulation and process factors impact on product performance.

Under the traditional manufacturing model, drug developers submitted extensive chemistry, manufacturing, and controls data (CMC) to the regulatory authorities that set tight product specifications. The aim being to develop commercial manufacturing processes to meet those specifications and to avoid changes later. However, this approach has resulted in frequent manufacturing failures and product recalls, leading to drug shortages and higher manufacturing costs due to low manufacturing efficiency, considerable waste, and low

Table 1 Traditional Product Development Compared with the QbD Approach

Aspects	Traditional	Quality by design
Product optimization	Empirical; mostly univariate experiments	Structured; multivariate experiments
Manufacturing process	Fixed	Adjustable within the design space
Process control	In-process testing and off-line analysis, with slow response for go/no-go response	Utilization of PAT for rapid feedback and real-time response
Product specification	Relatively tight limits and primary means of quality control based on batch data; difficult to justify decreased testing based on limited data	Part of overall quality control strategy
Control strategy	Reliance mainly on end-product testing; not appropriate for real-time release	Risk-based control strategy associated with better process and product performance understanding; real-time release possible
Life cycle management	Reactive to problems and out-of-specification changes; could lead to more postapproval changes needing regulatory approval	Continual improvement with changes enabled within the design space

Abbreviations: PAT, process analytical technology; QbD, Quality by Design.
Source: From Nasr (2006).

facility/equipment utilization rates. This in turn has resulted in a need for more regulatory oversight to deal with these issues. The new QbD approach encourages drug developers to use modern statistical and analytical procedures to define the critical sources of variability in the product/process and to establish appropriate quality controls. The intention is to demonstrate to regulatory authorities a sufficiently high level of understanding of the design space and quality control (QC). The expectation is that there will be significant benefits to drug developers of reduced costs, a smoother application approval process, and the potential to gain regulatory relief when making changes within the design space post registration and over-the-product life cycle. It is anticipated that the regulatory authorities will also benefit from a reduction in post-registration manufacturing supplements for modifications and changes to the production process. They should also see a reduction in the time spent on inspecting companies to review massive amounts of information because risk management is intended to identify areas that require closer monitoring and also those that require less attention. According to the shared vision, patients should also benefit because they are more likely to get improved access to high-quality affordable and innovative treatment options.

The situation prior to these ICH guidances was disparate regulatory requirements in the United States, Europe, and Japan for product development and registration. In the United States, pharmaceutical development information was submitted in Investigational New Drugs (INDs) and New Drug Applications (NDAs) at minimal levels mostly, and a Pharmaceutical Development Report was produced to summarize the development history to aid preapproval inspection (PAI). Whereas, in the European Union (EU) the development pharmaceutics sections describe formulation development and critical attributes and provide some information on the manufacturing design. In Japan, there was very limited product development information unless it involved a complex dosage form. Through these ICH initiatives there is greater harmonization of international agreement on key quality and Good Manufacturing Practice (GMP) principles, so narrowing the gap between regional expectations. The key differences between the traditional approach to product development and the QbD approach is summarized in Table 1 (Nasr, 2006).

ICH Guideline Q8 "Pharmaceutical Development"

The purpose of the ICH Q8 guidance on pharmaceutical development is to provide harmonized guidance for the suggested contents of section 3.2 P.2 (pharmaceutical development) contained in Module III of the Common Technical Document (CTD) for new drugs and biologics (FDA, May 2006). It was adopted as an ICH topic in October 2003 (International

Conference on Harmonization of Technical Requirements for Registration of Pharmaceuticals for Human Use), was finalized in November 2005, and came into effect in May 2006. ICH Q8 recommends that drug developers present the knowledge gained from pharmaceutical studies, which provide scientific understanding to support the establishment of the drug product and its specifications and manufacturing controls in the pharmaceutical development section of the drug marketing application. ICH Q8 adopts the FDA principles of QbD, also known as "building quality in" and "right first time." This deeper understanding of process control allows for the development of an expanded design space, which is defined as: "... the multidimensional combination and interaction of input variables (e.g., material attributes) and process parameters that have been demonstrated to provide assurance of quality. Working within the design space is not considered as a change. Movement out of the design space is considered to be a change and would normally initiate a regulatory post-approval change process. Design space is proposed by the applicant and is subject to regulatory assessment and approval" (FDA, 2006). Section 2 of the Q8 document states how the design space is established through product/process design. By making changes to formulations and manufacturing processes during development, drug developers should generate the scientific knowledge that supports "establishment of the design space." The Q8 document implies that both positive results and negative results are important to understanding the design space.

ICH Q8 (R1), the first revision of Q8, provides an annex to the already approved Q8 guideline and shows how the concepts and tools outlined in the parent document can be put into practice (ICH, 2008). This annex describes the principles of QbD and elaborates on the concept of design space with guidance on the selection of variables, defining and describing a design space in a regulatory submission, unit operation design space, relationship of design space to scale of equipment, design space versus proven acceptable ranges, and design space and edge of failure. Appendix 1 of ICH Q8 (R1) contains a useful table that compares a "minimal" approach with pharmaceutical development with an "enhanced" QbD approach. At a minimum, the pharmaceutical development report for a submission should provide information to support the formulation and manufacturing process proposed. To achieve this, pharmaceutical studies should identify properties of the active ingredient(s), excipient(s), and manufacturing process "that are critical and that present significant risk to product quality, and therefore should be monitored or otherwise controlled." However, although not mandatory, there is an opportunity for drug developers to perform additional pharmaceutical development studies that can enhance "knowledge of product performance over a wider range of material attributes, processing options and parameters" (Fig. 1). They can share this information with the regulatory bodies in the development report section of the marketing application to demonstrate a higher degree of understanding of the manufacturing process and process controls. By doing this, pharmaceutical companies can benefit from the possibility of risk-based review and inspection, being able to make manufacturing process changes within the approved design space without further regulatory oversight, and also, the potential for reduced end-product release testing through real-time QC.

Process Analytical Technology

The PAT guidance initiative was introduced by the FDA in 2004 to encourage the pharmaceutical and biotechnology industries to improve their production processes by implementing new monitoring and control technology (FDA, 2004), and the FDA definition of PAT has been broadly accepted by the industry and its regulatory partners. In the PAT guidance, FDA defines PAT as "a system for designing, analyzing and controlling manufacturing through timely measurements (i.e. during processing) of critical quality and performance attributes of raw and in-process materials and processes, with the goal of ensuring final product quality." The PAT initiative and design space are intricately linked, and it is the PAT tools described in the guidance that the FDA proposes should be used for gaining process understanding and can also be used to meet the regulatory requirements for validating and controlling the manufacturing process. For example, in traditional manufacturing processes, fixed blending times are specified, whereas in a PAT system mixing would continue until the system indicates that the blend is homogenous. A range of blending times may be specified on the basis of the variability of the process. A higher level of assurance of

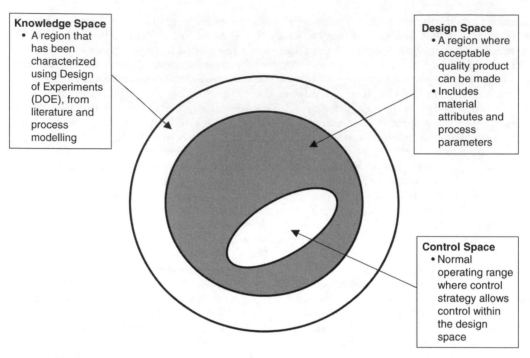

Knowledge Space
- A region that has been characterized using Design of Experiments (DOE), from literature and process modelling

Design Space
- A region where acceptable quality product can be made
- Includes material attributes and process parameters

Control Space
- Normal operating range where control strategy allows control within the design space

Figure 1   Representation of design space.

quality should be achieved by continuously monitoring, evaluating, and adjusting every batch, using validated in-process measurements, tests, controls, and process endpoints.

- *At line*: Measurements where the sample is removed, isolated from, and analyzed in close proximity to the process stream.
- *On-line*: Measurements where the sample is diverted from the manufacturing process and may be returned to the process stream.
- *In-line*: Measurements where the sample is not removed from the process stream and can be invasive or noninvasive.

The types of technologies that can be applied at-, in-, and on-line to measure, monitor, and control products and processes include near-infrared (NIR) spectroscopy, Raman spectroscopy, gas chromatography (GC)/liquid chromatography (LC) and acoustics, for example.

ICH Guideline Q9 "Quality Risk Management"
ICH Q9 was released as FDA guidance in 2006 (FDA, June 2006) and was later implemented in Japan and Europe. It outlines risk management principles and methods that can be applied to establish QRM systems, which can determine the appropriate level of control for a manufacturing process, from development to postmarketing manufacturing (the product life cycle). QRM involves identifying risks and then analyzing them, evaluating the consequences of a high-risk event, and establishing policies for risk reduction. The aim is not only to determine the most essential areas to monitor but also to evaluate where such efforts may not be necessary. The expectation is that drug developers will incorporate risk assessments during product development, utilizing any prior knowledge and experimental design data to determine the critical and noncritical parameters and attributes.

ICH Guideline Q10 "Pharmaceutical Quality Systems"
A third ICH guidance document (Q10) reached step-4 of the ICH process in June 2008. It is intended to harmonize the concept of quality systems for the pharmaceutical industry between

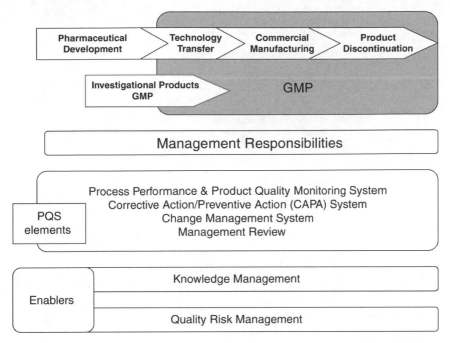

Figure 2 Diagram of the ICH Q10 pharmaceutical quality system model. *Abbreviation*: ICH, International Conference on Harmonisation.

the three regions: Europe, the United States, and Japan. This version contains a strong emphasis that one will only be able to achieve the aims of the new "quality paradigm" by implementing all three ICH guidelines Q8, Q9, and Q10. ICH Q10 enables the potential benefits from the other ICH guidance documents to be fully realized and links product development with risk management to assist drug developers in establishing PQSs. It encourages the industry to improve manufacturing processes, thus reducing undesired variability and leading to more consistent product quality, improved product robustness, and more efficient processes. Additionally, it recommends quality monitoring and review (e.g., data evaluation, statistical process control, and process capability measurements), which form the basis for continual improvement of processes. Figure 2 illustrates the major features of the ICH Q10 PQS model as defined in annex 2 of the ICH Q10 guidance.

The PQS covers the entire life cycle of the product, including pharmaceutical development, technology transfer, commercial manufacturing, and product discontinuation as shown in the upper part of the diagram. The PQS augments regional GMPs, including those applicable to the manufacture of investigational products. The next horizontal bar shows the importance of management responsibilities to all stages of the product life cycle as explained in section 2 of the ICH document. The following horizontal bar lists the PQS elements that support the PQS model. It is recommended that these elements be applied appropriately to each life cycle stage, recognizing opportunities to identify areas for continual improvement. The bottom set of horizontal bars shows the enablers the following: knowledge management and QRM that support the PQS objectives of achieving product realization, establishing and maintaining a state of control, and facilitating continual improvement.

ICH Q8 is a change from giving data to sharing knowledge with the regulatory authorities gained during product development, scale-up, and technology transfer from research and development (R&D) to Operations. Not every bit of information is mandatory, but it is understood that pharmaceutical development is a learning process, and it is acceptable to share information from both the successes and failures with the regulators. Discussions are ongoing between the regulators and the pharmaceutical industry using case studies and "mock" worked examples of regulatory submissions to illustrate the design space concept and to exemplify application of PAT, QbD, and QRM (ICH Q9) during the development process

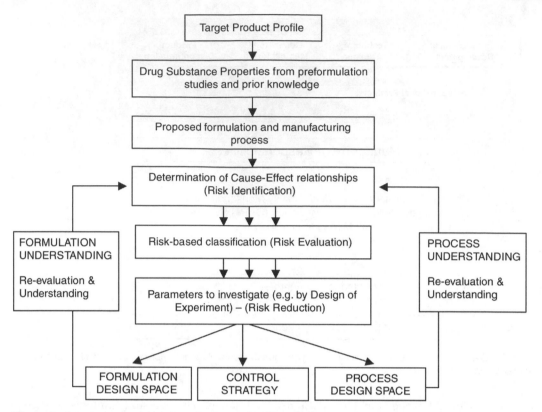

Figure 3 Iterative approach and application of ICH Q8 and Q9 to establish design space and control strategy. *Abbreviation*: ICH, International Conference on Harmonisation. *Source*: From Potter et al. (2006).

(Potter et al., 2006; Swanson, 2006). Figure 2 illustrates the iterative approach to formulation and process optimization of a pharmaceutical product using the scientific principles associated with the application of ICH Q8 and ICH Q9 to establish the design space and control strategy. Typically, the formulation and manufacturing process are developed first and then optimized by the iterative process described in Figure 3.

In July 2008, the FDA launched a QbD pilot program for biotechnology submissions to seek to define the clinically relevant attributes of biologics and link them to the manufacturing process. Many of the same fundamental QbD principles apply to both small molecules and biologics, but there is a greater challenge in characterizing complex proteins for routine QC. Through this program, the FDA will work with volunteer companies to gain the experience needed to implement a QbD, risk-based approach for complex biologics, and provide clear guidance to the industry. Additionally, ICH Q6B, Specifications: Test Procedures and Acceptance Criteria for Biotechnological and Biological Products, includes guidance for product characterization through the design of product specifications specifically aimed at controlling product heterogeneity. It allows for not testing certain impurities if supported by adequate process understanding and impurity clearance.

The approach to product optimization will depend on the nature of the product to be developed. It will always involve testing a range of options, for example, a variety of excipients from different sources, with different grades and concentrations, and in different combinations, or a range of pack sizes or different packaging materials. Additionally, it could involve testing a range of particle size distributions of the candidate drug or the excipients. Particle size may be critical for drug delivery or formulation processing. For example, material with a mean particle size distribution of 2 to 5 μm will be required for effective pulmonary delivery of aerosol suspensions and dry powders, whereas an even smaller particle size range (nanoparticles) may be required for the dissolution of poorly water-soluble drugs in parenteral formulations.

At the early stages of formulation optimization, preformulation studies are usually conducted to screen excipients or packaging materials and to select those compatible with the candidate drug, using accelerated stress-testing procedures. More details about the preformulation techniques, which can be employed for compatibility studies, are discussed in chapter 3. The importance of doing compatibility studies is for reducing the number of excipients and formulation options to test in further product optimization studies.

The final stage of formulation optimization will normally involve generating sufficient stability data on one or more variants to select the best variant. The optimal product will usually be selected on the basis of technical merit. However, there may be a need to consider other factors, such as the use of novel excipients and the associated safety/toxicological implications, supplier and sourcing issues, or the ability to patent the formulation or not. Some of these issues are discussed further below.

The manufacturing process used during product optimization should be designed with large-scale manufacture in mind. Ideally, the process should be as representative as possible to the eventual commercial-scale manufacture. This is because the manufacturing process may affect product performance characteristics and could influence the results of clinical studies. Although product and process design and optimization have been depicted as separate stages in the development framework, in practice they are often combined or closely linked. For example, it is important in pack optimization to select a pack that is suitable for use in production and will satisfy the demands of a high-speed automated filling line. Alternatively, the pack may have to be able to withstand stresses during processing, which could involve extremes of temperature or pressure, during autoclaving or freeze drying, for example. Process design and process optimization considerations are discussed later in this chapter.

At the completion of product optimization, when the best product variant has been selected, it is a good idea to summarize the work conducted in a Product Optimization Report. The report should reference the primary data from preformulation, product optimization, and stability studies, cross-referencing other investigational reports where necessary. It should clearly justify the recommendations for the quantitative formula, design space and the excipient, and component and product specifications. Such a document can be very useful to aid smooth technology transfer into production and for writing regulatory submissions.

EXCIPIENT AND PACK OPTIMIZATION CONSIDERATIONS

Excipient Selection
Historically, pharmaceutical excipients have been regarded as inert additives, but this is no longer the case. Each additive must have a clear justification for inclusion in the formulation and must perform a defined function in the presence of the active and any other excipients included in the formulation. Excipients are included for all sorts of reasons. They may function as an antimicrobial preservative, a solubility enhancer, a stability enhancer, or a taste masker, to name a few.

The International Pharmaceutical Excipients Council (IPEC) has defined a pharmaceutical excipient as any substance other than the active drug or prodrug that has been appropriately evaluated for safety and is included in a drug delivery system to

1. aid processing of the system during manufacture or
2. protect, support, or enhance stability, bioavailability, or patient acceptability or
3. assist in product identification or
4. enhance any other attribute of the overall safety and effectiveness of the drug product during storage or use.

In the 1960s, excipients were commodity items and tended to be of natural origin, but today many are synthetic or have been physically modified. Performance testing was done by the user, not the supplier. This has now changed with the introduction of recognized quality and performance standards for raw materials, which are defined in various pharmacopoeias (Moreton, 1999). The rationale for these changes is linked to the requirement to ensure that the patient is provided with the correct dose as safely and consistently as possible. This can only be achieved if the raw materials are of a consistent standard, together with the active and consistent processing.

Unfortunately, the standards for the same raw material can vary in different pharmacopoeias, and so the choice of pharmacopoeia will depend on the intended market for the product (see later comments about harmonization of standards). Suppliers should provide materials that comply with the specified pharmacopoeial standards. Monographs for excipients provide minimum tests and specifications, which can save time and resource negotiating new specifications with the regulatory authorities. Even so, the user may have to do additional tests to show that the excipient is suitable for use in a particular product or drug delivery system.

The basic selection and acceptance criteria for excipients to be used in a product being developed should have been defined in the Product Design Report section on "Design Specifications and Critical Quality Parameters." In practice, each excipient must be shown to be compatible with the formulation and pack and effectively perform its desired function in the product. At the same time, the product design acceptance criteria should be complied with, such as the following: the excipient should be well established, and its intended route of administration should be safe and acceptable to the regulatory authorities, and the excipient should comply with pharmacopoeial requirements, be globally acceptable, and meet the proposed design specification.

The case for using well-established excipients (and packs) that have already been administered to humans by the intended route, and in similar dosage forms, has been emphasized previously in the section on "Safety Assessment Considerations" in chapter 5. New chemical excipients (i.e., those that have not been used in registered pharmaceutical products before) usually require a full development program, including comprehensive toxicological testing, to gain "approval" by the regulatory authorities.

There are clearly cost and time savings of using well-established excipients that have already been approved for use in other registered products and that have an established safety profile. The regulatory status of excipients can easily be checked by consulting the FDA's *Inactive Ingredient Guide*, the *Japanese Pharmaceutical Excipients Directory*, or other similar sources of information (Table 1). These sources should provide information about registered products already approved, which contain a particular excipient with quantities used or a list of all products by dosage form that have contained a particular excipient.

Excipients are normally considered to be acceptable if they are listed in the major pharmacopoeias from the United States, Europe, and Japan. There has been much progress in harmonizing the monographs for key excipients in these pharmacopoeias. For products being developed for Japan, excipients must comply with the Japanese pharmacopoeia. If other pharmacopoeial grades are used, a detailed explanation of how these are equivalent or of better quality is usually required. However, even if the excipient is listed in all the major pharmacopoeias, additional toxicological studies may still be required to qualify an excipient under certain circumstances, such as (1) excipients used previously in humans but not by the intended route or (*ii*) increased concentration of an excipient above that previously used by the intended route. In either case, more extensive testing will be required so that the tests and specifications applied are shown to be capable of controlling the identity, strength, quality, and purity of the excipient to commensurate with its intended use. In Japan, excipients that have not been used previously will be treated as new excipients, even if they have been used in other countries.

Some assurance can be gained about the quality and safety of an excipient if a Drug Master File (DMF) is available and the DMF holder provides permission to reference it. The DMF is a document submitted to the FDA by a vendor that provides detailed information, including toxicological data and specification tests. Type III DMF is for packaging materials and type IV for excipients. A DMF is never approved, but it will be reviewed by the FDA if it is associated with a product license application. For more information about DMFs, refer to the FDA Guideline for Drug Master Files (FDA, September 1989) and the FDA Web site at www. fda.gov/cder/dmf/.

Some food and color additives may have GRAS (generally recognized as safe) status, which also gives some assurance that they could be used in pharmaceutical products with minimal additional safety testing. This is especially the case if the excipient is not likely to be absorbed systemically from the formulation.

However, there will always be situations where the introduction of a new excipient is inevitable. The candidate drug, for instance, may be incompatible with the current range of excipients. Another reason might be the phasing out of existing excipients for safety or environmental concerns, such as chlorofluorocarbons (CFCs) in metered-dose aerosols. There may be a need to introduce a new excipient for a novel drug delivery system or to overcome disadvantages with the currently available materials.

A common factor that often influences the selection of excipients and excipient suppliers is a company's historical preference for certain excipients based on proven technical, commercial, and quality criteria. Many pharmaceutical companies have a list of preferred suppliers that have already been audited and approved. There are significant advantages of selecting excipients that the company already uses, in terms of time and costs. Limiting the range of standard excipients on a company's inventory should minimize overhead because of the reduced auditing, analytical testing, and development required. Also, a greater knowledge can be developed about the characteristics of excipients that have been extensively used. Technology transfer from R&D to the final manufacturing site should be easier and faster if the excipients are already in the inventory, and the release specifications and analytical methods are already known to the QC department. However, a downside to having a limited company inventory is the reduced options of excipient choice placed on the formulator when faced with a new formulation or drug delivery challenge.

For products intended for global marketing, selection of excipients that meet the regulatory requirements can often be more challenging than the technical issues. Obtaining marketing approval for a new product requires the regulatory acceptance of the new candidate drug and the excipients used in the formulation. The specifications for excipients must comply with the pharmacopoeial standard for the particular country. Unfortunately, there is a diversity of specification tests and limits for the same excipients in the different pharmacopoeias. This issue has long been recognized, and there is an ongoing program to harmonize or unify the different requirements for some excipients in the three major pharmacopoeias—Europe, Japan, and the United States—through the ICH program. However, the process of establishing agreed international excipient specifications has proved to be extremely slow. Inevitably, some excipients for which pharmacopoeial standards are in conflict may be discounted from consideration, even though they perform well in terms of functionality.

Another issue for global marketing is the differences of opinion about the safety of some excipients in different countries. For example, ethylenediaminetetraacetic acid (EDTA) is permitted in most countries for use in intravenous (IV) injections as a metal ion–sequestering agent, but not in Japan. Colors, artificial sweeteners, and bovine-derived products are other examples where safety concerns vary significantly from country to country (Tovey, 1995). All dyes available for food and drug use are banned in at least one country. However, it may be essential to add a coloring agent to a product to distinguish one product from another or to differentiate among a number of product strengths.

Coloring agents may also be required for developing placebos to match colored products for blinding in clinical trials. Nedocromil sodium nasal, ophthalmic, and respiratory products are all examples that require color matching because of the inherent yellow color of the drug substance. This can be especially challenging when a range of drug concentrations is required, with each concentration having a different color intensity. For the above reasons, it is not always possible to develop a single formulation for the worldwide market.

The sourcing of excipients can be another important selection and optimization criterion. It is generally desirable to have excipient sources available in the country where product manufacture is taking place, to avoid stockpiling material to compensate for possible transport and import delays. Even better is if there are multiple sources of the same type of excipient so that if one supplier fails to deliver or discontinues delivery, an alternative can be used. This might rule out the use of some suppliers or excipients. To cater to different manufacturing sites in different countries, which might use slightly different equipment, it is important that the product and process developed are robust enough to cater to small differences in excipient characteristics and performance from different sources.

In conclusion, during product optimization, excipients will be selected on the basis of a variety of acceptance criteria. The quantities included in the formulation will be finalized on the performance characteristics of the excipient in the final product. At this stage it is important to fix the specifications of the excipients to ensure that the materials used, and hence the product, will be consistent throughout development. Setting product specifications is discussed in a following section.

Pack Selection and Optimization Considerations

A logical approach to packaging optimization is, first of all, to define the packaging function, followed by selection of the materials, and then testing the performance of the packaging to ensure that it will meet all the product design and functional requirements that were identified in the Product Design Report.

Product optimization of the pack should initially focus on defining the primary packaging (sometimes referred to as "primary container" or "immediate container"). This is most relevant to regulatory authorities because it is the primary packaging that is in direct contact with the drug product, including the closure, liner, and any other surface contacting the product.

The secondary packaging is the one outside the primary pack and, by definition, is not in direct contact with the drug product. Secondary packaging is often a carton or a blister, which may also function to protect the product from light or moisture. For example, it may be preferable to use a carton and a clear ampoule or vial, rather than an amber container for a photosensitive parenteral product, to allow users to inspect the contents of the primary package for contamination or signs of instability. There may be a requirement to have sterile secondary packaging, for example, for a sterile product likely to be used in an operating theater by a surgeon. The pharmaceutical company developing such a product should identify this requirement in the product design stage in the Target Product Profile to ensure that the pack and the sterilization process are considered during development. In the majority of cases, the purpose of the secondary packaging is simply to be elegant in its appearance, provide clear labeling instructions, and project a good marketing image.

Important selection and optimization criteria for the primary packaging may include the following:

- Satisfies environmental and legislative requirements for worldwide markets
- Availability of a DMF
- Ability to source from more than one supplier/country
- Acceptable cost of goods (particularly if a sophisticated device)
- Consistency of dimensions
- Consistency of pack performance
- Ability to meet function/user tests, customer requirements, and specifications

For some excipients, the global acceptability of some packaging materials varies from country to country. This can often stem from environmental concerns and the negative impact from the need to dispose of packaging waste. For example, polyvinyl chloride (PVC) is used widely to manufacture bottles and blisters for pharmaceutical products, but there is a growing concern about its safe use and disposal in some countries (Hansen, 1999). Incineration is the preferred method of disposal for PVC, with the downside that it emits toxic gases. Materials that are readily biodegradable, or that can be recycled, are preferred. This is not always possible with some types of synthetic materials.

Multiple sourcing of some synthetic polymeric materials may not always be possible, or desirable, because suppliers may have their own range of additives for the basic packaging material. It is therefore important that, once the packaging material has been established for a product, there is an understanding between the pharmaceutical company and the supplier not to alter the polymer formula or processing conditions without consultation. Any changes should become apparent if the supplier has filed a DMF with the regulatory authorities. Some sophisticated drug delivery systems, such as valves for metering pumps used for nasal and pulmonary delivery, can contain a multitude of components made of different materials and grades. It is important that the pharmaceutical company is made aware of any changes during development so that the implications for product performance and stability can be considered.

The role of the pack will include the following:

- Containment and protection of the product: to ensure stability over shelf life, protection to withstand the influences of climate, distribution, warehousing and storage during use, and protection for child safety.
- Presentation to the user (e.g., doctors, patients, parents): provides relevant information, identification, visually attractive appearance, and assurance against tampering.
- Administration of the product: provides convenient and consistent dose delivery.

Protection of the Product
The formulation must be protected from the environmental elements of heat, light, moisture, gaseous and sometimes chemical or microbial attack, as well as physical protection during transport and handling. A product license will not be granted unless the quality, safety, and stability of the formulation in the commercial pack of choice over the declared shelf life have been demonstrated to the regulatory authorities. They will be looking for acceptable stability data when the product is stored under anticipated normal conditions, in addition to acceptable data from "accelerated" or stressed conditions. This might include, for example, storage of the product in different orientations or in adverse conditions of extremes of temperature and humidity. Even though products will have recommended storage conditions on the label, there will be times when they are challenged to extremes outside of this, for example, during transportation. In the United States, it is common to post medicines to patients, and the product may be retained in postboxes that are very hot or humid. Appropriate stressed stability studies should demonstrate the integrity of the container and closure and any possible interaction between product and container. However, there is a possibility that components may be leached from packaging under accelerated/stressed conditions, which may not occur under normal conditions of use. Accelerated studies can be very useful for compatibility testing and screening materials, but they should be accompanied by long-term stability studies under normal conditions of use to confirm the suitability.

Other stress tests worth considering to establish the robustness of the product and pack include vibration and impact testing. Successful testing should instill confidence that the product can be transported and, to some extent, be physically abused (dropped) in the hands of users.

Two specific instances where the regulatory authorities will usually request extensive information are sorption of active(s) or excipient(s) from liquid and semisolid formulations and leaching of pack components into liquid or finely divided solid preparations, over the proposed shelf life of the product.

Plastics and rubber materials used in containers and closure systems can contain certain additives, for example, plasticizers, stabilizers, lubricants, and mold-release agents. It is worth asking the material suppliers what polymer additives are involved so that these can be analyzed when conducting compatibility studies. The regulatory authorities require that these additives should not be capable of extraction into the formulation or leach from the container/ closure to contaminate the product. Mercaptobenzothiazole (MCBT) is a common additive to rubber compositions used in closures for multidose parenteral containers, which is extremely toxic. For synthetic polymeric materials, the leaching of additives can result in morphological changes to the packaging materials. These changes may in turn affect physical properties such as hardness, stiffness, tensile strength, or viscoelasticity, which can be vital for pack performance. Leaking can be a problem because of the viscoelastic nature of some injection closure compositions. Other less obvious properties may also be affected, such as gas permeability and absorption. Permeation of gases or water vapor through the container material can affect formulation stability if the candidate drug is susceptible to hydrolysis or oxidation.

Drug and excipient interactions with the container may involve leaching, permeation, sorption, chemical reaction, or modification of the physical characteristics of the polymer or the product. During product optimization, formulation factors, such as the pH, concentration of ingredients, composition of the vehicle (solvents and surface active agents), area of contact, and contact time, will need to be evaluated. Also, processing variables such as temperature might be important. There are cases where the drug may absorb into components of the pack. This can be a particular problem with protein/polypeptide drugs onto glass and plastic packaging components. The best-known example of excipient adsorption or absorption is the loss of antimicrobial preservative from solutions to container/closure systems, most notably the rubber bungs of multidose injection containers, or the rubber gaskets used in metered-dose nasal pumps. The effective concentration in solution can be reduced to such an extent that the product is no longer protected from microbial growth.

There is also the possibility of constituents from label adhesives migrating through polyethylene or polypropylene containers. This is something to be aware of when carrying out stressed compatibility testing and long-term stability testing.

Packaging for sterile products must be effectively contained and sealed to prevent microbial contamination, and must be robust enough to withstand any sterilization process required. The sterilization process can affect the leaching of components from the container into the product or affect the physical properties of the container. For example, autoclaving can soften plastic containers, and γ-irradiation can cause certain polymers to cross-link.

Other protective elements have also become important in recent years, namely, those of child resistance and tamper evidence. Child-resistant packaging originated in the United States in the 1970s and was then introduced into Europe, where it was adopted mainly in the United Kingdom and Germany. There has been an ongoing debate between pharmaceutical manufacturers, container suppliers, and regulatory authorities on how to ensure that there is a practical balance between child safety and the pack being sufficiently user-friendly so that the elderly and arthritic can obtain their medication. Tamper-evident containers are closed containers fitted with a device that shows irreversibly whether the container has been opened. Tamper evidence is particularly important for sterile products and has become increasingly desirable for other products to demonstrate that the product has not been interfered with.

The FDA has published comprehensive information on container closure systems in a guidance for industry document, "Container Closure Systems for the Packaging of Human Drugs and Biologics: Chemistry, Manufacturing, and Controls Documentation" (FDA, May 1999).

Presentation to the User/Administration of the Product

For traditional dosage forms, such as tablets and capsules, the role of the pack is mainly for protection of the product during storage and presentation to the user. The design is not so critical for administration of the dose or performance of the product in the hands of the administrator (doctor or patient). For other dosage forms, such as inhalers for respiratory drugs and self-injection devices for parenteral products (e.g., insulin), the pack is an integral part of the drug product. These are often referred to as "drug delivery systems" because the packaging system or device in the hands of the administrator provides a means of ensuring that the correct amount of active drug product is delivered to the site of action as easily, reliably, and conveniently as possible.

With metered-dose inhalers (MDIs), for example, the FDA considers the drug product to be the canister, the valve, the actuator, the formulation, any associated accessories (e.g., spacers), and any protective secondary packaging. This is because the clinical efficacy of MDIs may be directly dependent on the design, reproducibility, and performance characteristics of the packaging and closure system. For these types of products, and other more sophisticated drug delivery systems, it is important that these product performance aspects are addressed during the product optimization stage. During development and before initiating critical clinical studies, the performance characteristics of the MDI (e.g., dosing and particle size distribution of the spray), in addition to the compatibility with the formulation, need to be thoroughly investigated.

When developing a product for Europe, which uses both device and medicinal product components (such as MDIs or powder-filled inhalers or prefilled syringes), the pharmaceutical company must establish whether the product will have to conform to the Essential Requirements of European legislation applied to medical devices (Medical Device Directive 93/42/EEC). If the medicinal product has a separate device element that could be refilled/reused, or the device and medicinal substance are presented separately, the device component will be subject to medical device controls, in addition to an application being made to the medicines authority (Tarabah and Taxacher, 1999). The letters "CE" are the abbreviations of the French phrase "Conformité Europeéne" which literally means "European Conformity" and is a declaration from the manufacturer that the product complies with the essential requirements of European health, safety and environment legislation. To obtain a CE mark for a medical device registered in Europe, there will be implications for the pharmaceutical company (and its suppliers) to have suitable quality systems in place (e.g., EN46001). Obviously, this should be established early on in product design to enable the appropriate routes for authorization to be obtained. Similar regulations apply for medicinal devices that will be marketed in the United States (cGMP, 21 CFR Part 820).

The packaging must also be convenient to use to promote good patient compliance, which is to encourage patients to take their medication at the correct times. User acceptance of the pack and/or delivery device can lead to that product being preferred in the market place. Product optimization studies may involve testing a range of pack options using a volunteer panel to establish the most user-friendly or patient-compliant packs that can be easily opened and closed. If a novel pack has been designed in-house by the pharmaceutical company, there is the possibility of filing a patent to gain market exclusivity for a number of years. Some examples of new innovations in pharmaceutical packaging development to improve drug delivery systems are described by Williams (1997).

SOURCES OF INFORMATION

Knowing where to find information about excipients and packaging materials as well as development and regulatory guidelines is critical to the preformulation and formulation scientist during the product design and optimization stages of development. Typical information that is often required for excipients and packaging materials include the chemical composition, function, chemical and physical properties, regulatory and safety status, manufacturers and suppliers, qualitative and quantitative composition of marketed products, stability data, known incompatibilities, and so on. Having this information can save much valuable time in the laboratory, generating the data from scratch.

There are also a lot of guidelines and regulations from various regulatory authorities and standard organizations to be aware of that affect product development. Some of the regulatory documents are legal requirements (regulations) such as the Code of Federal Regulations by the FDA, and some are regulatory requirements, which are stipulated within license applications, such as pharmacopoeial monographs. Others are guidelines, which must be followed or, if not, a very strong scientific argument must be provided for justification. For example, many of the documents published by the FDA as guidance are being held up by the assessors as a regulatory requirement. Companies have ignored these to their peril!

There is a host of reference sources available from literature, reference books, Web sites, and publications from various regulatory authorities and standard organizations. This section is not meant to be exhaustive, but should provide some general guidance to those developing new formulations.

If the excipient or packaging material has been used previously in marketed products by one's own pharmaceutical company, and the supplier has been audited, most of the information about these materials should already be available within the company. More often than not, excipients not listed in the company inventory will have to be considered. Some useful reference sources that may provide details of specific excipients and packaging materials are given in Table 2. These sources can be used to gain information about the choice and status of materials available. It should be possible to easily check whether the material of interest is well established, safe, and meets regulatory authorities' requirements or not. Some

Table 2 Sources of Information for Excipients and Packaging Materials

Source	Information	Comments
Various pharmacopoeias, e.g., United States/National Formulary; British, European, Japanese pharmacopoeias; Martindale, The Extra Pharmacopoeia; The Merck Index; The British Pharmaceutical Codex	Include standards and monographs for drugs, excipients, containers/closures, and medical devices	Updated regularly; many available in book format or CD-ROM; can be obtained through various publishers including Informa Healthcare
FDA Inactive Ingredient Guide	Lists excipients used in FDA-approved drug products marketed for human use by route administration and dosage form	Published by FDA, DDIR; available through FDA Web site; updated regularly
Handbook of Pharmaceutical Excipients	Excipient monographs containing data on uses, properties, safety, excipient interactions, standards; also a supplier's directory	A joint publication of the American Pharmaceutical Society and the Royal Pharmaceutical Society of Great Britain
Handbook of Pharmaceutical Additives	Excipients used in prescription and OTC products approved by the FDA or recommended by USP/NF, BP, and Ph. Eur., details manufacturers, composition, properties, function, and applications, toxicology and regulatory status of additives	Compiled by M. and I. Ash; Published by Gower, Aldershot, U.K, and Vermont, U.S.A.
Japanese Pharmaceutical Excipients Directory	Monographs on excipients used in pharmaceutical and cosmetic products	Edited by the Japan Pharmaceutical Excipients Council
Le Dictionnaire VIDAL	A codex of French-approved medicines includes quantitative composition of many products	
ABPI Compendium of Data Sheets and Summaries of Product Characteristics	Data sheets prepared by pharmaceutical companies on prescription and OTC products, including quantitative details of formulation ingredients and packaging used	Published annually by Datapharm Publications Ltd., London. Available electronically
Physicians' Desk Reference	Compendium of FDA approved pharmaceutical products; details formulation, pack, administration and use; identification guide	Published by Medical Economics Co., N.J., U.S.A., in participation with individual manufacturers; also PDRs for ophthalmology and nonprescription drugs; CD-ROM or hard copy or available electronically

Abbreviations: FDA, Food and Drug Administration; DDIR, Division of Drug Resources.

of the reference sources reveal quantitative compositions of products, giving an indication of acceptable levels that have been used previously in approved products.

Other leads can be found by browsing pharmaceutical and packaging technology journals or visiting trade shows and exhibitions.

Once a lead has been found on an excipient or packaging material of interest, the next useful step often is to contact the supplier for further information. It is usually in their interest to persuade pharmaceutical companies to use their materials because of the potential commercial return if the product is successful. Often, suppliers will assist customers with any enquiries and provide any missing information. They may provide small amounts of samples to try in attempts to satisfy the customers that their materials should be used. However, if a new supplier or material is seriously anticipated, it is wise to arrange for an audit of the supplier to ensure that it meets your company's appropriate quality standards, before becoming too committed. Also, it is advisable that more than one batch be evaluated to ensure

Table 3 IT Sources of Information and Development Guidelines

Source	Information	Comments
Food and Drug Administration (FDA)	Guidance for industry notes on various aspects of pharmaceutical product development, registration in the U.S.A., and inspections	Web site: http://www.fda.gov/
Committee for Proprietary Medicinal Products (CPMP) and European Medicines Evaluation Agency (EMEA)	Guidance for industry notes on various aspects of product development and registration in Europe, e.g., "Excipients in the dossier for application for marketing authorization of a medicinal product (III/3196/91)"	Web sites: http://www.eudra.org/emea/cpmp and http://www.eudra.org/w3/emea.html
National Institute of Health Sciences, Japan	Guidance notes on registration of pharmaceutical products in Japan	Web site: http://www.nihs.go.jp/
International Conference on Harmonisation (ICH)	Guidelines and information on harmonized requirements for product development and registration	Web sites: http://www.ifpma.org and http://www.chugai.co.uk
Web site for other regulatory authorities	Local regulatory guidance	Web site: http://www.pharmweb.net/
UK Medical Devices Agency (MDA)	Medical device regulations and guidance notes for industry on European Directives for medical devices	Web site: http://www.medical-devices.gov.uk/
International Medical Device Registration	A compilation of all the regulations affecting medical device registration worldwide	Book edited by M. E. Donawa Published by Interpharm
Parenteral Drug Association (PDA) and Pharmaceutical and Healthcare Sciences Society (PHSS)	Technical reports and guidelines prepared by industry on various parenteral topics, e.g., Sterile Pharmaceutical Packaging, compatibility and stability (PDA)	PDA Archive containing research papers, technical reports and conference proceedings available on CD-ROM; updated annually
International Federation of Pharmaceutical Manufacturers (IFPMA)	Information on pharmaceutical manufacturers	Web site: http://www.mcc.ac.uk/pharmweb/ifpma.html

Abbreviation: IT, information technology.

that the material is consistent. Be aware that sample materials are not always representative of purchased materials. They may have a different impurity profile, for example, or might have slightly different physicochemical properties that might give misleading performance results.

The rapid development in information technology (IT) in recent years has revolutionized the availability and speed of retrieval of information. Many reference sources are now available on CD-ROM, which are generally much easier to store, access, and search than books and journals. The introduction of the World Wide Web (WWW), with a user-friendly graphical interface based on hypertext links, provides easy access via the Internet to a wealth of information and databases, which are kept continually updated (D'Emanuele, 1996). Some of the useful Web sites for sources of information about pharmaceutical development and regulatory guidelines are listed in Table 3. The Web site addresses are correct at the time of this writing.

ARTIFICIAL INTELLIGENCE

Artificial intelligence (AI) technologies have been applied in the pharmaceutical field since the early 1990s. AI is defined as the ability of a machine to learn and "think" for itself from experience and perform tasks normally attributed to human intelligence, for example, problem solving, reasoning, and process understanding. Expert systems, neural networks, genetic algorithms (GAs), and neurofuzzy logic have been used to assist with formulation design and to obtain improved understanding of formulation and process optimization. They are widely used in situations where tasks are multidimensional and where relationships are nonlinear and extremely complex, for example, the underlying relationships between formulation components, manufacturing process conditions, and drug product quality. AI has become important in helping to make better use of information, increasing efficiency, and enhancing productivity. Many AI technologies are available as commercial software applications or computer-based programs for applications that include predictive models for various formulation types, and also, to model manufacturing processes and predict relationships between formulation properties and various process parameters (de Matas et al., 2007; Rowe and Roberts, 1998).

The development of a new medicinal product from a new molecular entity is a very time consuming and costly process. The formulator will usually start with a design specification. This could be very general, or it could be quite specific, perhaps expressed in terms of performance levels to be met in a number of predefined tests. To develop the formulation that will meet the product specification, the formulator will have to take into account several different technical issues such as the physicochemical properties of the candidate drug, the compatibility of the drug with pharmaceutical excipients, and packaging and the manufacturing process to be used. The formulator might have to go through several iterative formulation optimization steps before the ideal product is achieved.

Pharmaceutical formulation development is thus a highly specialized and complex task that requires specific knowledge and often years of experience. This type of knowledge is very difficult to document and is therefore often passed on by word of mouth from experienced senior formulators to new personnel. The loss of senior formulators from a company through retirement or transfers to other companies can lead to the loss of irreplaceable knowledge. Formulation "expert systems" have been developed to provide a mechanism of capturing and utilizing this knowledge and expertise.

Several different definitions for an expert system have been used (Partridge and Hussain, 1994; Turban, 1995). They all state that an expert system is an advanced computer program that mimics the knowledge and reasoning capabilities of an expert in a particular discipline.

In essence, the programmer will build a system based on the expertise of one or more experts so that it can be used by the layperson to solve difficult or ambiguous problems. The intent of an expert system is not to replace the human expert but to aid or assist that person.

An expert system consists of three main components:

1. *The user interface,* which is necessary for the expert system to interact with the user and vice versa.
2. *The inference engine,* the procedure, which generates the consequences, conclusions, or decisions from the existing knowledge extracted from the knowledge base.
3. *The knowledge base,* the set of production rules that is supplied by the human expert and encoded into rules so that the system can understand the information.

Expert systems can be developed using various techniques, including conventional computer languages (PASCAL and C), artificial intelligence languages (PROLOG, LISP, and SMALLTALK), and specialized tools known as shells or toolkits.

Expert systems shells are computer programs written in both conventional and specialized languages, which are capable of forming an expert system when loaded with the relevant knowledge. The development time of an expert system using a shell is much faster than using conventional languages and has therefore proved to be the method of choice. Shells used in product formulation vary from the relatively small and simple systems, such as Insight 2+ and Knowledge Pro, to the large and flexible Product Formulation Expert System (PFES) from Logica (UK). PFES was developed from research work conducted by a consortium of Shell Research, Logica (UK) and Schering Agrochemicals under the UK Alvey Programme, 1985 to 1987 (Turner, 1991).

To build a pharmaceutical formulation expert system, the formulation process has to be broken down into a number of discrete elements to provide distinct problem-solving tasks, each of which can be reasoned about and manipulated. However, as the formulation process is so complex, none of these tasks can be treated independently. A means of representing interactions and communicating information between tasks is therefore required. For example, one task may result in certain preferences that must be taken into account by subsequent tasks. To achieve this level of communication between tasks, the information in an expert system has to be highly structured and is therefore often represented as a series of production rules. An example of a production rule is as follows:

- IF (condition)
- THEN (action)
- UNLESS (exception)
- BECAUSE (reason)

Using a pharmaceutical example, this production rule would read:

- IF the drug is insoluble
- THEN use a soluble filler
- UNLESS the drug is incompatible with the filler
- BECAUSE instability will occur

The knowledge used in the production rules can come from many sources, including human experts, textbooks, past formulations, company standard operating procedures (SOPs), and development reports. The knowledge contained within these can be broken down into different types: facts, which are the objects and concepts about which an expert reasons, and rules and heuristics, which are often referred to as the expert's rules of thumb. The difference between rules and heuristics is that rules are always true and valid, whereas heuristics are the expert's best judgment in a particular situation and therefore may not always be true (Rowe, 1997). The knowledge will be put into the expert system shell by a knowledge engineer. The knowledge engineer is an IT expert who, through a series of interviews with the formulation experts, will capture all the steps involved in the formulation process. The knowledge engineer will then encode these tasks into a series of production rules, which he or she will build into the expert system. This process of knowledge acquisition can be very time consuming and therefore very expensive.

Reference to the use of expert systems in pharmaceutical product formulation first appeared on April 27, 1989, in the London's *Financial Times* (Bradshaw, 1989). This article was closely followed by one in the same year by Walko (1989). Both these authors described the work being undertaken by ICI (now Zeneca) Pharmaceuticals and Logica UK Ltd. to develop an expert system for formulating pharmaceuticals using PFES. Since these first publications, many companies and academic institutions have published on work being conducted in this area, as shown in Table 4.

A flow diagram of the AstraZeneca tablet formulation expert system is shown in Figure 4. The formulator enters the physicochemical information known about the drug, the

Table 4   Published Work on Pharmaceutical Formulation Expert Systems

Formulation	Company	System	Reference
Tablets	ICI (now AstraZeneca)	PFES	Rowe (1993a,b)
	Cadila Laboratories	PROLOG	Ramani et al. (1992)
	University of Heidelberg (GSH)	C/SMALLTALK	
Tablet film coating	GlaxoSmithKline (GSK) & AstraZeneca (AZ)		
Capsules	Sanofi Research Division	PFES	Bateman et al. (1996)
	Capsugel/University of London	C	Lai et al. (1995,1996)
	University of Heidelberg (GSH)	C/SMALLTALK	
Parenterals	ICI (now AstraZeneca)	PFES	Rowe et al. (1995)
	University of Heidelberg (GSH)	C/SMALLTALK	
Aerosols	University of Heidelberg (GSH)	C/SMALLTALK	

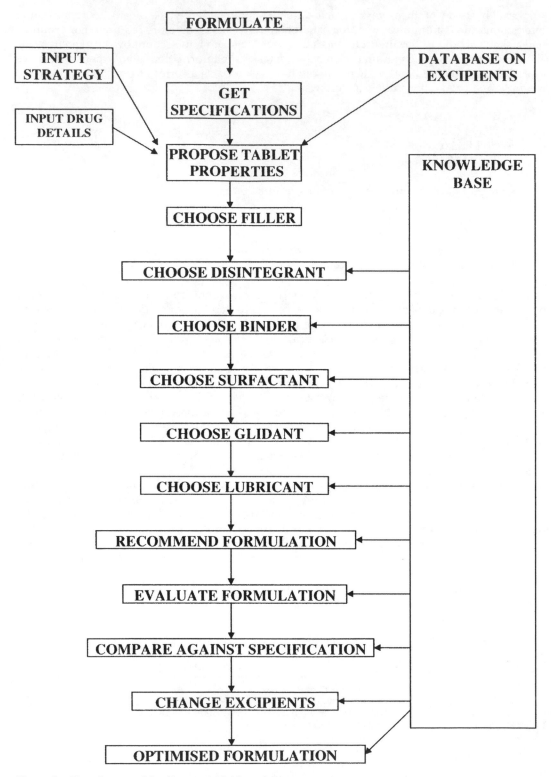

Figure 4   Flow diagram of the Zeneca tablet formulation.

specification for the formulation, and the formulation strategy (e.g., whether to use 1 or 2 fillers in the product). The system then goes through a series of steps from which the filler, the binder, the lubricant, the disintegrant, the glidant, and the surfactant and their relative proportions will be chosen. A formulation will then be recommended to the formulator. A series of defined tests can be carried out on the formulation to ensure that it meets the original specification. If it fails to satisfy the necessary requirements, the formulation can be optimized by feeding back the results into the system. The system has been designed to give a report on the decision processes used, which is the production rules that fired during the development of the formulation.

The following benefits have been seen from the development and use of formulation expert systems (Rowe and Upjohn, 1993):

- Protection of commercial knowledge. The expert system acts as a knowledge archive for formulation information, thereby overcoming the problems of staff turnover.
- Harmonization of formulation processes and excipient usage, giving a guarantee of a consistent approach to formulation within the same company.
- Training aid for novice formulators. Inexperienced formulators can quickly learn about a product or formulation area using an expert system. A spin-off from this is to release the time of more experienced formulators currently involved in the training process.
- Cost reduction. On the basis of the reduced time required for formulating and speed of development, Boots claim that they have saved 30 formulator days per year since the introduction of their sunscreen formulation expert system (Wood, 1991).
- Improved communication. The formulator and decision-making process is transparent to everyone in the company.

In spite of the many perceived benefits, the development of expert systems per se over recent years has been surprisingly slower than one would expect. One possible explanation for this is that when the systems were first introduced, their capabilities were overestimated, and they were seen as the panacea to all formulation problems. This was obviously not the case, but as a result, the systems are viewed with some degree of skepticism. Several reviews on the issues and limitations with the development of an expert system have been published (Dewar, 1989; Tinsley, 1992; Rees, 1996).

Other AI technologies that have been developed include neural networks, neurofuzzy logic, and GAs (Rowe and Roberts, 1998). Artificial neural networks are computer-based programs designed to mimic the process of the human brain's cognitive learning and work by building up a network of interconnecting processing units or nodes, which are the artificial equivalent of biological neurons. They can be used to find cause-effect relationships that may be hidden in experimental data and to generate predictive models, for example, to link important factors to measurable outputs such as the effect of drug particle size on tablet dissolution. Fuzzy logic is a powerful problem-solving technique based on mathematical theory that can be applied to control and decision making. It derives its power from being able to draw conclusions and to generate responses from vague, ambiguous, incomplete, and imprecise information. GAs are adaptive search algorithms, which are loosely derived from the principles of genetic variation and the Darwinian concept of natural selection. They provide another means of optimizing multivariant systems by identifying and evolving solutions until the desired combination of properties (e.g., formulation components or process parameters) giving optimum product performance is found. With the new regulatory paradigm where drug developers are expected to generate greater understanding of their products, the use of experimental design (see sect. "Experimental Design") coupled with AI technologies present a good opportunity to generate sufficient formulation and process understanding and build reliable predictive models. AI systems cannot be a substitute to an expert formulator, but can act as excellent decision-making tools.

EXPERIMENTAL DESIGN

The concept of experimental design originated in the agricultural industry and was developed by Sir Ronald Fisher. His first article appeared in the *Journal of the Ministry of Agriculture* in 1926, followed by a book *The Design of Experiments* in 1935. The concept of experimental design gradually spread to other industries, with the first publication of pharmaceutical relevance appearing in 1952 (Hwang, 1998). More recently, design of experiments (DOEs) techniques are being applied to formulation and process optimization because this is the most efficient means for identifying and studying the effect and interaction of product and process variables.

Pharmaceutical scientists are now almost universally aware of the disadvantages of traditional "one factor at a time" experimentation and recognize the advantages of a structured statistical approach to product development, as described below. Despite this, the routine use of experimental design in pharmaceutical development has only recently become widespread. The slow uptake of DOE techniques may have been a consequence of the lack of suitable user-friendly software packages. Until recently, scientists were forced to rely on SAS-literate statisticians, with the mechanics of data analysis being something of a "black box." This situation is changing with a number of easy-to-use software packages, such as Modde and Design Expert, being available. The impact of this development cannot be overstated; with relatively little statistical training, scientists are able to build their own experimental designs and analyze their data. Good statistical support remains of paramount importance, however, for all but the simplest of experimental designs, so that potential pitfalls are not overlooked. The key message from experience of using experimental design in pharmaceutical development is the importance of the pharmaceutical scientist and the statistician working side by side.

Benefits of Experimental Design

The potential benefits of using a structured statistically valid experimental design rather than using traditional one factor at a time experimentation are summarized below and are illustrated by the examples given later in this section.

- *Savings in time, money, and drug substance.* This is particularly important in early formulation development when both time and drug substance are usually at a premium. The use of a suitable screening design, such as a fractional factorial, can allow the main effects of a number of variables to be evaluated in a minimal number of experiments.
- *Identification of interaction effects.* One of the most important benefits of experimental design is that interaction effects between variables as well as the main effects of the individual variables can be identified and quantified. This is vitally important in instances where the effect of one variable is dependent on the level of another.
- *Characterization of response surface.* By defining how a response variable responds to changes in process variables, a process that is in a plateau region can be selected, thus avoiding carrying out a process close to an optimization precipice. In addition, knowledge of how a process responds to changes in one or more operating variables is invaluable in defining the design space and normal operating range.

The Practical Use of DOE Techniques

A detailed discussion of the statistical principles underlying DOE techniques is beyond the scope of this book. Rather, some literature examples are presented that serve to illustrate the potential utility of DOE in all stages of pharmaceutical development.

Screening Studies

Partial factorial designs are widely used in early preformulation and formulation development, since they allow a large number of variables to be evaluated using a relatively small number of experiments. Variables may be either quantitative or qualitative; for example, the presence or absence of a particular component at a fixed level could be an experimental variable. In full factorial experimental designs, every combination of variables is evaluated. This can lead to a large number of experiments, for example, a design that included four variables each at two levels would require 16 experiments. In a half factorial design this number would be reduced to eight. Clearly, there is a price to pay for this resource saving; some information on interaction effects will be lost by the process of confounding interaction effect terms with main effect terms. Nevertheless, the experiment can be structured such that those two-way interaction effects, which are suspected to be most significant, can be included in the model. Furthermore, fractional factorial experiments can be easily expanded by addition of the missing experimental runs. Hwang et al. (1998) described a tablet formulation optimization study in which a fractional factorial design was used to identify the formulation factors that were critical to achieving a high-quality product. Nine experimental factors were evaluated with only 16 experiments. Only main effects could be detected using such a small number of experimental runs, but statistical analysis of the data showed that only one factor required further optimization. This factor was then studied in detail in a subsequent optimization study. Plackett–Burnham designs, which are based on the two-level factorial approach, are widely used for screening studies where the main effects of a larger number of variables require evaluation in a limited number of experiments.

Optimization Studies

The use of a full factorial experimental design can provide a detailed understanding of the experimental response surface or design space. This type of design can be used when the number of variables to be investigated is small. Fransson and Hagman (1996) describe the use of a three-factor, two-level full factorial experimental design to evaluate the effects of light intensity, oxygen level, and phosphate content on methionine oxidation of human insulin-like growth factor. Although the basic design required eight experiments, a further four were carried out to provide an estimate of the inherent experimental variability. An interaction term was identified between the phosphate concentration and light intensity, with the effect of light being much greater when the phosphate concentration was high. The same technique was used by Bodea and Leucuta (1997) in the optimization of a sustained-release pellet formulation. Again, significant interaction effects were detected.

One of the limitations of two-level factorial designs is the assumption of linearity of the effects. In reality, it is rather unlikely that the factor/response relationship will be linear. This relationship can be characterized more fully by the use of three-level factorial experiments, but this adds considerably to the number of experimental runs required. Various other experimental designs can be used to obtain a detailed knowledge of the response surface. For example, Vojnovic et al. (1996) describe the use of a Doehlert experimental design in the optimization of a high shear granulation process. In this case, the authors were using experimental design to identify an experimental region in which the quality of the product was relatively insensitive to small changes in processing variables, thus verifying the robustness of the process.

An alternative method of optimization is the simplex search method. This is a model-independent procedure in which the results of earlier experiments are used to define subsequent experiments. This type of optimization is based on a systematic "trial and error" search for the optimum rather than statistical principles but can nevertheless be a useful method for defining the experimental region of interest.

Mixture Designs

Mixture designs are used in situations where the levels of individual components in a formulation require optimization, but where the system is constrained by a maximum value for the overall formulation. This is most easily illustrated by considering the optimization of a solution formulation containing a number of components each at a given percentage w/w. Clearly, the sum of all the components of the formulation, including water, must equal 100%. The experimental runs to be carried out depend on the model to be fitted. Marti-Mestres et al. (1997) describe the use of a simplex centroid design to optimize the relative proportions of three surfactants in a shampoo formulation. In this case, the total surfactant concentration was fixed at 18%, with the remainder being water and a number of minor components whose concentrations were also fixed and therefore not considered as experimental variables. Seven experimental runs were used to generate a quadratic model; a further three runs were carried out using other combinations of variables within the experimental region to check the fit of the model. Three response factors were used to evaluate the quality of the formulations, and contour plots were developed illustrating acceptable formulations in terms of the individual responses. These contour plots were superimposed to yield a relatively small area of the experimental region in which all three response factors were satisfactory. Vojnovic and Chicco (1997) used a similar approach but employed an axial design to evaluate the solubility of theophylline in a four-component solvent system.

It is evident that the use of suitably designed experiments can be an invaluable aid to the optimum use of resource at all stages of product development. In early development, screening studies enable the rapid assessment of the effect of several variables on the key characteristics of the product. More elaborate experimental designs can be used at the formulation, pack, and process optimization stages to ensure that the effect of all components and process variables are fully understood. Finally, prior to process validation, the use of experimental design techniques is invaluable in ensuring that the process is robust and that the operating region is not close to an "optimization precipice." The software tools are now available to enable the pharmaceutical scientist to exploit the potential benefits of DOE, and the regulatory authorities are now expecting DOE to be used in support of QbD.

STABILITY TESTING

The purpose of stability testing is to provide evidence of how the quality of a drug substance or formulated product varies with time under the influence of a variety of environmental factors such as temperature, light, and humidity. The ultimate goal of stability testing is the application of appropriate testing to allow the establishment of recommended storage conditions, retest periods, and shelf lives.

It is necessary to establish the "fitness for purpose" of the product throughout a proposed shelf life, which is to establish that all those attributes affecting product performance in use are not unacceptably changed during the period of storage up to the proposed expiry date. Testing must include factors affecting drug potency, formation of degradation products, and the microbiological and physical integrity of the product. It may also be required to measure other quality parameters considered important, such as the organoleptic and aesthetic properties of the product.

Stability studies are carried out during all stages of development of new drug substances, formulated products, and where appropriate, novel formulation excipients. However, the stability design and type of testing will depend on the stage of the development process and the nature of the drug and product under test. The types of stability studies carried out during development will typically include the following:

- Accelerated stress stability testing
- Stability to support safety and clinical studies
- Stability to support product license applications

Accelerated Stress Stability Testing

These are studies in which samples are stored under conditions designed to stress the drug substance or product. Techniques and test conditions that can be used are further discussed in chapter 6, "Preformulation Studies as an Aid to Product Design in Early Drug Development." Generally, samples are exposed to extremes of temperature or humidity. Also, exposure to intense light, metal ions, and oxygen may be investigated. The aim of these studies is to provide information about the possible routes of degradation of the drug substance and what chemical and physical factors will affect degradation. For the drug product, the compatibility of the candidate drug with potential formulation excipients and packaging, routes of degradation in potential formulations, and the identity of the major degradation products can be established. This information will provide important guidance to the formulator on the formulation factors that will affect product stability. Stability data from accelerated studies can also be used to predict shelf lives at ambient conditions as discussed below.

Stability to Support Safety and Clinical Studies

Although real-time data provide the ultimate test of the defined shelf life, the prediction of stability by the use of accelerated stress stability studies is vital in reducing the time to establish shelf lives for products used in safety and clinical studies. By applying the principles of chemical kinetics to data from accelerated storage tests, predictions can be made of the rate of decomposition at ambient temperatures. The Arrhenius relationship is often assumed for this modeling. However, this approach can sometimes fail to give good predictions when applied, because more complex decomposition is occurring, involving both chemical and physical factors. In these cases, more complex predictive models can be applied, but it may be that only real-time data can be used.

The regulatory authorities recognize that modifications are likely to be made to the method of preparation of the new drug substance and formulation and to the formulation itself during the early stages of development (phases I and II). The emphasis should generally be placed on providing information to develop a stable formulation and to support a shelf life suitable for the duration of the initial clinical studies.

During phases I and II, stability testing is required to evaluate the stability of formulations used in these clinical studies. The duration of the stability study will depend on the length of the clinical studies, usually one to two years. Data generated should be of the appropriate quality for submission to regulatory authorities, to support a Clinical Trials Application (CTA) or IND submission, for example. The information may also be used to provide supporting data for a product license application. These stability studies will monitor changes in product performance characteristics and identify formulation degradants produced under actual conditions of storage. Stability data should be sufficient to obtain the additional information needed to develop the final formulation and to select the most appropriate primary container and closure.

Stability to Support Product License Applications

In stability testing to support a product license application (usually conducted during phase III), the emphasis should be on testing the proposed commercial formulation stored in the proposed market packaging and using the final manufacturing process at the proposed commercial production site. Alternatively, the process must be representative of the final manufacturing process at a scale that should be at least 10% of that proposed for full commercial scale manufacture. Ideally, drug substance used should be synthesized using the final process. Stability data will be required on at least three batches of drug substance and for product batches made from three different batches of drug substance and different batches of excipients and packaging materials. If packaging components in contact with the product are obtained from more than one supplier and they are not considered to be equivalent, then product packed in components from both suppliers should be tested.

Detailed regulatory guidelines are available to provide assistance to companies making regulatory submissions, including recommendations regarding the design, conduct, and use of stability studies. Information is readily available from the Internet Web sites of various national and international regulatory authorities and manufacturers' associations:

- FDA (http://www.fda.gov/cder/guidance/index.html)
- CPMP (http://www.fda.gov/cder/guidance/index.html)
- ICH (http://www.ifpma.org)

Much progress has been achieved by ICH in harmonizing the requirements for stability testing in the three areas, namely, Europe, Japan, and the United States. Thus, information generated in any one of these three areas should be mutually acceptable in both of the other two areas, thereby avoiding unnecessary duplication of effort. ICH Q1 "Stability Testing of Drug Substances and Drug Products" was initially published in 1994, but has been revised in 2001 and 2003. This guidance defines what stability data package is required for a new drug substance or drug product registration application in the three regions. Additional published guidance on "Q1D Bracketing and Matrixing Designs for Stability Testing of New Drug Substances and Products" (2003) is intended to address recommendations on the application of bracketing and matrixing to stability studies conducted in accordance with principles outlined in the ICH parent guidance Q1A. The parent guidance notes that the use of matrixing and bracketing can be applied, if justified, to the testing of new drug substances and products, but provides no further guidance on the subject. In the Q1D guidance specific principles are defined for situations in which bracketing or matrixing can be applied. Examples are included where bracketing or matrixing could be acceptable for different strengths of the same product, different pack sizes, and different batch sizes, for example. A bracketing design can be usefully adopted to reduce the number of product strengths to be tested, but still cover the range of commercial product strengths. Similarly, a carefully designed matrix of testing can be used to reduce the number of product variants and time points tested, saving a lot of time and resource.

DEVELOPING SPECIFICATIONS

A specification is defined by ICH as a list of tests, references to analytical procedures, and appropriate acceptance criteria, which are numerical limits, ranges, or other criteria for the tests described. It establishes the set of criteria to which a drug substance or drug product should conform to be considered acceptable for its intended use.

Specifications will be required for the pharmaceutical active ingredient, any excipients used in the formulation, the packaging components, and the finished product (at the time of manufacture and over the shelf life). In all cases, the specifications tests and limits will evolve during development, as illustrated in Table 5. It is clearly beneficial to have full specifications in place for the start of the phase III pivotal clinical studies, when the product and process should have been optimized to ensure that there is equivalence between the product used in phase III and the commercial product.

Raw Material Specifications

The requirements for developing, testing, and setting of specifications for raw materials, whether they are new chemical entities (NCEs), pharmacopoeial active materials, excipients, or packaging materials, are essentially the same. Most emphasis is placed on establishing

Table 5 Development of Specifications

	Phase I	Phase II	Phase III	Commercial product
Active	Batch analysis; CofA; test methods developing	Draft specification; test methods developed and validated	Full specification; test methods developed and validated	Full specification; test methods developed and validated
Excipient	CofA and test methods developing on functional properties	Draft specification; test methods developed and being validated	Full specification; test methods developed and validated	Full specification; test methods developed and validated
Packaging	CofA and limited testing depending on functional properties	Draft specification; test methods developing and being validated	Full specification; test methods developed and validated	Full specification; test methods developed and validated
Finished product	Batch analysis; draft specification; test methods being developed	Refined draft specification; test methods developed (provisional) and partially validated	Full specification; test methods developed and validated	Full specification; test methods developed and validated

Abbreviation: CofA, certificate of analysis.

excipient and packaging specifications here because this usually involves an external supplier and the pharmaceutical company working together.

The initial concept and basic requirements for both excipient and packaging specifications should have been identified at the product design stage. For example, the design requirements for an antioxidant to be used in an IV injection may be of parenteral grade, GRAS status, or previously approved for use by regulatory authorities but must be compatible with the active pharmaceutical ingredient under development. Similarly, the primary pack should meet the basic product design requirements and be acceptable to regulatory authorities, should be available from multiple sources and reputable suppliers, should have a suitable volume for use, and should be sealed to maintain sterility; the container closure system should be compatible with the formulation.

If compatibility testing of the pharmaceutically active ingredient, excipients, and primary packaging components are satisfactory, development specifications are prepared for excipients and packaging materials to be used. These will contain essential information about the materials to be used, including the grade, proposed use, specific physical properties, and any testing required for investigational purposes. The quality of the raw materials used is vital to the effectiveness and quality of the finished product.

At the early stages of development, for example, to support phase I studies, pharmaceutical companies often accept excipient and packaging raw materials on the basis of a certificate of analysis (CofA) or certificate of conformance provided by the supplier. This is especially the case if it is a reputable supplier of an established material used by the industry. This reduces the pressure on the pharmaceutical company's analytical department to develop methods to test the materials at this early stage. The supplier may also provide useful information such as details of the critical dimensions and drawings for packaging materials.

With a new supply source or a new material, a pharmaceutical company will usually want to audit the supplier prior to accepting the material on a CofA. They may even want to repeat some of the tests on the CofA until there is confidence on compliance with the specification. The pharmaceutical company will want to seek assurance from the supplier that they are quality conscious at every stage of their process and have the facilities and internal systems and procedures in place to support this.

As product development progresses, the critical qualities of the raw materials will be identified, which affect final product quality, and results of investigational studies will be obtained to enable the specifications to be developed and refined.

Typical tests performed on raw materials, including the active pharmaceutical ingredient, excipients, and packaging components, are as follows:

- Appearance, for example, visual inspection, free from visible contamination.
- Identity tests, for example, comparison with a standard or by direct analysis, conformance with supplier's drawing.
- Chemical tests where appropriate, for example, for active, related substances, impurities.
- Microbiological tests where appropriate, for example, bioburden, absence of specific microorganisms.
- Relevant physical properties, for example, leak test, tensile strength, moisture vapor transmission, closure removal torque.
- Dimensional analysis, for example, for filling tolerances.
- Investigational tests, for example, reproducibility of dosing devices, particle size distribution of excipients.

Official compendia may provide tests and standards for listed excipients and for glass and plastic containers.

Packaging and excipient specification functional tests are developed on the basis of the functional requirements of these in the product. For example, the pack may have to prevent liquid loss and moisture ingress and maintain sterility or deliver a defined dose. An excipient such as an antimicrobial preservative must be able to preserve the formulation in the presence of the active and other formulation ingredients and in the intended pack. Excipient and packaging optimization must satisfy performance criteria, ensuring that packaging dimensional specifications and performance specifications can be consistently met at the extremes of the limits and during processing, handling, and transport. The evaluation of the sterilization process is particularly important for sterile products. Robustness to the sterilization process should be assessed, because it is possible that the thermal, electromagnetic, or chemical energy could adversely affect the properties of the materials in question. For example, there may be an irreversible loss in product viscosity, the embrittlement of polypropylene, or the loss in thermoplastic quality of polyethylene.

Once several batches of raw materials have been reviewed and tested to demonstrate that they will conform to the functional and quality requirements, the full excipient and packaging specifications can be finalized. Excipient and pack performance should be evaluated from a stability evaluation of the product and feedback from experience in clinical trials. Ideally, the specifications should be finalized for the start of phase III clinical trials. If for some reason, the excipient or packaging material has to be changed for phase III supplies, then some or all of the steps involved in the selection of materials, compatibility, and stability studies may have to be repeated.

Product Specifications

Product specifications will also evolve during development (Table 5). In the early stages, testing is typically performed on only a small number of samples due to the small scale of manufacture available. There may only be one or two product batches made to support phase I and early phase II studies. The specification limits also tend to be wide because of the limited data available. The specification limits are tightened as more information is gained from testing more batches, and the scale of manufacture is increased.

The product release specification contains tests and limits that apply after manufacture to release the product for use, whereas the product specification contains tests and limits with which the product must comply throughout its shelf life. The limits may differ from the product release limits to allow for changes during storage, for example, to allow for some drug degradation. Both product release and shelf life specifications are required for European regulatory submissions, but in Japan and the United States they are currently only interested in shelf life specifications. Some companies have internal or in-house specifications, which are different (usually tighter) from regulatory specifications. However, this can lead to confusion about which specification the product must comply with. Since the FDA only accepts the existence of the regulatory specifications, it is better to have "action limits" corresponding to the internal specification, rather than two sets of specifications.

When developing product specifications, test methods, and limits, the critical parameters must be identified and controlled, which affect the quality, safety, performance, and stability of the drug product. Several issues have to be considered, such as appropriate regulatory requirements and guidelines, for example, ICH, relevant compendial monographs and standards, and the capability of the manufacturing process and analytical methods used. Appropriate limits will also be influenced by safety/toxicology considerations. For example, impurities, degradation products, extractables and leachables, and preservatives should be qualified in safety studies.

Regulatory authorities such as the FDA publish specification guidelines with the expectation that pharmaceutical companies will comply with them. If there are difficulties in achieving the guideline requirements, or in the interpretation of them, it is advisable to discuss those points with the FDA. The internal regulatory group is usually the point of contact with external regulatory bodies. There are helpful ICH guidelines available on specifications, test procedures, and acceptance criteria, which describe the attributes that should usually be included for a variety of dosage forms. In particular, ICH Q6A and ICH Q6B provide guidance on specifications for new drug substances and new drug products, chemical substances, and biotechnological/biological substances, respectively. Other ICH guidelines are available, which describe impurities and residual solvents.

There are various general compendial monographs available on dosage forms, such as tablets and inhalation dosage forms, as well as compendial test methods and limits listed in the various pharmacopoeias. In spite of the progress made with harmonization, there are still some significant differences in the test procedures and limits recommended in the major pharmacopoeias. Often, the testing applied is aimed to cover the most stringent requirements.

During process optimization, the capability and robustness of the manufacturing process is assessed (as described later in this chapter on process robustness) to confirm that the specifications can be met at the extremes of the limits to define the design space. The capability of the test method, accuracy, precision, and reproducibility will also affect the limits that can be achieved.

With all test methods and limits there must be a sound technical justification to support them based on data generated for product and process optimization, clinical batches, and stability studies. A specification set too wide is more likely to be challenged by regulatory authorities. However, if the specification is too tight, it may result in some batches failing. It is considered best to freeze the specifications as late as possible so that considerable confirmatory data are available from all batches made to justify the limits. It is also very important to document the justifications for the specifications, and any changes during development, so that the complete specification development can be accounted for. This information will be required for the development report to support FDA PAI and regulatory submissions.

PROCESS DESIGN, PROCESS OPTIMIZATION, AND SCALE-UP

The primary objective of the process design and optimization stages of product development is to ensure that manufacturing operations supporting phase III studies and ultimately commercial manufacture are carried out under optimal conditions. The product should consistently comply with specifications.

Process design is the initial stage of process development where an outline of the clinical trial and commercial manufacturing processes are identified on paper, including the intended scale(s) of manufacture. This should be documented in a process design report.

The process design report should include all the factors that need to be considered for the design of the process, including the facilities and environment, equipment, manufacturing variables, and any material handling requirements. A list of typical factors to consider is given in Table 6.

Table 6 Process Design Considerations

Factor	Requirement	Purpose
Facility	Organization and layout	GMP
	Space	Health and safety
	Environmental control	Product sensitivity to:
	Temperature	Temperature
	Humidity	Moisture
	Air quality	Particulates/microorganisms
	Electrical zoned (flameproof)	Allow solvents for cleaning
	Barrier protection	Operator protection
Equipment	Type and design, e.g., bottom- or top-mounted mixing elements, baffles, heating/cooling jacket, etc.	Suitability for process mixing efficiency
	Materials of construction	Compatibility, extractives
	Range of sizes	Ease of scale-up
	Access to internal parts	Ability to clean/maintain
Material transfer	Product protection	Clean/sterile products
	Operator protection	Hazardous materials
Manufacturing variables	Order of addition of active and excipients	Mixing effectiveness
	Temperature	Stability/dissolution
	Speed	Mixing effectiveness
	Time	Mixing effectiveness
	Differences in excipient batches	Robustness of process

It is important to involve Production during the product design stage in the selection of equipment and the process. The eventual technology transfer is likely to be smoother if the same type of equipment employed by R&D is also available in Production on a larger scale. If a completely novel approach to manufacture is being considered, it is important that Production is made aware of this and can plan ahead to deal with the new process. This might involve the purchase of new equipment, which will have to be validated and which are needed to allow the technology transfer plans.

Other process design factors to consider are the need for any in-process controls during manufacture, with details of the tests and proposed limits. For example, the thickness, hardness, friability, and weight of tablets might be measured during the filling of a tablet product. The tests and limits applied will be based on experience gained from product development, optimization, and stability studies. Depending on the product being developed and type of process, it may be necessary to conduct preliminary feasibility studies before the process design report can be written.

Process Optimization

Process optimization will define and investigate critical process parameters, varying these within practical constraints to establish limits for the process parameters, within which acceptable product can be manufactured. Depending on the product being developed and type of process, it may be necessary to conduct preliminary feasibility studies before proceeding to process optimization. In a traditional approach to process understanding, every process parameter could potentially receive the same degree of scrutiny. However, this is not a very efficient way to evaluate all the possible permutations of process steps, process parameters, and raw material components. Process optimization can be streamlined by using existing data and knowledge, incorporating risk assessment and risk management tools, and applying statistically designed experiments (DoE) to define the acceptable operating ranges for both critical and noncritical process parameters. The QbD concept refers to a product and process that consistently delivers a product with the desired product quality attributes and provides a more structured approach to the identification of critical product quality attributes and how the process parameters (both critical and noncritical), which define the design space, affect them.

A useful approach to process optimization is to identify all the critical process parameters (CPP) that could potentially affect product quality or performance and prepare a process optimization protocol. The definition and concept of "criticality" with respect to process variables, for example, parameters, material attributes, and conditions, is a current topic of debate. The criticality task team within the ISPE Product Quality Lifecycle Implementation (PQLI) initiative has provided a concise, coherent, and universal approach for determining criticality to facilitate the consistent implementation of QbD principles and ICH Q8, Q9, and Q10 guidelines in the development of pharmaceutical manufacturing processes. The work is illustrated by useful case studies to increase understanding (Nosal and Schultz, 2008; Garcia, et al., 2008). A regulatory definition for a "critical process parameter" is: "A process input that, when varied beyond a limited range, has a direct and significant influence on a CQA, where a CQA is a quantifiable property of an intermediate or final product that is considered critical for establishing the intended purity, efficacy, and safety of the product." Risk is controlled for a CQA by establishing a product specification for the affected attribute.

From a business perspective, process parameters may have implications for optimizing yield, reducing costs, or improving process efficiency, but these should not be regarded as critical from a regulatory perspective. Typically, data used to identify CPPs will be derived from laboratory or pilot-scale batches and do not need to be confirmed on full-scale batches unless the control of the particular parameter can only be evaluated on a production scale (i.e., scale is a critical factor). There is good incentive to use the production facilities at the earliest opportunity, drug availability permitting, to iron out any transfer difficulties. Manufacture of the stability batches to support phase III studies, and also the phase III clinical batches, at the final commercial site should minimize any questions from the FDA during PAI about possible differences between R&D and Production process used.

The process optimization protocol should outline the program of work required to evaluate the effect of changes in the critical variables on product quality. This is to establish the working limits within which the process consistently produces product, which meets the CQAs. CPPs may include

- defining the order of addition of the active and excipients;
- defining the optimum equipment settings, for example, mixing speed;
- optimizing time-dependent process parameters, for example, mixing speed;
- defining the optimum temperature range;
- evaluating the effects of different excipient/active batches (within specification);
- setting in-process targets and controls; and
- developing cleaning procedures for the process.

Once the experiments have been completed, multiple regression analysis on the results can be performed using widely available statistical software to determine the effects of these process variables on the CQAs, their interactions, and their statistical significance. From this, a multidimensional picture of the design space can be produced. In the design space in which the process variables can consistently produce in-specification results, an area in the center can be selected as the operating space in which the process should be in control and should not drift into inoperable regions (Fig. 1).

On completion of the work program, a process optimization report should be written. This will summarize the results and evaluation of the activities specified in the protocol and also provide a rationale to define the operating limits for the process and the critical parameters affecting product quality or performance. The report should also conclude that the CQAs, including the specifications for the active excipients, components, in-process, and product can be met within the design space. The report and development data generated to establish process understanding provide the knowledge base to support and justify flexible regulatory relief for postapproval changes.

Process Capability and Robustness

Several pitfalls that are sometimes encountered with process development can hinder successful technology transfer to production, that is, if the process has not been designed or optimized with production in mind or a representative scale of production has not been used for the optimization studies. For example, the sterilization of a viscous ophthalmic gel by autoclaving at R&D on a 2-kg scale did not require any mixing of the bulk product for efficient heating and cooling. However, when transferred to production at a 100-kg scale, the heating and cooling times were found to be extensive, and the bulk contained hot spots because no stirring mechanism had been specified in the vessel.

Another pitfall is to design a process where the operating limits for one or more critical parameters are too narrow and cannot be consistently achieved. It is not acceptable if the process can be performed only by "experts" in R&D. Many pharmaceutical companies apply some measurement of process and equipment capability to demonstrate the reproducibility and consistency of the process in meeting specification limits. The process capability index (CpK) is often used to measure the reproducibility as a function of the specification limits. It is normally calculated from either of the two equations below, whichever gives the lowest number:

$$CpK = \frac{\text{upper limit of specification} - \text{mean}}{3 \times \text{standard deviation}}$$

or

$$CpK = \frac{\text{mean} - \text{upper limit of specification}}{3 \times \text{standard deviation}}$$

Some generally accepted rules, determined from experimental data, relate the CpK value with robustness. For example, a CpK of less than 0.8 is an indication that the process is not capable, as the acceptance criteria cannot be met routinely. Further work will need to be done to develop a more robust process. CpK values between 0.9 and 1.0 indicate a marginal process, between 1.0 and 1.25 are satisfactory, between 1.25 and 1.5 are good, and greater than 1.5 are excellent. Using these measurements, it is possible to evaluate process variables and identify which variable has the least or most effect. However, a possible pitfall is to obtain excellent CpK values, but not to have an acceptable process because the mean value is not on target. The process developed needs to be reliable and consistently meet product specifications to demonstrate it is manufacturable. Another pitfall is to aim for a CpK value much higher than 1.5, which is probably a waste of effort. The process does not have to be "bombproof."

Scale-Up

In reality, product and process development and scale-up will be progressing concurrently to meet the demands of phases I and II clinical and long-term safety supplies. The process used for initial clinical supply manufacture will probably be relatively small scale (laboratory scale). As more drug substance becomes available and the clinical requirements increase, the product batch size will increase to pilot scale, and the process may have to be modified during scale-up. If drug substance is available and very large phase III studies are anticipated, it may be essential to scale-up to production scale and transfer the process to the commercial production site at the earliest opportunity.

The objective of scale-up is to ensure that the process is scaled up to provide product, which will comply with specification and CQAs. Scale-up may encompass changes in process equipment and operation, with an associated increase in output, for example, in the following situations:

- An increase in batch size of 10-fold or greater on identical equipment
- Use of larger or high-speed versions of identical types of equipment
- Increase in output rate by more than 50% for identical equipment changes in equipment type for a given process step

Whenever scale-up is to be undertaken, it is strongly recommended that an experimental batch is manufactured to demonstrate that the process is still acceptable and the product is manufacturable on the increased scale. It must meet all the appropriate in-process and product specifications acceptance criteria.

Technology Transfer

The actual transfer of the manufacturing process from R&D to Production, along with the necessary knowledge and skills to be able to make the product, is referred to as "technology transfer." The ultimate objective for successful technology transfer is to have documented proof that the process is robust and effective in producing product complying with the registered specifications and GMP requirements.

The approach taken by different pharmaceutical companies to technology transfer varies widely from a "hand over the wall" to a more structured team approach. Clearly, the latter approach is more likely to result in successful technology transfer. In some companies, a third party is involved in the process, a specialized technology transfer group, which liaises between R&D and Production to ensure a smooth transfer. Companies vary in the way they divide responsibilities for technology transfer and the point of handover of responsibility, but there do not appear to be any clear advantages, provided the guidelines below are followed:

- Responsibilities are clear and well defined.
- Representation from Production and the technology transfer group are involved early, for example, during product and process design/optimization.
- Good communications are maintained with good R&D/Production interface. Time is spent face to face in factory and laboratory.
- There is good scientific basis for product/process design.
- Equipment used at laboratory/pilot scale is similar to production equipment.
- There is good documentation of product/process development and technology transfer.

A more comprehensive overview and guide to the technology transfer process for drug substance and drug product and the corresponding analytical tests and methods from R&D to Production can be found elsewhere (Gibson, 2005).

VALIDATION AND LAUNCH

The impact of QbD on traditional process validation to establish improved process understanding and the design space is a current topic of discussion. So much has changed since the FDA issued its "Guideline on General Principles of Process Validation" in 1987 (FDA, updated in 1999 and new draft available 2008), describing the principles and practices that are acceptable to the FDA and containing a section that describes the types of activities that should be considered when conducting process validation. Likewise, in Europe in 1999, the European Agency for the Evaluation of Medicinal Products (EMEA) and the Committee for Proprietary Medicinal Products (CPMP) issued a guidance on process validation with the aim of drawing together and presenting more clearly the requirements for effectively validating pharmaceutical manufacturing processes. With new levels of process understanding, and since the design space "assures quality" of the drug product, the value of conducting three arbitrary process validation batches to register a new product is being challenged (Bush, 2005). The design space limits should provide the basis of the validation acceptance criteria, and so once created, process validation becomes an exercise to demonstrate that the process will deliver a product of acceptable quality if operated within the design space and also that the smaller-scale systems used to establish the design space in R&D represent the performance of the commercial production scale process. It is anticipated that once the design space has been established and validated, the regulatory filing would include the acceptable ranges for all the CPPs within the design space and the control strategy. Although approaches to process validation may be changing, the principles of process validation have not changed:

- Identifying and controlling what is critical
- Using in-process measurements as part of evaluation
- Demonstrating a state of control
- Demonstrating reproducibility over time
- Identifying and documenting changes in controls

Clinical Trials Process Validation
At early clinical stages (phases I and II), where only limited GMP batches of product will have been produced and where product and process changes make batch replication difficult, only limited process validation may be possible. In such cases, the regulatory authorities will expect to see data from extensive in-process and end-product testing to demonstrate that the batch is adequately qualified, yielding a finished product that meets specification and quality characteristics.

For critical processes such as sterilization or aseptic manufacture, even for the earliest human studies, the regulatory authorities will expect the process to be qualified to attain a high degree of assurance that the end product will be sterile. If drug availability is an issue, the aseptic processing of sterile products may be validated using media fills to simulate the process (FDA 2004).

At later development stages, when process optimization has been completed and the design space and control strategy have been established, if clinical batches are being manufactured under replicated conditions, the regulatory authorities will expect process validation to be conducted. The actual process used and results obtained must be documented so that it can be duplicated. Normally, the product must meet predetermined product specifications and acceptance criteria on three occasions. The benefit of validating the process successfully is to reduce the amount of product testing.

Validation of Commercial Process

Process validation is currently still a requirement of the FDA Current Good Manufacturing Practices Regulations for Finished Pharmaceuticals, 21 CFR Parts 210 and 211, and of the Good Manufacturing Practice Regulations for Medical Devices, 21 CFR Part 820, and therefore is applicable to the manufacture of pharmaceuticals and medical devices intended for the United States.

The FDA's definition of process validation is to establish documented evidence, which provides a high degree of assurance that a specific process will consistently produce a product, meeting its predetermined specifications and quality characteristics.

As discussed earlier, the approaches to process validation are changing, but at the time of writing, the following still applies. Documented evidence must be achieved by preparing written validation protocols prior to doing the work and writing final reports at the completion of the work. The process equipment used should undergo installation qualification (IQ) and operational qualification (OQ) to establish confidence that the equipment was installed to specification and purpose and is capable of operating within established limits required by the process. Performance characteristics that may be measured include uniformity of speed for a mixer or the temperature and pressure of an autoclave, for example.

Performance qualification (PQ) is to provide rigorous testing to demonstrate the effectiveness and reproducibility of the process. PQ should not be initiated until the IQ/OQ has been completed and the process specifications have been essentially proven through laboratory, pilot, and scale-up batch manufacture. The PQ protocol should specify the approved procedures and tests to be conducted and the data to be collected. Acceptance criteria should be defined prior to starting the work. To gain a high degree of assurance that the process is reproducible, the traditional approach has been to manufacture at least three successive replicated process runs to ensure statistical significance. This approach may not be meaningful if it does not validate the design space, so it is recommended that the validation strategy is discussed with the regulatory authorities prior to commencing the work. According to QbD principles, validation consists of process development, process confirmation, and continual verification. The validation package of work will be flexible depending on the level of process knowledge and understanding and risk-based considerations. It is expected that the conditions for the different runs will encompass processing limits, widely known as "worst-case" conditions, but inside the design space limits. This will demonstrate whether the process limits are adequate to assure that the product specifications are met. PQ should ideally be undertaken at the scale at which commercial production will take place, although it may be acceptable to use different batch sizes if scale has been shown not to be a critical factor.

Preapproval Inspection

Once the clinical and safety evaluation studies for a new medicinal product have shown it to be safe, effective, and of acceptable quality, the pharmaceutical company will usually want to submit a marketing authorization application (MAA) or NDA to the regulatory authorities. Through the implementation of ICH Q8 guidance on pharmaceutical development the new regulatory submission will be defined according to section 3.2 P.2 (pharmaceutical development) contained in Module III of the CTD for new drugs and biologics (FDA, May 2006). ICH Q8 recommends that drug developers present the knowledge gained from pharmaceutical studies, which provide scientific understanding to support the establishment of the drug product and its specifications and manufacturing controls, in the pharmaceutical development section of the drug marketing application.

A current prerequisite to NDA approval in the United States is to have successfully passed an FDA PAI. The PAI will essentially be targeted at the commercial manufacturing facility to gain assurance that the facilities, equipment, procedures, and controls to manufacture the product are in place and conform with the NDA submission. The FDA will also want to check for compliance with current GMP (cGMP).

The FDA may also want to audit R&D to gain assurance that the product development has been done satisfactorily. In particular, the FDA may wish to see data that support the manufacturing process and controls from preformulation, product/process optimization, clinical trials process validation, and stability studies.

The FDA will check for equivalence, for both the drug substance and pharmaceutical product, between that used in the pivotal clinical studies, the pivotal stability studies, and commercial production. This is usually achieved by inspecting product and control data such as clinical trial batch records; in-process and end-product test results; and raw material, component, and product specifications. During an R&D PAI the FDA will also check for general compliance with cGMP, inspect the facilities and equipment used, and check the appropriateness of control systems and procedures.

It is in the interest of pharmaceutical companies to be in a state of readiness for a PAI. Staff should be aware of all procedures, policies, and regulations and have current training records. A good documentation storage and retrieval system is essential to be able to locate and retrieve records and reports efficiently. It is considered essential to have prepared a development report for the FDA to aid the PAI. The purpose of the report is to summarize all the product development and to demonstrate the equivalence of the manufacturing process and controls used for the pivotal clinical and stability batches and the commercial product. The typical contents of the development report requested by the FDA are as follows:

- Active and key excipients: physicochemical characteristics, particle size, purity, batch analysis.
- History of formulation and pack development: design rationale with critical characteristics affecting manufacture.
- History of process development: design rationale with CPPs.
- Specifications: rationale and supporting data for in-process and product.
- Product stability summary: equivalence of controls with commercial.
- Technology transfer batch history: list all batches made for development, safety, clinical, and transfer.
- Evaluate cause of failures and remedies.

The development report should be concise and structured. Clearly, it cannot be finalized until development is complete, but the preparation is much easier if summary reports have been compiled during development, such as the product and process optimization reports. The development report needs to be available to the FDA prior to the inspection, ideally, to give the FDA inspection team confidence that the product has been developed satisfactorily, perhaps resulting in a shorter inspection.

Consistent with the FDA's GMPs for the 21st century initiative, FDA is adopting a risk-based approach to prioritizing and conducting PAIs. They have reduced the number of PAIs on the basis of the current knowledge and cGMP status of companies. For a more comprehensive guide to successfully preparing for and passing PAIs, the book *Pharmaceutical Pre-Approval Inspections. A Guide to Regulatory Success* is recommended (Hynes III, 2008).

A successful PAI and regulatory approval of the NDA is usually followed by product launch. Launch activities need to be planned carefully and well in advance to ensure that no time is wasted after approval to sell the product on the market. The product insert and label claim will also have to be approved by the regulatory authorities. It may be better to wait for confirmation of approval before printing the labels and pack inserts; everything else can be prepared in advance. The launch stock is then packaged and labelled and QC released and then distributed for sale. Leading pharmaceutical companies can achieve this in one to two weeks postapproval, with good preparation and planning.

Postapproval Changes

Looking forward, submission of enhanced QbD information in a NDA or biologic license application toward the establishment of design space should enable the applicant to propose flexible regulatory approaches for postregulatory manufacturing changes. Therefore, changes within the approved design space should not require traditional postapproval regulatory submissions. However, the current status is that pharmaceutical companies and the regulators are still discussing how this will work in practice. Various workshops have been set up to discuss the types of information to be submitted and the type of regulatory flexibility as a result of sharing more extensive pharmaceutical development information in a QbD-based application.

Historically, pharmaceutical companies have often acknowledged changes after regulatory submissions have been done. Requests for postapproval changes could be for reasons outside the company's control, for example, because the source of raw materials changed, compendial specifications were revised, or suppliers of processing equipment made modifications. Alternatively, the change could be because the company wants to transfer a product to another manufacturing site. Sometimes changes are forced because the manufacturing process has not been properly evaluated, and it is found not to be robust enough until a few production runs have been made. Such a situation may be a consequence of the company striving for the earliest submission date, with an attitude of "we'll fix it later"!

However, with the traditional product development approach, all these changes require regulatory approval, and this can take significant time and result in lost sales. There are guidelines on the process for making changes in an initiative known as SUPAC or "scale-up and postapproval changes". SUPAC is designed to enable changes to be made to manufacturing processes with reduced regulatory input by providing guidance on what additional testing is required for specific changes.

There are a number of SUPACs, some approved (e.g., Immediate-Release Dosage Forms, Modified-Release Dosage Forms, and Semisolid Dosage Forms) and some still being considered (e.g., Sterile Products). SUPAC establishes the regulatory requirements for making changes to the composition or components of the dosage form, the batch size, the manufacturing process or equipment, or the site of manufacture. Different levels of change are defined and require different actions, for example:

- Level I—unlikely to have a detectable impact on product quality, for example, a change in the mixing time within the validated range; action: notify FDA in the annual report.
- Level II—could have a significant impact, for example, a change of mixing time outside the validated limits; action: submit updated batch records, generate and submit long-term stability in annual report, generate dissolution profile data, and notify the FDA of changes for approval.
- Level III—likely to have a significant impact, for example, a change from direct compression to wet granulation; action: (*i*) submit updated batch records, three months' accelerated stability data, dissolution data, in vivo bioequivalence study (unless in vitro/in vivo correlation verified), and long-term stability data and (*ii*) notify the FDA of all changes for approval

In Europe, there are different arrangements from country to country when changes to MAAs are to be made. It is a legal requirement in the European Community (EC) that all marketed products comply with the details of the MAA. Changes may or may not require prior approval, depending on the type of change. For example, a type I variation or minor change, such as a change in batch size, may not require prior approval. Details are submitted to all member states where the product is sold and deemed approved if there are no objections within 30 days. Type II variations, or quite major changes, have to be submitted to all member states where the product is marketed, and the change must be approved or rejected within 90 days. A significant change such as a change of strength or indication would probably require a new application. Companies can make an early submission and avoid regulatory delays by knowing in advance what changes are allowed without preapproval.

In terms of the type of regulatory flexibility proposed or envisaged in a QbD application, it has been suggested that no postapproval filings should be required for the following changes (Nasr et al., 2008):

- Manufacturing site change, alternate packaging or packaging sites, alternate analytical methods, and testing sites, scale-up.
- Movement within the design space and/or proven acceptance ranges.
- Replacement of end-product testing with in-process testing.

It is clear that flexibility would be dependent on what information was submitted in the application, and although still early days, there is definitely opportunity for companies to benefit from the QbD approach.

REFERENCES

Bateman SD, Verlin J, Russo M, et al. The development and validation of a capsule formulation knowledge-based system. Pharm Technol 1996; 20(3):174–184.

Bodea A, Leucuta SE. Optimisation of propranolol hydrochloride sustained release pellets using a factorial design. Int J Pharm 1997; 154:49–57.

Bradshaw D. The computer learns from the experts. Financial Times (London). April 27, 1989.

Bush L. The end of Process Validation as we know it? Pharm Technol 2005; (August 2). http://www.pharmtech.com/pharmtech/content/printContentPopup.jsp?id=173672.

D'Emanuele A. The communications revolution. Int Pharm J 1996; 10(4):129–134.

Dewar J. Expert systems trends revealed. Syst Int 1989; 17(7):12–14.

FDA. Chemistry Guidance Document on Drug Master Files (1). Rockville, MD: Center for Drug Evaluation and Research Food and Drug Administration, 2004.

FDA. Guideline on General Principles of Process Validation. Rockville, MD: Food and Drug Administration, 1999.

FDA. Guidance for Industry: Container Closure Systems for Packaging Human Drugs and Biologics: Chemistry, Manufacturing, and Controls Documentation. Rockville, MD: Food and Drug Administration, May 1999.

FDA. Guidance For Industry on Sterile Products Produced by Aseptic Processing. Rockville, MD: Food and Drug Administration, 2004.

FDA. Guidance for Industry: "PAT—A Framework for Innovative Pharmaceutical Development, Manufacturing and Quality Assurance" in Center for Drug Development and Research (US Food and Drug Administration). 2004. Available at: www.fda.gov/cder/guidance/6419fnl.doc.

FDA, Guidance for Industry: ICH Q8 Pharmaceutical Development. Rockville, MD: Food and Drug Administration, May 2006.

FDA, Guidance for Industry: ICH Q9 Quality Risk Management. Rockville, MD: Food and Drug Administration, June 2006.

Fisher RA. The arrangements of field experiments. J Min Agr Engl 1926; 33:503–513.

Fisher RA. The Design of Experiments. 7th ed. Edinburgh: Oliver and Boyd, 1960.

Fransson J, Hagman A. Oxidation of human insulin-like growth factor I in formulation studies II. Effects of oxygen, visible light and phosphate on methionine oxidation in aqueous solution and evaluation of possible mechanisms. Pharm Res 1996; 13(10):1476–1481.

Garcia T, Cook G, Nosal R. PQLI Key Topics—Criticality, Design Space, and Control Strategy. J Pharm Innov 2008; 3:60–68.

Gibson M, ed. Technology Transfer: An International Good Practice Guide for Pharmaceutical and Allied Industries. Bethesda, MD: PDA; River Grove, IL: Davis Healthcare International Publishing LLC, 2005.

Hansen OG. PVC in Scandinavia. Med Device Technol 1999; 10:31–33.

Hynes MD III, ed. Pharmaceutical Pre-Approval Inspections. A Guide to Regulatory Success. 2nd ed. New York, USA: Informa Healthcare, 2008.

Hwang R. Formulation/process optimisation using design of experiments. Paper presented at WorldPHARM 98, September 22–24, 1998, Philadelphia, PA.

Hwang R, Gemoules MK, Ramlose DS, et al. A systematic formulation optimisation process for a generic pharmaceutical tablet. Pharm Technol 1998; 5:48–64.

ICH Q8 (R). Annex to ICH Q8 Guidance on Pharmaceutical Development, 2008. Available at: http://www.ich.org.

Lai S, Podczeck F, Newton JM, et al. An expert system for the development of powder filled hard gelatin capsule formulations. Pharm Res 1995; 12(9):S150.

Lai S, Podczeck F, Newton JM, et al. An expert system to aid the development of capsule formulations. Pharm Technol Eur 1996; 8(9):60–68.

de Matas M, Shao Q, Shukla R. Artificial Intelligence The key to process understanding. Pharm Technol Eur 2007; 19(1):44–48.

Marti-Mestres G, Nielloud F, Marti R, et al. Optimisation with experimental design of nonionic, anionic and amphoteric surfactants in a mixed system. Drug Dev Ind Pharm 1997; 23(10):993–998.

Moreton CR. Aspects relating to excipient quality and specifications. Pharm Technol Eur 1999; 12:26–31.

Nasr M. FDA's Quality Initiatives—An Update. Presented at the 10th APIC/CEFIC Conference, Warsaw, Poland, October 2006.

Nasr M, Migliaccio G, Alle B, et al. FDA's Pharmaceutical Quality Initiatives—Implementation of a Modern Risk-Based Approach. Pharm Technol 2008; 5:54–72.

Nosal R, Schultz T. PQLI definition of criticality. J Pharm Innov 2008; 3:69–78.

Partridge D, Hussain KM. Knowledge Based Information Systems. London: McGraw-Hill, 1994.

Potter C, Beerbohm R, Coupe A, et al. A guide to EFPIA's Mock P.2 document. Pharmaceutical Technology Europe 2006; 12:39–44.

Ramani KV, Patel MR, Patel SK. An expert system for drug preformulation in a pharmaceutical company. Interfaces ; 22(2):101–108.

Rees C. Neural Computing—Learning Solutions (user survey). London: UK Department of Trade and Industry, 1996.

Rowe RC. An expert system for the formulation of pharmaceutical tablets. Manuf Intell 1993a; 14:13–15.

Rowe RC. Expert systems in solid dosage development. Pharm Ind 1993b; 55:1040–1045.

Rowe RC. Intelligent software systems for pharmaceutical product formulation. Pharm Tech 1997; 21: 178–188.

Rowe RC, Roberts RJ. Intelligent Software for Product Formulation. London: Talyor and Francis Ltd, 1998.

Rowe RC, Upjohn NG. Formulating pharmaceuticals using expert systems. Pharm Tech Int 1993; 5:46–52.

Rowe RC, Wakerly MG, Roberts RJ, et al. Expert system for parenteral development. PDA J Pharm Sci Technol 1995; 49:257–261.

Swanson A. A guide to EFPIA's Mock P.2. document. Pharm Technol Eur 2006; 12:39–44.

Tarabah E, Taxacher G. Drug-device products. Med Device Technol 1999; 5:44–48.

Tinsley H. Expert systems in manufacturing, an overview. Manuf Intell 1992; 9:7–9.

Tovey GD. Excipient selection for world-wide marketed dosage forms. In: Karsa DR, Stephenson RA, eds. Excipients and Delivery Systems for Pharmaceutical Formulations. London: The Royal Society of Chemistry, 1995.

Turban E. Decision Support Systems and Expert Systems. Englewood Cliffs, NJ: Prentice-Hall, 1995.

Turner J. Product formulation expert system. DTI Manuf Intell Newsl 1991; 8:12–14.

Vojnovic D, Chicco D, El Zenary H. Doehlert experimental design applied to optimisation and quality control of granulation process in a high shear mixer. Int J Pharm 1996; 145:203–213.

Vojnovic D, Chicco D. Mixture experimental design applied to solubility predictions. Drug Dev Ind Pharm 1997; 23(7):639–645.

Walko JZ. Turning Dalton's Theory into Practice, Innovation. London: ICI Europa Ltd, 1989:18–24.

Wechsler J. Quality standards to reshape manufacturing. BioPharm Int 2007; 2:16–18.

Williams DE. Pharmaceutical packaging—its expanding role as a drug delivery system. Pharm Technol Eur 1997; 9(4):44–46.

Wood M. Expert systems save formulation time. Lab Equip Dig 1991; 11:17–19.

9 | Parenteral Dosage Forms

Joanne Broadhead and Mark Gibson

AstraZeneca R&D Charnwood, Loughborough, Leicestershire, U.K.

INTRODUCTION

The dictionary definition of parenteral is nonenteral or nonoral and, therefore, strictly speaking, the term parenteral includes all products administered other than by the oral route. The pharmaceutical convention, however, is to use the term parenteral to describe medicines administered by means of an injection. The most common routes of parenteral administration are intravenous (IV), subcutaneous (SC), and intramuscular (IM), but there are also a variety of lesser-used routes, such as intra-arterial and intra-vitreal. In addition, products such as subcutaneous implants are usually classed as parenterals.

Although oral administration of drugs is a more widely accepted route of drug delivery, bioavailability often varies as a result of gastrointestinal absorption and degradation by the first-pass effect. Alternative routes of drug delivery also have their limitations, such as the impermeable nature of the stratum corneum for the percutaneous absorption of drugs in transdermal administration and degradation by enzymes present in the eye and nose for ophthalmic and nasal drug delivery. The parenteral route is the most popular and viable approach in many cases and remains the primary route for the administration of peptide and protein drugs (Pawer et al., 2004). These biopolymers have traditionally been administered via intramuscular or subcutaneous routes. Major progress has been made in recent years in the development of parenteral sustained-release systems to achieve long-term parenteral drug delivery, as evidenced by the regulatory approval and market launch of several new products. With the formulation challenges associated with peptides and proteins, new delivery systems have been developed to address the unmet needs in the parenteral sustained release of these biopolymers (Shi and Li, 2005).

There are, arguably, a greater variety of formulations administered by the parenteral route than by any other. These include emulsions, suspensions, liposomes, particulate systems, and solid implants as well as the ubiquitous simple solution. To develop a parenteral product the formulator must consider challenges such as drug solubility, product stability (particularly with biopharmaceuticals), drug delivery (particularly with sustained/controlled-release formulations after intramuscular or subcutaneous injection), and manufacturability. What sets parenteral products apart from most other dosage forms (with the exception of ophthalmic products) is the absolute requirement for sterility, regardless of the formulation type. This requirement must be uppermost in the pharmaceutical scientist's mind from the first stages of formulation conception, so that the formulation and manufacturing process can be developed in tandem to produce an optimized sterile product.

This chapter aims at providing a practical guide to the development of parenteral products, initially reviewing the basic principles of formulating a straightforward parenteral solution. Subsequent sections will examine the formulation options available when a more sophisticated formulation is warranted, for example, when the candidate drug exhibits poor aqueous solubility, is a macromolecule, or requires a more sophisticated delivery system. In vitro and in vivo testing methods for parenteral products will be touched on and the chapter concludes with a discussion of the manufacturing and regulatory issues unique to parenteral products. While, of necessity, the individual topics will be covered only briefly, the objective is to provide the reader with the basic information necessary to evaluate the formulation options available and to provide appropriate references to sources of further and more detailed information.

GUIDING PRINCIPLES FOR SIMPLE PARENTERAL SOLUTIONS

This section summarizes the principles that should be followed when developing simple solution formulations; these, after all, comprise the majority of marketed parenteral products. The information presented has been gleaned from standard textbooks and references, but where appropriate an attempt has been made to summarize the industry "norms." For further detailed information on the concepts discussed in this section, the reader is referred to Avis et al. (1992).

Selection of Injection Volume

Pharmacopoeias classify injectables into small-volume parenterals (SVPs) and large-volume parenterals (LVPs). The U.S. Pharmacopeia (USP) defines SVPs as containing less than 100 mL and LVPs as containing more than 100 mL. Many regulatory standards, for example, those for subvisible particulates, have first been developed for LVPs prior to their later application to all parenterals. SVPs can be given rapidly in a small volume; this type of injection is known as a bolus. They may also be added to LVPs, such as 5% dextrose and 0.9% sodium chloride infusion/injection, for administration by IV infusion. Some antibiotics are sold as LVPs, which eliminates the need for the extemporaneous addition of the drug to the infusion fluid prior to administration. The selection of bolus or infusion will depend on the pharmacokinetics of the drug, and the distinction can be somewhat blurred. Infusions can be as brief as 15 minutes or may continue for several days. Generally speaking, if a medicament is to be administered by infusion, the simplest approach is to formulate it as a concentrate, which will subsequently be diluted by the practitioner or pharmacist prior to administration.

Intramuscular or subcutaneous injections are almost always administered as a bolus. Typically, the injection volume is less than 1 to 1.5 mL by the subcutaneous route and usually no more than 2 mL by the intramuscular route, although higher volumes (up to 4 mL) can be administered if essential (Ford, 1988). Jorgensen et al. (1996) have shown a correlation between pain and the volume of a subcutaneous injection, with volumes of 1 to 1.5 mL causing significantly more pain than volumes of 0.5 mL or less. Clearly, it is preferable to minimize injection volume wherever possible, particularly if chronic administration is anticipated. When the total volume to be administered cannot be reduced to an acceptable level, two or more injections at multiple sites may be required.

One of the first steps in the formulation of a solution product is, therefore, to select the administration volume and concentration. This may be dictated primarily by physiological considerations, such as maximum injection volume as discussed above, or by pharmaceutical considerations. For example, if solubility is low, a larger volume/lower concentration formulation may be required, whereas if stability were to improve at higher concentrations, then the converse would be true.

pH and Tonicity Requirements

pH Considerations

Clearly, a parenteral product should be formulated with a pH close to physiological, unless stability or solubility considerations preclude this. Often, the pH selected for the product is a compromise between the pH of maximum stability, solubility, and physiological acceptability.

The first step in selecting a suitable formulation pH will be the generation of pH/stability and pH/solubility profiles. This type of information is often available in the preformulation data package. The target pH for maximum physiological acceptability is approximately pH 7.4. In practice, however, a reasonably wide pH range can be tolerated, particularly when dosing is via the IV route and dilution with blood is rapid. In these circumstances pHs ranging from 2 to 12 can be tolerated (although formulations at the extremes of this range are not recommended). The dilution rate is slower when administration is via the intramuscular route and decreases further when the subcutaneous route is used. For this reason, pH ranges of 3 to 11 and 3 to 6, respectively, are recommended for these routes (Strickley, 1999). Many products are formulated at a slightly acidic pH because of solubility or stability considerations, and the vast majority of licensed products have a pH between 3 and 9. A pH outside this range should be avoided, if possible, since a pH of greater than 9 can cause tissue necrosis, whereas a pH of less than 3 may cause pain and phlebitis (DeLuca and Boylan, 1992). Nevertheless, products with extreme pH values are encountered; Dilantin injection (phenytoin sodium) is formulated at pH 12, whereas Robinul injection (glycopyrrolate) is formulated at pH 2 to 3. Both products are for intramuscular administration. When a pH at the extreme of the acceptable ranges is necessary, and administration is via the subcutaneous or intramuscular route, it is advisable to conduct in vivo studies to assess the level of pain on injection (see sect. "Pain"). An important consideration in terms of the tolerability of a formulation is its buffering capacity; this may be more important than the pH per se. The pH of commercially available 0.9% w/v sodium chloride infusion, for example, can be as low as 4, but the lack of any buffering capacity means that it will have negligible effect on the pH of the blood into which it is infused, even when administration is rapid.

The use of buffers often can (and should) be avoided if the active ingredient is itself a salt that can be titrated with acid or base to a suitable pH for parenteral administration. Buffers may legitimately be required when the pH must be controlled at that of maximum stability or solubility. In the former case, the buffer concentration should be kept to a minimum so that after injection, the buffering capacity of physiological fluids will outweigh the buffering capacity of the formulation. Where buffers are used to improve solubility, the buffer concentration may need to be a little higher to prevent precipitation after injection. In vitro models have been developed, which can be used to screen formulations for the potential to precipitate after injection. These are discussed further in the section "In Vitro and In Vivo Testing Methods."

The buffers most commonly encountered in parenteral products are phosphate, citrate, or acetate. Phosphate is useful for buffering around physiological pH, whereas acetate and citrate are used when the required pH is lower. Table 1 summarizes the buffers that are typically encountered in approved parenteral products. Typically, buffer concentrations are in the 10 to 100 mmol/L range. In most cases, the sodium salts of acidic buffers are used, although potassium salts are occasionally encountered. Hydrochloride salts of basic buffers are usually used. It is preferable to avoid the combination of anionic drugs with cationic buffers (or vice versa) because of the risk of forming an insoluble precipitate.

Tonicity Considerations

Wherever possible, parenteral products should be isotonic; typically, osmolarities between 280 and 290 mOsm/L are targeted during formulation. Isotonicity is essential for LVPs, but again, a wider range of osmolarities can be tolerated in SVPs, since either rapid dilution with blood will occur after injection, or the product itself will be diluted with an LVP prior to administration. Hypertonic solutions are preferable to hypotonic solutions because of the risk of hemolysis associated with the latter. Fortunately, hypotonic formulations can be easily

Table 1 Buffers Used in Approved Parenteral Products

Buffer	pH range
Acetate	3.8–5.8
Ammonium	8.25–10.25
Ascorbate	3.0–5.0
Benzoate	6.0–7.0
Bicarbonate	4.0–11.0
Citrate	2.1–6.2
Diethanolamine	8.0–10.0
Glycine	8.8–10.8
Lactate	2.1–4.1
Phosphate	3.0–8.0
Succinate	3.2–6.6
Tartrate	2.0–5.3
Tromethamine (TRIS, THAM)	7.1–9.1

Source: From Powell et al. (1998), Flynn (1980), and Strickley (1999).

avoided by the use of excipients, often sodium chloride, to raise osmolarity. Mannitol, dextrose, or other inert excipients can also be used for this purpose and may be preferable if the addition of sodium chloride is likely to have an adverse effect on the formulation. Gupta et al. (1994a), for example, found that the presence of 0.9% w/w sodium chloride reduced the solubility of their candidate drug (Abbott-72517.HCl) by a factor of 3. Tonicity adjusters frequently have dual functionality; for example, mannitol often functions both to increase the osmolarity and to act as a bulking agent in lyophilized formulations.

CHOICE OF EXCIPIENTS

As with all pharmaceutical products, the most important "rule" to bear in mind when formulating parenterals is the "keep it simple" principle. Wherever possible, formulations should be developed using excipients, which have an established use in parenteral products administered by the same route as the product under development. The excipient concentration, rate of administration, and total daily dose should fall within the boundaries established by precedent in existing marketed products. The FDA's Inactive Ingredient Guide (see Table 2 of chap. 8) is a good place to start a search for information about a potential excipient, as it consists of an alphabetical list of all excipients in approved or conditionally approved drug products and includes the route of administration of the products containing them. The *Physicians' Desk Reference* (PDR) provides an essential source of detailed information on products available on the U.S. market and includes the quantitative formulation of each product. This enables both the rate of administration and total daily dose of excipients in existing products to be calculated. The PDR can be obtained in a CD-ROM format, which has a word search facility, thus providing a convenient means of searching for products containing a specific excipient. In addition to these reference sources, two excellent recent publications have specifically examined excipient usage in parenteral products on the U.S. market. Powell et al. (1998) have developed a compendium, which provides a comprehensive list of excipients present in commercial formulations, together with their concentrations and the routes of administration of products containing them. Nema et al. (1997) carried out a similar review; their article presents the data as summary tables, enabling the frequency of use and concentration range of a particular excipient to be obtained at a glance. The first part of a review article entitled "Parenteral Formulations of Small Molecule Therapeutics Marketed in the United States (1999)" is also recommended reading (Strickley, 1999) as it provides information similar to the publications of Powell et al. and Nema et al., but collates the information in terms of formulation type and includes the structure of the active ingredients. It also lists the concentration of excipients administered following dilution as well as the concentration in the supplied preparation, thus saving formulators the trouble of performing these calculations themselves! Finally, another recommended book is the *Handbook of Pharmaceutical Manufacturing Formulations: Sterile Products* (Niazi, 2004). This book covers formulations of injections, ophthalmic products, and other products labeled as sterile. Information is gathered from FDA New Drug Applications, patents, and other sources of generic and proprietry formulations. Each entry describes the formulation and manufacturing process and the book provides a detailed discussion of the difficulties encountered in formulating and manufacturing sterile products.

The information sources described above thus provide an invaluable resource to the parenteral formulator. The publications of Nema et al. (1997), Powell et al. (1998), and Strickley (1999) provide an instant, comprehensive and up-to-date reference source on U.S. licensed formulations, which can save the formulator many hours of trawling through the PDR! It is unfortunate that the same level of detail is not available for products outside the United States where manufacturers are not obliged to disclose the quantitative details of their formulations.

When considering the use of unusual excipients, or exceptionally high concentrations of "standard" excipients, it is important to bear in mind the indication for which the product is intended. An excipient, which may be acceptable as a last resort in a treatment for a life-threatening condition, should not be considered for a product to be administered chronically or for a less serious condition. A good example of this is the use of the solvent Cremophor EL in parenteral formulations of cyclosporin. This surfactant is associated with a range of toxic effects, and its use would not be envisaged unless all other more acceptable formulation strategies had been exhausted and the potential benefit of the treatment is such that the risk associated with the excipient is outweighed.

Another important consideration for excipients to be used in parenteral products is their quality, particularly in microbiological terms. Commonly used parenteral excipients can often be obtained in an injectable grade, which will meet strict bioburden and endotoxin limits. Pharmacopoeial grades of other excipients may be acceptable, but it is prudent to apply in-house microbiological specification limits, where none are present in the pharmacopoeias. For nonpharmacopoeial excipients, the best approach is always to purchase the highest grade available and apply internal microbiological specification limits.

STERILITY CONSIDERATIONS

The requirement for sterility in parenteral products is absolute and must be borne in mind at all stages of formulation and process development. The regulatory environment now requires that parenteral products be terminally sterilized unless this is precluded, usually by reason of instability (see sect. "Manufacturing of Parenteral Products").

For a solution product, one of the earliest investigations carried out during formulation development will be a study of the stability to moist heat sterilization. The results of this study may impact the formulation selection; for example, the stability to autoclaving may be affected by solution pH. Where stability is marginal, attempts should be made through the formulation process to stabilize the product such that it can withstand the stresses of moist heat sterilization. The regulatory authorities will expect to see good justification for new products that are *not* terminally sterilized. In many cases, however, the product will simply not withstand the stresses associated with autoclaving, and in this case, the usual alternative is filtration through sterilizing grade filters followed by aseptic processing. This is likely to be the case for biologicals/biopharmaceuticals, where heat may denature and deactivate them (see section on macromolecules). For the formulation scientist, it is important to select a suitable filter early on in development and ensure that the product is compatible with it. A good review of the practical and regulatory issues associated with sterile filtration has been reported by Twort et al. (2008). On behalf of The Pharmaceutical and Healthcare Sciences Society's Working Group on Process Filtration, Twort and coworkers address an increasing number of questions related to double sterile filtration and generally the need to use two sterilizing grade 0.2 um filters in series in aseptic processes as well as the location and practicalities of using these filters.

While the vast majority of parenteral products are rendered sterile either by moist heat sterilization or by filtration through sterilizing grade filters, other methods of sterilization should be considered, particularly in the development of nonaqueous formulations or novel drug delivery systems. For implants, for example, γ-irradiation is an option that should be explored early on in development.

Preservatives should not usually be included in parenteral formulations except where a multi-dose product is being developed. The Committee for Proprietary Medicinal Products' Notes for Guidance on Inclusion of Antioxidants and Antimicrobial Preservatives in Medicinal Products states that the physical and chemical compatibility of the preservative (or antioxidant) with the other constituents of the formulation, the container, and closure must be demonstrated during the development process. The minimum concentration of preservative should be used, which gives the required level of efficacy, as tested using pharmacopoeial methods. Certain preservatives should be avoided under certain circumstances, and preservatives should be avoided entirely for some specialized routes. The guidelines also require that both the concentration and efficacy of the preservative be monitored over the shelf life of the product. In multidose injectable products, the efficacy of the preservative must be established under simulated in-use conditions. Table 2 shows some of the most commonly encountered preservatives in licensed products and their typical concentrations. A review by Meyer et al. (2007) provides a comprehensive summary of antimicrobial preservatives that are

Table 2   Preservatives Used in Approved Parenteral Products

Preservative	Typical concentration (%)
Benzyl alcohol	1–2
Chlorbutanol	0.5
Methylparaben	0.1–0.18
Propylparaben	0.01–0.02
Phenol	0.2–0.5
Thiomersal	≤ 0.01

Source: From Nema et al. (1997) and Powell et al. (1998).

currently used in licensed parenteral products and also discusses the future use of preservatives. The criteria commonly used for the selection in parenteral product formulations are presented. According to the review, phenol and benzyl alcohol are the two most popular antimicrobial preservatives used in peptide and protein formulations, while phenoxyethanol is the most frequently used preservative in vaccines. Benzyl alcohol or a combination of methylparaben and propylparaben are generally used in small molecule parenteral formulations. The key criteria for antimicrobial preservative selection are the preservative dose, antimicrobial functionality, and effect on the active ingredient.

STRATEGIES FOR FORMULATING POORLY SOLUBLE DRUGS

Increasingly, formulation scientists are being asked to develop parenteral formulations of compounds with solubilities in the order of nanograms or micrograms per millilitre. This presents enormous challenges, particularly given the limited range of excipients that have been used historically in injectable products. This section briefly describes some of the strategies that can be considered and highlights some of the issues associated with each. For a more detailed review of this area, the reader is referred to a review by Sweetana and Akers (1996).

pH Manipulation
As discussed in the section "Guiding Principles for Simple Parenteral Solutions," the acceptable pH range for parenteral products is reasonably wide. Where the poorly soluble compound is a salt, pH manipulation may be all that is necessary to achieve adequate solubility. The potential for precipitation after administration should be, however, considered when using this approach. When administration is via the intramuscular and subcutaneous routes, consideration must be given to the possibility of pain on injection, particularly when the product is intended for chronic use. This may preclude the use of pH extremes and favor alternative formulation strategies.

Cosolvents
Cosolvents are reportedly used in 10% of FDA-approved parenteral products, although the range is limited to glycerin, ethanol, propylene glycol, polyethylene glycol, and *N,N*-dimethylacetamide (Sweetana and Akers, 1996). Some marketed formulations containing cosolvents are shown in Table 3. The use of cosolvents is often one of the earliest options considered by the formulator when solubility is an issue. Quite often, mixtures of cosolvents are used so that the dose or concentration of individual solvents can be minimized, and any synergistic effects can be maximized. The concentration of cosolvent(s) that is acceptable will vary depending on the route, rate of administration, and whether the product is to be given chronically. Again, the formulator will do well to be guided by the established precedent in marketed products and is once again referred to the publications of Powell et al. (1998) and Strickley (1999).

Nonaqueous Vehicles
Poorly soluble drugs for intramuscular administration can be formulated in a nonaqueous vehicle; this can have the additional benefit of providing a slow release of the active moiety. Oily vehicles have been used historically; the most commonly encountered is sesame oil, and

Table 3 The Formulations of Some Cosolvent-Containing Marketed Products

Active ingredient	Route	Vehicle composition	Special instructions
Diazepam	IM/IV	40% Propylene glycol 10% Ethyl alcohol 5% Benzoate buffer 1.5% Benzyl alcohol	Inject slowly (at least 1 min/mL) if giving IV Do not use small veins.
Co-trimoxazole	IV	40% Propylene glycol 10% Ethyl alcohol 0.3% Diethanolamine 1% Benzyl alcohol 0.1% Sodium meta-bisulfite	Must be diluted with 5% dextrose infusion Discard if cloudy or if there is evidence of crystallization
Etoposide	IV	65% w/v PEG 300 30.50% w/v Alcohol 8% w/v Polysorbate 80 3% w/v Benzyl alcohol 0.2% w/v Citric acid	Must be diluted. At concentrations >0.4 mg/mL, precipitation may occur.
Loxapine	IM	70% Propylene glycol 5% Polysorbate 80	
Lorazepam	IV/IM	80% Propylene glycol 18% Ethanol 2% Benzyl alcohol	Dilute twofold for IV injection.

six products containing it are listed in the PDR (Nema et al., 1997). Federal regulations, however, now require the specific oil to be included in the product labeling, because of the risk of allergic reactions to certain vegetable oils. This and the irritancy of oily vehicles have led to their decreased use. Formulations consisting entirely, or almost entirely, of organic solvents have also been developed, and examples are included in Table 3.

Surfactants

Surfactants, generally the polysorbates, are frequently encountered in parenteral products but generally at very low levels (<0.05%) and most commonly to prevent aggregation in formulations of macromolecules (see sect. "Strategies for the Formulation of Macromolecules"). Few IV products contain significant levels of surfactant; two notable exceptions are Cordarone IV and Etoposide IV, which contain 10% and 8%, respectively, of polysorbate (Tween) 80. Both products require dilution before administration, such that the maximum concentration of polysorbate 80 in the infusion solution is 1.2% and 0.16%, respectively. It is worth noting, however, that the polysorbate component of Cordarone IV has been implicated in a few cases of acute hepatitis, which have developed within hours of the start of administration. Somewhat higher levels of surfactants can be tolerated in products intended for the subcutaneous or intramuscular route. Aquasol A (vitamin A palmitate as retinol) for intramuscular administration, for example, contains polysorbate 80 at a level of 12%.

Novel approaches have been developed to formulate poorly soluble drugs for parenteral delivery using solid nanoparticle technology. Refer to the reviews of Kipp (2004) and also Wissing et al. (2004) for the application of this technology. Small-particle suspensions (200–2 μm), consisting essentially of pure drug, require only a minimum amount of surface-active agent for stabilization. Such suspensions may be formulated for rapid dissolution, therefore achieving similar pharmacokinetic profiles to those of a solution. Alternatively, drug insolubility may be controlled using this approach to establish sustained-release parenteral delivery.

Complexing Agents

Complexing agents, in this context, are molecules that have the ability to form soluble complexes with insoluble drugs. The most well-known examples are the cyclodextrins, which have been widely studied as agents for solubilization and stabilization. They are able to increase the aqueous solubility of some poorly soluble drug molecules by orders of magnitude, as a result of their ability to form inclusion complexes. Cyclodextrins are oligosaccharides obtained from the enzymatic conversion of starch. Depending on the number of glucopyranose units, they are named as α (6 units), β (7 units), or γ (8 units). These parent molecules can then be further substituted at the hydroxyl groups to alter the properties of the molecule. The nature of the substituents and the degree of substitution will influence the aqueous solubility, complexing capacity, and safety of the molecules. An excellent review of the characteristics of cyclodextrins is recommended (Thompson, 1997). In addition, Stella and Rajewski (1997) have reviewed the use of cyclodextrins in drug formulation and delivery, and this provides an excellent summary of the "status quo" in terms of their toxicology and use in pharmaceutical formulations.

Although the potential of cyclodextrins as solubilizing and stabilizing excipients has been the subject of numerous research papers, it took some time before the FDA approved the first commercial parenteral products containing them. Edex (alprostadil) for injection contains α-cyclodextrin at a concentration of approximately 1 mg/mL. This product is unusual, however, in that it contains an unsubstituted cyclodextrin. In general, the unsubstituted α- and β-cyclodextrins are not considered suitable for parenteral use because they can cause severe nephrotoxicity. This has led to the development of modified cyclodextrins. Hydroxypropyl-β-cyclodextrin is the most popular of the cyclodextrin family for use as a solubilizer in parenteral solutions because of its low toxicity and high inherent solubility. The first parenteral product containing this derivative (itraconazole) was approved in 1999. This product contains 40% hydroxypropyl-β-cyclodextrin and is administered intravenously after a twofold dilution with saline (Strickley, 1999).

In the past few years, several new marketed products containing cyclodextrin components have been approved. They include hydroxyl-β-cyclodextrin used in Sporonox® Injection (Janssen Pharmaceutical, New Jersey, U.S.) and sulfobutylether-β-cyclodextrin (Captisol®) in Vfend® IV and Zeldox®/Geodon® for injection (Pfizer, New York, U.S.). Other injectable formulations containing cyclodextrins are currently in clinical studies (Akers et al., 2007).

Novel parenteral drug delivery systems have been evaluated using dendromers as drug carriers to achieve administration of poorly water-soluble drugs (Demetzos, 2006). Dendrimers are hyperbranched polymers with well-defined structure and molecular weight; they are composed of a central core and repeated branching units; they have a globular shape, low polydispersity, and large void internal spaces that can be used for the encapsulation and delivery of drugs. Like cyclodextrins, they show great promise for the future in being able to deliver poorly soluble molecules.

Emulsions

Parenteral emulsions were first introduced to provide an IV source of essential fatty acids and calories. This has developed into the extensive and routine use of products such as Intralipid, Lipofundin, and Liposyn in total parenteral nutrition. There are relatively few commercially available emulsions containing active compounds; the only example on the U.S. market is Diprivan® Injectable Emulsion, the formulation of which is shown in Table 4. Diazepam is also available as an injectable emulsion on the U.K. market (Diazemuls®). For a more detailed discussion of the issues involved in developing parenteral emulsions, the reader is referred to Collins-Gold et al. (1990).

Table 4 Diprivan® Injectable Emulsion Formulation

Component	Concentration
Propofol	10 mg/mL
Soybean oil	100 mg/mL
Glycerol	22.5 mg/mL
Egg lecithin	12 mg/mL
Disodium edetate	0.005%
Sodium hydroxide	qs
Water for injection	to 100%

All parenteral emulsions are oil-in-water formulations, with the oil as the internal phase dispersed as fine droplets in an aqueous-continuous phase. An emulsifier, usually egg or soy lecithin, is needed to lower the interfacial tension and prevent flocculation and coalescence of the dispersed oil phase. Mechanical energy, usually in the form of homogenization, is required to disperse the oil phase into droplets of a suitable size. For IV administration, the droplet size should be below 1 µm to avoid the potential for emboli formation.

Clearly, physical stability is of critical importance for emulsion formulations, and care must be taken to ensure not only that the product itself is physically stable but also that any infusion solutions that may be prepared by dilution of the emulsion are also physically stable over the required period of time. In addition, parenteral emulsions should be able to withstand the stresses associated with moist heat sterilization. Alternatively, if this cannot be achieved, it may be possible to prepare an emulsion aseptically from sterile components or by sterile filtration, provided the process can be suitably validated. For a good introduction to the formulation and preparation of IV emulsions, the reader is referred to Hansrani et al. (1983).

STRATEGIES FOR FORMULATING UNSTABLE MOLECULES

Water Removal

The most common mechanism of instability in parenteral formulations is hydrolysis. Regardless of whether the formulation is a true solution, cosolvent solution, emulsion, or contains a complexing agent, the largest component of the formulation is likely to be water. Frequently, the only formulation strategy that will result in adequate stability is water removal. This is usually (although not exclusively) achieved by means of lyophilization. Lyophilization has a number of advantages over other potential drying methods, such as the ability to obtain an elegant end product with very low moisture content, and significantly, the fact that it is amendable to being carried out in an aseptic environment.

Lyophilization is essentially a three-stage process. Following standard aseptic filling, partially stoppered vials are transferred to a sterilizable lyophilizer in which drying is carried out. Sterilization of the lyophilizer is usually achieved by steam, although it is possible to use chemical methods such as hydrogen pyroxide. Initially the product is frozen to a low temperature (typically, $-30°C$ to $-40°C$). During primary drying, a high vacuum is applied, and ice is removed via sublimation. In the secondary drying stage, the product is heated under vacuum to $20°C$ to $40°C$, and any remaining water is removed by desorption. Products with very low moisture contents ($<2\%$) can easily be achieved. The process also allows vials to be backfilled with nitrogen, usually to slightly less than atmospheric pressure, prior to stoppering, thus creating an inert environment within the vials. At the end of the lyophilization cycle, the stoppers are fully inserted into the vials before removal of the product from the chamber.

The development of lyophilized products is a specialized area and requires a detailed understanding of the thermal properties of the formulation. Sub-ambient differential scanning calorimetry studies are required to identify the eutectic melting temperature (Te) (in the case of a crystalline solute) or the glass transition temperature of the maximally concentrated solute (Tg) (for an amorphous solute). The latter is closely related to the collapse temperature (Tc), which effectively represents the maximum allowable product temperature during the primary drying or sublimation phase of the process. Both Tc and Te can be estimated using freeze-drying microscopy, a technique in which the freeze-drying process is observed on a microscale and the Tc or Te visually determined. Lyophilized products usually contain excipients to act as bulking agents and/or improve the stability of the product. When the requirement is principally for a bulking agent, mannitol tends to be the favorite choice of formulators. Mannitol is a crystalline material with a Te of about $-2°C$ and, as such, is easily freeze-dried to give a self-supporting cake with good aesthetic properties. On the other hand, where an increase in stability is desired, an amorphous excipient (such as sucrose) is preferred since, once dry, the unstable compound will be "dispersed" in an amorphous glass with often greatly improved stability. The downside of formulating with amorphous excipients is that their low Tg values (approximately $-32°C$ for sucrose) result in long lyophilization cycles.

The formulator must also ensure that the product reconstitutes rapidly and that reconstitution time as well as chemical integrity is not adversely affected by storage.

For a detailed discussion of lyophilization, the reader is referred to Jennings (1999) as well as an excellent book by Rey and May (2004). The latter not only discusses freeze-drying fundamentals, but also practical guidance from the latest theoretical research, technologies, and industrial procedures including the mechanisms and means of protein stabilization and lyophilization of pharmaceutical and biological products. In addition, a thorough review of the manufacturing and regulatory aspects of lyophilization is provided in *Good Pharmaceutical Freeze-Drying Practice* (Cameron, 1997).

Use of Excipients

Excipients may be useful in preventing chemical and physical instability. Antioxidants are included in parenteral formulations, although their use is now in decline, and EU guidelines discourage their use unless no other alternative exists (see sect. "Parenteral Products and the Regulatory Environment"). A preferred method of preventing oxidation is simply to exclude oxygen; this is usually achieved by purging the product with nitrogen and creating a nitrogen headspace within the container. Where this process is insufficient, a metal chelator, such as disodium edetate, or an antioxidant compound, such as ascorbic acid or sodium metabisulfite, may be considered. These are included in marketed products typically at levels of up to 0.05%, 1%, and 0.3%, respectively.

Nonaqueous Vehicles and Emulsions

For the intramuscular and subcutaneous routes, the use of nonaqueous vehicles may be considered as a method of avoiding hydrolysis. For IV administration, the use of an oil-in-water emulsion is a possible, although little used, option. These approaches are discussed in the section "Strategies for Formulating Poorly Soluble Drugs."

STRATEGIES FOR THE FORMULATION OF MACROMOLECULES

Macromolecules present unique challenges to both the formulator and the analyst. Their large size and complex structural nature make degradation difficult to detect and sometimes difficult to prevent.

Proteins are composed of an amino acid backbone, which defines their primary structure. The amino acid side chains hydrogen-bond to each other, creating areas of local order such as α-helices and β-pleated sheets. These types of arrangement are known as secondary structure. The overall folding of the molecule, which defines its three-dimensional- shape, is known as the tertiary structure. Finally, some proteins, such as hemoglobin, are composed of more than one subunit; the spatial arrangement of these subunits is known as the quaternary structure.

The challenge to the formulator is ensuring the preservation of both the chemical integrity of the constituent amino acids and the overall three-dimensional folding or conformation of the molecule. Several amino acids are susceptible to degradation by oxidation (e.g., methionine, cysteine, and histidine) and deamidation (e.g., glutamine and asparagine). Peptide bonds in the backbone can undergo hydrolysis, and disulfide bonds between amino chains can also be disrupted and refolded incorrectly (disulfide interchange). Chemical modification may be detected by high-performance liquid chromatography (HPLC) techniques, but it is often extremely difficult to pinpoint where in the molecule degradation is taking place. Protein molecules frequently undergo aggregation, both covalent (through disulfide bond formation) and noncovalent. Noncovalent aggregation cannot be detected by normal HPLC methods, and techniques such as sodium dodecyl sulfate–polyacrylamide gel electrophoresis (SDS–PAGE) and size exclusion chromatography are required to detect this type of instability. In addition, protein molecules have a tendency to adsorb to surfaces such as filters.

It is clear that the formulation of a macromolecule is far from simple and requires a good understanding of protein chemistry in order that degradation pathways can be understood and degradation prevented. However, one faces the same limitation as formulators of small

Table 5 Excipients Encountered in Formulations of Macromolecules

Excipient	Function
Polyhydric alcohols, e.g., mannitol	Stabilization, bulking agent
Carbohydrates, e.g., sucrose	Stabilization
Amino acids, e.g., glycine, arginine	Stabilization, buffer, solubilization
Serum albumin	Prevention of adsorption
Surfactants (e.g., Polysorbate 80, Pluronic F68)	Prevention of adsorption and aggregation
Metal ions	Stabilization
Antioxidants	Prevention of oxidation
Chelating agents (e.g., EDTA)	Prevention of oxidation

molecules, namely, a relatively small armoury of established excipients, which can be safely used in parenteral products. Some of the excipients commonly encountered in formulations of macromolecules are listed in Table 5. For further guidance on the formulation of macromolecules, the reader is referred to Wang and Pearlman (1993) and Pawer et al. (2004). This text provides some excellent examples of strategies that have been used to develop commercial formulations of proteins and peptides, such as human growth hormone and alteplase.

LIPOSOMAL DELIVERY SYSTEMS

Liposomes are single or multilayer phospholipid vesicles, typically less than 300 nm in size. They are capable of entrapping both water-soluble and lipid-soluble compounds. Their use in parenteral formulations has exploited their preferential distribution to the organs of the reticuloendothelial system (RES) and their ability to accumulate preferentially at the sites of inflammation and infection. Liposome encapsulated amphotericin B is considerably less toxic than the free drug because of the altered pattern of biodistribution (Betageri and Habib, 1994). A sophisticated approach has been developed (commercialized as Stealth® liposomes), in which polyethylene glycol is grafted to the surface of the liposome, resulting in prolonged circulation of the liposomes in the bloodstream. A doxorubicin product that uses this approach (DOXIL®) is an example of a commercially available product (Martin, 1999). There has been a steady increase in successful commercial liposomal formulations marketed in recent years to deliver small molecules and biologics (Akers et al., 2007). Earlier problems with economic and reproducible large-scale production of liposomes have been largely solved.

SUSTAINED-RELEASE PARENTERAL FORMULATIONS

The chronic administration of molecules, which have a short biological half-life and cannot be given orally, presents a difficult challenge to formulators. One strategy that might be considered is the development of a sustained-release intramuscular or subcutaneous injection. Other nonparenteral options could include the inhalation or intranasal route, both of which have their own unique challenges. Sustained-release parenteral formulations might also be required in circumstances where patient compliance is likely to be poor. This consideration has led to the development of some antipsychotics and contraceptives as sustained-release injections. Table 6 lists some of the sustained-release parenteral products that are available on the U.S. market and their respective formulations. The typical approaches used in the formulation of sustained-release parenterals are summarized in this section.

Oily Vehicles
The use of oily vehicles as an approach for the formulation of poorly soluble molecules is discussed in the section "Nonaqueous Vehicles." For molecules that possess good oil solubility, a sustained-release profile may also be achievable. The nature of the sustained-release profile will depend to a large extent on the oil/water partition coefficient of the

Table 6   Examples of Sustained-Release Parenteral Formulations

Compound	Route	Formulation
Penicillin-G benzathine	IM (aqueous suspension)	0.5% Lecithin 0.6% Carboxymethylcellulose 0.6% Povidone 0.1% Methylparaben 0.01% Propylparaben in sodium citrate buffer
Haloperidol	IM (oily vehicle)	1.2% Benzyl alcohol in sesame oil
Leuprolide acetate	IM (microsphere suspension)	After reconstitution 0.13% Gelatin 6.6% dl-Lactic and glycolic acid copolymer 13% Mannitol 0.2% Polysorbate 80 1% Carboxymethylcellulose in WFI
Dexamethasone acetate	IM/soft tissue (aqueous suspension)	0.67% Sodium chloride 0.5% Creatinine 0.05% Disodium edetate 0.5% Sodium carboxymethylcellulose 0.075% Polysorbate 80 0.9% Benzyl alcohol 0.1% Sodium sulfite in WFI

molecule in question. Molecules that are not oil miscible could also be formulated as oily suspensions. The latter will usually result in a longer duration of action, because the drug particles must dissolve in the oily phase prior to partitioning into the aqueous medium (Madan, 1985). The use of oily vehicles would not normally be considered as a first-line approach for new formulations, however, because of concerns over allergic reactions to the oils.

Aqueous Suspensions

This approach can be used to prolong the release of compounds with limited aqueous solubility. A suspension of a compound in its saturated solution can provide both immediate-release and sustained-release components of a dose (Madan, 1985). A number of water-insoluble prodrugs are also formulated as suspensions, including hydrocortisone acetate and medroxyprogesterone acetate. As with any other type of suspension, excipients will usually be required to ensure the physical stability of the formulation. Strickley's (1999) article provides a table of parenteral suspension formulations; the most popular excipient combinations are clearly polyethylene glycol/polysorbate (Tween, 80) and carboxymethylcellulose/polysorbate (Tween, 80).

Perhaps the most well-known example of a parenteral suspension formulation is insulin. Many insulin formulations also take advantage of the different physical forms that can be produced when insulin is complexed with zinc. Suspensions of the amorphous form of insulin zinc have a faster onset of action and shorter duration of action compared with those of the crystalline form. To provide both a rapid onset and a long duration of action, many formulations are composed of a mixture of amorphous and crystalline zinc insulin.

Emulsions

For a molecule with a high aqueous solubility, the use of a water-in-oil two-phase emulsion or a multiple phase water-in-oil-in-water emulsion may enable a measure of sustained release to be achieved. In either case, the nature of the sustained-release delivery profile will be a function of the partition coefficient of the molecule between the two phases, which will define the rate at which the molecule is available for absorption The implications of using oil-in-water lipid emulsions for parenteral drug delivery is discussed in a review by Tamilvanan (2004).

Microemulsions have evolved as a novel vehicle for parenteral delivery of hydrophobic drugs. They provide several advantages such as spontaneity of formation, ease of manufacture, high solubilization capacity and self-preserving properties. Date and Nagarsenker (2008) have produced a good review of the excipients available for formulation of parenteral microemulsions and investigations that have been carried out with different therapeutic agents.

Microspheres

Polymeric microspheres, particularly those prepared from the biodegradable polylactide/polyglycolide (PLGA) copolymers, have been widely investigated as a means to achieve sustained-release parenteral drug delivery. The advantage of formulating the polymeric matrix as microspheres is the ability to administer them via a conventional needle and syringe as a suspension formulation, rather than as an implant (see below). The release rate can be tailored to the needs of the patient and employing biodegradable microspheres, the release of the drug can be controlled over a predetermined time span, ranging from days to weeks or even months. Various commercial lactide/glycolide controlled-release parenteral formulations are available on the market (Tice, 2004), for example, Lupron® Depot, which can provide therapeutic blood levels of leuprolide acetate for up to four months. These products are presented as lyophilized polylactic acid microspheres, which are reconstituted to form a suspension prior to administration. Other microsphere formulations meeting clinical and commercial success in recent years are discussed by Akers et al. (2007), while Sinha and Trehan (2005) have comprehensively reviewed the latest trends in the use of biodegradable microspheres for parenteral drug delivery.

Implantable Drug Delivery Systems

Implantable delivery systems extend the concept of sustained release beyond the capabilities of the strategies discussed so far in this section. Continual drug delivery lasting for months or even years has been achieved. Because these products must be administered as a solid rather than a liquid, they are usually supplied with a customized injection device.

The number of marketed implantable products is relatively limited, probably in part because of the limited market for this type of product. The most well-known example of an implantable delivery system is the Norplant® contraceptive device, which can deliver levonorgestrel for up to five years. The device is composed of a number of capsules fabricated from Silastic® (dimethylsiloxane/methylvinylsiloxane copolymer).

The Norplant device has been somewhat controversial, however, due to difficulties associated with its removal. A second example of an implantable drug delivery system is Zoladex®, which is an implantable biodegradable lactide/glycolide polymeric delivery system for the administration of goserelin acetate. It is available in one-month and three-month presentations and can be injected through a wide-bore needle.

Pegylation

The effectiveness of combining polyethylene glycol and macromolecules has resulted in several relatively new commercial products (Akers, 2007). The first pegylated oligonucleotide (Mucagen®, Pfizer, New York, U.S.) was launched in 2005 for the treatment of macular degeneration by intravitreal injection. Another example is pegfilgrastim (Neulasta™), which increases the serum half-life of filgrastim and reduces the dosing frequency from up to 11 injections per chemotherapy cycle to only 1 injection.

IN VITRO AND IN VIVO TESTING METHODS

When developing formulations for compounds with limited solubility or stability, where extremes of pH or cosolvents might be used, it is desirable to carry out screening studies to assess their potential to cause pain or other adverse events following injection. Hemolysis and phlebitis may occur as a consequence of IV therapy, while pain may occur on administration of any type of injection. Several in vitro and in vivo models have been developed to evaluate the potential for adverse effects following parenteral administration; these are discussed briefly below. For a more detailed discussion of this subject, the reader is referred to the excellent review by Yalkowsky et al. (1998).

In Vitro Precipitation

Clearly, when a drug is formulated at a non-physiological pH, or using organic solvents because of low solubility, there is a real risk of precipitation immediately following injection into the bloodstream. Crude models have therefore been used in the past to assess formulations for their potential to result in in vivo precipitation. These have generally involved performing dilutions in a medium resembling blood and monitoring the formation of a precipitate by visual or other means. More recently, dynamic methods have been developed, which more realistically simulate the in vivo situation. Typically, these involve a continuously circulating system of plasma or a medium representing plasma. After "injection" of the test formulation, the resulting solution passes through a flow-through cell within a spectropho-tometer where light scattering associated with particle formation is monitored. Although it is obviously difficult to precisely mimic in vivo conditions, these models can prove useful in terms of discriminating among a number of potential formulations. In addition, they can be used to assess the effect of injection rate. Yalkowsky et al. (1983) have shown that, perhaps counter-intuitively, the degree of precipitation of diazepam injection is in fact *inversely* proportional to injection rate.

Hemolysis

Hemolysis occurs when the red blood cell membrane is disrupted, resulting in release of cell contents into the plasma. Severe adverse events can occur if high levels of hemoglobin are released into plasma. Clearly, hypotonic formulations have the potential to cause hemolysis, and as discussed earlier, the administration of such formulations should be avoided. Other excipients, such as surfactants and cosolvents, can cause hemolysis, as may the drug itself. In vitro models to evaluate hemolytic potential typically involve exposing the formulation to blood, either in a static or a dynamic configuration, and then assessing the quantity of free hemoglobin released. The contact time between blood and the formulation is critical, as an unrealistic contact time can result in a substantial overestimation of the hemolytic potential of a given formulation (Wakerley, 1999). Hemolysis can also be measured in vivo by the measurement of free hemoglobin in blood or urine, and Krzyzaniak (1997) has reported agreement between a dynamic in vitro method and in vivo results.

Phlebitis

Phlebitis refers to inflammation of the vein wall. It can result in clinical symptoms such as pain and edema, and can cause thrombus formation, which may have serious consequences. Particulate matter is the most widely implicated cause of phlebitis. It is not surprising, therefore, that a link has been proposed between precipitation and phlebitis. The in vitro precipitation models described above may therefore be a good indicator of the phlebitic potential of a formulation. Phlebitis can be tested in vivo, usually by means of a rabbit ear vein model in which the "test" ear is visually compared with the "control" ear.

Pain

Pain on injection is usually of greatest concern with intramuscular injections because of the long residence time of the formulation at the injection site. Not surprisingly, there are no in vitro models to test the potential of a formulation to cause pain. It is therefore necessary to test for the potential to cause pain by means of an in vivo model. Gupta et al. (1994b) describe the use of the rat "paw-lick" model for the assessment of pain in response to formulation pH and cosolvent concentration. The potential for muscle damage should also be evaluated when developing an intramuscular formulation, and the industry standard is the rabbit lesion volume model (Sutton et al., 1996).

PACKAGING OF PARENTERAL PRODUCTS

Pack Selection

The packaging of parenteral products presents unique challenges in terms of the requirements for the packaging components to withstand sterilization prior to use and the requirement for the complete primary pack to maintain sterility throughout the shelf life of the product. Traditionally, SVPs have been packaged in ampoules, which are heat sealed after filling. Because of the inherent variability in the sealing process, products packaged in ampoules must be 100% integrity tested after sealing, usually by means of a dye immersion test. The use of ampoules for new products is now diminishing, partly because of the desire to avoid exposing medical personnel to injury on opening. This has led to an increase in the use of glass vials sealed with rubber stoppers for the packaging of SVPs. Regardless of whether an ampoule or a vial is used, the glass quality must be type I neutral.

An increasing number of simple solutions are now being filled using blow-fill-seal technology, in which the (plastic) ampoule is molded, aseptically filled, and sealed in a continuous process. Blow-fill-seal technology has emerged as a preferred packaging for parenteral products because of unrivalled flexibility in container design, overall product quality, operational output, and low operational costs (Reed, 2002). These manufacturing systems operate to high levels of asepsis and are validated by media fills in the same manner as conventional filling processes. It is possible to incorporate a multistep process of blow molding, aseptic filling, and hermetic sealing of liquid products in one sequential operation on a compact automated machine with fill volumes ranging from 1 to 1000 mL.

For products packaged in vials, a suitable rubber stopper must be selected. The surface of a rubber stopper is inherently less inert than the glass of an ampoule, and it is therefore important that the formulator ensures that the product and stopper are compatible by conducting suitable testing.

For lyophilized products, it is advisable to select a stopper with a low capacity to absorb moisture during the autoclaving process, since this can subsequently be transferred to the product during storage, which may lead to product deterioration. Various other specialized stoppers are available, such as Teflon coated, which may be useful when a highly inert surface is required. Stoppers containing a desiccant are also available to maintain a dry internal environment for moisture-sensitive products. Stoppers cannot withstand the depyrogenation process and so are autoclaved prior to use, but the presterilization treatment should be designed to ensure a satisfactory level of endotoxin removal. Traditionally, stoppers usually require some degree of siliconization to allow them to be easily processed in automatic filling lines, and they can be purchased washed, presiliconized to an agreed level and packaged in ready-to-sterilize bags. Stoppers that are purchased in a ready-to-sterilize format should be tested by the supplier to a suitable endotoxin specification.

The silicone used to siliconize stoppers is not chemically bonded to the rubber surface and so can be a problem interacting with formulation components. Recent developments in rubber stoppers have replaced silicone with special silicone polymers to provide lubricity and also reduce the potential for formulation and stopper interactions. Commercial examples of coated stoppers are Flurotec® (Daikyo/West Pharmaceutical Services, Pennsylvania, U.S.) and Omniflex® (Helvoet Pharma, Liege, Belgium).

It is also necessary to ensure that the product does not extract an excessive quantity of leachables from the stopper or any other part of the primary packaging. Glass leachables are reduced by using "treated" glass or by using specially prepared coated glass that significantly reduces the extractables profile and improves the chemical resistance of the glass surface. Plastic leachables are reduced or removed by using plastic materials that contain low levels of potential extractable materials. For example, polyvinyl chloride (PVC) contains relatively high levels of the extractable plasticizer diethylhexylphthalate, but can be replaced with combinations of polyethylene, polypropylene, or other polyolefinic materials that do have low levels of extractable material. Extractables and leachables remain a hot topic for both formulators and regulators and are discussed in more detail by Akers et al. (2007).

Increasingly parenteral products are being presented in more sophisticated packages, such as pre-filled syringes. These reduce the potential for needle-stick injuries by reducing the degree of manipulation required and facilitate administration in an emergency situation. They also eliminate the need for overfilling thus reducing waste, compared to vials and other containers, particularly important for expensive biomolecules. A number of companies, such as Becton–Dickinson and Vetter, specialize in this technology, and can supply purpose-designed filling equipment or can provide contract manufacturing services to fill product into their devices. Alternatively, presterilized ready-to-fill syringes can be readily purchased and filled in a sterile facility in a pharmaceutical company. The use of plastic packaging for vials and prefilled syringes is increasing over glass because of the elimination of the risk of broken glass and also leachables from glass. They are also preferred for proteins because there is less surface adsorption. However, if plastic containers are used, the potential for interactions with the formulation needs to be carefully evaluated. Traditional plastic materials such as PVC and polyethylene are not as transparent as glass, and so, inspection of the contents is not possible. In addition, plastic materials will soften or melt under the conditions of thermal sterilization and so alternative methods such as ethylene oxide or radiation sterilization may have to be employed followed by aseptic filling.

With the recent escalation in new biological drugs, including antibodies and recombinant proteins, there has been a renewed emphasis on drug injection devices. A wide range of sophisticated, application-specific injection devices have been developed to address the limitations of new classes of therapeutic drugs and to satisfy the patient and caregiver. Table 7 lists some examples of marketed injection devices that are currently available.

Needle-free injection technology has been in development for many years to try and overcome the issues of needle phobia, needle stick injuries, patient discomfort, and needle safety. Safety needles, autoinjectors, pens, needle guards, and particularly needle-free injector technologies have been developed for noninvasive delivery and to solve these issues. With the availability of synthetic materials and computerized design software, reliable and cost-effective devices have become available in recent years. Needle-free injectors can administer

Table 7 Examples of Injection Systems Used for Parenteral Drug Delivery

Injection system type	Examples	Features
Dual vial	Vetter-Lyo-Ject® Vetter, Germany	The lyophilized drug is in one chamber and a second chamber contains a solvent that is mixed with the drug just prior to administration.
Prefillable syringe and cartridges	BD Readifill™, Becton–Dickinson, U.S.	Glass prefillable syringe with needle isolation (The liquid is isolated from the needle so that drugs sensitive to needle contact are not affected during storage).
	Schott Cartridges, Schott, Germany	Cartridges that can be administered in the form of pen or pump systems.
Safety Syringes	Eclam Auto-Needle and Syringe, Eclam Medical Inc., Israel	Single-use automatic needle insertion and protection device that can be attached to any conventional Luer syringe to address both needle phobia and prevention of accidental needle sticks and contamination. Needle is hidden before and after injection.
Reconstitution systems	ADD-Vantage Hospira Inc., U.S.	Liquid or powdered medication are provided in a threaded vial that mates with the top of flexible diluent in 50, 100, or 250 mL sizes. The design keeps drug and diluent separate until activated just prior to administration.
Injector pens	LEVA®, Bang & Olufsen Medicom AS, Denmark	Designed for subcutaneous injections of fixed doses, offering consistent precise doses.
Speciality syringes	Sagent Dual Chamber Syringe, Sagent Pharmaceuticals Ltd, U.S.	Dual-chamber syringe enables the sequential administration of two separate IV medications with a single push, thus replacing two syringes with one.
Autoinjectors	SNAP JET®, Cambridge Biostability Ltd, U.K.	Hand powered, disposable, safety auto-injector containing stabilized liquid vaccines. After injection, a spring retracts the syringe and needle and the system is locked and disabled.

liquid medication under sufficient pressure in a fine, high-velocity jet to penetrate the skin tissue without a hypodermic needle. These injectors typically have a chamber holding the medication, and a plunger/piston is actuated by an energy source, such as a coil spring, gas spring, gas cartridge, or gas generation system. Needle-free technologies can be used for difficult to deliver medications, such as vaccines, proteins, antibodies, etc. into the ID, IM, or SC part of the skin. Most devices available are designed specifically to inject liquid products, with fewer options for delivering formulated powder/solid products, for example, from PowderJect (currently owned by Anesiva, California, U.S., for small molecules and by PowderMed, Oxford, U.K./Pfizer, New York, U.S., for proteins) have protypes in development. Needle-free technologies do have some disadvantages such as causing pain/bruising and bleeding at the injection site because of the high pressure of the jet. Also, proving bioequivalence between the needle-free device and the needle-based injection can be more challenging and the costs are higher than conventional needle/syringe delivery. The most established companies providing needle-free devices are Anesiva, Antares, Bioject, Injex, National Medical Products, and The Medical House.

Container/Closure Integrity

Considerable emphasis is now placed on providing an assurance of container closure integrity during the shelf life of sterile products. Historically, this has been achieved by performing sterility tests as a component of stability testing, usually initially and at 12-month intervals, but this approach alone would not now be considered sufficient to validate the integrity of a new container/closure system. Most manufacturers usually perform media immersion tests in which media-filled vials are immersed in contaminated media and subjected to repeated vacuum/overpressure cycles. This provides an assurance of the integrity of specific pack configurations under highly challenging conditions. This test should also be conducted on stored media-filled vials to provide data on the integrity of "aged" packs. FDA guidelines now allow physical tests to replace microbiological tests in demonstrating container closure integrity, but only where those physical tests are suitably validated. This is by no means straightforward because of the difficulty in correlating leakage measured by a physical method with the potential for microbial ingress. Kirsch et al. have published a series of articles in which they have been able to correlate helium leak rates measured by mass spectrometry and vacuum decay methods with a probability of microbial ingress (Kirsch et al., 1997a–c, 1999).

MANUFACTURING OF PARENTERAL PRODUCTS

The manufacture of parenteral products is focused at all times on the requirement for sterility of the finished product. Despite the fact that the regulators are clear in their preference for products to be terminally sterilized, the vast majority of parenterals are filtered through sterilizing grade filters and filled aseptically, primarily because stability considerations preclude the use of moist heat sterilization. The statistical limitations of sterility testing a sample from a batch are well known, and attention is now well and truly focused on process validation. The validation program must encompass facilities, instrumentation, sterilization of container and closures, clean room garments, and gowning procedures as well as including regular media simulations of aseptic processes. Guidance on the frequency and numbers of units to be filled in media simulations can be found in the publications of the Parenteral Drug Association (PDA) and the Pharmaceutical & Healthcare Sciences Society (PHSS) (see sect. "Parenteral Products and the Regulatory Environment"). In a production environment, a simulation of each aseptic process will typically be carried out at six-month intervals. It is important that media fills include planned interventions, such as filter changes, so that such interventions can be permitted during a manufacture, if required. In addition, holding times after filtration should be validated. Where a product is lyophilized, the media simulation must include loading into and removal from the lyophilizer and should also include pulling and releasing partial vacuums. It is obviously essential to ensure that all personnel participating in aseptic processes are adequately trained and aseptic operators are required to participate in regular media fills. Another important element of aseptic process validation is environmental monitoring and particulate monitoring; manufacturers are expected to know the organisms that may be present in their facility and to establish acceptable limits.

With the majority of parenteral products sterilized by filtration, it is not surprising that the validation of filtration processes is receiving increasing regulatory interest. The 1998 PDA Technical Report No. 26 (revised 2008) discusses this topic in detail (see sect. "Parenteral Products and the Regulatory Environment"). The revised document was developed in response to enhancements in filtration technologies and recent additional regulatory requirements within the pharmaceutical industry. References to scientific publications and international regulatory documents are provided where more supportive data and detail can be found. There is a regulatory expectation that the bacterial retention capability of sterilizing filters is demonstrated in the presence of product rather than simply water. Fortunately, the major pharmaceutical filter companies now have specialized validation laboratories, which are able to provide filter validation services. All filters used in a process, including vent filters, must also be integrity tested before and after use. Integrity testing of sterilizing-grade membrane filters is a commonly used and needed nondestructive test to determine whether or not the filter performs as specified or contains a flaw, which would cause microbial penetration. Common integrity tests employed are diffusive flow, bubble point, or pressure hold, all these tests demonstrating reliability and accuracy (Meltzer and Jornitz, 2008).

Organisms have recently been identified, which are capable of passing through 0.22 μm filters, and the filter companies can now provide 0.1 μm filters. Manufacturers are required to have knowledge of the type of organisms that may be present in the solution to be filtered; provided that these do not have the ability to pass through a 0.22 μm filter, there is no compelling scientific argument for the use of a 0.1 μm filter.

For products that can withstand sterilization in their final container, the focus of the validation exercise will clearly be the sterilization process. A detailed discussion of sterilization is beyond the scope of this chapter [for this, the reader is referred to the text by Nordhauser and Olson (1998)], but the premise central to all methods of sterilization is the concept of a log-reduction in viable organisms. Pharmacopoeias now require an assurance that there is less than one chance in a million that viable microorganisms are present in a sterilized article or dosage form (Hall, 1994). Achieving the required sterility assurance level of 10^{-6} is of course dependent on the initial microbiological loading of the material to be sterilized, and so it is vital to have knowledge of the initial bioburden and to set limits for this. For terminally sterilized products, the focus of the validation exercise will be in providing an assurance that sterilizing conditions have been reached in all units. Thus only loads and loading patterns that have been validated, usually by means of biological indicators, can be used. The concept of validated loading patterns also applies to the sterilization of equipment and packaging components to be used in an aseptic process.

The final stage in the manufacture of a sterile product is inspection. A 100% inspection for particulates, cracks, and defects is a regulatory requirement. The inspection may be carried out visually using suitable illumination, but in a production environment, a semiautomated or automated system is usually used.

The recently published PDA Technical Report No. 44 "Quality Risk Management for Aseptic Processes" provides an overview of a quality risk management program and presents a model to facilitate the risk assessment of aseptic processing of sterile products. It provides a tool to assess and evaluate activities, conditions, and controls that impact establishing and maintaining aseptic conditions and endotoxin control.

Clearly, the manufacture of sterile products is a specialized area, and the above discussion simply serves to highlight some of the critical issues; it is by no means comprehensive. For a detailed discussion of the manufacture of sterile products, the reader is referred to Hall (1994) as well as the publications of the PDA and the PHSS, which are detailed in the section "Parenteral Products and the Regulatory Environment." In addition, the MHRA publication entitled "Rules and Guidance for Pharmaceutical Manufacturers and Distributors," or widely known as the "Orange Guide," provides a very readable annex, covering the manufacture of sterile medicinal products; this includes guidance on clean room classifications, gowning and sanitization, as well as the manufacture and sterilization of medicinal products (MHRA, 2007).

ADMINISTRATION OF PARENTERAL PRODUCTS

During product development, it is essential that the formulators keep in mind the manner in which their product will ultimately be used. This is particularly true for products intended for IV infusion, since these will require dilution with IV infusion fluids prior to administration. The formulator must ensure that the active compound is compatible with all diluents that are to be included in the product labeling and must provide stability data to demonstrate that the resultant infusion solutions are stable for the period of time specified in the labeling. During clinical trials, compatibility and stability must be assured at the maximum and minimum concentrations to be administered during the study; this data will be expected by the regulatory authorities as part of an Investigational New Drug (IND) submission. It is also important to consider other drugs that may be coadministered with the product in question. The practice of mixing more than one drug in a single infusion is diminishing rapidly, and the labeling of new IV products usually specifies that this should be avoided. One must still consider, however, the potential for incompatibilities to occur when different infusion solutions mix in the infusion line or indeed the cannula. In general, mixing prior to the cannula can be avoided by the use of a different line for each infusion, but clearly, mixing in the cannula is inevitable where patients are receiving multiple IV infusions. The labeling of some medications, notably alteplase, specifically instructs that they should be administered in a completely separate infusion line to any other medications. The nature of alteplase may justify this statement, but in practice, such restrictions should be avoided, since they will clearly cause difficulties for medical practitioners.

When compatibility or stability issues do arise, there are limited options available to the formulator. The diluent cannot usually be controlled unless the manufacturer incurs the additional cost associated with supplying a custom diluent. Leachables from infusion bags can cause degradation, particularly oxidation. In addition, the low concentrations to which drugs may be diluted for continuous infusion can result in adsorptive losses. A number of products, therefore, specify a minimum concentration to which they can be diluted, presumably to address stability or adsorption issues. The infusion set can also contribute to instability and/or adsorption and so should be evaluated during product development. Some product labeling, for example, that of glyceryl trinitrate infusion, specifies that PVC infusion lines should not be used. In extreme cases, it may be necessary to add an additional excipient to the product to prevent degradation on dilution, although this approach should only be considered as a last resort.

PARENTERAL PRODUCTS AND THE REGULATORY ENVIRONMENT

The requirement for sterility in parenteral products means that their manufacture is scrutinized perhaps more closely than that of any other product type. A number of regulatory guidelines specifically pertain to parenteral products, and these are listed below. Included in these lists are also some more general guidelines where these contain sections specifically relevant to parenteral products. European Agency for the Evaluation of Medicinal Products (EMEA) publications provide useful guidance in formulation decision making and are essential reading early on in the formulation development process. The "Decision Trees for the Selection of Sterilization Methods" document provides clear guidance on the selection of a sterilization strategy; this is discussed in detail in chapter 12. Similarly, the "Notes for Guidance on Inclusion of Antioxidants and Antimicrobial Preservatives in Medicinal Products" is prescriptive in terms of defining the circumstances under which antioxidants and preservatives should be used. The former, for example, should be included only where their use cannot be avoided and where the manufacturing process has been optimized to minimize the potential for oxidation.

FDA guidelines are in general directed more toward the required components of a registration dossier and do not offer much in the way of guidance to the formulator. One exception to this is the "Guide to Inspection of Lyophilization of Parenterals"; this provides a useful indication of areas of specific interest to the FDA, which the formulator would be well advised to address during the development program.

There is an expectation that pharmaceutical companies will adopt the FDA Quality-by-Design (QbD) approach to formulation and process development described in detail in chapter 8, "Product Optimization." However, most of the currently available case studies shared to date have involved solid oral dosage forms rather than parenteral formulations. Establishing the design space for a sterile aqueous solution should be relatively straightforward because there are only a few process variables, and scale-up should not be an issue. However, for more complicated parenteral dosage forms, such as freeze-dried products, this can be more challenging. Gieseler et al. (2008) present a QbD case study in freeze-drying, including the application of process analytical technology (PAT) to control the most critical process parameters during a freeze-drying cycle. They showed that safety margins for shelf temperature and chamber pressure for a given product could be preevaluated in the laboratory, using PAT tools.

In addition to the regulatory guidelines, more detailed advice on specific issues relating to the development and manufacture of parenteral products can be obtained from the publications of thePDA. This is an American parent organization representing those involved in all aspects of parenteral product development and manufacture and is very active in lobbying the FDA. The PDA produces a bimonthly journal, the *PDA Journal of Pharmaceutical Science and Technology*, which is essential reading for all those involved in the development and manufacture of parenteral products. In addition, the PDA regularly publishes technical reports, which provide a detailed discussion of pertinent issues within the parenteral field. While these reports are not regulatory guidelines, they do provide a good indication of the direction in which the industry and, indeed, the regulators are heading, and those working in the field should take their recommendations seriously. Some of the recently published technical reports are listed below. In the United Kingdom, the PHSS publishes a quarterly journal in conjunction with similar bodies in France, Germany, Scandinavia, and Spain. This journal covers topics similar to those in the PDA journal. The PHSS also publishes a number of monographs, some of which are listed below. These monographs provide a good indication of industry "norms" in the United Kingdom.

FDA Guidelines
Inspection Guidelines
- Guide to Inspection of Lyophilization of Parenterals

Guidance for Industry
- Sterile Drug Products Produced by Aseptic Processing—Current Good Manufacturing Practice
- Container Closure Systems for Packaging Human Drugs and Biologics: Chemistry, Manufacturing, and Controls Documentation
- Submission of Documentation for Sterilization Process Validation in Applications for Human and Veterinary Drug Products
- Container Closure Integrity Testing *in Lieu* of Sterility Testing as a Component of the Stability Protocol for Sterile Products
- Stability Testing of Drug Substances and Drug Products

EMEA Guidelines
- Note for Guidance on Maximum Shelf Life for Sterile Products for Human Use after First Opening or Following Reconstitution
- Decision Trees for the Selection of Sterilization Methods
- Notes for Guidance on Inclusion of Antioxidants and Antimicrobial Preservatives in Medicinal Products

PDA Technical Reports

- Technical Report No. 1: Validation of Moist Heat Sterilization Processes: Cycle Design, Development, Qualification, and Ongoing Control, 61, S1, 2007
- Technical Report No. 22: Process Simulation Testing for Aseptically Filled Products, 50, S1, 1996
- Technical Report No. 23: Industry Survey on Current Sterile Filtration Practices, 51, S1, 1997
- Technical Report No. 24: Current Practices in the Validation of Aseptic Processing, 51, S2, 1997
- Technical Report No. 25: Blend Uniformity Analysis: Validation and In-Process Testing, 51, S3, 1997
- Technical Report No. 26: Sterilization Filtration of Liquids, 52, SI, 1998 (revised 2008)
- Technical Report No. 27: Pharmaceutical Package Integrity, 52, S2, 1998
- Technical Report No. 28: Process Simulation Testing for Sterile Bulk Pharmaceutical Chemicals, 52, S3, 1998
- Technical Report No. 29: Points to Consider for Cleaning Validation, 52, 6, 1998
- Technical Report No. 30: Parametric Release of Sterile Pharmaceuticals Terminally Sterilized by Moist Heat, 1999
- Technical Report No. 31: Validation and Qualification of Computerized Laboratory Data Acquisition Systems, 53, 4, 1999
- Technical Report No. 44: Quality Risk Management for Aseptic Processes

REFERENCES

Akers JM, Nail SL, Saffell-Clemmer W. Top ten hot topics in parenteral science and technology. J Pharm Sci Technol 2007; 61(5):337–361.

Avis KE, Lieberman HA, Lachman L, eds. Pharmaceutical Dosage Forms: Parenteral Medications. Vol 1. New York: Marcel Dekker, 1992.

Betageri GV, Habib MJ. Liposomes as drug carriers. Pharm Eng 1994; 14:8,10,12–14.

Cameron P, ed. Good Pharmaceutical Freeze-Drying Practice. Buffalo Grove, IL: Interpharm Press, 1997.

Collins-Gold LC, Lyons RT, Bartholow LC. Parenteral emulsions for drug delivery. Adv Drug Delivery Rev 1990; 5:189–208.

DeLuca PP, Boylan JC. Pharmaceutical Dosage Forms: Parenteral Medications. Vol 1. In: Avis KE, Lieberman HA, Lachman L, eds. New York: Marcel Dekker, 1992.

Demetzos C. Dendrimers as drug carriers. A new approach to increase the potential of bioactive natural products (review). Nat Prod Commun 2006; 1(7):593–600.

Ford JL. Parenteral products. Pharmaceutics: The Science of Dosage Form Design. In: Aulton ME, ed. New York: Longman, 1988.

Flynn GL. Buffers—pH control within pharmaceutical systems. J Parenter Drug Assoc 1980; 34(2):139–162.

Gieseler H, Kramer T, Schneid S. Quality by design in freeze-drying; cycle design and robustness testing using advanced process analytical technology. Pharm Technol 2008; 10:88–93.

Gupta LS, Patel JP, Jones DL, et al. Parenteral formulation development of renin inhibitor Abbott-72517. J Pharm Sci Technol 1994a; 48(2):86–91.

Gupta PK, Patel JP, Hahn KR. Evaluation of pain and irritation following local administration of parenteral formulations using the rat paw lick model. J Pharm Sci Technol 1994b; 48(3):159–166.

Hall NA. Achieving Sterility in Medical and Pharmaceutical Products. New York: Marcel Dekker, 1994.

Hansrani PK, Davis SS, Groves MJ. The preparation and properties of sterile intravenous emulsions. J Parenter Sci Technol 1983; 37(4):145–150.

Jennings TA. Lyophilization: Introduction and Basic Principles. Denver, CO: Interpharm Press, 1999.

Jorgensen JT, Romsing J, Rasmussen M, et al. Pain assessment of subcutaneous injections. Ann Pharmacother 1996; 30:729–732.

Kipp JE. The role of solid nanoparticle technology in the parenteral delivery of poorly water-soluble drugs (review). Int J Pharm 2004; 284(1–2):109–122.

Kirsch LE, Nguyen L, Moeckly CS. Pharmaceutical container/closure integrity I: Mass spectrometry-based helium leak rate detection for rubber-stoppered glass vials. PDA J Pharm Sci Technol 1997a; 51(5):187–194.

Kirsch LE, Nguyen L, Moeckly CS, et al. Pharmaceutical container/closure integrity II: The relationship between microbial ingress and helium leak rates in rubber-stoppered glass vials. PDA J Pharm Sci Technol 1997b; 51(5):195–202.

Kirsch LE, Nguyen L, Gerth R. Pharmaceutical container/closure integrity III: Validation of helium leak rate method for rigid pharmaceutical containers. PDA J Pharm Sci Technol 1997c; 51(5): 203–207.

Kirsch LE, Nguyen L, Kirsch AM, et al. An evaluation of the WILCO "LFC" method for leak testing pharmaceutical glass-stoppered vials. PDA J Pharm Sci Technol 1999; 53(5):235–239.

Krzyzaniak JF, Alvarez Núñez FA, Raymond DM, et al. Lysis of human red blood cells. 4. Comparison of in vitro and in vivo hemolysis data. J Pharm Sci 1997; 86(11):1215–1217.

Madan P. Sustained-release drug delivery systems. Part V: Parenteral products. Pharm Manuf 1985; 2:50–57.

Martin FJ. Stealth liposomes: a pharmaceutical perspective. In: Arcady R, ed. Microspheres, microcapsules and liposomes. London: Cites, 1999.

MHRA. Rules and Guidance for Pharmaceutical Manufacturers and Distributors. Compiled by the Inspection and Standards Division of the Medicines and Healthcare products Regulatory Agency. London: Pharmaceutical Press, 2007.

Meltzer TH, Jornitz MW. Principles and considerations for bubble point and diffusive airflow integrity testing methods for sterilizing-grade filters. Eur J Parenter Pharm Sci 2008; 13(4):99–101.

Meyer BK, Ni A, Hu B, et al. Antimicrobial preservative use in parenteral products: past and present (review). J Pharm Sci 2007; 96(12):3155–3167.

Nema S, Washkuhn RJ, Brendel RJ. Excipients and their use in injectable products. PDA J Pharm Sci Technol 1997; 51(4):166–171.

Niazi KS. Handbook of Pharmaceutical Manufacturing Formulations: Sterile Products. Vol 6. New York: Informa Healthcare, 2004.

Nordhauser FM, Olson WP, eds. Sterilization of Drugs and Devices: Technologies for the 21st Century. Buffalo Grove, IL: Interpharm Press, 1998.

Pawer R, BenAri A, Domb AJ. Protein and peptide parenteral controlled delivery. Expert Opin Biol Ther 2004; 4(8):1203–1212.

Powell MF, Nguyen T, Baloian L. Compendium of excipients for parenteral formulations. PDA J Pharm Sci Technol 1998; 52(5):238–311.

Reed CH. Recent Technical Advancements in Blow-Fill-Technology. Business Briefing: Pharmagenerics. 2002. Available at: www.weilerengineering.com.

Rey L, May JC. Freeze-Drying/Lyophilisation of Pharmaceutical and Biological Products. 2nd ed. New York: Informa Healthcare, 2004.

Shi Y, Li LC. Current advances in sustained-release systems for parenteral drug delivery (review). Expert Opin Drug Deliv 2005; 2(6):1039–1058.

Sinha VR, Trehan A. Biodegradable microspheres for parenteral delivery (review). Crit Rev Ther Drug Carrier Syst 2005; 22(6):535–602.

Stella VJ, Rajewski RA. Cyclodextrins: their future in drug formulation and delivery. Pharm Res 1997; 14(5):556–567.

Strickley RG. Parenteral formulations of small molecule therapeutics marketed in the United States (1999)—Part I. PDA J Pharm Sci Technol 1999; 53:324–349.

Sutton SC, Evans LAF, Rinaldi TS, et al. Predicting injection site muscle damage. I: Evaluation of immediate release parenteral formulations in animal models. Pharm Res 1996; 13(10): 1507–1513.

Sweetana S, Akers MJ. Solubility principles and practices for parenteral dosage form development. PDA J Pharm Sci Technol 1996; 50(5):330–342.

Tamilvanan S. Oil-in-water lipid emulsions: implications for parenteral and ocular delivering systems (review). Prog Lipid Res 2004; 43(6):489–533.

Thompson DO. Cyclodextrins—Enabling excipients: their present and future use in pharma-ceuticals. Crit Rev Ther Drug Carrier Syst 1997; 14(l):1–104.

Tice T. Delivering with depot formulations. Drug Deliv Technol 2004; 4:44–47.

Twort C, Matthews B, Dunn G, et al. GMP and sterile filtration: a review of some practical and regulatory issues. Eur J Parenter Pharm Sci 2008; 13(3):65–69.

Wakerley Z. In vitro assessment of the haemolytic potential of marketed formulations. AAPS Pharm Sci Suppl 1999; 1(4):S-209.

Wang YJ, Pearlman R, eds. Stability and Characterization of Protein and Peptide Drugs, Case Histories. New York: Plenum Press, 1993.

Wissing SA, Kayser O, Muller RH. Solid lipid nanoparticles for parenteral drug delivery. Adv Drug Deliv Rev 2004; 56(9):1257–1272.

Yalkowsky SH, Krzyzaniak JF, Ward GH. Formulation-related problems associated with intravenous drug delivery. J Pharm Sci 1998; 87(7):787–796.

Yalkowsky SH, Valvani SC, Johnson BW. In vitro method for detecting precipitation of parenteral formulations after injection. J Pharm Sci 1983; 72:1014–1017.

10 | Inhalation Dosage Forms

Paul Wright

AstraZeneca R&D Charnwood, Loughborough, Leicestershire, U.K.

INTRODUCTION

Asthma and chronic obstructive pulmonary diseases (COPDs) such as bronchitis and emphysema are major and growing disease areas where the major route of administration is topically, at the site of action, in the lung. Asthma is a common, chronic disease with a prevalence of more than 5% in adults and 15% to 20% in children, and is increasing in many parts of the world. The prevalence of COPD is even higher, and mortality rates are 10 times higher than those for asthma. At present, similar drugs are used for both diseases, with steroids, short- and long-acting β2s, and anticholinergics being the most common therapies. Combination products with two actives are gaining importance. Inhalation allows the delivery of smaller doses directly to the lungs, with the advantage of reduced systemic side effects. There are also other illnesses in which pulmonary delivery is appropriate, such as cystic fibrosis, human immunodeficiency virus (HIV), lung cancer, pain, and infections. In addition, the lung is being viewed as a possible route to the systemic circulation for the treatment of non-respiratory diseases, where normal oral administration is not technically possible. This is especially relevant to the delivery of peptides and proteins. The latter has recently been shown to be technically possible with insulin, although the inhaled insulin product Exubera™ has surprisingly been withdrawn after only one year on the market for a variety of reasons.

Unlike most other drug delivery systems, those in the respiratory area can have a major influence on physician/patient acceptance. A wide range of devices are available in the three main categories of dry powder inhalers (DPIs) and metered dose inhalers (MDIs), that is, pressurized aerosols and nebulizers. The preferred type of inhaler varies considerably between countries (e.g., DPIs in Scandinavia and MDIs in the United States) and between patient groups (e.g., nebulizers for pediatrics).

Until the mid-1980s, the MDI was the dominant inhalation dosage form, but the Montreal Protocol lead to greatly increased activity in device development, for both existing drugs and new chemical entities. The propellants for the existing MDIs were chlorofluorocarbons (CFCs). CFCs were implicated in the depletion of the stratospheric ozone layer, and their phaseout was agreed upon internationally in the United Nations sponsored Montreal Protocol. CFC-propelled MDIs were given a time-limited essential use exemption. MDIs propelled by hydrofluoroalkanes (HFAs), also known as hydrofluorocarbons (HFCs), have been introduced to the market after extensive safety testing of the propellants, and the transition is almost complete in the developed world. However, HFAs do have a global warming potential, and they come under the reach of another international environmental agreement, the Kyoto Protocol. At present HFAs for MDIs are free of regulation, and it is expected that HFAs will remain available, since no other suitable propellants have been identified. The banning of CFCs has also led to a resurgence of DPI development.

A consequence of this development activity has been corresponding patent applications for both formulations and devices. The patenting process, together with oppositions, is a lengthy operation, and some major patents published in the early 1990s are only now being finally decided (e.g., the Boerhinger HFA 227 patents in 2008), leading to long periods of uncertainty. Hence, a current knowledge of the patent situation is essential before commencing any practical development studies, although many critical patents will expire around 2010/12. It should also be noted that, since this area is very competitive, much of the available information is in the patent literature rather than in the scientific journals. However, it should be noted that in this chapter the references are predominantly from the scientific literature, since these better illustrate points of interest.

A last general point to be made here is to emphasize the complexity of inhalation products. They all contain a high degree of engineering, and it could be argued that the device is more critical than the formulation. This engineering dimension adds considerably to development times, since an alteration to a device component can typically take two to three months, and for an MDI, there is an additional one month equilibration time required following manufacture and before testing (see later in chapter for more details).

While the product is in the aerosol can or nebulizer vial, the dosage form that the patient experiences is a dynamic aerosol cloud. For example, the quality of the cloud from a DPI is often dependent on the airflow through the device, and an MDI cloud rapidly evaporates as it travels through the air. These factors affect the particle size distribution in the aerosol cloud, and the particle size is the critical parameter for lung deposition.

LUNG DEPOSITION

Particles are deposited in the lung by three main mechanisms: impaction, sedimentation, and diffusion. Impaction is the primary mechanism, hence the relevance of impactors in particle sizing, which is discussed later. Deposition will vary, depending on the airflow and the disease state, as smaller airways due to bronchoconstriction or inflammation will increase impaction in the upper airways. An increased airflow will also lead to increased impaction in the throat and upper airways; hence patients are instructed to breathe slowly and deeply. Some DPIs may conflict with this, since a high airflow is required for powder deaggregation. Sedimentation is a secondary deposition mechanism, occurring in the low airflow region of the deep lung, hence the requirement for patients to hold their breath after inhalation. Diffusion is a relatively slow process and is not very significant in the timescales of a breathing pattern, even with breath holding.

The classic diagram of deposition versus particle size is shown in Figure 1, but it should be noted that this is for a normal breathing pattern at low airflows.

There is often a need to test the efficiency of a product's lung delivery, and then in vivo measurements must be made. Any study is complicated by the fraction (often the majority) of drug that is swallowed and passes into the gastrointestinal system. The normal methods are a pharmacokinetic study or a γ-camera study. For pharmacokinetic work, the drug either has no oral absorption or can be negated by charcoal-block absorption. This study will not give a picture of regional deposition in the lung, whereas a γ-camera study (either 2D or 3D) will show regional variations (Newman and Wilding, 1998; Newman et al., 2000). A typical picture

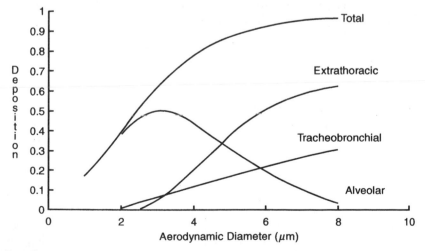

Figure 1 Lung deposition–deposition versus aerodynamic diameter.

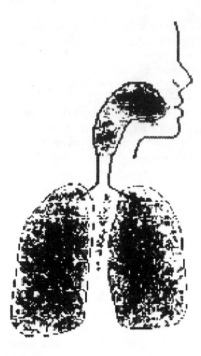

Figure 2   Deposition from a Turbuhaler®.

is shown in Figure 2 for deposition from a Turbuhaler®. Other technical approaches are urinary excretion and β2 drug challenge studies. In the challenge studies, the opening of the airways due to the β2 drug's pharmacological response can be measured by an increased ability to both inhale and exhale.

PARTICLE SIZING

The importance of particle sizing is that only small particles will reach the lung, since the nose and mouth will remove any larger particles. There is continuing debate as to what maximum size will reach the lung, but consensus is for around 5 to 7 µm. For alveoli penetration, a size of 3 µm is required, but very fine particles, below 1 µm, may be exhaled. It is the size of the droplets in the aerosol cloud that is important; for dry powders and fully evaporated liquid suspensions, this may be the original powder particle. Hence, it is essential to have powders in the micron range, and normal micronization will usually produce a size of 1 to 3 µm. Newer techniques, such as supercritical fluid extraction, can produce smaller particles. Naturally, if the product is a solution, the particle size formed on evaporation of the solvent will depend on solution concentration.

Impaction
As with most questions on particle size, the answer is very dependent on the definition used and the experimental technique. For a dynamic aerosol cloud, the correct definition is the aerodynamic particle size, which is the diameter of an equivalent sphere of unit density. An equivalent sphere is a conventional assumption in particle sizing, but for the aerodynamic size, the density is included to account for the momentum of the particle; that is, both mass and velocity are important. The technique chosen for measurement must include these parameters, and impaction is the normally chosen technique, which also reflects the major deposition mechanism in the lung. A schematic of an impaction plate is given in Figure 3.

The mathematics of fluid dynamics that define the parameters is quite complex, but the critical ones are airflow, jet diameter, and the jet-plate distance. A good analogy is driving a vehicle (the particle) around a sharp road bend (the change in airstream direction).

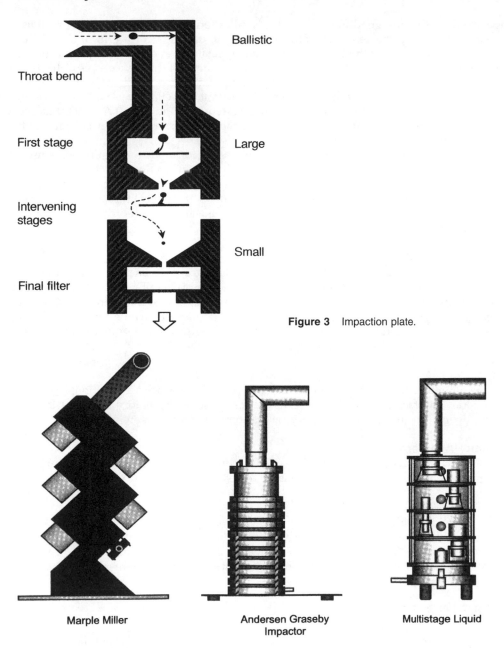

Figure 3   Impaction plate.

Figure 4   Commercial impactors.

A slow-moving car will navigate the bend, while a fast-moving car or a slow lorry will impact. In addition, impaction will measure a mass of drug on a particular plate, and hence is an unambiguous measurement.

A number of commercial impactors are built around this principle, the early ones being single stage, which have been superseded by multistage impactors, with both single and multiple jets. These are shown in Figure 4 for the Andersen-Graseby, Astra-Copley MSLI, and the less common Marple-Miller. All of these impactors will provide a particle size distribution. A more recent model is the result of an industry consortium and is the next generation impactor (NGI), which was designed for better productivity and the possibility of automation in analysis, together with improved operating characteristics.

Depending on the dosage, different experimental criteria will be important. For MDIs, the cloud evaporates; thus, the geometry of the entry port to the impactor is critical (LeBelle et al., 1997) and is well defined by the European Pharmacopoeia (EP) and the U.S. Pharmacopeia (USP). DPI performance will usually depend on the airflow through the device's aerosolization mechanism (de Boer et al., 1997); an airflow corresponding to the device's air resistance should be chosen. The rise time to peak steady state flow is important as well, because if it is too slow, the dose could be emitted as a bolus and not deaggregated to a fine cloud. Also the relative humidity (RH) of the air drawn through the device/impactor can have an influence, with high humidities reducing the deaggregation.

The discussion so far has related to the use of impactors for in vitro measurements used in formulation and/or device optimization, stability testing, or quality control. If the purpose of testing is to gain information on a potential in vitro/in vivo correlation, then modifications are sometimes made to the equipment. For MDIs, the use of an anatomical throat instead of the USP throat can improve correlation, while for DPIs, a lung machine that reproduces breathing patterns can be beneficial.

Light Scattering (Laser)

A number of commercial machines (e.g., the Malvern Mastersizer™) use the light-scattering technique, and for aerosol clouds, its main applicability is the sizing of essentially stationary clouds from nebulizer solutions. Here again, definitions are important, as different theories of light scattering may give different results. It is vital to distinguish between number and mass average, as the presence of relatively few large particles can give a low number particle size, but a high mass particle size, which is the important parameter.

Microscope

Microscopy is not relevant to aerodynamic particle size, since the particles are stationary on the microscope slide. The technique is, however, asked for by some regulatory agencies. It is of value during development for examining deaggregation or Ostwald ripening.

Phase Doppler Anemometry

Phase Doppler anemometry is a specialized research technique that gives information on both particle size and velocity of single particles within the cloud.

High-Speed Camera

By image analysis of single photographs, a particle size distribution can be established, but only the physical diameter is measured, not the aerodynamic component. However, it is of great value to see the establishment and decay of an aerosol cloud in slow motion. High-speed video is also possible, which gives an excellent picture of the changing aerosol cloud.

DRY POWDER INHALERS

Fisons introduced the first DPI with the capsule-based Spinhaler®. This was followed by a number of other capsule devices and then by unit dose blisters and multidose systems. DPIs are very diverse in their design and operation, since each product manufacturer has developed their own proprietary devices for their own drugs.

Formulation

The main formulation challenges come from the need to use very cohesive micronized powders, which presents problems in powder flow (Feeley et al., 1998) on filling machinery. These powders also aerosolize poorly in an airstream and give a deaggregated cloud. Unfortunately, the formulation approaches are severely limited by the very restricted number of excipients available because of a lack of lung administration safety data. Lactose is the only excipient commonly used (Zeng et al., 2000). Other sugars maybe considered (Naini et al., 1998) if the drug contains primary amine groups, which will give the Maillard reaction, which leads to a brown discoloration with lactose (for example, see sect. "Compatibility," chap. 6).

The objective is an ordered mix of the micronized drug with larger particle size lactose (Larhrib et al., 1999), typically 60 μm, but it can be in the range of 40 to 100 μm. Mixing such a cohesive system is difficult, and often a high-energy mixer is required, together with sieving(s) to aid homogeneity (Zeng et al., 2000).

Determination of homogeneity is challenging at the level of a single dose, for example, 5 to 20 mg of powder, and sampling errors with thief systems are possible (Muzzio et al., 1997). Often the best sampling system is the device itself, since further powder handling will occur during device filling. The balance of interparticle forces is very important, because a drug particle needs to be strongly attached to the lactose carrier during mixing, filling, and on stability, yet becomes easily detached on aerosolization to form a fine particle cloud (Podczeck, 1998). Hence, attention must be paid to surface morphology and surface energies (Kawashima et al., 1998). A method of improving fine particle fraction is to add an excipient such as magnesium stearate as a second micronized powder, and this blocks the more active and strongly binding sites on the lactose (Kippax and Morton, 2008). If the powder mix is to go into a unit dose system, such as a capsule or blister, then the particle need not be so strongly attached as for a free-flowing reservoir system where segregation could occur.

A second approach is to spheronize the micronized particles, which gives a free-flowing powder, which should break down easily on aerosolization. The advantage is that there is no risk of poor homogeneity or segregation, but this is balanced by the difficulty of metering minute quantities of powders (spheres are typically 100–250 μg).

During unit operations, such as milling and mixing, at pilot plant or at full production scale, it is very easy to produce a powder cloud. Since the particles in this cloud can be inhaled, it is vital to protect the operator's safety by appropriate containment measures and personal protection equipment.

Devices

As stated earlier, there is little commonality between devices, although some are now available for in-licensing. This diversity makes general comment difficult, but there are three main categories:

1. Pre-metered single dose, for example, capsule
2. Pre-metered multidose as single units, for example , blisters on a card or in a strip
3. Multidose bulk reservoir

Examples of these classes are shown in Figure 5.

The aerosolization operation depends on effective turbulence being created in the airstream, which lifts the powder from its metering position and carries it to the device's mouthpiece. This can be done by a number of mechanisms, such as a mesh, an orifice, or a swirl chamber. All of these methods introduce turbulence to provide the energy to remove the individual drug particle from the charge carrier particle surface or the spheronized aggregate. Computational fluid dynamics (CFD) is being increasingly used to model airflows in devices, with the consequent saving in time and expense of manufacturing models, and of testing them. Each program must be tailored to a specific device, however, and the results validated by experimental results.

Naturally, the development of the device must involve the formulation, as the engineering cannot be optimized in isolation, and close collaboration is required between formulators and design engineers.

Device design often commences with the aerosolization mechanism, since the fine particle dose reaching the lung is the critical therapeutic dose. This is often a crude mechanism to show proof of principle. However, for regulatory constraints, the metering system is more important, and this is often given insufficient attention in the early stages of a project.

The next stage is to produce a working model, which may be produced by a craftsman or, more probably, with modern technology, by soft moulds linked to a computer-aided design (CAD) system. At this stage, the project becomes complex, as almost always the engineering aspects are dealt with by an external company, even if the design work is internal.

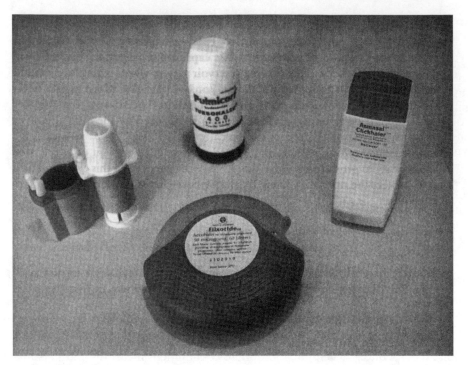

Figure 5   Device categories (clockwise from left): single-capsule, Spinhaler™ (Aventis), multi-dose reservoir, Pulmicort™ (AstraZeneca), multi-dose reservoir, Asmasal™ Clickhaler™ (Medeva), and multi-dose pre-metered, Flixotide™ Accuhaler™ (GlaxoWellcome).

It is essential to involve the eventual plastic molder at this stage, since any design must be capable of production, and mold design together with plastic flow is a very specialized activity. Also, an early involvement from market research, industrial design, and ergonomics is required, since the operation of the device should be heavily influenced by the user's opinion. This is the same for any consumer market product, for example , a hair-dryer. In market research, doctors, asthma nurse practitioners, patients, and parents of pediatrics should all be consulted in a number of countries, since they have very different requirements for a device. Nonworking models produced by stereoligography can often be used for these studies. For large quantities of working models, a single hard tool will be used.

Operation
In optimizing the product, both device and formulation are modified, and the normal product release tests are evaluated. Extra investigations are also carried out, such as a standard drop test to ensure that the device is robust. Other major areas for investigation are the dependence of fine particle dose on airflow rate (Srichana et al., 1998), the effect of humidity both on storage (Naini et al., 1998; Maggi et al., 1999) and in-use, drug retention within the device, and the effect of orientation and electrostatics (Carter et al., 1998).

Scale-up/Technology Transfer
For the formulation, there is a significant problem of increasing the mass of powder during blending and especially for spheronization, since a large mass can break down fragile spheres. Powder processing is usually carried out at controlled RH, usually <50% RH.

Devices are assembled typically from 15 to 20 individual components, and each will be produced on a multi-cavity mold with four or eight moulds. Until this stage is reached, with devices being assembled from these production moulds, and then tested, the final variability between devices cannot be fully established. However, during development, appropriate engineering and tolerance analyses can give good confidence. The device will be delivered from the molders with a minimum number of subassemblies and will be filled with the formulation at the pharmaceutical company. In the case of unit dose devices, the capsule or blister will usually be filled at the pharmaceutical company.

The transfer of analytical methodology is a major part of technology transfer, especially when robotics are involved.

Future Developments
At present, most DPI products are dependent on being operated by the patient. This will be reduced by the introduction of powered devices, for example, compressed air, a fan, or a hammer, and, in this way, they will be independent of airflow rate. Such an increase in complexity, however, will probably require the introduction of a breath activation feature. Breath activation may also be incorporated in passive devices to remove the variable of airflow rate through the device. Powder spaces may also be introduced.

A major question is how much market share DPIs will capture, balancing their environmental friendliness with patient acceptance and cost. In last decade the growth in the inhalation market has been taken up predominately by DPIs, with MDIs remaining constant in terms of number of units.

METERED DOSE INHALERS

Riker Laboratories, now 3M Health Care, invented the pressurized MDI in 1955 when they combined the atomizing power of CFCs and a metering valve design. The great majority of valves still use this basic retention valve principle, and hence pressurized MDIs (pMDIs) are all similar in appearance and operation when used with a standard actuator in the normal "press and breathe" manner.

Formulation
Environment
The transition to HFAs (or HFCs) is well under way and should be essentially complete by 2010 in the developed countries, while local production in the developing countries may take longer. The reason for this transition is that all CFCs are implicated in the destruction of the ozone layer due to a reaction between the ozone and the chlorine radical (Table 1, Fig. 6). Consequently the production and use of CFCs have been banned by the United Nations Montreal Protocol, but medicinal aerosols have been given an essential use exemption due to their vital performance in asthma and COPD therapy (Forte and Dibble, 1999). The transition to HFAs has been slower than expected, as the change from CFCs to HFAs was not just a drop-in excipient change, as was first believed (Leach, 2005). A major development program has been necessary involving the valve. This has taken approximately 10 years for most companies, and HFA products did not begin to reach the market in Europe until 1999, and the major salbutamol transition in the United States has only been in August 2007.

Because CFCs are being relegated to history, this chapter will concentrate on the new HFAs. Three main factors control formulation approaches, and only one of these is pharmaceutical in nature. HFA 227 and HFA 134a are very poor solvents; hence the existing CFC surfactants/valve lubricants are not soluble in the HFAs. The second factor that is related

Table 1 Environmental Actions of Propellants

Propellant	Ozone depletion potential	Global warming potential[a]
CFC11	1.0	4000
CFC 12	1.0	8500
CFC114	1.0	9300
HFA 134a	0	1300
HFA 227	0	2900

[a]Carbon dioxide = 1.
Abbreviations: CFC, chlorofluorocarbon; HFA, hydrofluoroalkane.

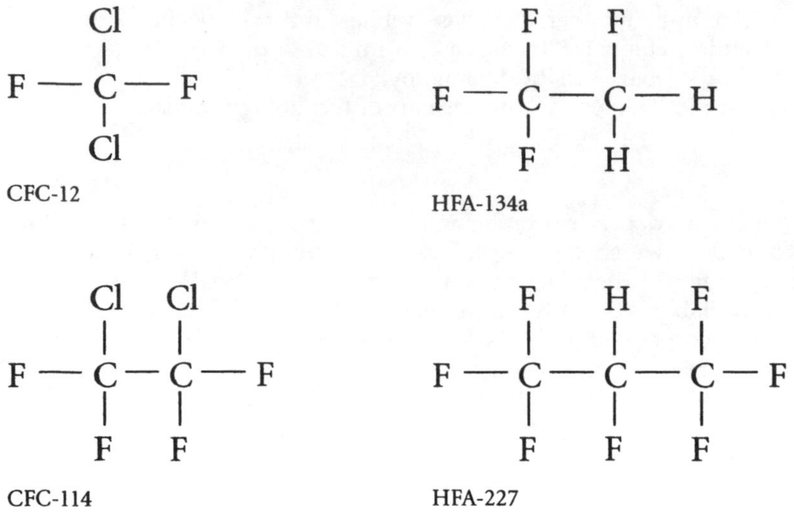

Figure 6 Formulae of CFCs and HFAs. *Abbreviations*: CFCs, chlorofluorocarbons; HFAs, hydrofluoroalkanes.

Table 2 Important Formulation Patents

Ethanol/HFA-134a EP 0372777	3M Health Care Priority date 06/12/88
HFA-227 and mixtures EP 513099	Boehinger Ingelheim Priority date 03/02/90
EP 514415 HFA propellant only WO 93/11744	Glaxo Priority date 12/12/91
PVP/PEG/HFA WO 93/05765	Fisons (Aventis) Priority date 25/9/91

is that any new surfactant must have adequate drug safety data, and this could mean a full New Chemical Entity (NCE) type safety-testing program. The third factor is the large number of often conflicting and overlapping patents in this area (Bowman and Greenleaf, 1999). The worldwide patent situation must be considered, since although a patent may have been revoked in Europe, it could have been granted in Australia and still be the subject of prosecution in the United States. Important examples are shown in Table 2, but the list is definitely not exhaustive.

Propellant Properties
The properties of the propellants are the dominant factors in formulation development for an MDI. Many formulation approaches are dictated by the fact that the HFAs are poorer solvents than the CFCs, which in absolute terms are already poor solvents, for both drugs and excipients. However, the main purpose of the propellant, as its name suggests, is to provide the energy to propel the drug from the valve in the form of droplets, which rapidly evaporate to leave the drug particles. Certain propellant properties are shown in Table 3.

Solution Formulations
Because of the very poor solvent properties of HFAs, only a very limited number of drugs, for example , beclomethasone diproprionate, may dissolve completely in the propellant with or without an ethanol cosolvent (Williams et al., 1999). For a solution, the crucially important factor of suspension homogeneity is almost guaranteed, but other problems increase, relating to drug adsorption into valve rubbers and drug reactivity leading to degradation. When the valve is actuated, the propellant will evaporate, leaving a precipitated particle, which may be

Table 3 Propellant Properties

Name: HFA	Formula	Pressure (psig @ 20°C)	Density (kg/L @ 20°C)	Water solubility (ppm)
11	CCl_3F	−1.8	1.488	∼100
114	$CC1F_2CC1F_2$	11.9	1.471	∼100
12	$CC1_2F_2$	67.6	1.329	∼100
12/114	60:40	49.0	1.387	
134a	CF_3CH_2F	68.0	1.226	∼2000
227	CF_3CHFCF_3	41.9	1.415	∼600

of smaller size than that from a suspension prepared from a micronized drug. This, in turn, may lead to higher fine particle fraction and increased lung deposition (Leach, 1999). For a new drug, this potential increased efficiency is excellent, but it may be a problem for a generic match to an existing suspension product, as the label dose will be less, leading to possible confusion. One way of avoiding this situation is to add a nonvolatile miscible liquid, for example , polyethylene glycol, which will maintain an aerosol drop in the micrometer-size range (Brambilla et al., 1999).

Suspension Formulations

Many of the principles here are the same as for normal oral aqueous suspensions, except that the liquid is essentially nonpolar; hence steric stabilization is thought to be more important than by electrostatic means (DLVO theory). A stabilizing agent is normally added to give an adequate suspension. The agent may also act as a valve lubricant, which may be necessary for this mechanical device, or a second excipient may be added for this function. The potential effect of water ingress through the valve rubbers by Fickian diffusion should be investigated, since this may well destabilize the suspension.

Moisture may well be preferentially adsorbed at the particle surface, leading to a microenvironment in this region that can alter the performance of the surfactant. Another important attribute is to density match the drug particle, by blending HFA-227 and HFA-134a, where possible, since a homogeneous (Williams et al., 1998a) suspension is vital for filling uniform aliquots into the dispensing valve. Fast aggregation into loose flocs is not always a problem, since the turbulence in the aerosol stream when the valve is actuated is high, and often enough to deaggregate any such floc.

There are three main approaches to suspension formulation. The first is to add a co-solvent to the propellant to increase its solvency power and enable the dissolution of conventional CFC surfactants such as oleic acid or sorbitan trioleate (Span) (Fedina et al., 1997). This is usually only employed with HFA 134a, since the addition of a co-solvent, usually ethanol, will lower the vapor pressure of the system and lead to larger droplets in the aerosol cloud, which may then be too large to be inhaled (Steckel and Muller, 1998; Williams et al., 1998b). Investigations must be made to ensure that the co-solvent for the surfactant is not also acting as a co-solvent for the drug, since even a slight solubility of the drug will lead to particle growth through Ostwald ripening.

A second approach is to use a new excipient that is soluble in the propellant only (Blondino and Byron, 1998). HFA-227 is a better solvent than HFA-134a, hence most references to new surfactants (e.g., polyvinylpyrrolidone) relate to HFA-227. A third approach is not to use any excipients, the formulation here being only drug and propellant. In such a system, the suspension is expected to be more sensitive to challenges than in a more robust one containing surfactants. In these excipient-free systems, the ability of the propellant to wet the drug surface may be crucial.

Devices

The hardware for a pMDI (Fig. 7) is as crucial as, or perhaps even more important than, the formulation. A normal "press and breathe" MDI consists of the can, valve, and actuator (also sometimes called an adapter). The three components are sourced externally.

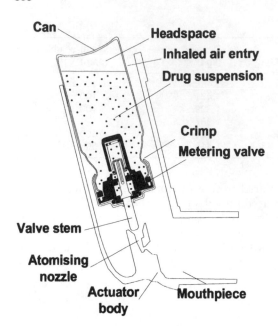

Figure 7 pMDI. *Abbreviation*: pMDI, pressurized metered dose inhaler.

Can

The container is normally made of aluminum, and although plastic-coated glass is available, it is normally only used for experimental work where direct observation of the contents is required. Stainless steel is also available, but this is too expensive for production. Drug particles in HFA suspensions have a much greater tendency to stick to the can walls than in CFC systems (Traini et al., 2006), and for this reason, certain formulations require the aluminum to be coated with a polymer, usually a fluoropolymer, to reduce or remove this deleterious phenomenon.

Valves

Retention valves all have a similar design and are normally bought from Valois (Fig. 8), Bespak, or 3M Neotechnic. The retention valve operates in a manner analogous to canal lock gates, with an opening either to the bulk formulation in the can or to the atmosphere via the actuator.

When the valve is depressed for firing, a direct pathway is opened to the atmosphere, and the vapor pressure of the propellant drives the boiling formulation out of the valve chamber to form the aerosol cloud. When the valve is released, this pathway to the atmosphere is closed; and in the "at rest" position, a small passageway of varying design is opened to the bulk formulation. This then fills the valve chamber, again driven by the propellant vapor pressure. This small passageway remains open to the can, but its narrow bore is designed to prevent emptying of the valve chamber due to surface tension.

Other valve designs exist, which do not have a retention chamber, but the metering chamber is formed to collect an aliquot of bulk suspension as the valve is being operated. These designs are relatively uncommon in marketed products, but development is progressing in this area.

Although valves appear to be standard items, each must be individually optimized for the particular formulation, in detailed design and, very importantly, with regard to the rubbers, where swell characteristics can control valve performance (Tiwari et al., 1998).

Actuator

The actuator can be obtained as a standard item or is often designed to give a company house style. The critical parameters are the expansion chamber where evaporation commences and

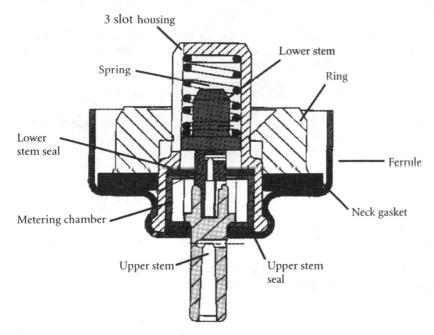

Figure 8 Retention valve (Valois RCS).

the orifice diameter, which controls the droplet particle size (Steckel and Muller, 1998). If orifice diameter is too large, the droplet particle size is too great, and if too small, excessive drug deposition and blockage can occur.

Operation

On operation, the interaction of the formulation and the valve must be considered. A major area is the performance of the valve rubbers, which can be determined only when their swelling due to propellant has reached equilibrium, which may take up to four weeks. If the rubber seals grip the valve stem too tightly, then the valve will stick, and excessive force will be required to actuate it. It may return to its rest position only under the spring force, but slowly. Alternatively, if the rubber seal to the valve stem is too loose, an alternative pathway for escape of propellant is formed, and on actuation, liquid escapes around the metering chamber (Cummings, 1999). Leakage is also possible, such as gross leakage from a poorly crimped valve or low losses, on storage, from Fickian diffusion through the rubber seals. Because of its smaller molecular weight, HFA-134a has a higher loss rate than HFA-227.

There is also the possibility of loss of drug from the metering chamber on storage (Cummings, 1999). This can occur if propellant drains out of the metering chamber and is known as "loss of prime," since the valve has to be primed before it is ready for use.

Another factor is that, on storage, the drug in the metering chamber may sediment, and even with shaking, may not re-disperse. Since the valve chamber is full there is very little turbulence possible, and hence little energy to aid re-dispersion of the sedimented drug.

Suspension stability is very important since the valve refills after actuation, and, depending on patient use, a varying time can elapse from the can being shaken to the valve being actuated. An informative experiment is to shake the can, leave it for varying periods up to 60 seconds, and then actuate and collect the dose. With increasing time lapses, the drug may increase (sedimentation) or decrease (creaming). This is important for patient usage, because patients can take a considerable time to coordinate breathing, or assemble a spacer (Blondino and Byron, 1998).

An alternative experiment is to use the optical suspension characterization (OSCAR) technique, where the turbidity at the bottom and/or top of a transparent vial is measured with time to obtain a plot of sedimentation or creaming.

Scale-up

Initial formulation work, when tens of cans are required, is often carried out by cold filling, where the propellants are cooled to below their boiling point, and can then be processed as liquids without any pressure implications. This method was often used for full-scale production for CFCs, since propellant 11 has a boiling point of 23°C. However, both HFA-134a and HFA-227 have low boiling points; therefore, pressure filling is more common for the HFA propellants.

Here the formulation is made up to between a 500 and 1000 L scale in pressurized vessels and then filled into cans through the aerosol valve, precrimped onto the can. Naturally, appropriate safety precautions have to be made for working with large-scale pressurized systems. With increasing scale, there is the move to increasing automation of the filling process.

For the components, the move to hard tooling multicavity molds for the actuator has the same implications as for DPI components, for example, dimensions must be checked. Valves can be assembled by hand, semi-automatically, or on fully automated production lines. It is important to obtain valves during development from the production line, if this is possible. A valve is constructed of 15 to 20 individual items, plastic, metal, and rubber, and a number of different batches of an item may be used in a major production run. Hence, valves from a production run may well not be from the same item batches, and the definition of a production batch then becomes important.

Add-on Devices

As well as the standard actuator mouthpiece, sometimes known as "press and breathe," which describes its mode of action, there are a number of supplementary devices whose main function is to aid coordination. One of the major disadvantages of pMDIs is the need for the patient to coordinate firing the device with inhalation.

Breath-Activated Inhaler

Breath-activated inhalers (BAIs), developed by Norton and 3M Health Care, are now relatively common. Although each has a different mechanical design, both work by a trigger threshold of airflow activating the preloaded can, and hence firing the pMDI. This ensures that the patient is inhaling at a medium airflow when the aerosol is fired. Other designs are entering the market as well such as the K-Haler.

Spacer

A spacer or chamber is a second way to improve coordination (Fig. 9).

The MDI is actuated as normal, but into the spacer, not the patient's mouth. The patient then inhales from the other end of the spacer, sometimes through a one-way valve. This again ensures coordination. A pMDI plus spacer is a common system used for young children, sometimes with a face mask (Finlay, 1998). Most spacers are plastic, and an electrostatic charge can build up on the plastic and attract the aerosol cloud, depositing it on the walls and significantly reducing the dose. This is especially true for unused spacers but can be reduced by washing with detergents. A metal spacer is also available, which has negligible electrostatics.

A second advantage of spacers is that the large particles are deposited on the walls before finer particles; hence the dose inhaled consists of a higher percentage of fine inhalable particles. Conversely, a lower amount of nonrespirable particles are deposited in the mouth and throat, where local side effects can occur, especially for steroids.

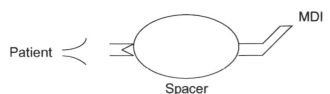

Figure 9   Spacer.

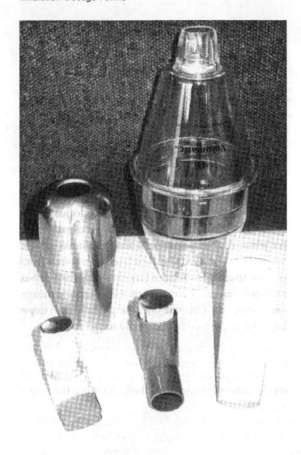

Figure 10 Auxiliary devices (from *left* to *right*): *rear*: Nebuchamber™ (AstraZeneca), Volumatic™ (Allen&Hanburys); spacers, front: Flutide™MDI (GlaxoWellcome), Qvar™ MDI (3M Health Care), Easi-breathe BAI (Baker Norton).

Dose Counter

The Food and Drug Administration (FDA) has issued guidance, requiring dose counters to be fitted on MDIs, and these are now reaching the market and are often on top of the can, but also can be incorporated in the actuator or a BAI. Dose counters will enable parents to check if their child has taken their medicine and will enable everyone to establish when the can is empty (Bradshaw, 2006). Patients should not be advised to float the can in water to gauge its contents, as potential water ingress is disastrous to formulation stability.

Future

An exhaustive search for new propellants was made at the time of the switch away from CFCs, and it is unlikely that new ones will be found with the necessary physicochemical properties combined with an excellent safety profile. However if possibilities do emerge they should be evaluated. New surfactants are possible, but there is the major cost hurdle of drug toxicity studies to NCE standards. Particle engineering may provide benefits, for example, production by supercritical fluid technology or hollow particles.

Devices are starting to appear, which contain electronics and batteries (e.g., BAI and Aradigm), and this allows the possibilities for extensive feedback to both patient and physician (see Fig. 10 for auxiliary devices).

NEBULIZERS

Nebulizer therapy is different, from the developer's perspective, to DPIs or pMDIs, in that nebulizer formulations and machines are developed and sold by independent companies. Hence, the formulator will take an existing commercial nebulizer machine(s) and will ensure that the formulation performs satisfactorily. Also, the target population is different, with nebulizers often being used in the hospital setting and for pediatric and geriatric patients.

Phase I Studies

It can take many months to develop an acceptable DPI or pMDI for early clinical studies, but an expeditious route is to use an extemporaneously prepared nebulizer solution of the drug and a matching placebo. This can be developed relatively quickly with only 24-hour stability required (drug and microbiology) and the performance of the solution in the nebulizer established. Naturally, the drug must have suitable physicochemical properties, for example, solubility. Sterility is not specifically required for phase I formulation. Instead, sterile water for injection is used, and the shelf life restricted to one working day, for example, eight hours.

Formulation

The formulation techniques and approaches are essentially similar to those for sterile products such as parenterals or ophthalmics (chaps. 9 and 12, respectively); hence the issues surrounding the production and validation of sterile solutions will not be considered here. Formulations are usually solutions, often giving a higher unit dose than the corresponding DPI or pMDI. Suspensions can also be formulated, although these are rare and usually relate to steroids. It is more difficult to get a drug particle taken up into a nebulized/aerosolized droplet; thus, a small particle size is essential (Ostrander et al., 1999), as it must naturally be significantly smaller than the droplet size, which itself has to be small to reach the lung. There are also major sterility difficulties with suspensions, since they cannot be produced asceptically using sterile filters. Because of their potential to cause bronchoconstriction, preservatives are not good practice and hence most formulations are unit dose unpreserved. Isotonicity of the solution, however, is favored for the same reason. If the drug itself is not sufficient, normal isotonicity agents are added, for example, sodium chloride. Naturally, if the drug solution is already hypertonic, little can be done.

The unit dose is either glass or plastic, with the use of plastic "form-fill-seal" equipment being dominant. However, glass is considered more elegant pharmaceutically in some markets and can be terminally sterilized where this is a requirement. With "form-fill-seal" processes, a strip of ampoules is produced, with the neck being much easier to break than glass. The plastic is pervious to moisture transmission, which will occur on storage, especially in dry environments; thus an aluminum overwrap may be necessary.

In clinical practice, nebulizer solutions are mixed, and it is essential to check if the product interacts with any of the common commercial products.

Nebulizer Devices

Conventional nebulizers are designed and supplied by medical equipment manufacturers, not by pharmaceutical companies. They range considerably in their effectiveness (Le Brun et al., 1999a), some producing droplets at around 3 μm for delivery to the deep lung, while others have such large particle sizes that they are only useful as room humidifiers. It is essential during clinical trials to ensure that all investigators are using an acceptable nebulizer, and, preferably, standardization has occurred to a number of units. These machines should span the normal performance of nebulizers; otherwise the product may be limited to the one nebulizer used in the clinical trials by a regulatory authority. There are two types of nebulizers: pneumatic and, more recently introduced, ultrasonic (Flament et al., 1995).

Nebulizers continue to improve, both in shortening the nebulization time and increasing the fine particle fraction.

There has also been the development of a number of small multidose nebulizers where the formulation is integral in the device, as in an MDI, for example, Boehringer's Respimat and the inhalation cycle is one breath (Steed et al., 1997).

Operation

The pharmaceutical company sells only the sterile ampoule, and release tests are really restricted to a sterile unit dose. Dose uniformity is for the contents of the vial, while aerosolization is not considered for any release tests. How well the ampoule empties must be considered.

In operation, the liquid is placed into the nebulizer chamber, the machine is switched on and the aerosol cloud is produced (Dunbar and Hickey, 1999). An important aspect of operation is the rate of nebulization, which controls how long the patient will take to receive the maximum dose (Le Brun et al., 1999b). A short time is preferable, since long times lead to poor compliance, with 10 to 20 minutes being typical. The volume of solution left in the nebulizer cup (dead volume) is also important, as this will control the dose available to the patient. Available dose is often approximately 1 mL; 50% of a 2-mL vial, but only 25% of a 4-mL vial (or 2 x 2 mL). During nebulization, concentration can increase, and the liquid temperature can rise. For nebulizers, the aerosol cloud is produced by a power source and is almost stationary. Hence, laser diffraction (e.g., Malvern) methods can be used to size solutions where a homogeneous distribution of drug will occur. It is important to distinguish between number average and mass average, since many small drops will only carry a small percentage of the dose. Impactors can be used, but water drops will evaporate in the airstream, giving an erroneous particle size.

A face mask is often used with a nebulizer, to promote compliance over the 10 to 20 minute of dosing, and any lengths of tubing between machine and face mask should be minimal, to prevent excessive wall losses.

STANDARDS

Regulatory and pharmacopoeial standards are always important in any development program. Normally, they are limited to the main parameters and change only slowly, and the technology available at the present enables the standards to be achieved relatively easily. However, for inhalation dose forms, the regulatory and pharmacopoeial standards have been under constant revision since the late 1980s and continue to be so. In addition, they can be very extensive and are at, or perhaps sometimes beyond, the limit of current technology. This activity is occurring in Europe and North America (Canada is quite active), while Japan at present is dormant in this area, probably reflecting the unpopularity of DPIs and MDIs in Japan. As well as regulatory standards there are other tests of value, especially patient-type usage tests (Harris, 2007).

It is essential to know the present official standards and to be aware of the draft guidelines at any time in the future. Draft guidelines can be obtained from the FDA, the European Agency for the Evaluation of Medicinal Products (EMEA), and the Committee for Proprietary Medicinal Products (CPMP) Web sites and from the publications *Pharmaceutical Forum* and *Pharm. Europa*. There is relatively good harmonization between the EP, USP, and CPMP, but not the FDA. Terminology is also important, with dose in the United States often expressed as exactuator, while in Europe it can be ex-valve. Naturally, the universal definition of dose uniformity also applies to respiratory systems, with the United States defining it around the target/label claim, while Europe defines it around the practically found mean. The former is perhaps more relevant, while the latter is more meaningful statistically. Dose and dose uniformity are always important parameters but are critical for MDIs and DPIs, since these are very challenging to achieve. Other parameters are excessively time consuming, for example, extractives testing, or perhaps unnecessary, for example, microscope tests for particle size.

Two new industry organizations have been formed to deal with these issues; the International Pharmaceutical Aerosol Consortium for Regulation and Science (IPAC-RS) for the United States and European Pharmaceutical Aerosol Group (EPAG) for Europe. Naturally the move to Quality by Design also covers inhalation dosage forms (Rignall et al., 2008).

There is also a parallel regulatory route for freestanding inhalation devices, which are supplied without the drug, for example, nebulizer machines, spacers, and some BAIs. In this case, they are controlled by a different division of the regulatory bodies. It is important to recognize early in development if your product will require device authorization, since the regulations are different following an International Organization for Standardization (ISO) pathway and not Standard Operating Procedures (SOPs) and Good Manufacturing Practice (GMP), and it is not easy to integrate the two systems.

FUTURE

Disease Types

At present, inhalation is known mainly for treating asthma, but its use in COPD, caused mainly by smoking, is gaining greater recognition, since there are significantly more patients in this group. Here, delivery systems may be tailored for the elderly. Other forms of lung treatment, such as the delivery of antibiotics or drugs for cystic fibrosis will continue.

An advancing area is the use of inhalation for systemic delivery via the alveoli in the deep lung (Gonda, 2006). This avoids "first-pass" metabolism and the acid environment of the stomach, and hence is particularly suitable for biopharmaceuticals, which otherwise would be delivered parenterally. However, the recent withdrawal of insulin inhalation products for a number of reasons (only prescribed for "needle-phobia patients," costs, side effects) has put questions over the delivery of large molecular entities by this route. There is interest from other areas for systemic delivery such as fentanyl for fast pain relief.

Delivery Systems

Technical attributes of DPIs and MDIs may converge, as BAIs become standard for MDIs, thus overcoming coordination problems, and as power sources are fitted to DPIs, they will become then independent of a patient's inspiratory ability. In addition, more information will be available to the patient and doctor, ranging from simple dose counters to sophisticated electronic recording and payback facilities for compliance, measuring peak flows or firing a device at a particular point in the inspiratory cycle to maximize lung deposition in a particular area of the lung.

Combination DPIs may be developed with each active in a separate container or blister, so making the development from a single active product easier.

REFERENCES

Blondino FE, Byron PR. Surfactant dissolution and water solubilization in chlorine-free liquified gas propellants. Drug Dev Ind Pharm 1998; 24(10):935–945.

Bowman PA, Greenleaf D. Non-CFC metered dose inhalers: the patent landscape. Int J Pharm 1999; 186:91–94.

Bradshaw DRS. Developing dose counters: an appraisal based on regulator, pharma, and user needs. Respiratory Drug Delivery. Boca Raton, FL: Davis Healthcare International Publishing, 2006.

Brambilla G, Ganderton D, Garzia R, et al. Modulation of aerosol clouds produced by pressurised inhalation aerosols. Int J Pharm 1999; 186:53–61.

Carter PA, Rowley G, Fletcher EJ, et al. Measurement of electrostatic charge decay in pharmaceutical powders and polymer materials used in dry powder inhaler devices. Drug Dev Ind Pharm 1998; 24(11):1083–1088.

Cummings RH. Pressurized metered dose inhalers: chlorofluorocarbon to hydrofluoroalkane transition—valve performance. J Allergy Clin Immunol 1999; 104(6):S230.

de Boer AH, Bolhuis GK, Gjaltema D, et al. Inhalation characteristics and their effects on in vitro drug delivery from dry powder inhalers. Part 3: the effect of flow increase rate (FIR) on the in vitro drug release from the Pulmicort 200 Turbohaler. Int J Pharm 1997; 153:67–77.

Dunbar CA, Hickey AJ. Selected parameters affecting characterisation of nebulized aqueous solutions by inertial impaction and comparison with phase-Doppler analysis. Eur J Pharm Biopharm 1999; 48:171–177.

Fedina LT, Zelko R, Fedina LI, et al. The effect of surfactant and suspending agent concentration on the effective particle size of metered-dose inhalers. J Pharm Pharmacol 1997; 49:1175–1177.

Feeley JC, York P, Sumby BS, et al. Determination of surface properties and flow characteristics of salbutamol sulphate, before and after micronisation. Int J Pharm 1998; 172:89–96.

Finlay WH. Inertial sizing of aerosol inhaled during pediatric tidal breathing from an MDI with attached holding chamber. Int J Pharm 1998; 168:147–152.

Flament M-P, Leterme P, Gayot AT. Factors influencing nebulizing efficiency. Drug Dev Ind Pharm 1995; 21(20):2263–2285.

Forte R, Dibble C. The role of international environmental agreements in metered-dose inhaler technology changes. J Allergy Clin Immunol 1999; 104(6):S217.

Gonda I. Systemic delivery of drugs to humans via inhalation. J Aerosol Med 2006; 19:47–53.

Harris D. Testing inhalers. Pharm Tech Eur 2007; 29–35.

Kawashima Y, Serigano T, Hino T, et al. Effect of surface morphology of carrier lactose on dry powder inhalation property of pranlukast hydrate. Int J Pharm 1998; 172:179–188.

Kippax P, Morton D. Unlocking the secrets of the DPI plume. Drug Deliv Technol 2008; 8:53–58.

Larhrib H, Zeng XM, Martin GP, et al. The use of different grades of lactose as a carrier for aerosolised salbutamol sulphate. Int J Pharm 1999; 191:1–14.

Leach C. Effect of formulation parameters on hydrofluoroalkane-beclomethasone dipropionate drug deposition in humans. J Allergy Clin Immunol 1999; 104(6):S250.

Leach C. The CFC to HFA transition. Respir Care 2005; 50:1201–1208.

LeBelle MJ, Graham SJ, Ormsby ED, et al. Metered-dose inhalers. II. Particle size measurement variation. Int J Pharm 1997; 151:209–221.

Le Brun PPH, de Boer AH, Gjaltema D, et al. Inhalation of tobramycin in cystic fibrosis. Part 1: the choice of a nebuliser. Int J Pharm 1999a; 189:205–214.

Le Brun PPH, de Boer AH, Gjaltema D, et al. Inhalation of tobramycin in cystic fibrosis. Part 2: optimization of the tobramycin solution for a jet and an ultrasonic nebulizer. Int J Pharm 1999b; 189:215–225.

Maggi L, Brunni R, Conte C. Influence of the moisture on the performance of a new dry powder inhaler. Int J Pharm 1999; 177:83–91.

Muzzio FJ, Robinson P, Wightman C, et al. Sampling practices in powder blending. Int J Pharm 1997; 155:153–178.

Naini V, Byron PR, Philips EM. Physicochemical stability of crystalline sugars and their spray-dried forms: dependence upon relative humidity and suitability for use in powder inhalers. Drug Dev Ind Pharm 1998; 24(10):895–909.

Newman SP, Wilding IR. Gamma scintigraphy: an in vivo technique for assessing the equivalence of inhaled products. Int J Pharm 1998; 170:1–9.

Newman SP, Wilding IR, Hirst PH. Human lung deposition. Int J Pharm 2000; 208:49–60.

Ostrander KD, Bosch HW, Bondanza DM. An in-vitro assessment of a NanoCrystal™ beclomethasone dipropionate colloidal dispersion via ultrasonic nebulisation. Eur J Pharm Biopharm 1999; 48:207–215.

Podczeck F. The relationship between physical properties of lactose monohydrate and the aerodynamic behaviour of adhered drug particles. Int J Pharm 1998; 160:119–130.

Rignall A, Christopher D, Crumpton A, et al. Quality by design for analytical methods for use with orally inhaled and nasal drug products. Pharm Tech Eur 2008; 20:24–31.

Srichana T, Martin GP, Marriot C. Dry powder inhalers: The influence of device resistance and powder formulation on drug and lactose deposition in vitro. Eur J Pharm Sci 1998; 7:73–80.

Steckel H, Muller BW. Metered-dose inhaler formulations with beclomethasone-17,21-dipropionate using the ozone friendly propellant 134a. Eur J Pharm Biopharm 1998; 46:77–83.

Steed KP, Towse LJ, Freund B, et al. Lung and oropharyngeal depositions of fenoterol hydrobromide delivered from the prototype III hand-held multidose Respimat nebuliser. Eur J Pharm Sci 1997; 5:55–61.

Tiwari D, Goldman D, Dixit S, et al. Compatibility evaluation of metered-dose inhaler valve elastomers with Tetrafluoroethane (P134a), a non-CFC propellant. Drug Dev Ind Pharm 1998; 24(4):345–352.

Traini D, Young PM, Rogueda P, et al. Use of AFM to investigate drug-canister interactions. Aerosol Sci Technol 2006; 40:227–236.

Williams RO III, Liu J. Influence of formulation additives on the vapour pressure of hydrofluoroalkane propellants. Int J Pharm 1998b; 166:99–103.

Williams RO III, Repka M, Liu J. Influence of propellant composition on drug delivery from a pressurized metered-dose inhaler. Drug Dev Ind Pharm 1998a; 24:(8):763–770.

Williams RO III, Rogers TR, Liu J. Study of solubility of steroids in hydrofluoroalkane propellants. Drug Dev Ind Pharm 1999; 25:(12):1227–1234.

Zeng XM, Pandhal KH, Martin GP. The influence of lactose carrier on the content homogeneity and dispersibility of beclomethasone dipropionate from dry powder aerosols. Int J Pharm 2000; 197:41–52.

BIBLIOGRAPHY

Byron PR, ed. Respiratory Drug Delivery. Boca Raton, FL: CRC Press, 1990.

D'Arcy PR, McElnay JC, eds. The Pharmacy and Pharmacology of Asthma. Ellis Horwood Series in Pharmaceutical Technology. Chichester: Ellis Horwood, 1989.

Gennaro AR, ed. Remington's Pharmaceutical Sciences. 18th ed. Part 8: Aerosols. Easton, PA: Mack Publishing, 1990.

Hickey AJ, ed. Inhalation aerosols: physical and biological basis for therapy. Lung Biology in Health and
   Diseases. Vol 94. New York: Marcel Dekker, 1992.

Johnsen MA, ed. The Aerosol Handbook. New Jersy: Wayne Dorland Company, 1983.

Lachman L, Lieberman HA, Kanig JL, eds. The Theory and Practice of Industrial Pharmacy. 3rd ed.
   Pharmaceutical Aerosols. Philadelphia: Lea and Febiger, 1986.

Moren P, Dolovich M, Newman S, et al. Aerosols in Medicine: Principles, Diagnosis and Therapy. 2nd ed.
   New York: Elsevier, 1993.

Purewal TS, Grant DJW, eds. Metered Dose Inhaler Technology. Buffalo Grove, IL: Interpharm Press, Inc,
   1998.

11 | Oral Solid Dosage Forms

Peter Davies
Shire Pharmaceutical Development Ltd., Basingstoke, U.K.

INTRODUCTION

In the last 25 to 30 years, a huge resource in both academia and industry has been devoted to the development of drug delivery systems that target drugs more effectively to their therapeutic site. Much of this work has been successful, and is reported in this text. In spite of this, oral solid dosage forms such as tablets and hard gelatin capsules, which have been in existence since the 19th century, remain the most frequently used dosage forms. This is not simply a reflection of the continued use of established products on the market; tablets and capsules still account for about half of all new medicines licensed (Table 1).

There are several reasons for the continued popularity of the oral solid dosage form. The oral route of delivery is perhaps the least invasive method of delivering drugs; it is a route that the patient understands and accepts. Patients are able to administer the medicine themselves. For the manufacturer, solid oral dosage forms offer many advantages: they utilize cheap technology, are generally the most stable forms of drugs, are compact, and their appearance can be modified to create brand identification.

Tablets and capsules are also very versatile. There are many different types of tablets, which can be designed to fulfill specific therapeutic needs (Table 2). It is beyond the scope of this chapter to cover all these dosage forms, instead it will review the common principles, with more specific detail being given for those most commonly used.

For drugs that demonstrate good oral bioavailability and do not have adverse effects on the gastrointestinal (GI) tract, there may be very little justification for attempting to design a specific drug delivery system. It is likely, therefore, that tablets and capsules will continue to remain one of the most used methods of delivering drugs to the patient in the future.

This chapter reviews the science behind the development of solid dosage forms, particularly tablets and hard gelatin capsules. Solid dosage forms are one of the most widely researched areas of pharmaceuticals and, given the space allowed, this chapter can only cover the science at a very basic level. It is an area that is served by a number of excellent texts, and these will be referenced at the appropriate points.

POWDER TECHNOLOGY

Virtually all solid dosage forms are manufactured from powders, and an understanding of the unique properties of powder systems is necessary for their rational formulation and manufacture. Powders consist of solid particles surrounded by spaces filled with fluid (typically air) and uniquely possess some properties of solids, liquids, and gases. Powders are not solids, even though they can resist some deformation, and they are not liquids, although they can be made to flow. Still further, they are not gases, even though they can be compressed. Powder technology is concerned with solid/fluid interactions, interparticle contact, and cohesion between particles. These are strongly influenced by particle size and shape and by adsorption of the fluid or other contaminants onto the surface of the particles.

While tablets and capsules, the two most common solid dosage forms, have their own unique requirements, there are similarities between them. They both require the flow of the correct weight of material into a specific volume, the behavior of the material under pressure is important; and the wetting of the powder is critical for both granulation and subsequent disintegration and dissolution of the dosage form.

While it is not possible to deal with all aspects of powder technology in a textbook covering such a diverse range of formulations, some basic principles of powder flow, mixing

Table 1 Number of FDA Drug Approvals for New Molecular Entities Presented as Tablet and Capsules Between 2003 and 2008

Year	No. of tablets approved	No. of capsules approved	No. of other dosage forms approved	Proportion of tablets and capsules (%)
2003	8	5	8	62
2004	11	3	16	49
2005	4	2	13	34
2006	9	4	6	68
2007	7	2	7	56
2008	7	2	6	60

Source: www.accessdata.fda.gov/scripts/cder/drugsatfda/index.cfm?fuseaction=Reports.ReportsMenu.

Table 2 Types of Solid Dosage Forms

Formulation type	Description
Immediate release	The dosage form is designed to release the drug substance immediately after ingestion.
Delayed release	The drug substance is not released until a physical event has occurred, e.g., time elapsed, change in pH of intestinal fluids, change in gut flora.
Chewable tablets	Strong, hard tablets to give good mouth feel.
Lozenges	Strong, slowly dissolving tablets for local delivery to mouth or throat. Often prepared by a candy molding process.
Buccal tablets	Tablets designed to be placed in buccal cavity of mouth for rapid action.
Effervescent tablets	Taken in water, the tablet forms an effervescent, often pleasant-tasting drink.
Dispersible tablets	Tablets taken in water, the tablet forms a suspension for ease of swallowing.
Soluble tablets	Tablets taken in water, the tablet forms a solution for ease of swallowing.
Hard gelatin capsules	Two-piece capsule shells, which can be filled with powders, pellets, semisolids, or liquids.
Soft gelatin capsules	One-piece capsules containing a liquid or semisolid fill.
Pastilles	Intended to dissolve in mouth slowly for the treatment of local infections. Usually composed of a base containing gelatin and glycerin.

and compaction, and compression properties will be described. For those interested in a more in-depth treatment of the topic, there are a number of excellent texts available (Rhodes, 1990; Alderborn, 1995).

Particle Size and Shape

A knowledge of the particle shape and size distribution is essential to the understanding of the behavior of powders, as it will contribute to knowledge of the secondary properties of a powder, such as flow and deformation, which influence the processability. This topic is dealt with in detail in chapter 6.

Density

When a powder is poured into a container, the volume that it occupies depends on a number of factors, such as particle size, particle shape, and surface properties. In normal circumstances, it will consist of solid particles and interparticulate air spaces (voids or pores). The particles themselves may also contain enclosed or intraparticulate pores. If the powder bed is subjected to vibration or pressure, the particles move relative to one another to improve their packing arrangement. Ultimately, a condition is reached where further densification is not possible without particle deformation.

The density of a powder is, therefore, dependent on the handling conditions to which it has been subjected, and there are several definitions that can be applied either to the powder as a whole or to individual particles.

Particle Densities

British Standard 2955 (1958) defines three terms that apply to the particles themselves. Particle density is the mass of the particle divided by its volume. The different terms arise from the way in which the volume is defined.

1. True particle density is when the volume measured excludes both open and closed pores, and is a fundamental property of a material.
2. Apparent particle density is when the volume measured includes intraparticulate pores.
3. Effective particle density is the volume "seen" by a fluid moving past the particles. It is of importance in processes such as sedimentation or fluidization but is rarely used in solid dosage forms.

Powder Densities

The density of a powder sample is usually referred to as the bulk density, and the volume includes both the particulate volume and the pore volume. The bulk density will vary depending on the packing of the powder, and several values can be quoted.

- Minimum bulk density is when the volume of the powder is at a maximum, caused by aeration, just prior to complete breakup of the bulk.
- Poured bulk density is when the volume is measured after pouring powder into a cylinder, creating a relatively loose structure.
- Tapped bulk density is, in theory, the maximum bulk density that can be achieved without deformation of the particles. In practice, it is generally unrealistic to attain this theoretical tapped bulk density, and a lower value obtained after tapping the sample in a standard manner is used.

The porosity of a powder is defined as the proportion of a powder bed or compact that is occupied by pores, and is a measure of the packing efficiency of a powder.

$$\text{Porosity} = 1 - \left(\frac{\text{bulk density}}{\text{true density}}\right) \tag{1}$$

Relative density is the ratio of the measured bulk density divided by the true density.

$$\text{Relative density} = \frac{\text{bulk density}}{\text{true density}} \tag{2}$$

POWDER FLOW

Good flow properties are a prerequisite for the successful manufacture of both tablets and powder-filled hard gelatin capsules. It is a property of all powders to resist the differential movement between particles when subjected to external stresses. This resistance is due to the cohesive forces between particles. Three principal types of interparticle force have been identified (Harnby et al., 1985): forces due to electrostatic charging, van der Waals forces, and forces due to moisture.

Electrostatic forces are dependent on the nature of the particles, in particular, on their conductivity. For nonconducting particles, high cohesive stresses in the range of 10^4 to $10^7 \, \text{N/m}^2$ have been reported.

Van der Waals forces are the most important forces for majority of pharmaceutical powders. The forces of attraction between two spherical particles is given by

$$F = Ad\left(\frac{Ad}{12x^2}\right) \tag{3}$$

where A is the Hamaker constant ($A = 10^{-19} \, \text{J}$), x is the distance of separation of the particles, and d is the particle diameter. The forces are inversely proportional to the square of the distance between the two particles, and hence diminish rapidly as particle size and separation increases. Powders with particles below 50 μm will generally exhibit irregular or no flow because of van der Waals forces. Particle shape is also important; for example, the force between a sphere and plane surface is about twice that between two equal-sized spheres.

At low relative humidity (RH), moisture produces a layer of adsorbed vapor on the surface of particles. Above a critical humidity, typically in the range 65% to 80%, it will form liquid bridges between particles. The attractive force due to the adsorbed layer may be about 50 times the van der Waals force for smooth surfaces, but surface roughness will reduce the effect. Where a liquid bridge forms, it will give rise to an attractive force between the particles due to surface tension or capillary forces.

The role of the formulator is to ensure that the flow properties of the powder are sufficient to enable its use on modern pharmaceutical equipment. Two types of flow present the formulator with particular challenges: flow from powder hoppers and flow through orifices.

Powder Flow in Hoppers

Tablet machines and capsule-filling machines store the powder to be processed in a hopper above the machine. It is important that the powder flows from the hopper to the filling station of the machine at an appropriate rate and without segregation occurring. There are two types of flow that can occur from a powder hopper: core flow and mass flow (Fig. 1).

The flow pattern of a core flow is shown in Figure 1A. When a small amount of powder is allowed to leave the hopper, there is a defined region in which downward movement takes place and the top surface begins to fall in the center. As more material leaves the hopper, the area that moves downward begins to widen, and the upper surface becomes conical. In the areas of the hopper outside the falling region, near the walls, the material has not moved. Even when the hopper has almost emptied, there will be regions where the powder is undisturbed. A core flow hopper is characterized by the existence of dead spaces during discharge. A mass

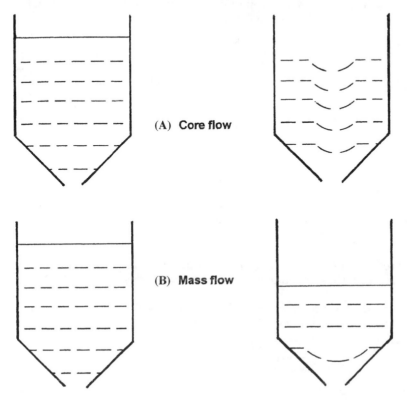

Figure 1 Powder flow patterns in hoppers.

flow hopper is one in which all the material is in motion during discharge, in particular the areas adjacent to the hopper wall (Fig. 1B). As a small amount of powder is discharged, the whole bulk of the powder moves downward.

Core flow hoppers have two significant disadvantages. First, flow from the hopper can stop for no apparent reason. The stoppage may be due to the formation of an arch between the walls of the hopper that is strong enough to support the weight of powder above it. Alternatively, it may be the result of piping or rat holing, in which the material directly above the outlet falls out, leaving an empty cylinder. The second disadvantage is that the flow pattern is likely to encourage segregation, and there may be a considerable loss of mixing quality.

Whether core flow or mass flow is achieved is dependent on the design of the hopper (geometry and wall material) and the flow properties of the powder. For most pharmaceutical applications, the hopper design for a particular machine will be fixed; thus, it is incumbent on the formulator to ensure that mass flow is achieved by modification of the powder properties.

Powder Flow into Orifices

Flow into orifices is important when filling dies in tablet machines and in certain types of capsule-filling machines. For a given material, the flow into or through an orifice is dependent on the particle size, and typically, a plot of flow rate versus particle size will display the trend shown in Figure 2. At the lower end of the particle size range, cohesive forces will result in poor flow. As the particle size increases, the flow rate increases until a maximum is achieved, at an orifice diameter/particle diameter ratio of 20 to 30. As the particle size continues to increase, the rate decreases because of mechanical blocking or obstruction of the orifice. Flow stops completely when the orifice/particle ratio falls below 6.

Measuring Powder Flow Properties

There are several different methods available for determining the flow properties of powders, and there are many literature examples demonstrating correlations between a test method and the manufacturing properties of a formulation. Listed below are some of the more commonly used tests, together with references, detailing their use in pharmaceutical applications.

Shear Cell Methods

Developed to aid silo and hopper design, shear cells provide an assessment of powder flow properties as a function of consolidation load and time. There are a number of types of shear cells available, the most common type being the Jenike shear cell (Fig. 3).

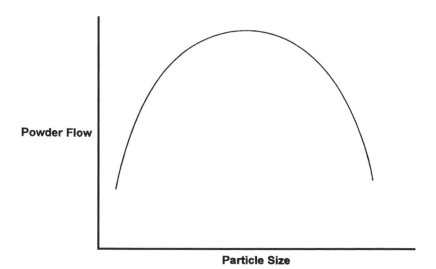

Figure 2 Effect of particle size on the rate of powder flow through an orifice.

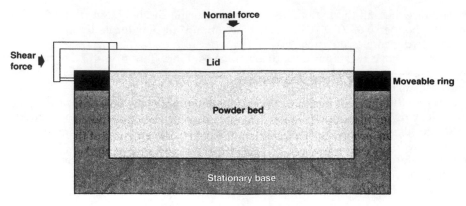

Figure 3   Jenike shear cell.

The shear cell is filled in a standard manner to produce a powder bed with a constant bulk density. A vertical (normal) force is applied to the powder bed and a horizontal force applied to the moveable ring. As the powder bed moves because of the horizontal shear stress, it will change volume, either expanding or contracting depending on the magnitude of the vertical force. A series of tests are performed to determine the vertical load under which the bed remains at constant volume when sheared, referred to as the critical state. Once the critical state has been determined, a series of identical specimens are prepared, and each is sheared under a different vertical load, with all loads being less than the critical state.

The test results are used to produce a graph referred to as a Jenike yield locus in which the shear stress required to initiate movement is plotted against the normal stress (Fig. 4). The line gives the stress conditions needed to produce flow for the powder when compacted to a fixed bulk density. If the material is cohesive, the yield locus does not produce a straight line, and it does not pass through the origin. The intercept OT is the tensile strength of the consolidated specimen, and OC is the cohesion of the specimen, that is, the shear stress needed

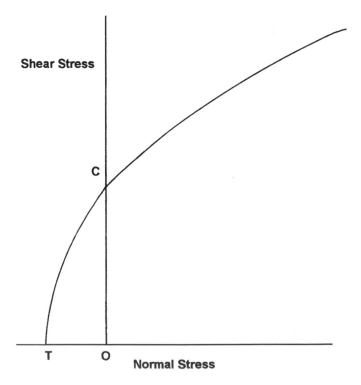

Figure 4   Jenike yield locus.

Table 3 Carr Indices

Carr index (%)	Flow
5–12	Free flowing
12–16	Good
18–21	Fair
23–35	Poor
33–38	Very poor
>40	Extremely poor

to initiate movement of the material when it is not subjected to normal force. The application of the yield loci to pharmaceuticals is well documented in the literature (Kocova and Pilpel, 1972, 1973; Williams and Birks, 1967).

The limitations of the Jenike shear cell are that it is not very useful for measuring bulk solids with large shear deformations, for example, plastic powders. The level of consolidation stresses required are inappropriate for pharmaceutical materials, and the quantity of material required is often beyond that available in the early stages of development. Alternative shear cells that have been used include annular shear cells (Nyquist and Brodin, 1982; Irono and Pilpel, 1982) and ring shear testers (Schulze, 1996).

Changes in Bulk Density

The increase in bulk density of a powder is related to its cohesiveness. Ratios of the poured to tapped bulk densities are expressed in two ways to give indices of flowability.

$$\text{Hausner ratio} = \frac{\text{tapped bulk density}}{\text{poured bulk density}} \tag{4}$$

$$\text{Compressibility (Carr index)} = \frac{100 \times (\text{tapped bulk density} - \text{poured bulk density})}{\text{tapped bulk density}} \tag{5}$$

The Hausner ratio varies from about 1.2 for a free-flowing powder to 1.6 for cohesive powders. The Carr index classifications are listed in Table 3.

Compressibility indices are a measure of the tendency for arch formation and the ease with which the arches will fail and, as such, is a useful measure of flow. A limitation of the bulk density indices is that they only measure the degree of consolidation; they do not describe how rapidly consolidation occurs.

Angle of Repose

If powder is poured from a funnel onto a horizontal surface, it forms a cone. The angle between the sides of the cone and the horizontal surface is referred to as the angle of repose. The angle is a measure of the cohesiveness of the powder, as it represents the point at which the interparticle attraction exceeds the gravitational pull on a particle. A free-flowing powder will form a cone with shallow sides, and hence a low angle of repose, while a cohesive powder will form a cone with steeper sides.

This method is simple in concept, but not particularly discerning. As a rough guide, angles less than 30° are usually indicative of good flow, while powders with angles greater than 40° are likely to be problematic.

Avalanching Behavior

If a powder is rotated in a vertical disc, the cohesion between the particles and the adhesion of the powder to the surface of the disc will lead to the powder following the direction of rotation until it reaches an unstable situation where an avalanche will occur. After the avalanche, the powder will again follow the disc prior to a further avalanche. Measurement of the time between avalanches and the variability in time is a measure of the flow properties of the powder.

MIXING

Mixing of powders is a key step in the manufacture of virtually all solid dosage forms. A perfect mixture of two particles is one in which any group of particles taken from any position within a mix contains the same proportions of each particle as the mixture as a whole (Fig. 5). With powders, unlike liquids, this is virtually unattainable. All that is possible to achieve is a maximum degree of randomness, that is, a mixture in which the probability of finding a particle of a given component is the same at all positions in the mixture (Fig. 6).

To determine the degree of mixing obtained in a pharmaceutical operation, it is necessary to sample the mixture and determine the variation within the mix statistically. In assessing the quality of a mixture, the method of sampling is more important than the statistical method used to describe it. Unless samples that accurately represent the system are taken, any statistical analysis is worthless. Furthermore, to provide meaningful information, the scale of scrutiny of the powder mix should be such that the weight of sample taken is similar to the weight that the powder mix contributes to the final dosage form.

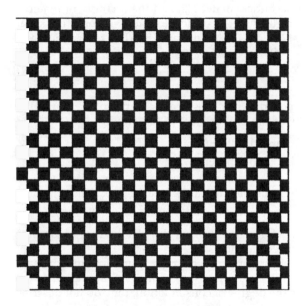

Figure 5   Perfect mix.

Figure 6   Random mix.

A large number of statistical analyses have been applied to the mixing of powders. These tend to be indices where the variance of the actual mix is compared to the theoretical random mix. The statistics are beyond the scope of this text and can be found in a number of standard texts on powder technology (Rhodes, 1990).

Segregation

If a powder consisting of two materials, both having identical physical properties, is mixed for sufficient time, random mixing will eventually be achieved. Unfortunately, most pharmaceutical powders consist of mixtures of materials with differing properties. This leads to segregation, where particles of similar properties tend to collect together in part of the powder. When segregating powders are mixed, as the mixing time is extended, the powders appear to unmix, and equilibrium is reached between the action of the mixer, introducing randomness and the resistance of the particles due to segregation.

While a number of factors can cause segregation, *differences in particle size* are by far the most important in pharmaceutical powders. There are a number of mechanisms by which segregation of different-sized particles can occur, and consideration should be given to these when designing pharmaceutical processes. *Trajectory segregation* occurs when a powder is projected horizontally in a fluid or gas; larger particles are able to travel greater horizontal distances than small particles before settling out. This could cause segregation at the end of conveyor belts or vacuum transfer lines. When a powder is discharged into a hopper or container, air is displaced upward. The upward velocity of this air may be sufficient to equal or exceed the terminal velocity of some of the smaller particles, and these will remain suspended as a cloud after the large particles have settled out. This process is known as *elutriation segregation*. The most common cause of segregation is due to *percolation* of fine particles. If a powder bed is handled in a manner that allows individual particles to move, a rearrangement in the packing of the particles occurs. As gaps between particles arise, particles from above are able to drop into them. If the powder contains particles of different sizes, there will be more opportunities for the smaller particles to drop, so there will be a tendency for these to move to the bottom of the powder, leading to segregation. This process can occur whenever movement of particles takes place, including when vibrating, shaking, and pouring.

Ordered Mixing

As stated above, differences in particle size are the most common cause of segregation in pharmaceutical powders. One exception to this is when one component of a powder mix has a very small particle size (< 5 mm) and the other is relatively large. In such circumstances, the fine powder may coat the surface of the larger particles, and the adhesive forces will prevent segregation. This is known as ordered mixing, and using this technique, it is possible to produce greater homogeneity than by random mixing.

COMPACTION

The manufacture of tablets, and to a lesser extent powder-filled hard gelatin capsules, involves the process of powder compaction, the purpose of which is to convert a loose incoherent mass of powder into a single solid object. Knowledge of the behavior of powders under pressure, and the way in which bonds are formed between particles, is essential for the rational design of formulations.

Powder in a container subjected to a low compressive force will undergo particle rearrangement until it attains its tapped bulk density. Ultimately, a condition is reached where further densification is not possible without particle deformation. If, at this point, the powder bed is subjected to further compression, the particles will deform elastically to accommodate induced stresses, and the density of the bed will increase with increasing pressure at a characteristic rate. When the elastic limit is exceeded, there is a change in the rate of reduction in the bed volume as plastic deformation or brittle fracture of particles begins (Fig. 7). Brittle materials will undergo fragmentation, and the fine particles formed will percolate through the bed to give secondary packing. Plastically deforming materials will distort to fill voids and

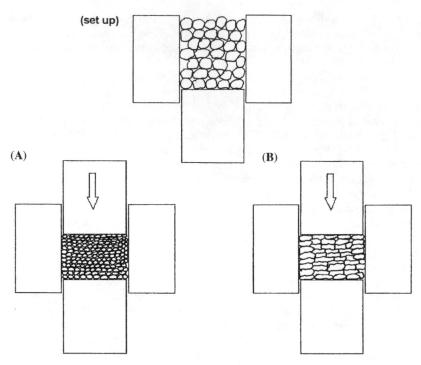

Figure 7 The behavior of powders subjected to a compaction force: (**A**) brittle fracture and (**B**) plastic deformation.

may also exhibit void filling by percolation when the limit of plastic deformation is reached and fracture occurs. Either mechanism, therefore, consists of at least two submechanisms, and the processes could be repeated on the secondary particles produced by the fracture until the porosity is at a minimum and the internal crystalline structure supports the compressional stress.

Both processes will aid bonding to form a single compact, as plastic flow increases contact areas between particles irreversibly and fragmentation produces clean surfaces that bond strongly. The successful production of compacts depends on achieving high contact areas between uncontaminated surfaces.

To fully understand the compaction behavior of a material, it is clear that it is necessary to be able to quantify its elasticity, plasticity, and brittleness.

Measurement of Compaction Properties

To characterize the compaction properties of a material or formulation, it must be possible to measure the relationship between the force applied to a powder bed and the volume of the powder bed. A typical instrumentation will consist of measurement of the forces on the upper and lower punches by means of strain gauges or load cells together with a measure of the punch movement, which is performed using displacement transducers, the most common type being linear variable-differential transducers (LVDTs). The positioning and installation of the load and displacement transducers are critical to obtain meaningful information. The topic of instrumentation is comprehensively covered by Ridgway and Watt (1988). There are three approaches that have been used to generate compaction information, as discussed below.

Conventional Testing Machines

Testing machines are widely used in materials science and engineering laboratories for the measurement of physical properties of various materials. Many of the basic principles of compaction and the test methodologies currently employed in pharmaceutical formulation have been developed on testing machines by the metallurgy and ceramic industries. The drawback with testing machines is that the compression speeds that can be achieved are well below those encountered on tabletting machines, so while they are of value in fundamental studies, they are not necessarily useful for predicting the behavior of a material or formulation in the factory.

Conventional Tablet Machines

The first tablet machines to be instrumented were single punch eccentric presses. While these provide useful information, the compression profiles differ from those of rotary tablet machines used for commercial production. The profile of a single punch involves the powder bed being compressed between a moving upper punch and a stationary lower punch, while on a rotary machine, both punches move together simultaneously. Consequently, rotary machines have been instrumented, even though this is technically more challenging than single punch machines. The instrumented rotary press provides information that is directly relevant to production conditions, although it should be borne in mind that profiles do vary between machines, and any results obtained may be peculiar to that machine. A major advantage of instrumented machines is that they provide information not only on the compaction properties but also on flow and lubrication. The disadvantage of using instrumented rotary machines is the quantity of material required to perform tests, making them unsuitable for preformulation activities, when material is in short supply.

Compaction Simulators

Compaction simulators are a development of testing machines. They consist of single punch machines in which the upper and lower punches are driven individually by hydraulic rams. The movement of the hydraulic rams is controlled by computer and can be programmed either to simulate the movement of any tablet machine or to follow a simple profile similar to a testing machine. The big advantage of the compaction simulator is that it can be used to prepare a single compact using a profile that might be encountered on a production machine, so only small quantities of material are required.

Quantitative Compaction Data

There are two principal types of compaction studies used to characterize material: pressure/volume relationships and pressure/strength relationships. While ultimately it is the strength of a tablet that is important, the pressure/volume relationships provide the information about the compaction properties of a material that allows an appropriate formulation to be developed.

Heckel Plots

A large number of equations have been proposed to describe the relationship between pressure and volume reduction during the compaction process. Many of these have an empirical basis and may relate to a particular material or range of pressures, while others attempt to define the complete process of densification. The equation that has been most widely used to describe the compaction of pharmaceutical powders is the Heckel equation (Heckel, 1961). This equation, originally used to describe the densification of ceramics, is essentially a curve-fitting equation that provides reasonable correlation with the observed facts over a wide range of pressures.

The equation is based on the premise that compaction is a first-order process where the rate at which pores within a powder can be eliminated is proportional to the number of pores present. As the compaction process continues, the number of pores continue to drop, and consequently, the rate of volume reduction per unit increase in pressure drops. This was expressed mathematically as

$$\ln\left(\frac{1}{1 - D_r}\right) = kP + A \tag{6}$$

In a system where there was no rearrangement of particles, and compaction was achieved solely by plastic deformation, a plot of $\ln(1/1 - D_r)$ versus P would yield a straight line (Fig. 8).

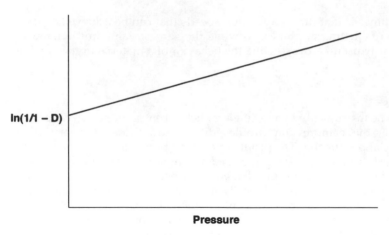

Figure 8 Theoretical Heckel plot.

Pharmaceutical powders do not produce perfect straight lines, and the type of deviation provides information about the compaction behavior of the material. A typical Heckel plot for a pharmaceutical powder is illustrated in Figure 9. A straight-line portion is obtained over a certain pressure range with a negative deviation at low pressures and a positive deviation at high pressures.

The curved portion at low pressures is due to particle rearrangement and possibly fragmentation, the deviation from a straight line (A–B) is a measure of its extent (Fig. 9).

The gradient of the straight-line portion of the plot is related to the reciprocal of the yield pressure of the material, and as such is a measure of the plasticity of the material. While the absolute values obtained for the yield pressure will be dependent on the equipment and test conditions employed, the relative values obtained under given test conditions will provide information about the compaction properties of materials. Table 4 displays the values for yield pressure obtained for excipients, known to have differing compaction properties, tested using a compaction simulator.

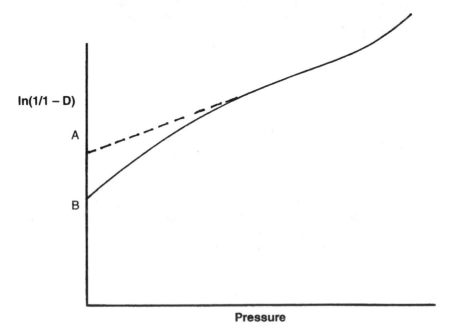

Figure 9 Heckel plots of pharmaceutical powders.

Table 4 Yield Pressure for Excipients

Excipient	Yield pressure (Mpa)	A–B	Deformation mechanism
Microcrystalline cellulose	54	0.15	Plastic/deforming
Anhydrous lactose	174	0.5	
Calcium phosphate dihydrate	396	0.95	Brittle/fragmenting
Starch 1500	53	0.1	

The densification behavior of powders has been categorized into types A, B, and C (York and Pilpel, 1973). Type A (plastic) exhibits parallel but distinct graphs for different size fractions, type B (fragmenting) exhibits particulate fragmentation at low pressures, with graphs becoming coincident at higher pressures, and type C (extremely plastic) is characterized by a small initial curved section, a low value of mean yield pressure, and a rapid approach to zero porosity at low pressure.

The effect of compression speed on the yield pressure of a material has been suggested as a method of determining the time-dependent nature of materials compression properties (Roberts and Rowe, 1985). Heckel plots are produced at two punch velocities, 0.03 and 300 mm/sec, and the yield pressures determined. The strain rate sensitivity (SRS) is calculated as

$$\mathrm{SRS} = \frac{P_{Y2} - P_{Y1}}{P_{Y1}} \times 100 \tag{7}$$

where P_{Y1}, = the yield pressure at 0.03 mm/sec and P_{Y2} = the yield pressure at 300 mm/sec. Materials that exhibit plastic deformation have larger SRS than values fragmenting materials.

Elasticity
While Heckel plots are able to distinguish between plastic and fragmenting mechanisms, they do not readily distinguish between plastic and elastic deformation. The data presented in Table 4 would suggest that microcrystalline cellulose and starch 1500 have very similar properties, yet the elastic nature of starch and its derivative products is well documented in the literature. Additional methods are, therefore, required to measure elasticity.

Elasticity can be determined either by monitoring the elastic energy during the decompression phase of a compact within the die or by comparing the dimensions of the ejected compact with the dimensions of the compact within the die at peak compaction pressure.

The elastic energy is determined by plotting a force-displacement curve. If punch force is plotted against punch tip displacement or punch tip separation, a curve with a progressively increasing slope is obtained, reaching a maximum force at the point of minimum separation. As the punch begins to retract, the compact will expand because of elastic recovery and will remain in contact with the punch. This recovery is apparent from the force-displacement curve. If the material being compressed is truly elastic, the curve for the decompression phase will overlay the compression phase. For a truly plastic material, the force will fall to zero immediately as the punch begins to retract. Pharmaceutical materials tend to show a combination of elastic and plastic deformation.

Integrating the force-displacement curves gives a measure of the energy involved in the compaction process (Fig. 10), it being possible to calculate both the elastic energy and the net energy of compaction.

An alternative measure of elasticity is the percentage elastic recovery ($ER_\%$) (Armstrong and Haines-Nutt, 1972):

$$ER_\% = \frac{H - H_c}{H_c} \times 100 \tag{8}$$

where H = thickness of compact after ejection and recovery and H_c = minimum thickness under load.

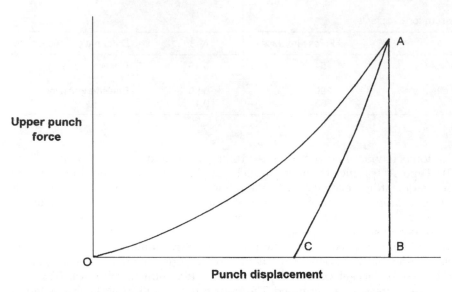

Figure 10 Force-displacement curve for a pharmaceutical powder. The total work of compaction is represented by the area defined by OAB; elasticwork by CAB. The network of compaction is the area defined by OAC.

This measure differs from the elastic energy in that it includes the viscous contribution to elastic recovery as well as the purely elastic behavior during the unloading period of compression. Whichever method is used to calculate the elasticity, it should be borne in mind that the punches will also display a degree of elasticity, and this must be allowed for when calculating punch separations at pressure.

Indentation Hardness
An alternative method of determining the plasticity and elasticity of a material is indentation hardness testing. The principle of indentation hardness testing is that a hard indenter of specified geometry, either a sphere or square-based pyramid, is pressed onto the surface of the test material with a measured load and the size of the indentation produced measured. The hardness of a material is the load divided by the area of the indentation to give a measure of the contact pressure.

There are two types of hardness tests: *static tests* that involve the formation of a permanent indentation on the surface of the test material and *dynamic tests* in which a pendulum is allowed to strike the test material from a known distance. Vickers and Brinell tests, two examples of static methods, are the most commonly used methods for determining the hardness of pharmaceutical materials. In the Brinell test, a steel ball of diameter D is pressed on to the surface of the material, and a load F is applied for 30 seconds and then removed. The diameter d_I of the indentation produced is measured, and the Brinell Hardness Number (BHN) calculated by

$$\text{BHN} = \frac{2F}{\pi D_I \left(D_I - \sqrt{D_I^2 - d_I^2} \right)} \tag{9}$$

The Vickers hardness test uses a square-based diamond pyramid as the indenter. The Vickers hardness, H_v is calculated by

$$H_v = \frac{2F \sin 68}{d^2} \tag{10}$$

where d is the length of the diagonals of the square impression.

Traditionally, it has been necessary to perform indentation testing on compacts because of the size of the indenters. The surfaces of compacts are not homogeneous, and this introduced variability. Recently, nanoindentation testers have been developed, which are capable of performing indentation tests on single crystals. Such testers offer significant potential for characterizing the mechanical properties of materials at an early stage of development.

Pressure/Strength Relationships

The strength of tablets has traditionally been determined in terms of the force required to fracture a specimen across its diameter, the *diametral compression test*. The fracture load obtained is usually reported as a hardness value, an unfortunate use of a term that has a specific meaning in materials science, associated with indentation. The use of the fracture load does not allow for compacts of different shapes, diameters, or thicknesses to be directly compared. For flat-faced circular tablets, a complete analytical solution exists for the stress state induced during the test (Carneiro and Barcellos, 1953), allowing the tensile strength to be determined from the fracture load:

$$\sigma_x = \frac{2P}{\pi Dt} \tag{11}$$

where P is the fracture load, D the tablet diameter, and t the tablet thickness. The solution for tensile stresses can only be used for tablets that fail in tension, characterized by failure along the loaded diameter.

The stresses developed in the tested convex tablets undergoing the diametral compression test have been examined by Pitt et al. (1989), who proposed the following equation for the calculation of the tensile strength:

$$\sigma_f = \frac{10P}{\pi D^2} \times \left(\frac{2.84t}{D} - \frac{0.126t}{C_L} + \frac{3.15C_L}{D} + 0.01 \right) \tag{12}$$

where P is the fracture load of the convex tablet, D the diameter, C_L the cylinder length, and t the overall thickness of the tablet.

Typical plots of tensile strength versus compaction pressure are illustrated in Figure 11. Initially, most materials demonstrate an increase in tensile strength proportional to the compaction pressure applied. As the compaction pressure is increased, the tablet approaches zero porosity, and large increases in pressure are required to achieve small volume reductions, and consequently, small increases in bonding. Some materials will attain maximum strength, and subsequent increases in pressure will produce weaker tablets.

Other materials also display an initial increase in strength proportional to the applied pressure, but the strength reaches a maximum before falling off sharply. This is due to capping or lamination, which results in tablets failing in a characteristic manner (Fig. 12). Capping is the partial or complete removal of the crown of a tablet from the main body, while lamination

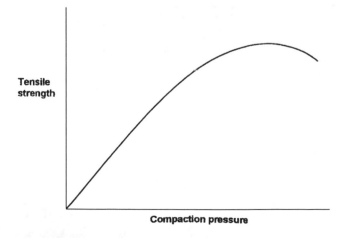

Tensile strength

Compaction pressure

Figure 11 Compaction pressure/tensile strength profile. Typical plot for a pharmaceutical material.

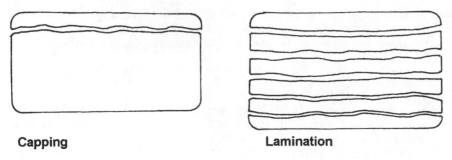

Capping   **Lamination**

Figure 12 Tablet flaws: capping and lamination.

is the separation of a tablet into two or more distinct layers. The problem may be apparent on ejection of the tablet or may manifest itself when the tablet is subjected to further stress, for example, mechanical strength testing or film coating.

Capping

Capping and lamination can affect both individual substances and formulations and constitute one of the most common problems facing the formulator. It occurs when a material is unable to relieve stresses present within a compact following compression by plastic deformation (Hiestand and Smith, 1984). When a material is compressed within a die by means of two opposing punches, the axial load that is applied through the upper punch is transmitted to the die as a shearing force. In addition, force is transmitted radially to the die wall. The nature of this radial force is determined by the elastic or plastic behavior of the compact. When an axial force is applied to a column of powder in a die, the pressures developed within the powder vary with depth. This phenomenon is attributed to the development of friction between the powder and the die wall and leads to density variations within the final compact. The nature of such variations has been the subject of a number of investigations (Train, 1957; Kamm et al., 1949; Charlton and Newton, 1985). These studies have been performed on a number of materials that have been compressed in dies with one moving and one stationary flat-faced punch. The results obtained in each study indicated a similar density distribution within a compact, high-density region being present on the perimeter of the compact adjacent to the moving punch and low-density regions near the stationary punch. In addition, there was a second high-density region remote from the moving punch (Fig. 13). An explanation for the density distribution has been proposed on the basis of the development of high-density wedges of material at the die wall adjacent to the moving punch. Figure 14 represents the forces developed in the compact. At equilibrium, the axial force is supported by the punch in direction *a* and by the powder in direction *b*. The radial component is supported by the die wall in direction *c* and by the powder bed in direction *d*. The resultant force acting on the mass

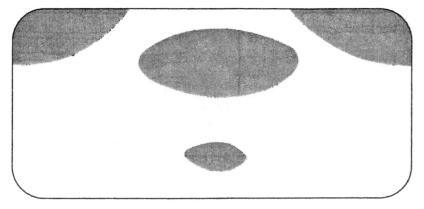

Figure 13 Regions of high density within a compact.

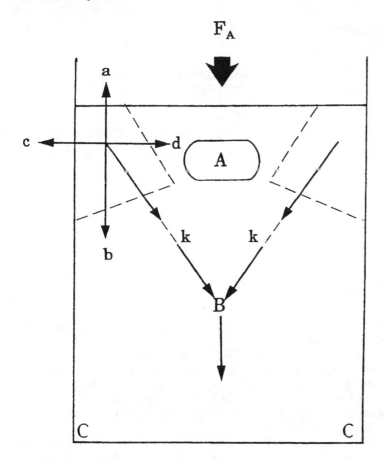

Figure 14 Development of the pressure pattern within a compact. *Source*: From Train (1957).

is denoted by k. The pressure front can be considered as a conical surface with its focal point B. The region around point B will be exposed to the greatest pressure and will have a greater density than the surrounding areas. The wedge-shaped areas bounded by the dotted lines adjacent to the moving punch will be highly densified due to the high shearing forces that they are exposed to. The central area, A, will be subject to negligible shearing forces and will be protected from normal axial pressures by the vaulting effect of the high-density wedges resulting in an area of low density. The area C, adjacent to the stationary punch, will undergo no movement relative to the die wall, and thus will not be subject to shearing forces. Density in this region will be low, as consolidation will depend solely on transmitted axial forces.

On removal of the upper punch, there will be a degree of axial elastic recovery resulting in expansion of the compact within the die. Following ejection, expansion may also occur in the radial direction. This elastic recovery is considered to be the most likely cause of capping. Train (1956) attributed capping to the strain imposed by elastic recovery of the areas of high density within the compact on ejection (Fig. 15). The elastic recovery of the dense peripheral ring would be larger than that of the adjacent, less dense, part of the tablet. The differential stress in this region is exacerbated by both axial and radial relaxation of that part of the tablet extruded from the die during the early stages of ejection.

Attempts have been made to predict the capping tendencies of materials. Malamataris et al. (1984) examined the plastoelasticity of mixtures of paracetamol and microcrystalline cellulose and showed that the tensile strengths of compacts were inversely proportional to the ratios of the samples' elastic recovery: plastic compression (as defined in Fig. 10). Lamination and capping occurred when this ratio exceeded 9. Nyström et al. (1978) measured the tensile strength of compacts in both the radial and axial directions and found that the values were not equal, the axial strength often decreasing at high compaction pressures. It was proposed that

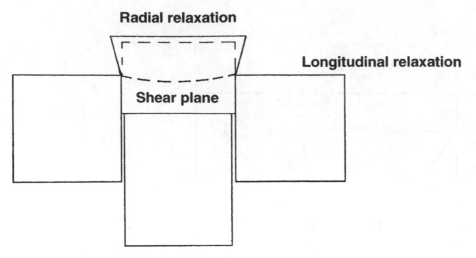

Figure 15   Elastic recovery of compact during ejection from die leading to capping. *Source*: From Train (1956).

the ratio of axial to radial tensile strength should be close to unity for a good formulation. Krycer et al. (1982) examined the capping tendencies of three grades of paracetamol and proposed a capping index defined as the slope of the $ER_\%$ versus residual die wall pressure (the pressure exerted on a die by a compact after removal of the upper punch). The higher the values of the capping index, the greater the tendency for capping. The residual die wall pressure relates to the irreversible deformation undergone during compaction. Low values for residual die wall pressure indicate that the compact had recovered axially and contracted radially, which would induce strain within the compact.

The methods of predicting capping discussed so far have been measures of the degree of elastic recovery occurring in the compact. For capping to occur, the stresses produced by the elastic recovery during decompression must be sufficient to disrupt the bonds that are formed during compression. Hiestand and Smith (1984) proposed a measure of the ability of a material to relieve localized stresses called the brittle fracture index (BFI). This test involves comparing the tensile strength value obtained using the diametral compression test of a compact that contains a central, axial hole with one that does not. Under the conditions of the test, the hole acts as a stress concentrator; elasticity theory predicts that the stress concentration factor is approximately 3.2 for a hole in an isotropic solid. However, for most pharmaceutical materials, the ratio of tensile strengths obtained is less than 3 due to the relief of the highly localized stresses by plastic deformation. The BFI is defined as

$$\mathrm{BFI} = \frac{\sigma_s - \sigma_0}{2\sigma_0} \tag{13}$$

where σ_s is the tensile strength of the compact without the hole and σ_0 is the tensile strength of the tablet with the hole. A BFI of 1.0 would correspond to a purely brittle material; a value of zero would indicate that the stresses at the hole had been completely relieved by plastic deformation.

Hiestand and Smith (1984) proposed that a material with a high BFI would be less able to relieve the stresses occurring during decompression and ejection and would therefore be more susceptible to capping and lamination. Experiments showed that problems were likely to occur with materials having a BFI of 0.8 or more. The BFI will be dependent on the relative density of a material; at low densities, pores may act as stress concentrators in the same way as the central hole, so the measurements should be made at fixed, high relative densities. Roberts and Rowe (1986) determined the BFI of compacts produced at a range of relative densities using a range of compaction speeds. Magnesium carbonate, a brittle material, displayed increasing BFI values with increases in compaction speed and relative density, while microcrystalline cellulose showed little change.

Summary

It is clear from the preceding discussions that there is not one single technique that can be used to fully characterize the compaction properties of a powder. A number of tests have been widely applied to pharmaceutical materials, but used in isolation, they will not provide the formulator with all the data required to fully understand their behavior when tabletted. Two sets of workers have tried to address this problem by suggesting a range of tests that, used in combination, will give a more complete picture of the materials properties.

Hiestand and Smith (1984) proposed three indices referred to as Tabletting Indices. The three indices are a strain index, bonding index, and the BFI, which was described in the section "Capping." The strain index is a measure of the strain present in a material following compaction and is a measure of elastic recovery calculated by a dynamic indentation hardness test. The bonding index is a measure of the material's ability to deform plastically and form bonds and is the ratio of a compact's tensile strength and indentation hardness.

Roberts and Rowe (1987) have proposed a material classification on the basis of the knowledge of Young's modulus of elasticity: yield stress, hardness, and SRS.

Rational formulation relies on a thorough understanding of the physicochemical properties of the material. Ideally, the mechanical properties should be determined at an early stage in the development process. It must, however, be borne in mind that the properties are sample dependent, and changes in particle size, morphology, and so on during development will affect the compaction properties.

SOLID DOSAGE FORMS

When formulating any pharmaceutical dosage form, it is important to remember that there is equilibrium between the bioavailability of the product, its chemical and physical stability and the technical feasibility of producing it.

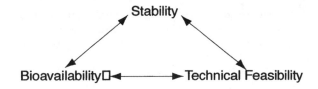

Any changes made to a formulation in an attempt to optimize one of these properties is likely to have an effect on the other two parameters, which must be considered. This is especially true of immediate-release solid dosage forms. Many of the properties required to optimize the bioavailability through rapid disintegration and dissolution of the active constituent, for example, small particle size, must be balanced with the manufacturability, where the fluidity and compatibility of a powder will often be enhanced by an increase in particle size.

Tablets and hard gelatin capsules form the vast majority of solid dosage forms on the market. While the actual processes involved of filling capsules and compressing tablets differ, the preparations of the powders to be processed are, in many cases, very similar.

TABLETS

Tablet Machines

Tablets are produced using tablet presses. While these presses vary in their output, from approximately 3000 tablets per hour to more than 1 million per hour for the fastest machines, the principle of manufacture remains the same. Powder is filled to a specified depth in a die and compressed between two punches. The compression force is ended by removal of the upper punch, and the lower punch then moves upward in the die to eject the tablet. Presses can be divided into two types, single punch (or eccentric) presses and rotary presses.

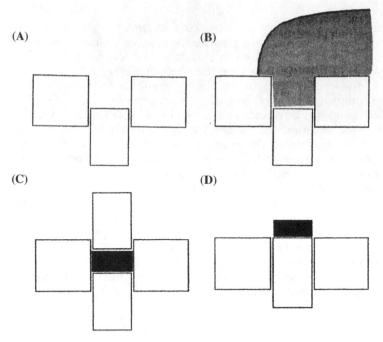

Figure 16 Schematic representation of a single punch tablet machine. (**A**) The upper punch is raised out of the die, and the lower punch drops to a set position. (**B**) The feed shoe oscillates above the die, filling it with powder. (**C**) The upper punch enters the die and compresses the powder. (**D**) The upper punch is removed, and the lower punch rises in the die to eject the tablet.

Single Punch Presses

Single punch presses are sometimes referred to as eccentric presses because the movement of the punches is controlled by an eccentric cam. The tabletting cycle of a single punch machine is represented schematically in Figure 16. The powder hopper is attached to a feed shoe, which oscillates horizontally.

The compression cycle starts with die filling. The lower punch descends in the die. The depth of the descent can be controlled, and this determines the tablet weight. The feed shoe then passes over the die a number of times, allowing the die to be filled with powder. As the die shoe moves away, it removes all excess powder away from the die table, leaving the die filled to an even level.

The upper punch then descends into the die, compressing the powder. The depth to which the punch descends into the die is adjustable, and this controls the compaction pressure applied. The lower punch remains stationary during the compression phase.

As the upper punch moves upward at the end of the compression phase, the lower punch rises in the die until it is level with the die table. The feed shoe then begins its oscillatory phase and knocks the tablet off the lower punch and down a collection chute. The lower punch then descends to its filling position as a second cycle commences.

Single punch presses are rarely seen in production environments because of their relatively slow production rates, although there are still a number of old products that can only be successfully produced on this type of machine. They are still used in development laboratories because they require only relatively small amounts of material to produce tablets compared with most rotary machines.

Rotary Tablet Machines

Commercial manufacture of tablets is performed almost exclusively on rotary tablet machines due to their higher output. On a rotary machine, the punch and dies are positioned on a rotating turret, and output depends on the number of stations positioned around the turret and the speed of rotation. Machines are available with anything from 4 stations for a development machine to 79 stations for the largest production machines. All such machines operate using virtually identical principles that are represented in Figure 17.

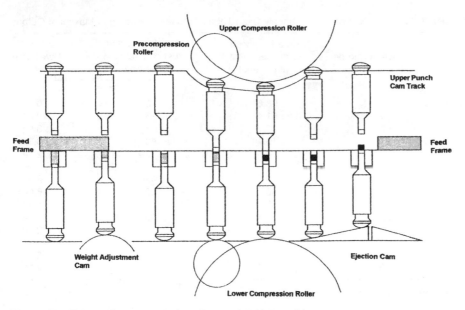

Figure 17 Schematic representation of a rotary tablet machine.

The powder hopper is positioned above a feed frame, a frame that retains a powder bed above the dies when the lower punch is in the filling position. As the lower punches pass below the feed frame, they descend within the die to their lowest possible position so the whole die cavity can be filled with powder. The powder is filled into the dies by the suction effect caused by their descent and gravity from the feed frame above. To optimize filling, the feed frame is designed so that the powder in contact with the die table and following the rotary action of the table is directed in a manner that makes it pass to and fro across the dies. Some machines also have mechanical paddles in the feed frame. As the lower punches approach the end of the feed frame, they pass over a weight-control cam; this causes the punch to rise, ejecting some of the powder that is scraped off by the edge of the feed frame. Adjusting the height of the cam controls the amount of material remaining in the die as the punch moves toward the compression stage.

Compression takes place when the upper and lower punches pass between compression rollers. During compression, the upper and lower punches move together, in contrast to the single punch machine, where only the upper punch moves. The compression force is controlled by moving the lower compression roller up or down, thus adjusting the distance between the punches at the point of maximum compaction. Some machines are fitted with two sets of rollers, a small roller being positioned between the feed frame and the main compression roller allowing a small degree of compression to take place. This is termed precompression, and was introduced to minimize capping and lamination by removing air from the powder bed and effectively increasing the dwell time of the compression phase.

Following compression, the upper punches are removed by the upper punch cam track, and the lower punches pass over an ejection cam, a gentle ramp that moves the lower punches vertically within the die until the tablet is fully ejected. The tablets are removed from the punch tip by a scraper blade positioned on the edge of the feed frame, and the punch then descends to allow die filling to occur for the next cycle.

When developing formulations, it is usual for the early batches to be manufactured on either single punch machines or small rotary machines due to the batch sizes being produced and the limited availability of new drug substances. It should be borne in mind that the formulations that are being developed may ultimately be required to run on larger rotary machines, and there are great differences in the rate of compression between the machines generally found in formulation laboratories and those found in production. These differences are summarized in Table 5.

The differences in punch speed at initial contact and dwell times, the period at which the compact is held at maximum compression, are likely to affect the nature of those tablets that

Table 5   Speed-Related Data for a Number of Commonly Used Tablet Presses Operating at Maximum Output

Tablet press	Production rate per die (tablets/min)	Time for punch to descend last 5 mm (msec)	Punch speed at first contact with powder (mm/sec)	Dwell time (msec)
Manesty				
F3 [Single punch)	85	68.6	139	0
B3B	44	61.4	163	10.84
Express	100	26.7	416	3.94
Unipress	121	19.1	485	3.16
Novapress	100	10.0	720	2.14
Kilian				
Tx	105	19.0	494	2.96
F1000	55	36.4	232	6.60
F1000	75	26.6	317	4.84
F2000	75	23.1	402	3.68
F2000	100	17.3	526	2.76
Korsch				
300	80	21.7	419	3.44
300	100	17.3	526	2.76

Source: Adapted from Armstrong, 1989.

have any viscoelastic components. Compaction simulators that are able to reproduce the punch speeds of production machines, yet only require small quantities of powder for testing, can have a valuable role to play in formulation development.

Tablet Formulation

A tablet formulation should possess the following properties to optimize the technical feasibility, stability, and bioavailability of the formulation:

- Compatibility of drug substance with excipients
- Flowability
- Compactibility
- Lubricity
- Appearance
- Disintegration
- Dissolution

Compatibility

Compatibility studies have been discussed in detail in chapter 6. The solid-state compatibility is of particular importance in tablets due to the compaction process increasing the contact area between particles, and hence the potential for reactivity.

Flowability

The importance of powder flow was emphasized in the section Powder Flow. The formulation should have sufficient flowability to ensure that the appropriate quantity of powder flows into the dies of the tablet machine on a consistent basis. While the tests described for powder flow are useful development tools, the ultimate test of a formulation is the uniformity of weight of tablets manufactured on a production tablet machine.

There is bound to be some variability in tablet weight during manufacture due to variation in the particle size of the material being compacted, flow property variation, and machine parameters (e.g., small differences in the lengths of the lower punches). To allow for such variability, pharmacopoeias set tolerances to ensure adequate control without providing a specification that is impossible to achieve in production. The European Pharmacopoeia (EP) test is to weigh 20 individual tablets and calculate the mean. The individual tablet weights are then compared to the mean. The sample is acceptable if no more than two tablets are outside

Table 6 European Pharmacopoeia Uniformity of Weight Limits

Average tablet weight (mg)	Percentage deviation
≤80 mg	10.0
>80 mg and <250 mg	7.5
≥250 mg	5.0

the stated percentage limit and no tablet is outside twice the stated limit (Table 6). The pharmacopoeial limits are generous, and typically much more stringent limits will be applied as in-process controls. The in-process controls will also apply strict limits for the value of the mean tablet weight.

Uniformity of weight does not guarantee that there is uniformity of active ingredient throughout a batch of tablets. If there is segregation of the active ingredient occurring, the weights may remain uniform, while the potency varies. For this reason, the U.S. Pharmacopeia (USP) only allows a uniformity of weight test for tablets containing 50 mg or more of an active ingredient comprising 50% or more, by weight, of the tablet. In all other instances, a content uniformity test must be performed.

Uniformity of weight is also important in achieving consistency of tablet strength, as there is a relationship between the quantity of powder in the die and the compaction pressure required to compress it to a given thickness, which is what the tablet machine is effectively doing. If the quantity of powder in the die is reduced to a lower compaction, pressure will be applied, producing a weaker tablet. Variation in tablet strength may in turn lead to variability in the disintegration and dissolution properties of the product.

With low-dose drugs, it may be possible to influence the flow properties by combining the drug substance with excipients possessing good flow properties. Where a formulation is prepared by simply dry mixing the drug with excipients prior to compaction, the process is referred to as direct compression. With high-dose drugs, the quantity of such excipients that would be needed to achieve suitable flow and compaction properties may result in the final weight of the dosage form being unrealistically high. In such cases, the usual formulation approach is to granulate, a process that imparts two primary requisites to formulations: compactibility and flowability. Granulation is a process of size enlargement, whereby small particles are gathered into larger, permanent aggregates in which the original particles can still be identified. The direct compression and granulation processes and their relative merits are discussed in greater detail in the section "Processing of Formulations."

The flow properties of a powder can be enhanced by the inclusion of a glidant. These are added to overcome powder cohesiveness by interposing between particles to reduce surface rugosity, thus preventing interlocking of particles and lowering the interparticulate friction. Commonly used glidants are listed in Table 7.

Talc is traditionally one of the most commonly used glidants, having the additional benefit of being an excellent anti-adherent. The level of talc that can be added to a formulation

Table 7 Commonly Used Glidants

Glidant	Typical percentage
Talc	1–5
Fumed silicon dioxide	0.1–0.5
Aerosil	–
Cab-O-Sil	–
Syloid	–
Starch	1–10
Calcium silicate	0.5–2.0
Magnesium carbonate (heavy)	1–3
Magnesium oxide (heavy)	1–3
Magnesium lauryl sulfate	0.2–2.0
Sodium lauryl sulfate	0.2–2.0

is restricted by its hydrophobic nature, too high levels resulting in decreased wetting of the tablet and a subsequent reduction in the rate of dissolution.

The *fumed silicon dioxides* are perhaps the most effective glidants. These are materials with very small (10 nm) spherical particles that may achieve their glidant properties by rolling over each other under shear stress. They are available in a number of grades with a range of hydrophobic and hydrophilic forms.

Starch has been used as a glidant, though relatively large amounts are required. The use of large amounts of starch has also aided the disintegration properties.

Compactibility

The aim of the formulator is to design a formulation that will reliably compact to form a strong tablet. The production manager wants a formulation that achieves the appropriate strength at a low compaction pressure, to reduce wear and tear on the tablet machine and increase the life of the punches.

The compaction properties of a formulation will largely be governed by its major components. For high-dose drugs, the active ingredient will strongly influence the compaction, while for low-dose drugs, it will be necessary for the tablet to be bulked out with an inactive material termed a diluent. High-dose formulations may also use a diluent to overcome compaction problems experienced with an active substance. The selection of the diluent will depend to an extent on the type of processing to be used. A direct compression formulation will require a diluent with good flow and compaction properties. While a granulated formulation can be more forgiving, some degree of compactibility is desirable.

There are a number of general rules for selecting a diluent. The compaction properties of the active ingredient should be considered. If the material is extremely plastic, it is appropriate to add a diluent that compacts by brittle fracture; similarly, a brittle drug substance should be combined with a plastic filler. The solubility of the drug substance should also be considered. A soluble drug is normally formulated with an insoluble filler to optimize the disintegration process.

Apart from their flow and compaction properties, all diluents, and indeed other tablet excipients, should have the following properties:

- They should be inert and physically and chemically compatible with the active substance and the other excipients being used in the formulation.
- They should be physiologically inert.
- They should not have an unacceptable microbiological burden.
- They should not have a deleterious effect on the bioavailability.
- They should have regulatory acceptability in all countries where the product is to be marketed.

There will also be commercial factors in the selection of the diluent. There are hundreds of different brands and grades of diluents available, but it would be unrealistic for the formulator to expect to have a totally free choice. Most manufacturing companies wish to limit the inventory that they carry, and will try to rationalize the excipients used in the factory. This inventory will have been selected on the basis of cost, availability, and performance and will provide the formulator with a starting point.

Table 8 lists the more commonly used diluents. These have been listed in terms of their chemical nature. For each of the substances listed, there will be several suppliers offering branded goods that may or may not be equivalent. Most products will be available with a range of particle sizes.

As can be seen from the table, the excipients all have pharmacopoeial monographs, but it is important to understand that compliance with a monograph does not indicate equivalence between different grades or suppliers. The monographs confirm the chemical identity and purity of the excipients but do not measure the performance of the materials as diluents. To establish the equivalency of excipients obtained from different sources, it is necessary to perform some kind of functionality testing. The *Handbook of Pharmaceutical Excipients*, a joint publication between the Pharmaceutical Press and the American Pharmaceutical

Table 8 Common Tablet Diluents

Diluent	Pharmacopoeia	Comments
Lactose	USP, Ph Eur, JP	Available as anhydrous and monohydrate. Anhydrous material used for direct compression due to superior compressibility.
Microcrystalline cellulose	USP, Ph Eur, JP	Originally a direct compression excipient, now often included in granulations due to its excellent compressibility.
Dextrose, glucose	USP, Ph Eur, JP	Direct compression diluent, often used in chewable tablets.
Sucrose	USP, Ph Eur, JP	Was widely used as a sweetener/filler in effervescent tablets and chewable tablets. Less popular nowadays due to cariogenicity.
Starch and derivatives	USP, Ph Eur, JP	Versatile material can be used as diluent binder and disintegrant.
Calcium carbonate	USP, Ph Eur, JP	Brittle material
Dicalcium phosphate	USP, Ph Eur, JP	Excellent flow properties. Brittle material.
Magnesium carbonate	USP, Ph Eur, JP	Direct compression diluent.

Association, contains some details of functional tests carried out on a wide range of excipients, but the onus on establishing equivalency of excipients still remains with the user (Kibbe, 2000).

Lubricity

The section "Flowability" discussed the role of glidants in tablet formulation. Glidants are one of the three interrelated types of lubricants employed in solid dosage form manufacture. The two other classes of lubricants are anti-adherent excipients, which reduce the friction between the tablet punch faces and tablet punches, and die-wall lubricant excipients, which reduce the friction between the tablet surface and the die wall during and after compaction to enable easy ejection of the tablet.

When two contacting solids are displaced relative to each other and parallel to the plane of contact, the resistance to the movement is termed friction. Contacting surfaces initially touch at points on the asperities of the two surfaces. If a force is applied, these asperities deform to form a contact area. For relative movement of the materials to occur parallel to the contact area, the materials must be sheared. The higher the shear strength of the materials in contact, the greater the force that will be required to produce movement. Die-wall lubricants work by reducing the shear force necessary to promote movement.

The level of a lubricant required in a tablet is formulation dependent and can be optimized using an instrumented tablet machine. On a single punch machine, strain gauges or load cells on the lower punch can directly measure the force required to eject the tablet. An alternative method of measuring lubrication is to measure the ratio of the maximum forces on the upper and lower punches during the compaction cycle (Hölzer and Sjøgren, 1978). On a single punch machine, the lower punch remains stationary during the compaction phase, and the compaction pressure is exerted by the movement of the upper punch. If there were no resistance to the movement of particles in the die, the force transmitted through the powder bed to the lower punch would be the same as the force applied by the upper punch. In practice, the interparticle friction and friction between the particles and the die wall result in a lower force being transmitted to the lower punch. The ratio of the upper to lower punch forces, termed the *R*-value, has been used as a measure of the lubricant efficacy. The *R*-value cannot be used on a rotary machine because the compaction pressure is applied from both the upper and lower punches simultaneously. The ejection force can be measured either by instrumenting the punch tips or by positioning load cells or strain gauges below the ejection cam. If an instrumented machine is not available, the signs of inadequate lubricity are the presence of scoring around the tablet circumference and screeching during ejection. While these problems can be overcome by increasing the level of lubricant added, the aim should be to use the minimum level of lubricant required to produce an acceptable product, for reasons discussed later.

Die-wall lubricants can be divided into two classes, fluid and boundary lubricants. *Fluid lubricants* work by separating moving surfaces completely with a layer of lubricant. These are typically mineral oils or vegetable oils, and they may be either added to the mix or applied directly to the die wall by means of wicked punches. Tablets containing oily lubricants may have a mottled appearance due to uneven distribution. When added to the mix, they have an adverse effect on powder flow due to their tacky nature, and have been reported to reduce tablet strength (Asker et al., 1973). Low-melting-point lipophilic solids can also act as fluid lubricants because the heat generated at the die wall is sufficient to cause them to melt, forming a fluid layer, which solidifies on ejection. Fluid lubricants include stearic acid, mineral oils, hydrogenated vegetable oils, glyceryl behenate, paraffins, and waxes. Low-melting-point lubricants should be used with caution in tablets that are to be film coated. Lubricants can melt on the tablet surface during the film-coating process, resulting in tablets with a pitted appearance (Rowe and Forse, 1983). Their use tends to be restricted to applications where a suitable boundary lubricant cannot be identified.

Boundary lubricants work by forming a thin, solid film at the interface of the die and the tablet. Metallic stearates are the most widely used boundary lubricants, and their activity has been attributed to adherence of polar molecular portions on their surface to the surfaces of one particle species and of nonpolar surface components to the other species' surface. Such lubricants should have low shear strength of their own and form interparticulate films that resist wear and reduce surface wear. A list of lubricants with typical ranges for their usage is given in Table 9.

Magnesium stearate is the most widely used lubricant; it forms dense, high-melting-point films between the powder and the die wall to reduce friction and has low shear strength between its own surfaces. Despite its popularity, which is a reflection of its excellent lubricant properties, the material is far from ideal, and has had problems associated with product consistency, its effect on tablet strength, and its hydrophobicity.

The magnesium stearate used in the pharmaceutical industry is not a pure substance but a mixture of magnesium salts of fatty acids, though predominantly magnesium stearate and magnesium palmitate. The USP requires that the stearate content should account for not less than 40% of the fatty acid content of the material, and the stearate and palmitate combined should account for not less than 90%. Within this definition, there is clearly scope for a range of materials to be supplied as magnesium stearate. Furthermore, there is no pharmacopoeial particle size specification for the material. As the lubrication activity of the material is related to its surface area, substantial decreases in ejection force are noted when using sources of

Table 9 Lubricants and Their Usage

Lubricant	Level required (%)	Comments
Boundary lubricants		
Magnesium stearate	0.2–2.0	Hydrophobic, variable properties between suppliers.
Calcium stearate	0.5–4.0	Hydrophobic.
Sodium stearyl fumarate	0.5–2.0	Less hydrophobic than metallic stearates, partially soluble.
Polyethylene glycol 4000 and 6000	2–10	Soluble, poorer lubricant activity than fatty acid ester salts.
Sodium lauryl sulfate	1–3	Soluble, also acts as wetting agent.
Magnesium lauryl sulfate	1–3	Acts as wetting agent.
Sodium benzoate	2–5	Soluble.
Fluid lubricants		
Light mineral oil	1–3	Hydrophobic, can be applied to either formulation or tooling.
Hydrogenated vegetable oils	1–5	Hydrophobic, used at higher concentrations as controlled-release agents.
Stearic acid	0.25–2	Hydrophobic.
Glyceryl behenate	0.5 –4.0	Hydrophobic also used as controlled-release agent.

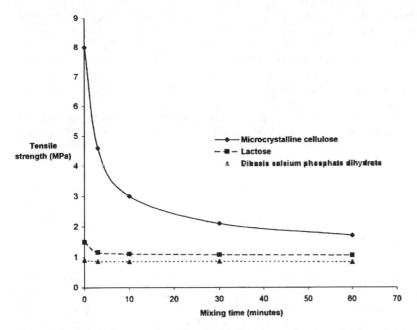

Figure 18 Effect of magnesium stearate mixing time on the strength of compacts.

magnesium stearate with larger surface areas. For a given formulation, it is important that a single source of magnesium stearate is used for all batches. A new supplier should not be used until the effect on the compaction properties and dissolution rates have been assessed.

The lubricant activity of magnesium stearate is related to its readiness to form films on the die wall surface. When it is mixed in a tablet formulation, it displays the same film-forming propensity on the surfaces of the drug and excipient particles, which can have two consequences: a reduction in the ability of the powder to form strong compacts and, due to its hydrophobicity, a deleterious effect on the dissolution rate of the tablets. Figure 18 illustrates the effect of mixing time on the mechanical strength of compacts produced using a range of excipients. While the strength decreases with increasing mixing time for all the materials tested, the effect is far more marked for materials that deform plastically. When plastic-deforming materials are compressed, the film of magnesium stearate around the particles remains relatively intact, so the interparticulate bonds are primarily between magnesium stearate particles, which, by virtue of its lubricant properties, are inherently weak. Materials that compact by fragmentation are less sensitive to the lubricant because the fragmentation process produces a number of clean, uncontaminated surfaces that are able to form strong bonds.

The hydrophobic surfaces created by magnesium stearate have been shown to reduce the rate of dissolution and bioavailability of several tablet formulations. To minimize this effect, the manufacturing process should be designed to ensure that the lubricant is the last excipient to be added. When both lubricant and disintegrant are being added to a granulated formulation, the disintegrant should be blended with the granules prior to the addition of the lubricant to minimize the risk of forming a hydrophobic film around the disintegrant. The mixing time for the lubricant should be set as the minimum time required to produce the desired effect.

The third class of lubricant activity is the anti-adherent. Some materials have adhesive properties and can adhere to the punch surfaces during compression. This will initially manifest itself as sticking, with a film forming on the surface of the tablets, leading to dull tablet surfaces. A more extreme version of sticking is picking, where solid particles from the tablet stick to the punch surface. This will often be evident in the intagliations on the tablet surface, resulting in poor definition of the surface markings.

Attempts have been made to assess picking tendencies using instrumented tablet machines. Load cells have been fitted to the edge of feed frames of rotary machines to monitor the force required to knock tablets off the lower punch following ejection. Shah et al. (1986) postulated that the magnitude of the residual force remaining on the lower punch of a single punch machine following removal of the upper punch was inversely related to the degree of adherence to the upper punch. In practice, sticking tends to be monitored during extended runs on tablet machines.

Most die-wall lubricants have anti-adherent actions, and in many formulations the addition of a specific anti-adherent is not required. Materials that can be added include talc, maize starch, and microcrystalline cellulose.

Appearance
The appearance of a tablet is of great importance to the way it is perceived by the patient. The macroscopic appearance of a tablet, its shape, size, color, and markings can all contribute to the patients' expectations of a medicine, while the microscopic appearance, such as surface roughness and color homogeneity, are easily perceived as measures of quality. It is now the norm to be able to identify new products because of their unique appearance achieved by a combination of shape, size, color, and surface markings.

The size of a tablet is very often governed by the dose being administered. The compression weight of a high-dose drug will usually be determined by the level of filler required to impart the appropriate compactibility on the formulation, the aim being to produce the smallest possible tablet for ease of swallowing. For low-dose drugs, the quantity of filler added is determined by the minimum acceptable size for a tablet. The actual minimum acceptable size for a tablet will vary between pharmaceutical companies but is generally in the region of 6 or 7 mm diameter for a circular tablet, which would equate with a compression weight of 80 to 100 mg. Tablets below this range tend to be difficult for the patients to handle.

Early tablets were produced in cylindrical dies with flat-faced, flat bevel-edged, or concave punches. While the majority of tablets are still circular, over the last 20 years, there has been an increasing shift away from circular to shaped tablets for new products. The tablet identification section of the *Chemist and Druggist Directory* (2000) describes 274 noncircular tablet products that are on the market in Britain, while the *Physicians' Desk Reference* (PDR) (1998) contains illustrations of 502 noncircular tablets that are available in the United States. After round tablets, the most common presentation is the capsule-shaped tablet, sometimes referred to as a caplet. This shape is particularly popular for high-dose products where the compression weight is necessarily high, as the elongated shape makes the tablet easier to swallow than round tablets of equal weight. A survey performed on the reaction of patients to the appearance of tablets has indicated that the tablet shape can influence patients' expectations of a medicine in terms of its potency, side effects, and suitability for a particular ailment (Anon, 1989). The studies found that tablets with highly angular appearances were universally disliked on the basis that they would be hard to swallow. Less predictable was the finding that other elements of tablet design, such as the number and depth of scorelines, the degree of rounding of corners, and the hardness of the finish indicated by surface shine, appeared to play a role in determining how easy or hard to swallow a tablet might be. When designing a tablet shape, consideration should also be given to the processes following compression, such as coating and packaging. These processes depend on tablets being able to move relative to each other, and if the tablet shape allows tablets to form "structures" (e.g., due to straight sides), it may be problematic.

The coloring of tablets can be achieved either by incorporating a dye or pigment into the powder prior to compression, or by applying a colored coat to the tablet following compression. Coating methods, which are dealt with in the section "Tablet Coating," tend to provide a more uniform color than inclusion of pigments in the compression mix but have the disadvantage of requiring an additional manufacturing process.

Colorants come in three forms: soluble dyes, insoluble pigments, and lakes. Lakes are formed by adsorbing dyes onto the surface of an inert substrate, usually aluminum hydroxide. If the colorant is being added to a granulate, soluble dyes can be dissolved in the granulating fluid to ensure a uniform mix. When adding colorants as solids, the mixing process needs to be very efficient to achieve a uniform color with no mottling. The usual method of inclusion is to form a premix with a portion of the powder mix, and to mill this prior to incorporating the remaining ingredients. The problem can be reduced by the appropriate selection of colors, mottling being less evident with pastel shades. The insoluble pigments tend to be more light, stable, and less prone to fading than the soluble dyes.

The choice of color is severely restricted by the number of regulatory acceptable dyes and pigments available to the formulator. This is particularly true when trying to achieve a globally acceptable formulation, due to the lack of international harmonization of permitted colorants. Table 10 lists the commonly used pigments and dyes together with their international acceptability. It can be seen that for an international formulation, the choice of colorants is restricted to the iron oxide pigments and indigo carmine, and as a result, there are large

Table 10 Pharmaceutical Colorants and Their Regulatory Acceptability

Color	Other names	Regulatory acceptability				
		EU	USA	Japan	Canada	India
Azorubine	Carmoisine	+	−	−	+	+
Ponceau 4R	Cochineal Red A Brilliant Scarlet 4R	+	−	+[a]	+	+
Canthaxanthin	Food Orange 8	+	+	−	+	−
Sudan 3	Toney Red	−	+	−	−	+
FD&C Red 2	Amaranth Bordeaux S	+	−	+[a]	+	−
FD&C Red 3 lakes are prohibited	Erythrosine	+	+[b]	+	+	+
FD&C Red 4	Ponceau SX Naphtalone Red B	−	+	− ADI 0–0.75 mg	−	−
FD&C Red 40	Allura Red	+	+[b]	−	+	−
D&C Red 6	Lithol Rubin B	−	+	−	+	−
D&C Red 7	Lithol Rubin Ca	−	+	−	+	−
D&C Red 21	Tetrabromo Fluorescein	−	+	−	−	−
D&C Red 22	Eosin Y	−	+[b]	−	+	+
D&C Red 28	Phloxine B	−	+[b]	+ AL-lake only	+	−
D&C Red 30	Helindone Pink CN	−	+	−	+	−
D&C Red 31	Brilliant Lake Red R	−	+	−	−	−
D&C Red 33	Acid Fuchsin D	−	+	−	+	−
D&C Red 34	Lake Bordeaux B	−	+	−	−	−
D&C Red 36	Flaming Red	−	−	−	+	−
D&C Red 39	Alba Red	−	+	−	−	−
Cochineal Extract	Natural Red 4 Carmine	+	+	+	+	+
Iron Oxide–Red		+	+	+ ADI 0–0.5 mg elemental iron	+	+
Anthocyanin		+	−	−	+	−
Lutein		+	−	−	−	−
Lycopene		+	−	−	−	−
Paprika Extract		+	−	−	−	−
Beetroot Red	Betanin	+	−	−	−	−
FD&C Yellow 5	Tartrazine	+[c]	+[b,c]	+	+	+
FD&C Yellow 6	Sunset Yellow FCF Yellow Orange S	+	+	+	+	+
D&C Yellow 7	Fluorescein	−	+	−	−	−
D&C Yellow 8	Uranine	−	+	−	−	−
D&C Yellow 10[d]	Quinoline Yellow WS	−	+[b]	−	+	+

(Continued)

Table 10 Pharmaceutical Colorants and Their Regulatory Acceptability (*Continued*)

Color	Other names	Regulatory acceptability				
		EU	USA	Japan	Canada	India
Quinoline Yellow[d]	China Yellow	+	−	−	−	−
Fast Yellow	Acid Yellow G	−	−	−	−	−
Yellow 2G		−	−	−	−	−
D&C Orange 4	Orange II	−	+	−	−	−
D&C Orange 5	Dibromofluorescein	−	+	−	−	−
D&C Orange 10	Diiodofluroscein	−	+	−	−	−
D&C Orange 11	Erythrosine Yellowish Na	−	+	−	−	−
β-Carotene		+	+	+	+	+
Turmeric	Curcumin Natural Yellow 3 Indian Saffron	+	−	−	−	+
Annatto		−	−	−	−	+
Orange G		−	−	−	−	+
Iron Oxide–Yellow		+	+	+ ADI 0–0.5 mg elemental iron	+	+
Riboflavin	Lactoflavin Vitamin B$_2$	+	−	+	+	+
Gold		+	−	+	−	−
Patent Blue V		+	−	−	−	−
FD&C Blue 1	Brilliant Blue FCF	+	+[b]	+	+	+
FD&C Blue 2	Indigotine Indigo Carmine	+	+	+	+	+
Naphthol Blue		−	−	−	−	+
D&C Violet 2	Alizurol Purple SS	−	+	−	−	−
FD&C Green 3	Fast Green FCF	−	+[b]	+	+	+
D&C Green 5	Alizarine Cyanine Acid Green	−	+	−	−	+
D&C Green 6	Quinazarine Green	−	+	−	−	+
D&C Green 8	Pyranine Conc.	−	+	−	−	−
Acid Brilliant	Green S	+	−	−	−	−
Chlorophyllin		+	−	+	+	+
Powdered Green Tea		−	−	+	−	−
Rye Green Leaf Extract		−	−	+	−	−
Brilliant Black BN	Food Black 1	+	−	−	−	−
Carbon Black	Medicinal Vegetable Charcoal	+	−	+	+	−
Iron Oxide–Black		+	+	− ADI 0–0.5 mg elemental iron	+	+
Caramel	Burnt Sugar	+	+	+	+	+
Glycyrrhiza Extract		−	−	+	−	−
D&C Brown 1	Resorcin Brown	−	−	−	−	+
Brown HT		+	−	−	−	−
Titanium dioxide		+	+	+	+	+

Note: + Permitted; − Not permitted.

[a]Manufacturers have imposed a voluntary ban on this color.

[b]Requires FDA certification on each lot of dye.

[c]Requires label declaration.

[d]The quinoline yellow approved for use in the EU is not the same as D&C Yellow 10, the dyes differ in composition. Quinoline Yellow is primarily the disulfonated quinoline dye, whereas D&C Yellow 10 is the monosulfonated color.

numbers of tablets with varying shades of red, yellow, orange, and brown being introduced onto the market.

The easiest way to give a tablet a unique identity is to mark the surface with a code or unique identifier. This can be achieved by applying a printed logo to the surface of the tablet or by compressing the powder with punches that are embossed with the code, producing tablets with intagliations. Printing is performed with ink jet printers applying approved inks to the surface of tablets. The advantage of printing is that it is possible to fit more information on to the surface than is possible with embossed punches, but it is an additional process, and not all tablet surfaces are suitable for printing. The use of embossed punches does not increase the manufacturing time, but it does stress a formulation. The embossing of the punches will exacerbate any tendency for punch adherence, and this should be considered when selecting the levels of lubricant and anti-adherent in the tablet. The intagliations will also highlight the presence of any abrasion on the crown of the tablet, and care must be taken to ensure that the surfaces are sufficiently robust, particularly if they are to be subsequently film coated.

Disintegration

The chapter to date has concentrated on ensuring that it is possible to produce a tablet of sufficient strength that it can withstand the stresses of subsequent manufacturing operations, such as coating and packaging, and will reach the patient in an acceptable condition. However, once an immediate-release tablet is taken by the patient, it is important that it breaks up rapidly to ensure quick dissolution of the active ingredients.

To maximize the dissolution rate of a drug substance from a tablet, it is necessary to overcome the cohesive strength produced by the compression process and break the tablet into the primary particles as rapidly as possible (Fig. 19). This is achieved by adding disintegrants, which will induce this process.

Starch was the first disintegrant used in tablet manufacture and is still used, although it has largely been superseded by the so-called super disintegrants, croscarmellose sodium,

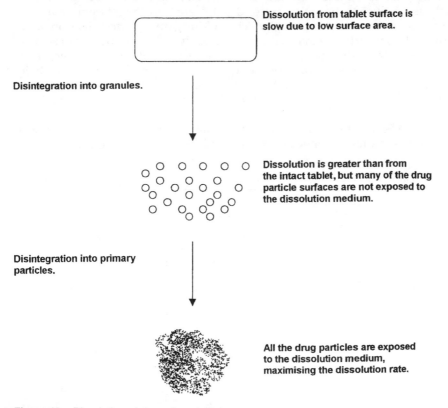

Dissolution from tablet surface is slow due to low surface area.

Disintegration into granules.

Dissolution is greater than from the intact tablet, but many of the drug particle surfaces are not exposed to the dissolution medium.

Disintegration into primary particles.

All the drug particles are exposed to the dissolution medium, maximising the dissolution rate.

Figure 19 Dissolution of drugs from tablets.

sodium starch glycolate, and crospovidone, which display excellent disintegrant activity at low concentrations and possess better compression properties than starches.

Traditionally, swelling and rate of swelling have been regarded as the most important characteristics of disintegrants. Rudnic et al. (1982) quantified the rate of swelling and force generated by the swelling of disintegrants, and found no simple relationship between the maximum disintegrating force and disintegration time. It was the ability to develop a significant swelling force rapidly that appeared to be more important. The other important factor in a formulation is that as the swelling develops, it should not be accommodated within the tablet, which prevents a significant disruptive force from being generated. If the tablet displays elasticity to the swelling, the force will be expended on the system, and disintegration will not take place. Similarly, if the tablet is composed entirely of soluble components, their dissolution will deprive the disintegrant of a matrix to push against. As a general rule, soluble drugs are formulated with insoluble fillers to maximize the effect of disintegrants.

The positioning of disintegrants within the intragranular and extragranular portions of granulated formulations can affect their efficacy. Placing the disintegrant in the extragranular portion results in rapid disintegration to granular particles, while the disintegrant present in the granule will promote further disintegration to the primary particles, thus aiding dissolution. Studies performed to determine the optimum location of disintegrant (Shotton and Leonard, 1972; Rubenstein and Bodey, 1974) suggest that dividing it between the two portions, with between 20% and 50% being in the extragranular portion, produces the best results.

Optimizing the level of disintegrants in a formulation is a good example of a situation where there are a number of opposing factors to consider, and the final formulation needs to be a compromise. To optimize the biopharmaceutical properties of the formulation, the tablet should disintegrate rapidly, which can be achieved by increasing the level of disintegrants. The particle size of most disintegrants is too small to maximize the surface area, and thus increase the rate of water uptake. The addition of large quantities of such materials could have an adverse effect on the flow properties of the formulation. The compaction properties of many disintegrants, including starch, are less than ideal, and high concentrations could also reduce the strength of tablets produced. By their nature, disintegrants are hygroscopic materials and will absorb moisture from the atmosphere, which could negatively affect the stability of water-sensitive drugs. The super disintegrants, if used at excessive concentrations, can actually absorb sufficient moisture from the atmosphere to initiate disintegration on storage, if the packaging does not provide adequate protection from the environment. Disintegrant activity can be affected by mixing with hydrophobic lubricants, so care needs to be taken to optimize the manufacturing process as well as the formulation. The commonly used disintegrants are listed in Table 11.

For a disintegrant to be able to function properly, the tablet surface must be amenable to wetting. If the tablet contains a high proportion of a hydrophobic drug that has a high contact

Table 11 Commonly Used Disintegrants

Disintegrant	Normal usage concentration (%)	Comments
Starch	5–10	Probably work by wicking; swelling is minimal at body temperature.
Microcrystalline cellulose		Strong wicking action. Loses disintegrant action when highly compressed.
Insoluble ion exchange resins		Strong wicking tendencies with some swelling action.
Sodium starch glycolate	2–8	Free-flowing powder that swells rapidly on contact with water.
Croscarmellose sodium	1–5	Swells on contact with water.
Gums—agar, guar, xanthan	<5	Swell on contact with water; form viscous gels that can retard dissolution, thus limiting concentration that can be used.
Alginic acid, sodium alginate	4–6	Swell like the gums but form less viscous gels.
Crospovidone	1–5	High wicking activity.

angle, it may be wise to include a wetting agent or surfactant in the formulation, which will aid not only the disintegration time of the tablet but also the subsequent dissolution of the drug substance. The most commonly used wetting agents are sodium lauryl sulfate and the polysorbates.

An alternative mechanism of disintegration is used in effervescent tablets, which utilizes a gas-liberating chemical reaction to effect rapid disintegration. These tablets contain an organic acid and an alkali metal carbonate, which, when added to water prior to administration, react to produce carbon dioxide, for example,

$$RCOOH + NaHCO_3 \rightarrow RCOONa + CO_2 + H_2O \qquad (14)$$

Most pharmacopoeias include a disintegration test, which can be applied to tablets and capsules. The USP test consists of six glass tubes, 3 in long and open at the top, with a 10-mesh screen at the bottom and immersed in a beaker of disintegration fluid that is maintained at 37°C. The tubes are raised and lowered 5 to 6 cm at 30 cycles per minute, such that the bottom of the tubes remain 2 to 5 cm below the liquid surface at the top of the stroke and are no closer than 2 to 5 cm from the base of the beaker at the lowest point. One tablet is placed in each tube, and the disintegration time is the time taken for all six tablets to break up sufficiently for all material to pass through the mesh at the bottom of the tube. If the dosage form floats, it is permitted to place perforated plastic discs in the tubes to ensure that they remain submerged during the test. Pharmacopoeial tests use water as the disintegration fluid for nonenteric-coated tablets, but during development, it is prudent to test the tablets over a range of pH values.

Disintegration testing is an important part of in-process control testing during production to ensure batch-to-batch uniformity, but its role in end-product testing has largely been superseded by dissolution testing.

Dissolution

Drug materials administered orally are required to dissolve in the GI fluids before absorption can take place. Dissolution occurs most rapidly from the primary particles of the drug substance, hence the importance of rapid disintegration to this state. However, disintegration studies only demonstrate that a tablet will break up when immersed in fluid; there are many other factors that can influence the dissolution of a material. A carefully designed dissolution test will, therefore, be a better indication of the performance of a dosage form. The design of dissolution tests and the correlation between in vitro dissolution and in vivo performance is discussed in chapter 7, "Biopharmaceutical Support in Formulation Development." The optimization of the dissolution of a substance is discussed in chapter 8.

Processing of Formulations

The performance requirements of a tablet were discussed in the previous section, and it is clear that most tablets contain several ingredients. The drug substance, probably a filler, a disintegrant, and a lubricant will be common to most formulations, while glidants, colorants, and wetting agents may also be included. The quality of the final product will be as dependent on the way in which the components are combined as it is on the components selected. Traditionally, tablet formulations have been prepared by one of two methods: direct compression or granulation.

Direct compression is the term used to define the process where powder blends of the drug substance and excipients are compressed on a tablet machine. There is no mechanical treatment of the powder apart from a mixing process. Granulation is a generic term for particle enlargement, whereby powders are formed into permanent aggregates. The purpose of granulating tablet formulations is to improve the flow and compaction properties prior to compression. There are a number of different methods that can be used to granulate a powder blend, but the most common one for pharmaceuticals is wet granulation, where a liquid is added to aid agglomeration and then removed by drying prior to compression. Even from this short description, it is obvious that direct compression is a much simpler process; yet it is not universally adopted. This section will review the advantages and disadvantages of the two techniques in an attempt to explain why granulation still plays an important role in tablet manufacture.

Direct Compression

The term *direct compression* was initially applied to the formation of compacts from materials that required no pretreatment and the addition of no additives or excipients. As such, it was only used for inorganic materials such as potassium bromide. Today, within the pharmaceutical industry, the term is used for tablet manufacture that does not involve the pretreatment of the drug substance apart from blending with excipients.

Advantages of direct compression. The most obvious advantage of direct compression is its simplicity and subsequent economy. The manufacture requires fewer operations, and the omission of a drying step results in lower energy consumption. If a new production line is being built for a product, there will be considerable savings in the plant required, equipment such as granulators and driers being unnecessary. The reduced processing times will produce savings in labor costs, and the simplicity of the process should make process validation simpler. However, some of these savings will be offset by the need to use specialized, more expensive, excipients.

Direct compression can provide technical, as well as economic, benefits. Stability of certain drugs can be improved, and the elimination of a wetting and drying process can be beneficial when formulating drugs that are thermolabile or moisture sensitive.

For certain drugs, the dissolution rate can be improved by utilizing direct compression. In the section "Disintegration," it was stated that for optimal dissolution, the tablet must disintegrate into its primary particles as quickly as possible. With no agglomeration stage involved in direct compression, the tablets will disintegrate directly to the primary particles.

Disadvantages of direct compression. The main limitation of direct compression is that it cannot be used for all drug substances; the technique depends on the major components of the formulation having appropriate flow and compaction properties. While it is possible to modify the properties of drug substances by particle engineering, this is usually outside the scope of the formulator, and the formulation must be designed to accommodate the limitations imposed by the drug substance. For low-dose drugs, it is usually possible to overcome such limitations through careful selection of excipients, but there will be a dose level at which it becomes impractical to produce a tablet of acceptable size.

The challenges facing the formulator of low-dose drugs by direct compression are related to achieving and maintaining a homogeneous mix. Very low-dose drugs can be formulated to form ordered mixes that reduce the risk of segregation. Consideration must be given to the entire manufacturing process to minimize the possibility of segregation.

Direct compression places greater demands on the excipients, particularly the fillers. This has resulted in the introduction of a number of excipients that have been designed specifically for use in direct compression formulations, although they tend to be expensive.

Armstrong (1998) described the following requirements for direct compression fillers:

- Have good flow properties
- Possess good compaction properties
- Have high capacity (defined as the ability to retain their compaction properties when mixed with drugs substances)
- Have appropriate particle size distribution to minimize the segregation potential
- Have high bulk density
- Be capable of being manufactured reproducibly to minimize batch-to-batch variation

Jivraj et al. (2000) have classified the direct compression fillers in terms of their disintegration and flow properties (Table 12).

Table 12 Direct Compression Fillers

Classification	Examples	Comments
Materials that act as disintegration agents with poor flow characteristics	Microcrystalline cellulose	Probably the most widely used direct compression excipients. Excellent compactibility at low pressures, high-dilution capacity.
	Directly compressible starch	
Free-flowing materials that do not disintegrate	Dibasic calcium phosphate dihydrate	Excellent flow properties. Very brittle material, and is best used in combination with microcrystalline cellulose or directly compressible starch.
Free-flowing powders that disintegrate by dissolution	Lactose	Anhydrous β-lactose possesses excellent compaction properties. Picks up moisture at elevated humidity and may be less compatible with moisture-sensitive compounds than the monohydrate form (Jain et al., 1998).
	Sorbitol	Good compactibility. Popular in chewable tablets due to its cool mouth feel.
	Mannitol	Hygroscopic.

In addition to these excipients, there are also a number of proprietary preparations that combine two or more materials to optimize the flow and compaction properties. Examples of such excipients include the following:

- Ludipress—a combination of a-lactose monohydrate, polyvinylpyrrolidone, and crospovidone
- Cellactose—microcrystalline cellulose and lactose
- Cel-O-Cal—coprocessed microcrystalline cellulose and calcium sulfate
- Silicified microcrystalline cellulose—coprocessed microcrystalline cellulose that has been silicified with colloidal silicon dioxide

A number of active drug substances are also available in coprocessed forms for use in direct compression formulations. While such materials might not be considered direct compression in its purest form, they do pass on the advantages of direct compression technology to the tablet manufacturers.

Granulation
Granulation is the most widely used technique to prepare powders for compaction. The term *granulation* is a generic description for a process of particle enlargement in which particles are agglomerated while retaining the integrity of the original particles. A number of methods can be used to achieve the agglomeration; these are normally classified as either wet granulation, where a liquid is used to aid the agglomeration process, or dry granulation, where no liquid is used.

The purpose of granulating is to transform the powdered starting materials, which would otherwise be unsuitable for tabletting, into a form that will run smoothly on a tablet machine. This is achieved in a number of ways. The most obvious benefit of granulation is the improved flow properties resulting from the increase in particle size.

In forming granules, individual particles of the starting ingredients are agglomerated together. If a homogeneous powder mix is achieved before commencing agglomeration, the granules will consist of a homogeneous mix of those ingredients. More importantly, the particles of drug substance will be bound to the particles of the excipients, thus reducing the potential for segregation, and improving the chances of content uniformity.

The granulation process usually involves the addition of a polymeric binder that sticks the individual particles together. It has been demonstrated with paracetamol (Armstrong and

Morton, 1977) that this process can reduce the elasticity of starting materials, thus improving the compactibility.

The polymers used as binders are usually hydrophilic in nature. This can have a beneficial effect on the dissolution of hydrophobic drugs. During the granulation process, a film of hydrophilic polymer will form over the surface of hydrophobic drug particles, which will aid wetting.

One of the advantages of granulation is that it results in the densification and subsequent volume reduction of the starting material. This is particularly useful in the case of voluminous starting materials. A further benefit is that the densified, coarse material will reduce the amount of air entrapment.

A number of methods are routinely used within the pharmaceutical industry to produce granulations. These are traditionally classified as dry granulation and wet granulation, depending on whether a liquid is used to aid the agglomeration.

Wet granulation. Wet granulation methods are the most commonly used in tablet manufacture. These methods involve the addition of a liquid and, usually, a polymeric binder to the powdered starting materials, and a form of agitation to promote agglomeration followed by a drying process. In most cases, the liquid used is water, although in certain circumstances organic solvents such as ethanol or ethanol/water mixes are used. Nonaqueous granulation will be considered when the active substance is particularly unstable in the presence of water, when water will not wet the powder or, possibly, if the drug substance forms a significant portion of the granulate, and demonstrates extreme solubility in aqueous media, and control of the granulation process becomes difficult due to the occurrence of significant dissolution. While there are a number of approaches to wet granulation used in the pharmaceutical industry, they all share the following basic principles:

- Dry mixing: The starting materials are mixed together. Prior to mixing, the ingredients may be deagglomerated by a milling or sieving process. If the granulate has a low drug content, the active substance may be premixed with one of the ingredients prior to being added to the granulation vessel to ensure good content uniformity.
- Addition of granulating liquid: The granulating fluid is added to the dry ingredients and mixed to form a wet mass. The mixing of the fluid with the dry ingredients leads to agglomeration of the powder. This agglomeration can be controlled by altering the amount of fluid added, the intensity of the mixing, and the duration of the mixing. Depending on the state of agglomeration achieved, this stage may be followed by a wet sieving process to break up the larger agglomerates.
- Drying: The fluid is removed by a drying process.
- Milling: The dried granulate undergoes a sieving or milling operation to obtain the desired particle size distribution.

To understand the granulation process, it is necessary to consider what is occurring at the particulate level during the process. The aim of granulation is to increase the particle size of a powder mix, and this is achieved in wet granulation by the formation of liquid bridges between the powder particles. If a liquid that is able to wet the powder is added, the system will minimize its surface-free energy by forming liquid bridges between the particles. The nature and extent of these bridges will be dependent on the amount of liquid added.

At low liquid levels, it is assumed that the liquid will distribute itself evenly through the bed, forming discrete liquid bridges at points of contact between particles (Fig. 20). This is known as the pendular state. The strength of an individual pendular bond, σ, between two spherical particles can be calculated as

$$\sigma = \frac{2\pi r T}{1 + \tan\frac{1}{2}\phi} \tag{15}$$

where r is the radius of the spherical particle, T is the surface tension of the liquid, and ϕ is the angle formed between the line joining the center of the spheres and the edge of the pendular

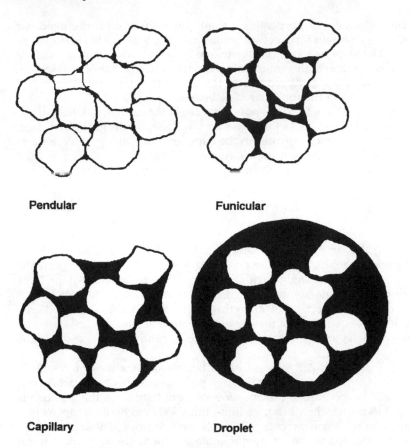

Pendular   Funicular

Capillary   Droplet

Figure 20   Stages involved in granulation.

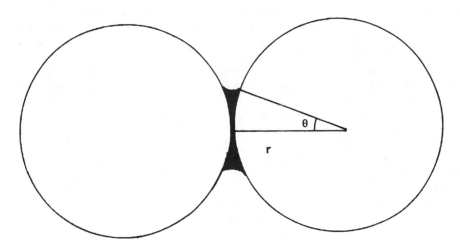

Figure 21   Calculation of the strength of a pendular liquid bridge.

bond (Fig. 21) (Eaves and Jones, 1972). This equation predicts that the bond strength will increase as the surface tension of the liquid increases and as the liquid content decreases. In practice, the strength of agglomerates tends to zero at very low liquid contents, and this has been attributed to the presence of dry joints occurring between particles, due to uneven distribution of the liquid throughout the powder bed.

As the liquid content is increased, the pendular state will remain until the pendular bonds start to coalesce and liquid bridges form between non-touching points. This is known as the funicular state (Fig. 20). The state depends on the degree of liquid saturation or voidage saturation, which is defined as the ratio of the liquid volume to the total volume of pores in the powder bed. Typically, a powder bed will remain in the pendular state until the liquid saturation reaches around 25%, and in the funicular state between 25% and 80%.

As the liquid saturation rises above 80%, the powder reaches the capillary state, and the granule is held together by capillary suction as the liquid air interfaces on the granule surface. While the tensile strength of the granule is greater in the capillary state, the granulate starts assuming a paste-like consistency, which is unsuitable for wet sieving.

The theoretical tensile strength of agglomerates in the funicular and capillary states has been derived by Rumpf et al. (1974)

$$\sigma = SC\left(\frac{1-\varepsilon}{\varepsilon}\right)\left(\frac{\gamma}{d}\right)\cos\theta \tag{16}$$

This equation applies to the strength of agglomerates formed from monosize spheres with diameter d that are packed to porosity ε. The degree of liquid saturation is S, and the liquid has surface tension γ and a contact angle θ with the solid. C is a material constant. Note that in these states, the strength of agglomerates now increases with decreasing particle size. The porosity of the powder also affects the strength; if the material is densified, the agglomerate strength will increase. Addition of further liquid converts the capillary state into the droplet state, where the particles are enclosed in a water droplet and the mass takes on the properties of slurry.

The gradual transition from pendular through funicular to capillary bonding assumes that there is always a uniform distribution of liquid throughout a powder bed. In practice, this is obviously not always the case because the dispersion of liquid through the powder is achieved by mechanical agitation, which will take a finite time. What actually happens in a powder bed during a typical granulation process will be the creation of small areas of high saturation that will lead to the formation of agglomerates, which, through mechanical agitation, are dispersed throughout the powder bed. The fate of the agglomerates will change as the degree of liquid saturation increases.

Three phases of agglomeration are recognized, and these will to an extent be occurring simultaneously within a powder bed as the liquid becomes distributed by agitation. The first stage of particle growth is nucleation, which occurs whenever a powder is wetted, particles being held together by liquid bridges. In practice, the liquid addition will lead to overwet agglomerates being formed, to which further powder adheres until the number of liquid bridges is saturated. At low saturation levels, interactions such as friction will also contribute to the strength of the agglomerates. The theoretical strength of the agglomerates is proportional to the degree of liquid saturation, so the initial agglomerates will tend to be weak, and in an agitated environment, agglomerates will constantly be formed and destroyed. The survival of the agglomerates will increase during the granulation process as the liquid saturation increases and as densification occurs, reducing the porosity of the powder bed.

The powder then undergoes a transition state as it takes up sufficient liquid for the effects of particle interactions to diminish, and the strength becomes controlled by the liquid bridges. The agglomerates become less brittle and more plastic in nature. At this stage, coalescence between colliding particles occurs, and particle growth takes place.

The final stage of granulation is ball growth, a period characterized by rapid growth in particle size. Large granules are formed by the fracture of smaller granules, and the resulting fragments build up in layers on the surface of the larger agglomerates.

The above description of the granulation process illustrates that the formulator is dealing with a complex system, and the quality of the final product will be influenced by a large number of factors, from the selection of the raw materials to the processing conditions employed.

While one of the stated advantages of granulation over direct compression is that the technique is better able to cope with variations in raw material, the agglomeration process will be affected by significant changes in the raw materials used. The particle size of the starting materials will affect the strength of granules produced, as predicted in equation 16. The quantity of granulating fluid required to achieve granulation is dependent on the particle size and shape. This additional requirement is partly related to the increase in surface area but also relates to the material-packing properties that affect the granule porosity and the degree of liquid saturation achieved. Granulation is essentially a wetting process and, as such, is dependent on the surface chemistry of the particles. It is well established that powder-handling processes such as milling and drying can significantly affect the surface properties of powders. Small areas of amorphous material on the particle surface produced by particle attrition, too small to be detected by techniques such as X-ray powder diffraction, can have dramatic effects on the wetting characteristics.

Granulating agents (binders). It is possible to granulate a powder simply by adding water or an organic solvent to a powder. Provided that the liquid is able to wet the powder surface, it will form liquid bridges. When the granulate dries, the crystallization of any solids that had dissolved in the liquid will form solid bonds between the particles. These bonds will usually be fairly weak, and friable granulates will be formed; often the granules will not be sufficiently robust to withstand the drying process. It is usual, therefore, to include granulating agents or binders to granulations to increase the granule strength. Granulating agents are usually hydrophilic polymers that have cohesive properties that both aid the granulation process and impart strength on the dried granulate.

For a granulating agent to be effective, it is vital that it is able to form a film on the particle surface. Rowe (1989) has suggested that binders should be selected on the basis of their spreading coefficients, where the spreading coefficient is defined as the difference between the "work of adhesion" of the binder and the substrate and the "work of cohesion" of the binder. The commonly used granulating agents are listed in Table 13.

The synthetic polymers such as polyvinyl pyrrolidine (PVP) and hydroxypropyl methylcellulose (HPMC) have almost totally superseded the use of natural products such as starch, acacia, and tragacanth in modern formulations. The most common method of adding binders is as a solution in the granulating fluid. It is possible to add some of the synthetic polymers such as PVP and HPMC as powders, and use water as the granulating agent. This approach, which has the advantage of not requiring a solution manufacturing step in production, is likely to result in incomplete hydration of the polymers during processing, which will affect the quality of the final granulate.

The level of binder used needs to be a balance between the level required to produce a robust, compressible granulate and the biopharmaceutical properties. As the granule strength increases, there is often an adverse effect on disintegration and dissolution. The binders form hydrophilic films on the surface of the granules, which can aid the wetting of hydrophobic

Table 13 Commonly Used Granulating Agents

Granulating agent	Normal usage concentration (%)	Comments
Starch	5–25	Was once the most commonly used binder. The starch has to be prepared as a paste, which is time consuming.
Pregelatinized starch	5–10	Cold water soluble, so easier to prepare than starch.
Acacia	1–5	Requires preparation of paste prior to use. Can lead to prolonged disintegration times if used at too high a concentration.
PVP	2–8	Available in range of molecular weights/viscosities. Can be added either dry or in solution. Soluble in water and ethanol.
HPMC	2–8	Available in range of molecular weight/viscosities. Soluble in water and ethanol.
MC	1–5	Low-viscosity grades most widely used.

Abbreviations: PVP, polyvinylpyrrolidone; HPMC, hydroxypropyl methylcellulose; MC, methylcellulose.

drugs; but if added in too great concentrations, the films can form viscous gels on the granule surface, which will retard dissolution. To optimize the dissolution of a drug from a granulated product, it is important that the granule should disintegrate into its primary particles as rapidly as possible, and it is usual to position at least a portion of any disintegrant inside the granules.

Wet granulation methods. A number of processing methods are commonly used within the pharmaceutical industry. Each method will impart particular characteristics and, as such, granulates produced by each method may not be equivalent in terms of either their physical properties (which will influence subsequent performance on tablet machines) or their biopharmaceutical properties. This latter point is well recognized by regulatory authorities that regard changes in the granulation method as potentially having a significant effect on the bioavailability of poorly soluble, poorly permeable compounds. The U.S. Food and Drug Administration (FDA) and industry representatives have outlined their expectations regarding the testing required when changing the method of granulation in *SUPAC-IR: Immediate-Release Solid Oral Dosage Forms: Scale-Up and Post-Approval Changes: Chemistry, Manufacturing and Controls, In Vitro Dissolution Testing, and In Vivo Bioequivalence Documentation*. This document concludes that changing the type of granulation process used can, for some drug substances, result in the need to perform a bioequivalence study prior to the change being granted regulatory approval.

The three main methods of producing pharmaceutical granulates are low-shear granulation, high-shear granulation, and fluid bed granulation. *Low-shear mixers* encompass machines such as Z-blade mixers and planetary mixers, which, as their names suggest, impart relatively low shear stresses onto the granulate. Widely used in the past, this approach has largely been superseded by high-shear mixers. The low level of shear applied is often insufficient to ensure good powder mixing, so a premix is often required. The process is forgiving in terms of the amount of liquid added, although it does result in long granulation times. The degree of ball growth tends to be uncontrolled because there is insufficient shear to break up the plastic agglomerates, so a wet screening stage is almost always necessary prior to drying to reduce the larger agglomerates.

High-shear granulators are closed vessels that normally have two agitators; an impeller, which normally covers the diameter of the mixing vessel, and a small chopper positioned perpendicular to the impeller. The powders are dry mixed using the impeller, and then the granulating fluid is added. Wet massing takes place using the impeller and the chopper, and granulation is usually completed in a number of minutes. The granulation process can be controlled using an appropriate combination of impeller and chopper speeds and time. The ability of the chopper to limit the size of the agglomerates can negate the need for a wet screening stage for many granulates. High-shear mixers provide a greater degree of densification than the low-shear mixers. This, combined with the relatively short processing times, can lead to the process being very sensitive to the amount of granulating liquid added.

In both high-shear and low-shear mixers, the mode of liquid addition can affect the quality of the final product. The liquid can either be added in one go or slowly sprayed onto the powders. Slow spraying leads to the most uniform distribution of liquid but can increase the overall processing time. Pouring the liquid onto the powder will result initially in large overwet granulates being formed. The mixer needs to impart sufficient energy to the system to break up the agglomerates to achieve uniform distribution of liquid.

Fluid bed granulation involves spraying the dry powder with a granulating fluid inside a fluid bed drier. The powder is fluidized in heated air and then sprayed with the granulating fluid. When all the granulating liquid has been added, the fluidization of the powder continues until the granules are dry. Advantages of this technique are that the granulation and drying are performed in a continuous manner in the same vessel, and there is no need for a wet screening operation. Nucleation occurs by random collisions between the droplets of granulating fluid and particles until all the individual particles have been incorporated into agglomerates. Densification of materials is limited due to the lack of shear forces.

Seager et al. (1985) produced a detailed analysis on the influence of manufacturing method on the tabletting performance of paracetamol granulated with hydrolyzed gelatin.

The main difference in the granules produced by different methods was their final density, high-shear mixers producing denser granules than low-shear granulators, which in turn produced denser granules than fluid bed granulations. Disintegration times were greater for tablets produced from the denser granulates.

Extrusion/Spheronization
One specialized method of particle agglomeration is extrusion and spheronization, to produce spherical or near-spherical particles. Such particles are suitable for coating with release, modifying coats to produce controlled-release formulations. The particles are usually filled into hard gelatin capsules for administration to patients. The process of extrusion/ spheronization is depicted in Figure 22.

The drug and filler are mixed with water to form a wet mass. This step is performed using equipment similar to that of conventional wet granulation, though the quantity of water added is greater, resulting in a plastic mass rather than granules. The mass is then extruded, that is, forced through a screen containing circular holes, to form a spaghetti-like extrudate. The extrudate is cut into lengths roughly twice the diameter of the holes and rolled by frictional and centrifugal forces on a rotating grooved plate known as a marumerizer or spheronizer. The rolling action compresses the cylinder along the length and rounds the ends, forming dumbbells, which become further compressed along their length to form spheres. The spheroids are discharged from the spheronizer and dried, usually by fluid bed drying.

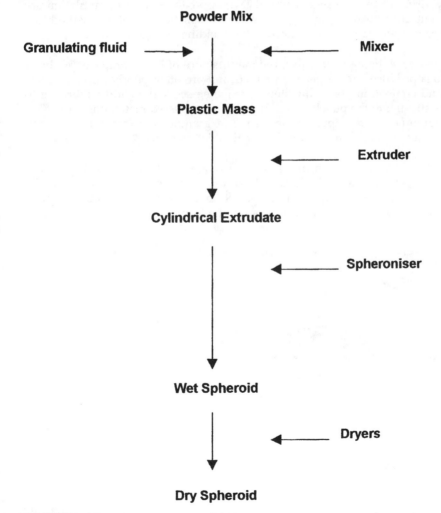

Figure 22 Schematic description of extrusion/spheronization.

The basic ingredients of most spheroids are the drug substance, microcrystalline cellulose, and water. Microcrystalline cellulose appears to be unique in its ability to form spheroids by this method due perhaps to its ability to hold onto the water during extrusion. The squeezing of the wet mass through a screen during extrusion forces most materials to lose water, and the resulting extrudates do not have the necessary plasticity to form spheroids.

The robustness of microcrystalline cellulose means that for most low-dose drugs, it is possible to make spheroids, certainly if the drug loading is below 10%. As the drug loading increases, the process becomes more difficult. Two factors appear to be required for success, the mass must retain the water during the extrusion process, and the extrudate must have the appropriate rheological properties.

There are many types of extruders available, with very different shear forces. The different shear forces will have an effect on the water distribution in the extrudates. As the water level is critical for optimizing the spheronization process, it is clear that the formulation development and process development need to be considered as one for this type of process.

Dry Granulation

It is possible to form granulates without the addition of a granulating fluid, by techniques generically referred to as dry granulation. These methods are useful for materials that are sensitive to heat and moisture, but which may not be suitable for direct compression.

Dry granulation involves the aggregation of particles by high pressure to form bonds between particles by virtue of their close proximity. Two approaches to dry granulation are used in the pharmaceutical industry: slugging and roller compaction. In either method, the material can be compacted with a binder to improve the bonding strength.

Slugging. Granulation by slugging is, in effect, the manufacture of large compacts by direct compression. The slugs produced are larger than tablets and are often poorly formed tablets exhibiting cracking and lamination. As with tablets, it may be necessary to add a lubricant to prevent the compacts sticking to the punches and dies. The compressed material is broken up and sieved to form granules of the appropriate size. The granules are then blended with disintegrant and lubricant, and compressed on a normal tablet machine.

Roller compaction. In roller compaction, the powder is compacted by means of pressure rollers (Fig. 23). It is fed between two cylindrical rollers, rotating in opposite directions. The rollers may be flat, which will produce sheets of compacted material, or they may be dimpled, in which case, briquettes in the shape of the dimples will be formed. If sheets are produced,

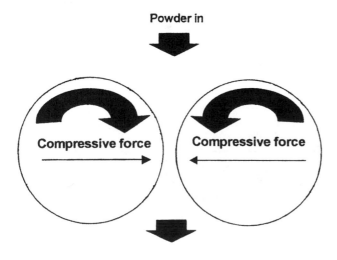

Powder in

Compressive force   **Compressive force**

Granulate out   **Figure 23**   Principles of roller compaction.

they are milled and screened to the required size. Roller compaction requires less lubricant to be added than does slugging.

Selection of the Appropriate Process
The methods of formulating and manufacturing tablets have been described in the preceding sections. Each method has certain unique benefits and advantages as well as drawbacks, and these are summarized in Table 14.

For any given compound, there will normally be more than one approach that is technically feasible, so how does one choose which approach to take? For most formulators, the choice is strongly influenced by the philosophy of the production department of the company in which they work. Different companies can have very different philosophies; some believe that the cost savings of direct compression are such that attempts should be made to formulate all tablets by this route, other companies feel that wet granulation is a more robust process, and should be used even when a compound looks amenable to the direct compression route.

Tablet Coating
For some tablets, compression marks the final stage of the production process, but many formulations involve coating the compressed tablet. There are several reasons for applying a coat:

- Protecting the drug from the environment (moisture, air, light) for stability reasons
- Taste masking
- Minimizing patient/operator contact with drug substance, particularly for skin sensitizers
- Improving product identity and appearance
- Improving ease of swallowing
- Improving mechanical resistance; reducing abrasion and attrition during handling
- Modifying release properties

There are three main methods used to coat pharmaceutical tablets: sugar coating, film coating, and compression coating. Sugar coating was the most commonly used method until the 1970s, when it was largely superseded by film coating.

Sugar Coating
Sugar coating, as its name suggests, involves coating tablets with sucrose. This is a highly skilled, multistep process that is very labor intensive. The process involves applying a number of aqueous solutions of sucrose, together with additional components, which gradually build

Table 14 Manufacturing and Formulating Tablets—Advantages and Disadvantages

Method	Advantages	Disadvantages
Direct compression	Simple, cheap process. No heat or moisture, so good for unstable compounds. Prime particle dissolution.	Not suitable for all drugs, generally limited to low-dose compounds. Segregation potential. Expensive excipients.
Wet granulation (aqueous)	Robust process suitable for most compounds. Imparts flowability to a formulation. Can reduce elasticity problems. Coating surface with hydrophilic polymer can improve wettability. Binds drug with excipient, thus reducing segregation potential.	Expensive: time- and energy-consuming process. Specialized equipment required. Stability issues for moisture-sensitive and thermolabile drugs with aqueous granulation.
Wet granulation (nonaqueous)	Suitable for moisture-sensitive drugs. Vacuum-drying techniques can remove/reduce need for heat.	Expensive equipment; explosion proof; solvent recovery.
Dry granulation (slugging)	Eliminates exposure to moisture and drying.	Dusty procedure. Not suitable for all compounds. Slow process.
Dry granulation (roller compaction)	Eliminates exposure to moisture and drying.	Slow process.

up into a smooth, aesthetically pleasing coat. The final coat can account for up to 50% of the final tablet weight, and will result in a significant increase in the tablet size. Traditionally, sugar coating has been performed in coating pans in which the tablets are tumbled. With the appropriate tablet load and rotation speed, the tablets are tumbled in a three-dimensional direction. The pan is supplied with a source of warm air for drying and an extraction system to remove moist air and dust.

The coating solution is ladled onto the tablet bed and is distributed around the tablets by their tumbling action. The tablets are then tumbled for a period of time to allow the coating to dry before a further quantity of solution is added. A dusting powder may be sprinkled onto the surface of the tablets during the drying phase to prevent the tablets sticking together. One of the skills of sugar coating is adding an appropriate quantity of solution. If too little is added, then not all tablets will pick up some of the coating, and an uneven distribution will result. If too much solution is added, the tablets will stick together. The cycle of wetting and drying is continued until the desired amount of coating has been applied to the tablets. Typically, a sugar coating will consist of three types of coat: a sealing coat, a subcoat, and a smoothing coat (Fig. 24).

One of the reasons for coating tablets is to protect the drug substance from environmental factors such as moisture, so it is important that the coating solution does not penetrate into the core. This is achieved by applying a sealing coat. Traditionally, a coating of shellac dissolved in ethanol was applied, but this has largely been replaced by the use of synthetic water-resistant polymers such as cellulose acetate phthalate or polyvinylacetate phthalate. The challenge for the formulator is to optimize the quantity of subcoat applied to ensure the core is protected while minimizing the effect on drug release.

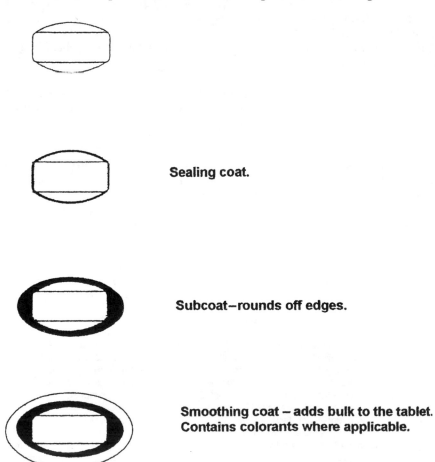

Sealing coat.

Subcoat–rounds off edges.

Smoothing coat – adds bulk to the tablet.
Contains colorants where applicable.

Figure 24   Stages of sugar coating.

The subcoat is an adhesive coat on which the smoothing coat can be built. A second purpose of the subcoat is to round off the sharp corners of the tablet to produce a smooth surface. The subcoat is a mixture of a sucrose solution and an adhesive gum, such as acacia or gelatin, which rapidly distributes over the tablet surface. A dusting follows each application of solution with a subcoat powder containing materials such as calcium carbonate, calcium sulfate, acacia, talc, and kaolin that help to produce a hard coat. The application of the subcoat continues until the tablets have a rounded appearance and the edges are well covered.

The smoothing coat consists of the majority of the tablet bulk, and provides the tablet with a smooth finish. The coat consists of sucrose syrup, which may contain starch or calcium carbonate. Each application is dried, and layers are added until the required bulk has been achieved. The last few coatings will consist of sucrose solution and colorants, where required. The colorants may be either soluble dyes or lakes, lakes often being preferred because a uniform color is easier to achieve with them.

The coated tablets are usually transferred to a polishing pan and coated with beeswax–carnauba wax mixture to provide a glossy finish to the surface.

Film Coating

Film coating involves the application of a polymer film to the surface of the tablet and, in contrast to sugar coating, only adds up to 5% weight to the final tablet, with a negligible increase in tablet size. It is a technique, which, while used mainly to coat tablets, can also be applied to hard gelatin capsules, soft gelatin capsules, and multiparticulate systems such as spheroids.

The method of application of the coat differs from sugar coating in that the coating suspension is sprayed directly onto the surface of the tablets, and drying occurs as soon as the coat hits the tablet surface. To achieve this, the tablet only receives a small quantity of coat at a time, and the coat is built up in an intermittent manner. While the coating can be applied using a number of methods, all share the following properties: a method of atomizing the coating suspension, the ability to heat large volumes of air (which heat the tablets and facilitate the rapid drying of the applied coat), and a method of moving the tablets that ensures all tablets are evenly sprayed. The main methods of coating are modified conventional coating pans, side-vented pans, and fluid bed coating.

When the technique of film coating was first applied to tablets, the coatings were suspended in organic solvents, and conventional coating pans were used. Additional air handling was required to provide the volume of air necessary to dry the tablets and to extract the vapors from drying. The nature of the pans was such that the drying air was only present on the surface of the tablet bed; there was no mechanism for it to percolate through it. Providing the volume of air required for such drying was difficult, and a number of modifications have been made to the pans. The limitation in drying efficiency, however, remains a constraint, particularly as most coating now uses aqueous suspensions, which impose even greater energy demands. A further limitation to the use of conventional coating pans is their poor mixing efficiency that results in dead spots in the tablet bed.

The side-vented pan, which is now the most commonly used equipment for film coating, was designed to maximize the interaction between the tablet bed and the drying air. In such apparatus, the coating pan is made of perforated metal. The drying air is introduced into the center of the pan but exhausted through the perforations in the pan beneath the tablet bed (Fig. 25). Mixing efficiency is achieved by the use of appropriately designed baffles on the pan surface.

Fluid bed coating offers an alternative to pan coating, and is particularly popular for coating multiparticulate systems. In fluid bed systems, the objects being coated are suspended in an upward stream of air, maximizing the surface available for coating. The coating is applied by an atomizer, and this is dried by the fluidizing air. There are three methods by which the coating can be applied (Fig. 26):

1. Top spraying involves the spray being applied from the top of the fluid bedchamber into the fluidizing air using equipment similar to that used for spray granulation.
2. Bottom spraying, sometimes referred to as the Wurster process, involves the spraying of the tablets at the bottom of the fluid bed. In this setup, there is a column

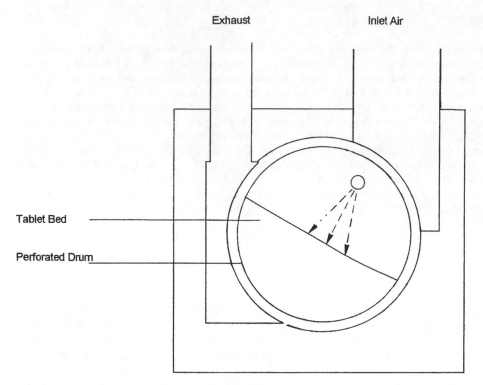

Figure 25 Schematic of the side-vented coating pan.

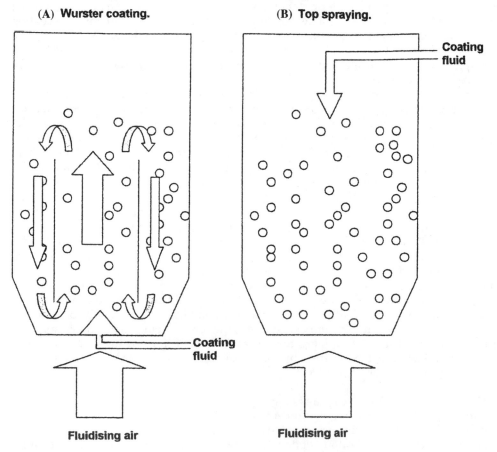

Figure 26 Fluid bed coating of tablets.

introduced into the fluid bedchamber, which ensures that tablets in the center of the chamber are directed upward. At the top of the column, the tablets descend the chamber at the edge of the chamber from where they will be redirected to the spraying region.
3. Tangential coating which is restricted to the coating of spheroids.

A polymer for film coating will ideally meet the following criteria:

- Solubility in the solvent selected for application. These days, the solvent will usually be water, although certain types of film coat may require organic solvents to be used. Commonly used solvents include alcohols (methanol, ethanol, and isopropanol), esters (ethyl acetate and ethyl lactate), ketones (acetone), and chlorinated hydrocarbons (dichloromethane and trichloroethane). The polymer should not only be soluble in the chosen solvent but should adopt a conformation in solution that yields the maximum polymer extension, which will result in films with the greatest cohesion strength. If mixed solvents are used, consideration should be given to the effect of the solvent ratios changing during the drying process. If the polymer is most soluble in the component with maximum volatility, it may precipitate out during the spraying before reaching the tablet surface.
- Solubility in GI fluids. Unless the coating is being applied for enteric coating or taste masking purposes, it should ideally be soluble across the range of pH values encountered in the GI tract.
- Capacity to produce an elegant film even in the presence of additives such as pigments and opacifiers
- Compatibility with film-coating additives and the tablet being coated
- Stability in the environment under normal storage conditions
- Free from undesirable taste or odor
- Lack of toxicity

Table 15 lists the most commonly used polymers. With the exception of HPMC, the polymers are rarely used alone, but are combined with other polymers to optimize the film-forming properties.

The actual film-coating process is described schematically in Figure 27. There are two important stages: droplet formation and film formation. The film formation is itself a multistage process involving the wetting of the tablet surface followed by spreading of the

Table 15 Commonly Used Polymers

Polymer	Comments
MC	Soluble in cold water, GI fluids, and a range of organic solvents.
EC	Soluble in organic solvents, insoluble in water and GI fluids. Used alone in modified-release formulations and in combination with water-soluble celluloses for immediate-release formulations.
HEC	Soluble in water and GI fluids.
MHEC	Soluble in water and GI fluids. Has similar film-forming properties to HPMC, but is less soluble in organic solvents, which limited its popularity when solvent coating was the norm.
HPC	Soluble in cold water, GI fluids, and polar solvents. Becomes tacky when dried, so is unsuitable for use alone, often used in combination with other polymers to optimize adhesion of coat.
HPMC	Soluble in cold water, GI fluids, alcohols, and halogenated hydrocarbons. Excellent film former, and the most widely used polymer. Can be used with lactose to improve adhesiveness.
NaCMC	Soluble in water and polar solvents.

Abbreviations: MC, methylcellulose; EC, ethylcellulose; HEC, hydroxyethylcellulose; MHEC, methyl hydroxyethylcellulose; HPC, hydroxypropyl cellulose; HPMC, hydroxypropyl methylcellulose; NaCMC, sodium carboxymethylcellulose; GI, gastrointestinal.

Droplets of the coating suspension wet the surface of the tablet.

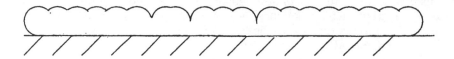

The droplets spread, forming a continuous film over the surface.

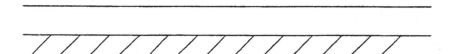

Eventually the droplets completely coalesce to form a smooth film.

Figure 27   Mechanism of film formation on the tablet surface.

film, and eventually coalescence of the individual film particles into a continuous film. For such coalescence to be able to occur, it is necessary for the polymer to be in a plasticized state, that is, above its glass transition temperature, the point at which a polymer goes from being a rigid, brittle material to a flexible material. Most film-forming polymers have glass transition temperatures in excess of the temperatures reached during the coating process (typically 40–50°C), so it is necessary to add plasticizers to the formulations, which act by reducing the glass transition temperature. The choice of plasticizer is dependent on the particular polymer (s) being used. The main factors to consider in selection are permanence and compatibility. Permanence is the duration of the plasticizer effect; the plasticizer should remain within the polymer film to retain its effect, so it should have a low vapor pressure and diffusion rate. Compatibility requires the plasticizer to be miscible with the polymer. Commonly used plasticizers include phthalate esters, citrate esters, triacetin, propylene glycol, polyethylene glycols, and glycerol.

Film coating provides an opportunity to color tablets, and most film coats will contain pigments or opacifiers. Insoluble pigments are normally preferred to soluble dyes for a number of reasons. Solid pigments produce a more opaque coat than dyes, protecting the tablet from light. The presence of insoluble particles in the suspension allows the rate of solid application to the tablet to be increased without having an adverse effect on the viscosity of the coating suspension, improving productivity. The pigments also tend to exhibit better color stability than dyes.

Film coating of tablets requires both the process and the formulation to be optimized if a uniform and intact coating is to be achieved. The most common flaws, their cause, and possible remedies are described in Table 16.

It has been emphasized to this point that the coat should not delay the release of the drug substance from the tablet. It is possible to design a coat that will modify the release of a drug substance for a beneficial effect.

Table 16 Film-Coating Defects

Flaw	Cause	Remedy
Wrinkling or blistering Film detaches from tablet surface, causing blister that can burst to form wrinkles.	Gases forming on tablet surface during coating; exacerbated by poor adhesion of film to tablet surface.	Reduce drying air temperature.
Picking Areas of tablet surface are not covered by film coat.	Overwet tablets stick together and pull film off surface as they move apart.	Decrease spraying rate. Increase drying temperature.
Pitting Holes appear on tablet surface.	Melting of lubricant on tablet surface. Most common with stearic acid.	Decrease coating temperature to below melting point of lubricant. Substitute lubricant.
Blooming Dulling of surface, normally after prolonged storage.	Migration of low-molecular-weight components of film to tablet surface.	Decrease temperature and length of drying process. Increase molecular weight of plasticizer.
Mottling Uneven color distribution in film.	Inadequate pigment dispersion. Color migration, a problem with dyes and lakes rather than pigments.	Alter suspension preparation to ensure pigment aggregates are dispersed. Replace dyes with pigments.
Orange peel Film surface has a rough finish resembling orange peel.	Film-coat droplets are too dry or too viscous to spread on tablet surface.	Reduce solids content of coating suspension. Reduce drying temperature. Reduce viscosity of polymer.
Bridging Film forms a bridge over intagliations, leaving them indistinct.	High internal stresses in film relieved by pulling the film off the Surface of the intagliation.	Increase adhesion of coat to tablet by changing core formulation. Add plasticizer or increase plasticizer concentration. Alter geometry of intagliations.
Cracking, splitting, peeling The film cracks on the crown of the surface or splits on the tablet edge. Can be differentiated from picking by presence of loose film around the flaw.	High stresses in the film that cannot be relieved due to the strong Adhesion of the film to the tablet surface.	Increase plasticizer concentration. Use stronger polymer.

The most common type of modified-release coating is the enteric coat, which is designed to prevent release of the drug substance in the stomach because the drug is either irritant to the gastric mucosa or it is unstable in gastric juice. The most common method of achieving an enteric coating is to apply a polymer that contains acidic substitutions, thus giving it a pH-dependent solubility profile. Examples of such polymers are listed in Table 17.

Film coating can also be used to delay the release of drugs. This is normally applied to multiparticulate systems where particles will be coated with differing thicknesses of water-insoluble polymers such as ethylcellulose.

Compression Coating

The third type of tablet coating used in pharmaceuticals is compression coating. This technique involves producing a relatively soft tablet core containing the drug substance and compressing

Table 17   Commonly Used Enteric-Coating Polymers

Polymer	Solubility profile	Comments
Shellac	Above pH 7	The original enteric-coating material, originally used in sugar-coated tablets. The high pH required for dissolution may delay drug release. Natural product that exhibits batch-to-batch variability.
CAP	Above pH 6	The high pH required for dissolution is a disadvantage. Forms brittle films, so must be combined with other polymers.
PVAP	Above pH 5	
HPMCP	Above pH 4.5	Optimal dissolution profile for enteric coating.
Polymers of methacrylic acid and its esters	Various grades available with dissolution occurring above pH 6	

Abbreviations: CAP, cellulose acetate phthalate; PVAP, polyvinylacetate phthalate; HPMCP, hydroxypropyl methylcellulose phthalate.

a coating around it (Fig. 28). This is achieved by placing the core in a large die that already contains some of the coating formulation. Further coating material is then added to the die and the contents compressed. The three types of coating have now been described, and the relative merits of each approach are summarized in Table 18.

HARD GELATIN CAPSULES

After tablets, hard gelatin capsules are the most common solid dosage form. Hard gelatin capsules are rigid two-piece capsules made from gelatin, water, and colorants. The capsules are produced as empty shells consisting of a cap and body, which during the manufacture of the finished product are separated, filled with the formulation, and then rejoined.

Hard gelatin capsules are generally considered to be more forgiving than tablets, from a formulator's perspective. While many of the challenges facing the formulator of tablets are still present, the need for a free-flowing material, powder homogeneity, lubricity, and optimizing the biopharmaceutical properties, the challenges of forming a robust compact have been removed. Capsules have traditionally been filled with solid formulations such as powder mixes and granulations, but increasingly, multiparticulate formulations, liquid, and semisolid fills are being developed.

Hard gelatin capsules have some disadvantages compared with tablets. The filling speeds of capsule machines are lower than the speeds of the fastest tablet presses, and the cost of the capsule shells makes them a more expensive dosage form. Certain materials are unsuitable for inclusion in capsule shells due to incompatibility with gelatin, or because of their affinity for water. One advantage sometimes claimed for capsules is ease of swallowing due to their elongated shape, but this may be countered by the fact that capsules are often larger than corresponding tablets due to the reduced compression of the powder and incomplete filling of the shells. Furthermore, there are concerns that capsules are more prone to sticking in the esophagus than tablets following swallowing.

The manufacture and formulation of hard gelatin capsules has not been the subject of as much research as tabletting, partly because encapsulation, unlike compression, is not a science shared by many other disciplines. Nevertheless, there has been important work performed on this dosage form, and much of it is captured in *Hard Capsules Development and Technology* (Ridgway, 1987).

Manufacture of Empty Capsule Shells

Gelatin is a heterogeneous product prepared by the hydrolysis of collagen, the principal constituent of connective tissue. The suitability of gelatin for capsule manufacture is due to the following properties:

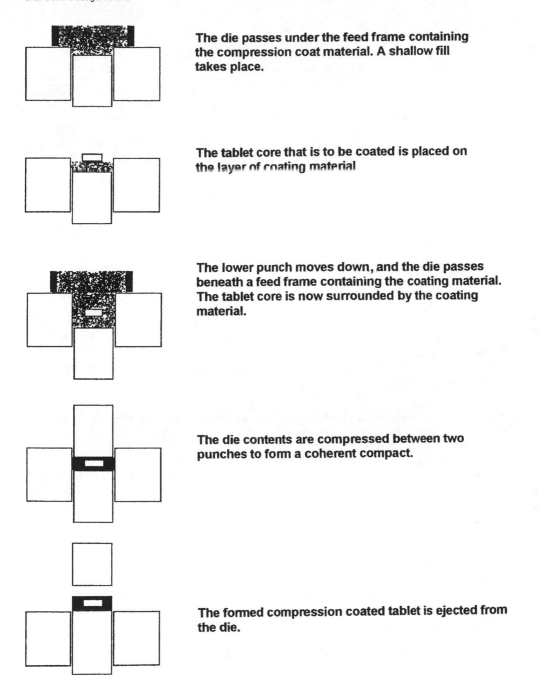

The die passes under the feed frame containing the compression coat material. A shallow fill takes place.

The tablet core that is to be coated is placed on the layer of coating material.

The lower punch moves down, and the die passes beneath a feed frame containing the coating material. The tablet core is now surrounded by the coating material.

The die contents are compressed between two punches to form a coherent compact.

The formed compression coated tablet is ejected from the die.

Figure 28　Schematic of the compression coating process.

- It is commonly used in foods and has global regulatory acceptability. However, because it can be derived from a number of animal sources, not all the gelatin is acceptable in all markets, and capsule manufacturers will produce capsules from different animal sources to allow for local religious restrictions. All pharmaceutical capsule manufacturers now use gelatin produced in accordance with current requirements relating to bovine spongiform encephalopathy.
- It is a good film former, producing a strong flexible film.

Table 18 Coating Methods

Coating method	Advantages	Disadvantages
Sugar coating	Elegant final product. Tablets can be printed for identification purposes. Cheap, readily available starting materials. Simple equipment requirements. Excellent protection from environment.	Long process time. Traditional manufacture more an art than a science; high operator dependency. Significantly increases tablet size.
Film coating	Quick process, easy to automate. Negligible increase in tablet size. Tablets can be identified either by printing or through intagliations. Minimal effect on drug release. Enteric coating feasible.	Finish not as elegant as sugar coating. Coating process stresses tablet formulation, cores must be robust to resist abrasion and edge chipping during coating.
Compression coating	It is a dry process; so suitable for moisture-sensitive compounds. Can be used for combination products where the active substances are incompatible.	Significant increase in tablet weight. Possible to produce tablets with no inner core.

- It is readily soluble in water and in GI fluids at body temperature, so will not retard the release of drugs.
- It changes state at low temperatures, enabling a homogeneous film to be formed at ambient temperature.

The properties of a given batch of gelatin are determined by a number of factors: the source of the parent collagen, method of extraction, the pH of the hydrolytic process, and its electrolyte content. The properties of most interest to capsule manufacturers are the bloom strength and the viscosity.

The bloom strength is a standard, but arbitrary, test of the rigidity of gel produced by a sample of gelatin. The test measures the force required to depress the surface of a 6.67% w/w gel, matured at 10°C for 16 to 18 hours, by a distance of 4 mm using a flat-bottomed plunger 12.7 mm in diameter. The force is applied in the form of a stream of lead shot, and the weight, in grams, is termed the bloom strength. Bloom strengths in the region of 230 to 275 are used for the manufacture of hard gelatin capsule shells. The standard viscosity is measured using a U-tube viscometer with a 6.67% w/w solution, and values in the range of 3.3 to 4.7 mPa sec being used for capsule shells.

Capsule shells are manufactured by dipping moulds into a gelatin solution, drying the gelatin to form a film, removing the dried film from the mould, and trimming the film to the right size. The moulds are made of stainless steel and are referred to as pins. The cap and body of the capsule shells are made on separate pins, with the body pins being longer than the cap. The external diameter of the body at its open end is slightly larger than the internal diameter of the cap at its closed end to ensure a snug fit when closed.

The empty capsule shells contain 13% to 15% water, a level that is important for optimum performance on capsule-filling machines. If the level falls below 13%, the capsules become brittle, while if they take up too much water, the gelatin becomes soft, and there are problems with capsule separation. The dimensions of the capsule shell will also change with variations in water content, typically increasing by 0.5% for every 1% increase in moisture content. It is important that capsule shells are both stored and filled in areas where the RH is controlled between 30% and 50%.

It is also important that the capsule fill not adversely affect the moisture content of the shell. This is not a suitable dosage form either for deliquescent materials, which will dry the capsules, making them brittle, causing cracking or splitting, or for efflorescent materials, which will soften the shells and may lead to capsules sticking together. Similarly, the presence of

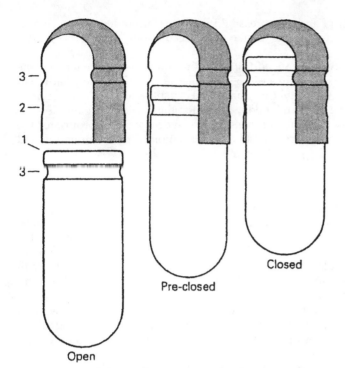

Figure 29 Locking mechanism of a hard gelatin capsule shell.

1. The tapered rim prevents faulty joins.
2. These indentations prevent the pre-closed capsules from opening too early.
3. These grooves lock the two halves together after filling.

moisture in the capsule shells makes them an unsuitable delivery form for drugs that are highly moisture sensitive.

Any fill materials must be chemically compatible with gelatin. Cross-linking of gelatin can be catalyzed by trace quantities of formaldehyde, rendering the gelatin insoluble in gastric fluids. Formaldehyde is sometimes present at trace levels in a number of excipients.

Capsules manufactured for use on automatic filling machines, which covers almost all pharmaceutical capsules, have locking devices molded into the side of the capsule (Fig. 29). There are two locking positions, a pre-lock to prevent premature opening prior to the filling process and a locked position, which forms an interference seal to prevent the capsule coming apart after filling.

There are a number of companies manufacturing capsule shells for use in the pharmaceutical industry, and all produce capsules to standard sizes, which enable them to be filled on standard filling machines. There are eight sizes of capsules commercially available, which are listed in Table 19. The largest capsule size normally considered for oral administration is size 0, with the 00 and 000 capsules being difficult to swallow due to their size.

Capsule Filling

Before considering how to formulate products for filling into hard gelatin capsules, it is necessary to understand the capsule-filling mechanisms available. All capsule-filling machines perform three basic operations: the orientation and separation of the empty capsule shell, the filling of the material into the shell, and finally rejoining the cap and the body. From the formulator's perspective, the important stage is the filling, as this will determine the properties required of the formulation. The requirements imposed by the filling mechanism will include

Table 19 Capsule Sizes

Capsule size	000	00	0	1	2	3	4	5
Fill volume (mL)	1.37	0.95	0.68	0.50	0.37	0.30	0.21	0.13

factors such as powder flow, lubricity, and compressibility, and as discussed in the section "Tablets," the optimization of these factors needs to take into consideration the effects on drug release from the formulation.

Drug release from capsules involves an additional step compared with tablets, the dissolution of the capsule shell. When placed in a dissolution medium at 37°C, the gelatin will begin to dissolve, initially retaining its integrity. Eventually, the capsule shell will rupture at its thinnest points, the shoulders of the cap and body, allowing the dissolution medium to penetrate into the capsule contents. The rate of penetration and, where appropriate, the disintegration of the capsule fill will be determined by a combination of the formulation and the processing method, including the filling mechanism.

Powder and Granulate Filling

The requirements of capsule formulations are very similar to those of tablets, and the general formulation principles described earlier apply equally to capsules. As with tablets, most capsules will contain a combination of ingredients including some or all of the following: the active drug substance, filler(s), disintegrant, binder, glidant, and lubricant. The main difference in the requirements is the demands placed on the compressibility of the formulation. With tablets, it is necessary to produce a compact capable of withstanding the rigors of subsequent handling. For capsules, it is often necessary to form a plug for ejection into the capsule body, but it is not necessary for the plug to retain its integrity beyond the filling stage. While good flow is necessary for the successful manufacture of both tablets and capsules, the filling mechanisms on certain capsule-production machines tend to be more forgiving than those on tablet-production machines.

Powder fills for capsules can be either simple blends of starting materials, analogous to direct compression formulations, or granulations. The reduced demands on compressibility and flow increase the options for powder mixes, making capsules a potential dosage form for active substances that do not possess the compression properties required for direct compression tablets, and are not amenable to granulation.

Powders account for the majority of capsule fills, and a number of quite disparate filling mechanisms have been developed unlike tabletting, where the principle of manufacture, compression between two punches in a die, is the same for all machines. The mechanisms can be divided into two broad groups, those that rely on the volume of the capsule shell to control the dose, known as capsule dependent, and those methods where the quantity of powder to be filled is measured away from the capsule, known as capsule independent. The dependent mechanisms require the capsule shell to be well filled to achieve weight uniformity and are less flexible than the independent methods.

Dependent Methods

The simplest method of dependent capsule filling is leveling, in which the capsule bodies are held flush with a dosing table, and powder is filled into the bodies by gravity. The powder within the capsule bodies may be consolidated by vibration or tamping, and additional powder added to fill the space generated. The final fill weight will depend on the bulk density of the powder and the degree of tamping applied. This method is popular in hand-filling devices such as the Tevopharm, Feton, Bonaface, and Zuma, which are amenable to most powder mixes. Poor flowing powders will take longer to fill, but with skilled operators, should be feasible. The major formulation challenge is to prepare a blend that will provide an appropriate fill for a standard-sized capsule.

Osaka Automatic Machine Co. produces a fluidization machine, which is an automatic dependent filling machine. The capsule body in its holder passes below the powder hopper. The powder is fluidized by a vibrating plate to aid flow into the capsule body. The capsule body can be held below the hopper base so that it becomes overfilled, and the fill can be compressed into the capsule by raising the body against a flat surface prior to the capsule closing. This technique has not been the subject of published formulation studies, but appropriate flow properties and lubrication are likely to be required.

Independent Methods

Auger or screw method. This was the first mechanism used in industrial-scale machines, although the dosator and piston-tamp mechanisms have now largely superseded it. The capsule body in its holder passes beneath the powder hopper on a turntable. The powder is fed into the capsule body by a revolving Archimedean screw. The auger rotates at a constant rate so the fill weight is related to the duration of filling that is related to the speed of rotation of the turntable.

Fomulation studies on auger machines have tended to concentrate on the optimization of fill weight uniformity. Reier et al. (1968) demonstrated that the variation in the capsule fill weight was influenced by the machine speed, capsule size, powder density, powder flow, and the presence of a glidant. Ito et al. (1969) determined that there was an optimum level of glidant for minimum weight variation. Powders still account for the majority of capsule fills, and a number of quite disparate filling mechanisms have been developed. Powders should be adequately lubricated to prevent build up of densified material on the auger.

Piston-tamp method. In piston-tamp machines, the powder passes over a dosing plate containing cavities slightly smaller than the internal diameter of the capsule. The powder falls into the holes by gravity, and is then tamped by a pin to form a soft plug. This procedure is repeated several times until the cavity is full. Excess powder is removed from above the cavity by a deflector plate. The cavity is then positioned over the capsule body and the plug ejected (Fig. 30). The dose is controlled by the thickness of the dosing plate, the degree of tamping applied, and the height of the powder bed above the dosing plate.

The uniformity of fill weight for the piston-tamp machines has been shown to correlate well with the angle of repose of the powders (Kurihara and Ichikawa, 1978) and the angle of internal flow (Podczech et al., 1999). Lubrication of formulations is important to prevent build up of material on the tamping pins, and to ensure smooth ejection of the plugs from the dosing plate. The ability of the material to compress into a plug is important; if a formulation does not form a plug, the ejection will not be as clean, and can lead to increased weight variation. Studies have shown that for certain formulations, the tamping pressure applied by the pins can affect the dissolution rate of the final product (Shah et al., 1983). The minimum tamping force necessary to obtain a plug that will fit inside the body of the capsule shell should be aimed for.

Dosator method. A dosator, consisting of a stainless steel cylinder containing a spring-loaded stainless steel piston, is lowered, open end first, into a flat powder bed. As the cylinder

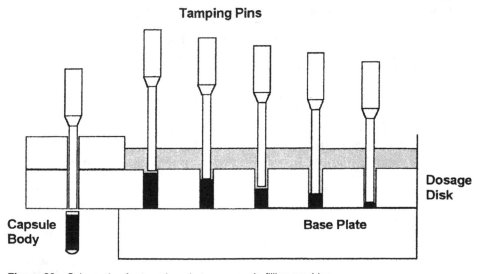

Figure 30   Schematic of a tamping pin-type capsule-filling machine.

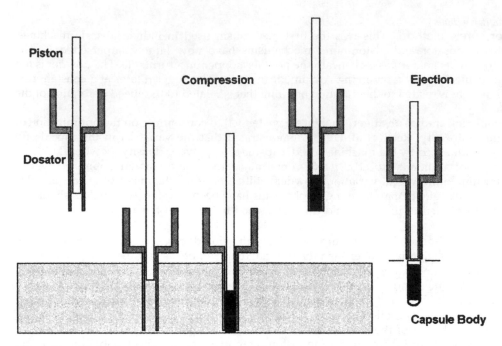

Figure 31 Schematic of a dosator-type capsule-filling machine.

passes into the bed, powder is forced up into the cylinder until it reaches the piston, forming a plug. Additional compression of the plug can be obtained by applying a downward pressure on the piston. The dosator is lifted from the powder bed and, if a suitable plug has formed, the powder will remain within. The dosator is positioned above a capsule body, and the plug ejected by lowering the piston. The dose is controlled by the dimensions of the dosator, the position of the piston within the dosator as it enters the powder bed, and the height of the powder bed (Fig. 31).

This mechanism is the most widely used one, and can be found on small pilot scale machines using an intermittent action similar to rotary machines, capable of production rates in excess of 120,000 capsules per hour. As a result of its popularity, there have been considerable studies into the formulation of powder for filling on these types of machines, and instrumentation of the dosators.

The fundamental requirements of a formulation to be filled on a dosator-type machine are good flow properties, compressibility, and lubricity. *Flow* is important in the powder bed: when the dosator dips into the powder, it leaves a void, which must be closed with material of the same bulk density prior to the next dosator entering that area of the hopper. Irwin et al. (1970) investigated the effect of powder flow on the uniformity of weight achieved on a Zanasi filling machine, and concluded that the better the rate of flow, the better the uniformity of fill.

Compressibility is necessary to form a plug of sufficient strength so that powder does not escape from the dosator as it leaves the powder hopper and position itself above the capsule body. Jolliffe and Newton (1982a,b) considered the theoretical aspects of powder retention using powder hopper design theory to calculate the forces required to hold a free powder surface in an open-end cylinder. The powder retention relies on the formation of a stable powder arch, which is dependent on the shear developed at the dosator walls and the unconfined yield strength. It was demonstrated that the angle of wall friction between the powder and dosator could have an important influence on powder retention. This was explored experimentally (Jolliffe and Newton, 1982a,b) by showing that the internal friction changed during manufacture as the powder fill coated the internal wall of the dosator. Furthermore, these authors proposed that the optimum design for a dosator would have two types of surface finish, a smooth finish with a low value of wall friction for the main body of the cylinder together with a higher value of wall friction at the outlet to promote arch formation. The dosator mechanism does permit high compressive forces to be applied to powder beds. The objective of a capsule formulation is not to make a mini tablet that can be filled into a capsule; the compression force should be restricted to the minimum level necessary to form a coherent plug. Whenever powders are compressed, there is the possibility of elastic recovery when the compressive stress is removed. The tolerance between the internal diameter of the dosators and the internal diameter of capsule shells is fairly tight, and any elasticity in capsule formulations can lead to the plugs not sitting properly in the capsule shells, resulting in powder loss as the cap is reunited with the body. In such circumstances, the pragmatic approach is to use dosators designed for the next smallest capsule size.

The *lubricity requirements* of formulations being filled with dosators has been examined by Small and Augsburger (1978) using a Zanasi machine on which strain gauges had been attached to the dosator pistons. The magnitude of the force required to eject the powder plug from the piston was shown to be dependent on the identity and level of lubricant, the height of the initial powder bed, the piston height, and the compression force applied.

Filling Capsules with Pellets

The use of multiparticulate systems to provide modified-release formulations is ever increasing, and hard gelatin capsules provide an ideal way of delivering unit doses of such formulations. The two most common approaches to pellet formulation are extrusion/ spheronization (discussed in an earlier section) and the coating of nonpareil seeds. Nonpareil seeds are sucrose beads, which can be film coated with a solution/suspension of the drug substance followed by layers of modified-release coatings to obtain the release profile required. The capsule-filling method has to be gentle enough on the pellets to retain the integrity of the coating.

As with powder filling, the filling of pellets into capsules can be dependent or independent. A dependent method often performed uses a modified augur-type machine, in which the pellets are simply poured by gravity into the capsule shells. The critical formulation aspect of this approach is ensuring that the required dosage of active substance is present in the volume of pellets taken to fill the capsule body.

An independent method uses a volumetric fill by a modified dosator method. The piston inside the dosator is narrower than that used for powder filling, and this allows air to flow between the piston and the dosator wall. The dosator is lowered into the pellet bed, but in this case, there is no compression applied. A vacuum source is applied from above the piston to retain the pellets as the dosator is moved above the capsule body. Once over the capsule body, the vacuum is removed and the ejection of the pellets is aided by an air jet.

Tablets

Capsules can also be filled with tablets, which can be of use when preparing blinded clinical trial materials. Tablets are fed from a hopper into a chamber that simply releases one or more tablets into the capsule body as it passes underneath. The optimum formulation for capsule filling is a biconvex film-coated tablet, the film coating reducing abrasion and material loss.

Capsugel produces a range of specially sized opaque capsules specifically for the encapsulation of tablets for double-blind clinical trial supplies. The capsules are wider than standard-sized capsules to allow larger diameter tablets to be filled but have shorter bodies to retain patient acceptability/tolerability.

Liquids and Semisolids

Two types of liquid formulations can be filled into hard gelatin capsules, those that are liquid at room temperature and those that are solid at room temperature. Such solid formulations can be liquefied either by heating to temperatures up to 70°C (the maximum temperature the gelatin shell can withstand) or by the application of shear stress. In the case of liquids that are mobile at room temperature, the capsules need to be sealed after filling to prevent leakage of the contents.

The filling of such formulations requires machines fitted with hoppers that can provide a heating and stirring system. For most formulations, the capsules are filled using a volumetric pump, although certain viscous preparations may require an extrusion pump. The pump must be designed to be non-drip, and the capsule handling needs to be modified to control product spillage. A sensing system is required to detect the presence or absence of caps or bodies so that the pump can be stopped and the bushes not contaminated with fill material. With powder fills, contamination of the exterior of capsules can be removed by vacuum dedusting. With liquids, if one capsule is covered with liquid, it can lead to major problems with capsules sticking together.

There are a number of applications for liquid/semisolid filled capsules:

- Improvement of bioavailabilty
- Safety—minimizing operator exposure to dusty processes
- Content uniformity—it is easier to achieve and maintain content uniformity in a solution system than a powder system
- Stability

These advantages are similar to those of soft gelatin capsules, and are dealt with in greater depth in a following section.

With soft gelatin capsule technology being so well established, what advantages does liquid filling of hard gelatin capsules provide the formulator? The major advantage is that it is a technology that can be installed in-house relatively simply, unlike soft gelatin capsule manufacture, which remains in the hands of a limited number of contract suppliers. This has been made possible by the development of techniques for sealing the capsules.

The approach taken to formulate a liquid-filled capsule will depend on the reason for selecting such a dosage form. The most important aspect of the formulation is to ensure that the fill is compatible with the gelatin shell. It is well known that the gelatin shell is sensitive to changes in moisture levels, and hence liquids that readily take up moisture such as the low-molecular-weight polyethylene glycols will be unsuitable. Capsugel, one of the main suppliers of capsule shells, performed extensive compatibility testing of liquid vehicles, and has published a list of those deemed to be compatible (Stegemann, 1999) (Table 20).

Table 20   Liquid Excipients Compatible with Hard Gelatin Capsule Shells

Lipophilic excipients	Hydrophilic excipients	Amphiphilic excipients
Vegetable oils	PEG 3000–6000 MW	Poloxamers
Peanut oil		Lecithin
Castor oil		PEG esters (e.g., Gelucir 44/14;
Olive oil		50/13; Labrafil)
Fractionated coconut oil		
Corn oil		
Sesame oil		
Hydrogenated vegetable oil		
Soybean oil		
Esters		
Glycerol stearate		
Glycol stearate		
Isopropyl myristate		
Ethyl oleate		
Fatty Acids		
Stearic acid		
Laurie acid		
Palmitic acid		
Oleic acid		
Oleic acid		
Fatty Alcohols		
Cetyl alcohol		
Stearyl alcohol		

Abbreviations: PEG, polyethylene glycol; MW, molecular weight.

Capsule Sealing

The filling of liquids into hard gelatin capsules has been thought about for many years, but was not commercially feasible until reliable methods for capsule sealing were available. The incidents involving the tampering of paracetamol capsules in the United States in the mid-1980s forced capsule manufacturers to develop a method of making capsules tamper evident. This, in turn, led to the development of the Quali-Seal capsule-banding machine. This machine applies a narrow band of gelatin around the joint of the cap and body of filled capsules, which can be dried without the application of heat. Heat would cause air expansion within the capsule, disrupting the seal.

A recent development in sealing technology has been liquid encapsulation microspray sealing (LEMS) in which a sealing fluid of approximately 50% water and 50% ethanol is sprayed onto the joint between the cap and body. This fluid penetrates the cap/body joint by capillary action and lowers the melting point of the gelatin; the capsule is then exposed to a short cycle of warm air, which melts and fuses the gelatin at the joint. This technique is an elegant method of sealing, as the seal is not visible to the user.

Alternatives to Gelatin Capsules

There have been a number of attempts to make capsules from materials other than gelatin. Initially, the attempts were aimed at overcoming the original patents filed by Mothe in the 19th century, and used materials such as starch, gluten, and animal membranes. However, the only material with the correct film-forming properties was gelatin.

More recently, the attention has moved to synthetic polymers, with the aim being to produce capsules that will overcome the shortcomings of gelatin, particularly its moisture content. Two alternative materials have been offered by capsule manufacturers, starch and HPMC.

The starch capsules are produced by an injection molding process using potato starch, and are produced in five sizes, all of the same diameter but with different lengths (Vilivalam et al., 2000). While the fill volumes are similar to gelatin capsules, the different dimensions necessitate specialized filling equipment. The capsule surface is less smooth than gelatin capsules, and the injection molding allows a smooth join between cap and body to be obtained. These properties make the capsules amenable to film-coating processes. The moisture content of the capsules is 14%.

HPMC capsules are made by the pin-dipping process used for gelatin capsules, and are made to the same size specifications, allowing them to be filled on conventional capsule-filling equipment. These capsules have a lower moisture content than gelatin capsules, and the moisture is tighter bound, making them more suitable for moisture-sensitive drugs and hygroscopic excipients. The capsule surfaces have rougher finishes than gelatin capsules, and coloring the capsules is more difficult. The rough coat leads to better adhesion with coating materials, so they could have applications for enteric coating.

SOFT GELATIN CAPSULES

Soft gelatin capsules are included in this chapter on oral solid dosage forms, although there is debate as to whether or not they are solid or liquid dosage forms. The drug is presented in a liquid encapsulated in a solid, thus combining advantages of liquid dosage forms with the unit dosage convenience of solid forms.

Manufacture

Unlike hard gelatin capsule shells, which are manufactured empty and subsequently filled in a separate operation, soft gelatin capsules are manufactured and filled in one operation. This is a specialized process, and tends to be performed by a limited number of companies. One consequence, therefore, of selecting a soft gelatin capsule formulation is that the product will probably be manufactured by a contract manufacturer. A desire to keep all manufacturing in-house is one of the reasons for companies considering the use of liquid-filled hard gelatin capsules as an alternative.

The shell ingredients of a soft gelatin capsule are gelatin, glycerol, which acts as a plasticizer, and potentially other ingredients, which could include additional plasticizers such as sorbitol or propylene glycol, dies or pigments, preservatives, and flavors. The glycerol-gelatin mix is dissolved in water, then heated and pumped onto two cooling drums to form two gelatin ribbons, which are fed into the filling machine. The liquid fill is pumped between the gelatin ribbons as they pass between the two die rolls of the filling machine, forcing the gelatin to adopt the shape of the die. The two ribbons are sealed together by heat and pressure, and the capsules are cut from the ribbon (Fig. 32). They then pass through a tumble drier to remove the bulk of the water and are conditioned at 20% RH.

The fill can be either a solution or a suspension, liquid or semisolid. The main limitation is that the fill must be compatible with the shell. The main incompatibilities are high concentrations of water or other solvents, which will dissolve the shell, high pH (>7.5) solutions, which will cause cross-linking of the gelatin, which will retard dissolution of the shell, low pH solutions, which may hydrolyze the gelatin, and aldehydes, which promote cross-linking. The types of vehicles that can be used in soft gelatin capsules are similar to those used for liquid-filled hard gelatin capsule shells listed in Table 20.

Benefits of Soft Gelatin Capsule Formulations

Soft gelatin capsules are a more expensive dosage form than either tablets or capsules, so they tend to be considered when they can offer a major benefit to the formulator. Justifications for

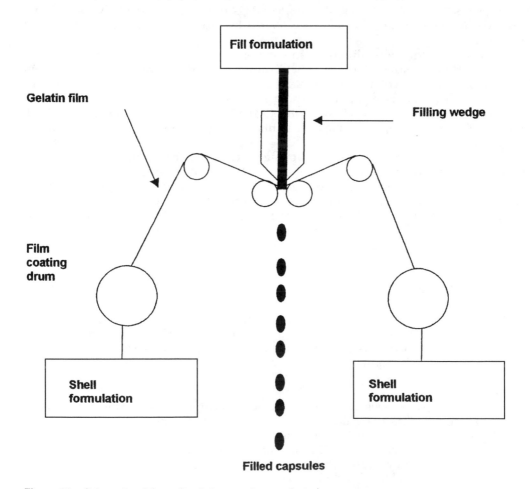

Figure 32 Schematic of the soft gelatin capsule manufacturing process.

their use include improved content uniformity, safety, improved stability, and improved bioavailability.

Improved Content Uniformity

Because soft gelatin capsules are filled with liquids or suspensions, excellent content uniformity can be achieved with even the most potent of drugs. The accuracy of the filling mechanism enables the dose to be filled to a tolerance of $\pm 1\%$ for solutions and $\pm 3\%$ for pastes.

Safety

Dissolving potent drugs in a liquid vehicle reduces the risk of operator exposure to dusts that is present with tablet and hard gelatin capsule–manufacturing operations.

Improved Stability

Varying the level of glycerol in the shell formulation will alter the permeability of the shell to oxygen. The filling process can be performed under nitrogen, so by appropriate selection of shell composition, this technology can provide excellent protection for oxygen-sensitive drugs.

Improved Bioavailability

Presenting the drug to the GI tract in a solubilized form overcomes the processes of disintegration and dissolution that are required from hard gelatin capsules and tablets before the drug substance is available for absorption. This has been utilized to improve the bioavailability of drugs with a range of solubilities.

Acid-soluble drugs can be dissolved or dispersed in water-miscible vehicles that rapidly distribute the drug throughout the stomach following administration. Acid-insoluble drugs can be dissolved in water-miscible vehicles, which results in the drug precipitating as a fine suspension in the stomach. The surface area of the solid in suspension is high, resulting in rapid dissolution.

Formulation of compounds that have very low aqueous solubility in lipid vehicles is an area that has seen the most growth in recent years. Two approaches can be used, depending on the solubility characteristics of the drug substance. For compounds with log P values in the region of 2 to 4, the preferred approach is to form self-emulsifying systems. These formulations comprise a lipid vehicle, typically a medium-chain triglyceride together with a surfactant, which, on contact with an aqueous environment, spontaneously form micelles. The drug remains solubilized in the micelles. Drugs with higher log P values can be dissolved in digestible oil such as medium-chain monoglycerides, which are immiscible with water. On release from the capsule, the drug remains solubilized in the immiscible oil. The precise mechanism by which the drug is absorbed from the oil is not fully understood, but there are a number of compounds on the market that have successfully demonstrated improved bioavailability by this route.

ORALLY DISINTEGRATING DOSAGE FORMS

One of the fastest growing categories of oral solid dosage forms is the orally disintegrating or rapidly dissolving dosage form. These dosage forms disintegrate in the mouth extremely rapidly and are thus swallowed without the need for water, making them extremely convenient to administer. The ideal properties for such formulations include

- Good stability—low sensitivity to temperature and humidity
- Robustness —requiring no special packaging
- Pleasant taste or, where the drug substance is unpalatable, delays dissolution of the drug until it reaches the stomach
- Ability to achieve a high drug loading

The first commercially available orally disintegrating dosage form was Zydis, a proprietary technology that involved filling solutions of the drug and excipients into blister packs and lyophilizing. This produced a porous wafer that rapidly dissolved when placed on the tongue. While this technology has been successfully applied to a number of products, there are limitations, particularly the amount of drug that can be incorporated into a formulation, which is typically less than 50 mg. The process also requires specialized equipment and protective packaging, as the wafers are very fragile.

The patient acceptability of the Zydis preparations prompted the development of a number of alternative technologies that have attempted to circumvent the intellectual property of Zydis or address one or more of its limitations.

The most productive approach to developing oral disintegrating tablets has been to utilize existing tabletting technology. The two main approaches have been to produce softly compressed tablets that require protective packaging and to optimize the disintegration properties by careful selection of disintegrants. Novel approaches include the use of spinning sugars to produce a candy floss–type structure that can be compressed into tablets and the manufacture of porous structures using 3D printing techniques.

An alternative approach that is gaining acceptance in the over-the-counter (OTC) markets is the use of rapidly dissolving films. Initially used as a delivery device for breath fresheners, a number of drugs are now being formulated in films. The films can be prepared by one (or a combination) of the following processes; solvent casting, semisolid casting, hot melt extrusion, or rolling. The films possess certain advantages over orally disintegrating tablets including portability and cost effectiveness but do themselves have limitations, the principal one being the drug loading that can be achieved.

SUMMARY

This chapter has summarized some of the key aspects of powder technology that are important to the development of the principal solid dosage forms, tablets, and capsules. Space restrictions have prevented this from being a very detailed review, and there are many specific types of tablets that have not been discussed at all. The area of solid dosage forms is very well served by the literature, and those interested in studying the subject area further are encouraged to consult the texts listed in the reference section.

REFERENCES

Alderborn G, Nystrom C. Pharmaceutical powder compaction technology. Drugs and the Pharmaceutical Sciences. Vol 71. New York: Marcel Dekker, 1995.

Anon, Can the appearance of medication improve compliance? Pharm J 1989; 281:88.

Armstrong NA. Time-dependent factors involved in powder compression and tablet manufacture. Int J Pharm 1989; 49:1–13.

Armstrong NA, Morton FSS. The effect of granulating agents on the elasticity and plasticity of powders. J Powder Bulk Solids Technol 1977; 1:32.

Armstrong NA. Direct compression characteristics of granulated Lactitol. Pharm Technol 1998; 22: 84–92.

Armstrong NA, Haines-Nutt RF. Elastic recovery and surface area changes in compacted powder systems. J Pharm Pharmacol 1972; 24(suppl):135P–136P.

Asker A, el-Nakeeb M, Motawi M, et al. Effect of certain tablet formulation factors on the antimicrobial activity of tetracycline hydrochloride and chloramphenicol. 3. Effect of lubricants. Pharmazie 1973; 28: 476–478.

Carneiro FLL, Barcellos A. Concrete tensile strength. RILEM Bulletin 1953; 13:97–123.

Charlton B, Newton JM. Application of gamma-ray attenuation to the determination of density distributions within compacted powders. Powder Technol 1985; 41:123–134.

Chemist and Druggist Directory and Tablet and Capsule Identification Guide. London: Benn Publications, 2000.

Eaves T, Jones TM. Effect of moisture on tensile strength of bulk solids. 1. Sodium chloride and effect of particle size. J Pharm Sci 1972; 61:256–261.

Food and Drug Administration (FDA), Guidance for Industry. Immediate Release Solid Oral. Dosage Forms. Scale-up and Postapproval Changes: Chemistry, Manufacturing, and Controls, In Vitro Dissolution Testing, and In Vivo Bioequivalence Documentation. Rockville, MD: Food and Drug Administration, Center for Drug Evaluation and Research, 1995.

Harnby N, Edwards MF, Nienow AW. Mixing in the Process Industries (Butterworth's Series in Chemical Engineering). London: Butterworth, 1985.

Heckel RW. Density-pressure relationships in powder compaction. Trans Metall Soc AIME 1961; 221:671–675.

Hiestand EN, Smith DP. Three indexes for characterizing the tabletting performance of materials. Adv Ceram 1984; 9:47–57.

Hölzer AW, Sjøgren J. The influence of the tablet thickness on measurements of friction during tabletting. Acta Pharm Suec 1978; 5:59–66.

Irono CI, Pilpel N. Effects of paraffin coatings on the shearing properties of lactose. J Pharm Pharmacol 1982; 34:480–485.

Irwin GM, Dodson GJ, Ravin LJ. Encapsulation of clomacron phosphate. 1. Effect of flowability of powder blends, lot-to-lot variability, and concentration of active ingredient on weight variation of capsules filled on an automatic filling machine. J Pharm Sci 1970; 59:547.

Ito K, Kaga SL, Takeya Y. Studies on hard gelatin capsules. II. The capsule filling of powders and effects of glidant by ring filling method. Chem Pharm Bull 1969; 17:1138.

Jain R, Railkar AS, Malick AW, et al. Stability of a hydrophobic drug in the presence of hydrous and anhydrous lactose. Eur J Pharm Biopharm 1998; 46:177–182.

Jivraj M, Martini LG, Thomson CM. An overview of the different excipients useful for the direct compression of tablets. Pharm Sci Technol Today 2000; 3(2):58–63.

Jolliffe IG, Newton JM. Practical implications of theoretical consideration of capsule filling by the dosator nozzle system. J Pharm Pharmacol 1982a; 34:293–298.

Jolliffe IG, Newton JM. An investigation of the relationship between particle size and compression during capsule filling with an automated mG2 simulator. J Pharm Pharmacol 1982b; 34:415–419.

Kamm R, Steinberg MA, Wulff J. Lead-grid study of metal powder compaction. Trans Am Inst Mining Met Eng 1949; 180:694–706.

Kibbe AH. Handbook of Pharmaceutical Excipients. 3rd ed. Washington D.C: American Pharmacists Association, 2000.

Kocova S, Pilpel N. Failure properties of lactose and calcium carbonate powders. Powder Technol 1972; 5:329–343.

Kocova S, Pilpel N. Failure properties of some simple and complex powders and the significance of their yield locus parameters. Powder Technol 1973; 8:33–35.

Krycer I, Pope DG, Hersey JA. The prediction of paracetamol capping tendencies. J Pharm Pharmacol 1982; 34:802–804.

Kurihara K, Ichikawa I. Effect of powder flowability on capsule-filling weight variation. Chem Pharm Bull 1978; 26:1250–1256.

Malamataris S, Bin Baie S, Pilpel N. Plasto-elasticity and tabletting of paracetamol, Avicel and other powders. J Pharm Phamacol 1984; 36:616–617.

Nyquist H, Brodin A. Ring shear cell measurements of granule flowability and the correlation to weight variations at tabletting. Acta Pharm Suec 1982; 19:81–90.

Nyström C, Malmqvist K, Mazur J, et al. Measurement of axial and radial tensile strength of tablets and their relation to capping. Acta Pharm Suec 1978; 15(3):226–232.

Physicians' Desk Reference. 52nd ed. New York: Medical Economics, 1998.

Pitt KG, Newton JM, Richardson R, et al. The material tensile strength of convex-faced aspirin tablets. J Pharm Pharmacol 1989; 41:289–292.

Podczechk F, Blackwell S, Gold M, et al. The filling of granules into hard gelatine capsules. Int J Pharm 1999; 188:49–59.

Reier G, Cohn R, Rock S, et al. Evaluation of factors affecting the encapsulation of powders in hard gelatin capsules. I. Semi-automatic machines. J Pharm Sci 1968; 57:660–666.

Rhodes M. Principles in Powder Technology. New York: Wiley, 1990.

Ridgway K. Hard Capsules Development and Technology. London: Pharmaceutical Press, 1987.

Ridgway K, Watt P. Tablet Machine Instrumentation in Pharmaceutics: Principles and Practise. Chichester, UK: Ellis Horwood, 1988.

Roberts RJ, Rowe RC. The effect of punch velocity on the compaction of a variety of materials. J Pharm Pharmacol 1985; 37:377–384.

Roberts RJ, Rowe RC. Brittle fracture propensity measurements on "tablet-sized" compacts. J Pharm Pharmacol 1986; 38:526–528.

Roberts RJ, Rowe RC. The compaction of pharmaceutical and other model materials—a pragmatic approach. Chem Eng Sci 1987; 42:903–911.

Rowe RC. Binder-substrate interactions in granulation: a theoretical approach based on surface free energy and polarity. Int J Pharm 1989; 38:149–154.

Rowe RC, Forse SF. Pitting—A defect on film coated tablets. Int J Pharm 1983; 17:343.

Rubenstein MH, Bodey DM. Disaggregation of compressed tablets. J Pharm Pharmacol 1974; 26:104P.

Rudnic EM, Rhodes CT, Welch S, et al. Evaluations of the mechanism of disintegrant action. Drug Dev Ind Pharm 1982; 8:87–110.

Rumpf H. Die wissenschaft des agglomerierens. Chem Ing Tech 1974; 46(1):1–11.

Schulze D. Comparison of the flow behaviour of easily flowing bulk materials. Schuettgut 1996; 2: 347–356.

Seager H, Rue PJ, Burt I, et al. Choice of method for the manufacture of tablets suitable for film coating. Int J Pharm Tech Prod Manuf 1985; 6:1–20.

Shah KB, Augsburger LL, Small LE, et al. Instrumentation of a dosing disc automatic capsule filling machine. Pharm Technol 1983; 7:42–54.

Shah NH, Stiel D, Weiss M, et al. Evaluation of two new tablet lubricants—sodium stearyl fumarate and glyceryl behenate. Measurement of physical parameters (compaction, ejection and residual forces) in the tabletting process and effect of the dissolution rate. Drug Dev Ind Pharm 1986; 12:1329–1346.

Shotton E, Leonard GS. The effect of intra- and extragranular maize starch on the disintegration of compressed tablets. J Pharm Pharmacol 1972; 24:798–803.

Small LE, Augsburger LL. Aspects of the lubrication requirements for an automatic capsule-filling machine. Drug Dev Ind Pharm 1978; 4:345–372.

Stegemann S. Liquid and semi-solid formulaion in hard gelatin capsules. Swiss Pharma 1999; 21(6): 21–28.

Train D. An investigation into the compaction of powders. J Pharm Pharmacol 1956; 8:745–761.

Train D. Agglomeration of solids by compaction. Trans Ins Chem Engrs 1957; 35:258–262.

Vilivalam VD, Illum L, Iqbal K. Starch capsules: an alternative system for oral drug delivery. Pharm Sci Technol Today 2000; 3(2):64–69.

Williams JC, Birks AH. The comparison of the failure measurements of powders with theory. Powder Technol 1967; 1:199–206.

York P, Pilpel N. The tensile strength and compression behaviour of lactose, four fatty acids and their mixtures in relation to tabletting. J Pharm Pharmacol 1973; 25(suppl):1P–11P.

12 | Ophthalmic Dosage Forms

Mark Gibson
AstraZeneca R&D Charnwood, Loughborough, Leicestershire, U.K.

INTRODUCTION

There are many diseases affecting the eye that are treated with various types of drugs and drug delivery systems. Table 1 lists some of the main therapeutic classes of drugs currently used to treat eye diseases and types of dosage forms commercially available. There are three main routes for delivery of drugs to the eye: topical, systemic, and intraocular injection. The dosage forms listed in Table 1 are intended for topical administration and include various eye drop solutions, suspensions, and ointments. Additionally, there are controlled delivery systems, such as ocular inserts, minitablets, and disposable lenses, that can be applied to the exterior surface of the eye for treatment of conditions affecting the anterior segment of the eye. Extended residence times following topical application have the potential to improve bioavailability of the administered drug, and additionally a range of strategies have been tested and patented to improve penetration including cyclodextrins, liposomes, and nanoparticles (Conway, 2008). Drugs such as antibiotics and corticosteroids can be administered systemically to treat certain eye conditions, but this route of administration is not often favored because of the poor drug penetration into the eye from the systemic circulation. Subsequently, high doses have to be administered, leading to systemic side effects and toxicity. Periocular injections are also used to administer anti-infective drugs, mydriatics, or corticosteroids, but these cannot be administered by patients themselves. Also, injections tend to be reserved for serious conditions affecting the posterior portion of the eye where topical therapy is ineffective.

The posterior eye segment is an important therapeutic target with unmet medical needs. Drug delivery to the posterior segment of the eye is important for potentially treating diseases such as age-related macular degeneration (AMD), posterior uveitis, and persistent macular edema due to diabetic retinopathy. AMD is a degenerative retinal disease that causes progressive loss of central vision and is the leading cause of irreversible vision loss and legal blindness in individuals over the age of 50 in the Western world (Birch and Liang, 2007). Historically, most of this pathology could only be dealt with surgically, and then only after much damage to the macula had already occurred. Because of anatomic membrane barriers and the lacrimal drainage, it can be quite challenging to obtain therapeutic drug concentrations in the posterior parts of the eye after topical administration. In recent years, there has been much research conducted in the field of drug delivery systems with emphasis placed on controlled release of drug to specific areas of the eye. The development of therapeutic agents that require repeated long-term administration is a driver for the development of sustained-release drug delivery systems to result in less frequent dosing and less invasive techniques. Current effective therapies for AMD include corticosteroids and anti-vascular endothelial growth factor compounds, with recent successes reported using anti-angiogenic drugs (Booth et al., 2007). Novel ophthalmic formulations developed to specifically target drug delivery to the posterior segment of the eye include polymeric controlled-release injections (microspheres and liposomes), implants (biodegradable and nonbiodegradable), nanoparticulates, micro-encapsulated cells, iontophoresis, gene medicines, and enhanced drug delivery systems, such as ultrasound drug delivery (Del Amo and Urtti, 2008; Loftsson et al., 2008; Fialho and Cunha, 2007; Hsu, 2007; Wagh et al., 2008). Such devices provide significant drug release over a period of days or weeks. However, currently, there is no "gold standard" for AMD therapy and/or drug delivery. Further work is required to improve the efficiency and effectiveness of drug delivery to the posterior chamber of the eye.

Table 1   Examples of Therapeutic Classes of Drugs Currently Used to Treat Ocular Diseases

Class	Drugs	Action	Clinical use	Dosage forms
Antibacterial	Chloramphenicol, framycetin	Bacteriostatic or bacteriocidal	Eye infections	Eye drop solution, viscous drops, eye ointment, liquid gel
Antiviral	Acyclovir	Antiviral	Control of viral infections	Eye ointment
Anti-inflammatory	Dexamethasone, sodium cromoglycate	Inhibition of inflammatory response	Inflammation, allergic conjunctivitis	Eye drop solution, suspension, eye ointment
Mydriatics and cycloplegics	Tropicamide, cyclopentolate	Dilation of pupil	Examination of the fundus of eye	Eye drop solution, eye ointment
β-Blockers	Timolol, betaxolol	Reduction in aqueous humor production	Treatment of glaucoma	Eye drop solution, suspension, gel-forming solution
Miotics	Pilocarpine, carbachol	Constriction of pupil	Treatment of glaucoma	Eye drop solution, viscous eye drops, ocular insert, gel
Local anesthetics	Oxybuprocaine, amethocaine	Irreversible blocking of pain sensation	Tonometry and prior to minor surgery	Eye drop solution
Diagnostics	Fluorescein sodium	Coloring of the eye	Locating damaged areas of cornea	Eye drops
Artificial tear preparations	Hypromellose, polyacrylic acid	Eye lubrication	Tear deficiency dry-eye syndrome	Liquid gel, viscous eye drops

By far, the most popular route of administration for drug treatment in ocular diseases and diagnostics is the topical route, and this route is therefore the main focus of this chapter.

In recent years, there have been increased efforts to find safer and effective drugs to treat various ocular conditions and diseases that are poorly controlled now, as well as to develop novel dosage forms and delivery systems to improve the topical delivery of existing drugs. There is an unmet demand for new products in some markets, such as anti-glaucoma products for patients that do not respond to currently available marketed products. There has been a steady increase in conventional new drugs to treat infections, glaucoma, anti-inflammatory and anti-allergic conditions, as well as the emergence of peptides and proteins.

The development of new ocular drug products, and more sophisticated delivery systems for the effective administration to the patient, poses several technical challenges to the formulator. These are discussed in more detail later in this chapter.

OCULAR TOPICAL DRUG DELIVERY ISSUES AND CHALLENGES

Ocular topical drug delivery is particularly challenging because of the inherent difficulties associated with absorption of topically applied drugs into the eye. Consideration of the anatomical and physiological features of the eye, as well as the physicochemical properties of the drug, is important when developing a topical ophthalmic delivery system.

Physiological Barriers

A good overview of the physiological features of the eye and the implications for ophthalmic drug delivery is presented in a review by Jarvinen et al. (1995). The most salient points are summarized briefly here.

Figure 1 shows the structure of the outside of the eye and a cross-section of the anterior segment of the eye. The front part of the globe of the eye is clear and colorless and is called the cornea. It contains no blood vessels but is rich in nerve endings. The cornea consists of three major layers: the outer epithelium, middle stroma, and inner endothelium. When topically applied products are administered to the eye, they first encounter the cornea and conjunctiva,

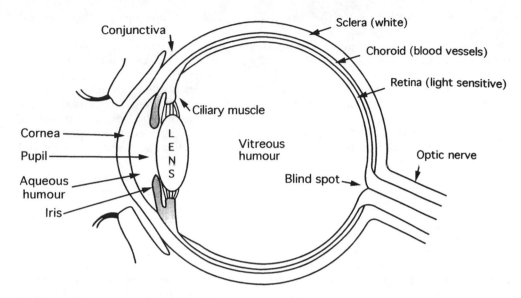

Figure 1 Structure of anterior segment of the eye (Glasspool, 1984).

representing the primary barriers to drug penetration. The epithelium and endothelium of the cornea are rich in lipid content, making them barriers to the permeation of polar, water-soluble compounds. The stroma, on the other hand, is a hydrophilic layer containing 70% to 80% water, presenting a barrier to the permeation of nonpolar, lipid-soluble compounds.

The other part of the boundary layer to the front of the eye is the sclera. This is white in color and opaque and contains most of the blood vessels supplying the anterior tissues of the eye. The outer surface of the schlera is loosely covered by the conjunctival membrane, which is continuous with the inner surface of the eyelids, and also presents a significant permeability barrier to most drugs. For drugs that permeate the vascular systems of the schlera and conjunctiva, transport tends to be away from the eye into the general circulation.

Other major physiological barrier mechanisms are due to tear production and the blink reflex. The conjunctival and corneal surfaces of the eye are continuously lubricated by a film of fluid secreted by the conjunctival and lachrymal glands. The lachrymal glands secrete a watery fluid called tears, and the sebaceous glands on the margins of the eyelids secrete an oily fluid, which spreads over the tear film. The latter reduces the rate of evaporation of the tear film from the exposed surface of the eyes. Blinking assists in evenly spreading the tear film over the surface of the eye and in draining the tears via the nasolachrymal duct into the nose, and ultimately down the back of the throat into the gastrointestinal (GI) tract.

Ophthalmic solutions are available for multidose or single-dose administration in a wide variety of glass and plastic dropper bottles, which deliver drops with a volume between 25 and 70 μL (Van Santvilet and Ludwig, 2004). Upon administration of topically applied eye drops, removal from the eye is rapid because of tear production and the blinking processes occurring simultaneously. The precorneal volume is about 7 μL, but volumes of up to 20 to 30 μL can be held in this area before spillage occurs. Instillation of volumes greater than this will result in simply spilling out onto the cheek or rapid loss with the tears through drainage into the nasolachrymal duct. Also, the instilled product is diluted by normal tear production, with tear production rates in man reported as 1 μL/min under resting conditions (Maurice and Mishima, 1984). In practice, the introduction of any eye drop product, but particularly products causing irritation, is likely to stimulate the tear production rate and increase the rate of drug removal from the eye. The removal of material by dilution is also aided by the blink reflex where each blink pumps approximately 2 μL of tear fluid into the nasolachrymal duct. It is estimated that the turnover for material instilled into the eye is approximately 16%/min of the total volume, indicating a rapid removal from the precorneal area (Schell, 1982). The net result is that less than 10%, and typically 1% or less, of the topically instilled dose into the eye actually permeates the cornea and is absorbed into the eye (Burstein and Anderson, 1985).

Other physiological factors affecting ocular delivery of topical drugs are protein binding and drug metabolism. Protein accounts for up to 2% of the total content of normal tears and can be higher under certain pathological conditions such as uveitis. The increased size of the protein–drug complex will render the bound drug molecules unavailable for absorption, and lachrymal drainage will rapidly remove them from the eye. Tears are known to contain a range of enzymes such as esterases, monoamine oxidases, and aminopeptidases, among others. Consequently, many ocularly applied drugs are metabolized during or after absorption in the eye. This can be detrimental if the enzyme is responsible for inactivating the topically applied drug, for example, pilocarpine being inactivated with esterases (Bundgaard et al., 1985). Alternatively, there are several examples, such as dipivalyl epinephrine, where metabolism by esterases is advantageously used to bioactivate a topically applied prodrug administered to the eye (Tammara and Crider, 1996).

Patient Compliance

Another factor that can affect the ocular bioavailability of a topically applied product is patient compliance and how the patient is using the medication. Patient compliance could be related to the acceptability of the product. Adverse effects such as irritation, burning, stinging or blurring of vision may provide a reason for patients to stop their medication. Local irritation is very common with many ophthalmic products, especially when high drug concentrations are involved. The design of the formulation and selection of excipients can influence the degree of irritation. For example, the use of cyclodextrins in eye drops has been shown to reduce ocular irritation by pilocarpine prodrugs (Suhonen et al., 1995). Formulation design can also be important in minimizing the amount of systemic absorption of the instilled drug and possible systemic side effects that may affect patient compliance. A variety of modified drug delivery systems have been developed to reduce systemic absorption and increase absorption into the eye. Some of these are discussed later in this chapter.

Finally, how the patient uses the product can affect ocular bioavailability. For example, applying more than one drop, or a larger drop by squeezing the dropper bottle harder, is not likely to be beneficial. The drug administered in the first drop is dramatically reduced when a second drop is instilled straight afterwards. Also, it has been shown that increasing the instilled solution volume actually reduces the fraction of dose absorbed because of a resultant increase in the drainage rate (Patton, 1980). The ideal volume of instilled drug is 5 to 10 μL, but this is not achievable with some conventional eye drop packs (Van Santvilet and Ludwig, 2004). There are, however, new pack devices that are able to accurately deliver such small quantities (see sect. "Packaging Design Considerations" later in this chapter).

DRUG CANDIDATE SELECTION

Physicochemical drug properties, such as solubility, lipophilicity, molecular size and shape, charge and degree of ionization, will affect the rate and route of permeation into the cornea.

For most topically applied drugs, passive diffusion along the concentration gradient, either transcellularly or paracellularly, is the main permeation mechanism across the cornea. Occasionally, a carrier-mediated active transport mechanism is indicated (Liaw et al., 1992). Lipophilic drugs tend to favor the transcellular route, whereas hydrophilic drugs usually permeate via the paracellular route through intercellular spaces (Borchardt, 1990).

Since the cornea is a membrane barrier containing both lipophilic and hydrophilic layers, drugs possessing both lipophilic and hydrophilic properties permeate it most effectively. The optimal range for the octanol/buffer pH 7.4 distribution coefficient (log P) for corneal permeation is 2 to 3 (Schoenwald and Ward, 1978), observed for a wide variety of drugs.

Drugs capable of existing in both the ionized and unionized form (weak acids and bases) tend to permeate the cornea the best. The unionized form usually permeates the lipid membranes more easily than the ionized form. The ratio of ionized to unionized drug in the eye will depend on the pK_a of the drug and the pH of both the eye drop and the lachrymal

Table 2 Examples of Prodrugs Used in Ophthalmic Drug Delivery

Parent compound	Prodrug moiety	Comments
Acyclovir	2'-O-Glycyl ester	Prodrug developed to increase solubility (30 times enhancement)
Pilocarpine	Acid diesters	Prodrug developed to increase aqueous stability
Terbutaline	Diisobutyl ester (ibuterol)	Prodrugs developed to increase efficacy: 100 times more potent to reduce intraocular pressure
Timolol	Aliphatic and aromatic amines, (acycloxy) alkyl carbomates	Increased corneal penetration and efficacy to treat glaucoma Prodrug developed to reduce systemic side effects
5-Fluorouracil	1-Alkoxycarbonyl, 3-acyl, and 1-acyloxymethyl	Significant enhancement in corneal penetration, resulting in reduction in dose and toxicity

fluid. Therefore, drugs formulated at a pH providing a higher concentration of unionized drug usually render the best corneal absorption.

For ionizable drugs, the nature of the charge, as well as the degree of ionization, will affect corneal permeability. The corneal epithelium is negatively charged above its isoelectric point (pI 3.2). As a result, charged cationic drugs permeate more easily through the cornea than do anionic species. Below the isoelectric point, the cornea is selective to negatively charged drugs, but in practice, the pH would be too acidic and irritating to use (Rojanasakul et al., 1992).

The molecular size of the drug does not seem to be a major factor for corneal permeability, provided the molecular weight is less than 500. Compounds larger than this are usually poorly absorbed when instilled into the eye and therefore are not a favorable option for biologicals/biopharmaceuticals.

The chemical form of the drug can be very important for ocular bioavailability. Changing the salt can affect the solubility and lipophilicity of the drug. For example, dexamethasone acetate ester has the preferred solubility and partition coefficient properties for corneal permeation compared with the very water-soluble phosphate salt or very lipophilic freebase.

During the candidate drug selection stage, preformulation studies should be performed to establish measurements of the physicochemical properties of potential compounds for development. Ideally, the compound with the preferred properties is selected. In cases where the physicochemical properties of the drug are not considered optimum to reach the site of action in the eye, it may be possible to design a suitable inactive bioreversible derivative (or prodrug) of the drug. The prodrug is then converted enzymatically or chemically to the parent drug in the eye in order to illicit a pharmacological effect (AlGhaneem and Crooks, 2007).

The prodrug approach has been used in ocular drug delivery not only to improve drug bioavailability but to increase solubility, stability, and potency and to decrease systemic side effects. The aim of the prodrug approach is to modify the physicochemical properties, such as solubility or lipophilicity, by making prodrug derivatives (Lee and Li, 1989). Some examples of prodrugs used in ophthalmic drug delivery are given in Table 2.

If the most appropriate physicochemical properties are not built into the candidate drug during candidate selection, the formulator faces a challenge in trying to overcome these deficiencies during formulation development. In practice, this is usually the case. Some of the formulation and drug delivery options that may be considered are discussed later in this chapter.

PRODUCT DESIGN CONSIDERATIONS

Formulation Design Options

Traditionally, topical ophthalmic dosage forms have been available as aqueous and oily solutions or suspensions, and administered as drops, gels, ointments, or solid devices. The selection of formulation type will be largely dependent on the properties of the drug such as its aqueous drug solubility. Other factors will be the target concentration of drug required in the dose to be delivered and the eye condition to be treated. In recent years, there has been a lot of research on novel ophthalmic delivery systems to try and improve corneal retention time, reduce the frequency of administration, and improve compliance. The scope and limitations of various ophthalmic dosage forms are discussed briefly below with the implications for formulation and pack design.

Solutions

Fortunately, many therapeutic agents used in eye products are water-soluble compounds or can be formulated as water-soluble salts, and a sufficiently high solution concentration can be achieved in the administered dose. In comparison with more sophisticated multiphase systems, solution products are preferred because they are generally easier to manufacture and potentially provide better dose uniformity and ocular bioavailability.

However, solution eye drops do have the disadvantage of being rapidly drained from the eye, with corresponding loss of drug. The inclusion of viscosity-increasing agents in the formulation, such as hypromellose, hydroxyethylcellulose, polyvinyl alcohol, povidone, or dextran, can be used to increase the tear viscosity, which decreases drainage, thereby prolonging precorneal retention of the drops in the eye. Various studies have shown that an increase in product viscosity increases the residence time in the eye (Li and Robinson, 1989; Chrai and Robinson, 1974), but there is a danger that high-viscosity products may not be well tolerated in the eye. For this reason, most ophthalmic products are formulated within the range of 10 to 25 cP by the addition of viscosity-increasing agents. Certain viscosity-increasing materials, such as hyaluronic acid and its derivatives, or carbomer, have been shown to be more effective in achieving precorneal retention because of their mucoadhesive properties (Seattone et al., 1991; Vulovic et al., 1989).

Water-Based Gels

Ophthalmic delivery systems can be developed containing polymers that undergo a phase change from liquid to semisolid as a result of changes in temperature (e.g., poloxamers), pH (e.g., cellulose acetate hydrogen phthalate latex), or ionic strength in the tear film (e.g., low-acetyl gellan gum, Gelrite^{TM}) (Rozier et al., 1989). These formulations are liquid formulations upon administration, but gel on contact with the eye to provide extended retention times. In situ gel formers also have the advantage of ease of administration, and improved patient compliance, because they can be instilled as a liquid drop (Robinson and Mylnek, 1995). Many drugs already in commercial use have been reformulated in longer acting liquid dosage form for once-daily application such as an in situ gelling preparation of timolol (Timoptic-XE^{TM}, Merck and Co., Inc., Whitehouse Station, NJ, U.S.).

Semisolid gel-type preparations have also been developed for ophthalmic delivery as an alternative to traditional ointments, based on the effect of increasing the viscosity to prolong the retention of drug in the eye (for example, Pilopine HS gel, Alcon Laboratories, Inc., Fort Worth, TX, U.S.). Several types of gelling agents have been used, such as polyacrylic acid derivatives, carbomer, and hypromellose.

Suspensions

Aqueous or oily suspension eye drop formulations may be considered for drugs that are poorly water soluble, or because of poor aqueous drug stability. The drug particle size must be reduced to less than 10 μm levels to avoid irritation of the eye surface, leading to blinking and excessive lachrymation. One possible advantage of ophthalmic suspensions is that they should prolong the residence time of drug particles in the eye, allowing time for dissolution in the tears and an increase in ocular bioavailability (Sieg and Robinson, 1975). This is only true if the dissolution rate of the particles and the rate of ocular absorption are faster than the rate of clearance of the drug from the eye. In practice, it is more likely that particles acceptable for ophthalmic suspensions, smaller than 10 μm, are removed from the eye as rapidly as drugs in solution.

Suspensions may also be used to overcome the chemical instability of the drug, but at the same time may pose physical instability problems. For example, there may be an increase in particle size with time (Ostwald ripening), or difficulties in resuspension after periods of storage. The latter may result in problems with homogeneity and dose uniformity. The selection of a suitable salt with a low aqueous solubility can be employed to minimize the risk of Ostwald ripening, but it is also important that the suspended particles dissolve reasonably quickly in the eye, or else bioavailability will be reduced.

Suspension products may pose challenges to the formulator in manufacturing to achieve a sterile product. The possibilities of either degradation or morphological changes occurring during the sterilization process exist and must be prevented.

Ointments

Eye ointments are sterile semisolid preparations intended for application to the conjunctiva. They are attractive because of their increased contact time and better bioavailability compared to solutions. They can be very useful for nighttime application; however, they are not always well accepted by patients because upon application they often cause blurred vision. A wide variety of ointments are available commercially.

The majority of water-free oleaginous eye ointment bases are composed of white petrolatum and liquid petrolatum (mineral oil), or a modification of the petrolatum base formula. They are designed to melt at body temperature. Other types of lipophilic ointment bases can also be used. An anhydrous vehicle can be advantageous for moisture-sensitive drugs. Alternatively, semisolid, anhydrous, water-soluble bases for ophthalmic use have been formulated from nonaqueous organogels, such as carbomer gelled with polyethylene glycols, and a suitable amine, providing good spreadability in the eye and low irritation potential. The drug can be incorporated in the vehicle as a solution or as a finely divided powder. For multidose products, a suitable antimicrobial preservative is required to prevent the potential contamination of the solution by microorganisms during use of the medication. The selection of antimicrobial preservatives is discussed later in this chapter.

Like suspensions, ointments can be more difficult to manufacture in sterile form. They can be terminally sterilized; alternatively, they must be manufactured from sterile ingredients in an aseptic environment. Filtration through a suitable membrane or dry heat sterilization is often used.

Ocular Inserts

Solid erodible (soluble) or nonerodible (insoluble) inserts have been commercially available for some time as a means of prolonging the release of drugs into the eye. The Ocusert[TM] nonerodible system developed by Alza Corporation was first marketed in the United States in 1974. It is a membrane-controlled reservoir insert containing pilocarpine alginate, enclosed above and below by thin ethylene vinyl acetate (EVA) membranes. Ocusert is used in contact with the surface of the eye and is capable of releasing the drug at a reproducible and constant rate over one week. Other nonerodible therapeutic systems are based on hydrogel contact lenses filled with drug. Merkli et al. (1995) have written a comprehensive review of the various erodible polymers currently available, and particularly on the use of biodegradable polymers for ophthalmic drug delivery. The authors discuss the different possible erosion mechanisms, which depend on the polymer type, and the type of drugs best suited for a particular polymer type. Ocular inserts incorporating a bioadhesive polymer, thiolated poly(acrylic acid), are promising new solid devices being developed for ocular drug delivery (Hornof et al., 2003).

Soluble insert products have also been developed in which the drug is bound to an erodible matrix such as hydroxypropyl cellulose (HPC), hyaluronic acid, carbomer, or polyacrylic acids. They are placed in the lower cul-de-sac and generally dissolve within 12 to 24 hours. The advantage over nonerodible systems is that the erodible polymeric device undergoes gradual dissolution while releasing the drug, and so the patient does not have to remove it following use. A commercially available example is the Lacrisert[®] insert (Merck and Co., Inc.), a sterile, translucent, rod-shaped, water-soluble form of HPC. The product is inserted into the inferior cul-de-sac of the eye of patients with dry eye states typically once or twice a day. It softens and slowly dissolves following administration to lubricate and protect the surface of the eye. Conventional hydrogel contact lenses have also being evaluated for topical drug delivery to the eye (AlvarezLorenzo et al., 2006).

Another example of a commercially available erodible insert is the soluble ophthalmic drug insert (SODI™), a soluble copolymer of acrylamide, *N*-vinylpyrrolidone, and ethyl acrylate, designated as ABE. It is in the form of a sterile thin film of oval shape, which is introduced to the upper conjunctival sac. Following application, it softens in 10 to 15 seconds, conforming to the shape of the eyeball, and then in the next 10 to 15 minutes, the film turns to a clot, which gradually dissolves while releasing the drug. SODI was developed as a result of a vast collaborative effort between Russian chemists and ophthalmologists in the 1970s (Khromow et al., 1976).

Saettone and Salminen (1995) provide a good review of the advantages, disadvantages, and requirements for success of ocular inserts, and examine inserts that are available on the market or are in development including Ocusert, SODI, Collagen Shields, Ocufit, Minidisc, and Nods. The limited uptake of inserts has been attributed to psychological factors, such as the reluctance of ophthalmologists and patients to abandon the traditional liquid and semisolid medications. Commercial failure may also be attributed to the relatively high cost of treatment compared to conventional liquid products, and to occasional therapeutic failures.

Novel Ophthalmic Drug Delivery Systems

The shortfalls of conventional topical liquid eye drops, discussed earlier, particularly the relatively short precorneal half-life, have resulted in several new ophthalmic drug delivery approaches being investigated. Promising systems have been evaluated employing small colloidal carrier particles such as liposomes, microspheres, microcapsules, nanoparticles, or nanocapsules. These systems have the advantage that they may be applied in liquid form, just like eye drop solutions, because of their low viscosity. Thus, they avoid the discomfort often associated with viscous gels and ointments but still provide a reservoir from which the drug can be delivered slowly.

Liposomes may increase the ocular bioavailability of certain drugs by increasing the association of the drug with the cornea by means of an increased lipophilic liposomal bilayer interaction with the corneal epithelium. Several other potential advantages of using liposomes as drug carriers for ophthalmic drug delivery have been reported (Meisner and Mezei, 1995). They can accommodate both hydrophilic and lipophilic drugs, they are biocompatible and biodegradable, they can protect the encapsulated drug from metabolic degradation; and they can act as a depot, releasing the drug slowly. Liposomes, however, have the disadvantages of reduced physical stability and difficulties in sterilizing the product. Temperatures required for autoclaving can cause irreversible damage to vesicles, while filtration is only applicable to vesicles less than 0.2 μm.

Microparticles (>1 μm) and nanoparticles (<1μm) are colloidal drug carriers in the micrometer and sub-micrometer range, respectively. Microspheres are monolithic particles possessing a porous or solid polymer matrix, whereas microcapsules consist of a polymeric membrane surrounding a solid or liquid drug reservoir. Nanoparticles, including nanospheres or nanocapsules, have a particle size in the nanometer size range from 10 to 1000 nm. Drugs can be incorporated into the core of the carrier, either dissolved in the polymer matrix in the form of a solid solution or suspended in the form of a solid dispersion. Alternatively, the drug may be adsorbed on the particle surface. Release of drug can be attributed to degradation of the polymer, drug desorption from the polymer surface, or diffusion through the polymeric matrix. Various synthetic and natural biocompatible polymers have been used to prepare microparticles and nanoparticles. Polylactic acid is an example of a biodegradable polymer, and poly(alkyl) cyanoacrylate derivatives with various lengths of alkyl chain are examples of nonbiodegradable polymers that can be used. The ocular bioavailability of a number of drugs has been demonstrated in animal models, compared to conventional aqueous eye drops (Zimmer and Kreuter, 1995). In addition, nanoparticles have been shown to adhere preferentially to inflamed precorneal tissues of the eye. Although there are currently no commercial formulations on the market using novel polymers, these carrier systems show a lot of promise for the future. The challenge will be to demonstrate safety and tolerability, and gain acceptance by the regulatory authorities. Amrite and Kompella (2006) report a good summary of ocular applications of these systems.

Other attempts to improve ocular bioavailability have focused on overcoming poor corneal permeability with penetration enhancers, or improving the lipophilicity of the drug through ion pair formation. Also, proposals have been made to improve packaging and device design to deliver the dosage form in a more precise manner. Ophthalmic packaging is discussed in more detail in the next section.

Packaging Design Considerations

The choice of packaging for ophthalmic products will depend on the type of dosage form, such as whether it is a liquid solution/suspension or semisolid gel or ointment. Also, choice will depend on how the product is to be used by the patient, such as whether it is intended to be a unit-dose or multidose application. For any formulation type, the packaging design acceptance criteria must ensure that the

- materials are compatible with the formulation and ensure product stability;
- sterility of the product can be achieved and assured for the entire shelf life;
- materials meet pharmacopoeial and regulatory standard requirements;
- containers should be tamper-evident; and
- pack design offers ease of administration to the patient.

Liquid Drops (Solutions/Suspensions)

Traditionally, ophthalmic liquid products were packed in glass containers fitted with rubber teats for the eye dropper. Glass containers have (limited) use today when there is product stability or compatibility issues, which exclude the use of flexible plastic containers, made of polyethylene or polypropylene. Most liquid eye products on the market are plastic containers fitted with nozzles from which, by gentle squeezing, the contents may be expressed as drops.

Plastic containers have several advantages over the glass dropper combination such as minimizing the risk of the contents being contaminated with microorganisms by the replacement of a pipette, which may have become contaminated by touching the infected eye. Also, plastic containers are cheap, light in weight, more robust to handle and easier to use than glass dropper-type containers. Multidose plastic bottles can be conventional dropper bottles or a form-fill-seal bottle where the dropper tip is an integral part of the bottle.

However, there are some disadvantages of plastic eye drop containers. Some plastic materials such as polyethylene can absorb some antimicrobial preservatives [e.g., benzalkonium chloride (BKC)], or some drugs. They may also leach plasticizers into the product or printing inks from the label through the plastic into the product. It is necessary to conduct compatibility and stability studies to ascertain whether this is likely to be a problem. For ophthalmic solutions that require the addition of a preservative because the drug product itself has no adequate antimicrobial properties, it may be necessary to use glass. Alternatively, a preservative-free product could be considered. The challenge is to develop a packaging system for preservative-free products, which maintains the sterility of the product throughout its shelf life and during use.

Unit-dose systems offer the easiest technical solution to this problem, but have the disadvantages of higher cost of manufacture and of not being as compact as a multidose product containing equivalent doses. Unit-dose products are usually made of low-density polyethylene (LDPE), with the formulated sterile solution being without a preservative, and sealed using the form-fill-seal process.

An alternative approach is to develop a multidose, preservative-free system. The container is required to be collapsible, and the suck-back of air, which could contain bacteria, has to be avoided. Containers are now available that contain a valve mechanism to achieve this. The ABAK® system (Transphyto, France) is a patented preservative-free, multidose eye drop dispenser that contains a 0.2 μm nylon fiber sterilizing membrane to filter the solution. The pressure exerted when squeezing the pack causes the solution to pass through the anti-bacterial filter forming a drop that falls from the tip of the dispenser. When pressure is released, the solution is re-absorbed and filtered. Each pack can deliver 300 sterile drops (10 mL) reproducibly, and stability studies show that the solution contained in the ABAK system remains sterile and preserved for up to eight weeks after opening.

BKC is the most common preservative used in commercial eye drops, and yet there are reports of side effects such as allergic reactions, irritation, decreased lacrimation, and damage to the corneal endothelium caused by its multiple use in eye products (Fraunfelder and Meyer, 1989). Also, BKC can accumulate in soft contact lenses and is therefore not recommended for these patients. Use of the ABAK device is a good way of avoiding the need for BKC in the eye drops to overcome these issues.

Plastic containers can also be permeable to water vapor and oxygen over prolonged periods of storage. This can lead to gradual loss of liquid product or oxidation of an unstable drug over time.

Polyethylene containers are not able to withstand autoclaving and are usually sterilized by ethylene oxide or by irradiation before being filled aseptically with presterilized product. Polypropylene containers can be autoclaved, but are not as flexible as polyethylene for eye dropper use. Guidance on the manufacture of sterile medicinal products from a number of regulatory sources suggests that there is an expectation that terminal sterilization will be employed in preference to aseptic manipulation during the manufacturing process (Matthews, 1999). The implication is that the type of container is not a satisfactory reason for not autoclaving the product, and the manufacturer should use a package that is currently available as a heat-stable alternative (such as polypropylene) and use standard terminal sterilization by heat as recommended in the European Pharmacopoeia (EP). If a non-heat-stable container is progressed, and terminal sterilization is not possible, a full justification will be required for this approach. This may put manufacturers off investing in novel packaging concepts that may offer advantages to the patient.

There are other novel ophthalmic liquid pack design features in development or have been developed in recent years. For example, the "Optidyne system" being developed by Scherer DDS is an atomized spray, which delivers a tiny volume (about 5 µL) directly to the front of the eyeball so fast that it beats the blink reflex. The volume is similar to the capacity of the precorneal volume in the eye. Unlike the traditional eye drops, the spray product can be directed more easily and should reduce the wastage associated with conventional eye drops, which have a typical volume of 40 µL.

Another device to aid administration is an eyecup fitted to a metered dose pump to help the patient position the product correctly over the eye during administration. Novel devices have been developed to accommodate moisture and/or oxygen-sensitive drugs, such as a dual-chamber container that can hold drug, or freeze-dried drug, and diluent separately in a single package. The drug, or lyophilized drug, is contained in a glass bottle, and the reconstitution liquid is contained in a plastic bottle. Prior to use, the liquid contents are transferred into the glass bottle by rupturing a membrane, and a drug solution is produced by mixing prior to administration.

Semisolid Gels and Ointments
Semisolid products have been traditionally packed in collapsible tin tubes. Metal tubes are a potential source of metal particles in ophthalmic products, and so the tubes have to be cleaned carefully prior to sterilization. Also, the final product must meet limits for the number of metal particles found. Plastic tubes are not suitable because of their noncollapsible nature, which causes air to enter the tube after withdrawal of each dose. However, collapsible tubes made from laminates of plastic, aluminum foil, and paper are a good alternative to tin tubes. Laminated tubes fitted with polypropylene caps can be sterilized by autoclaving, whereas tubes fitted with polyethylene caps are sterilized by gamma irradiation. The tubes are usually filled aseptically, sealed with an adhesive, and then crimped.

Design Specifications and Critical Quality Parameters
In addition to the design selection criteria, there are some other design specification criteria and critical quality parameters that should be emphasized.

Ophthalmic products should comply with compendial requirements specified for the territory in which the product is to be registered. Reference to the major pharmacopoeias (European, U.S., and Japanese) should highlight the majority of requirements. The EP offers the most detailed guidance for the different types of preparations, eye drops, eye lotions, semisolid preparations, or ophthalmic inserts. There are also pharmacopoeial requirements relating to the container to be used, which have already been discussed in the previous section on pack design considerations. One very important design requirement worth stressing is that the container/ delivery system be easy to use. Glaucoma is a common eye condition affecting many elderly patients who may have poor eyesight and manual dexterity, and thus are not capable of administering a complex delivery system. Design of a new delivery system should include consumer trials and customer feedback to ensure that the new device is acceptable.

All ophthalmic products are required to be sterile up to the point of use and must comply with the pharmacopoeial tests for sterility. Terminal sterilization is the preferred method from a regulatory point of view, as opposed to aseptic manufacture. If terminal sterilization is not used, for example, because the drug substance cannot withstand the processing conditions, good supporting documentation will be required to gain regulatory approval (also see a later section on ophthalmic processing).

The advantage of using established excipients, which have been used previously in registered ophthalmic products, has been emphasized previously in this book (see chap. 5). A list of excipients used previously in registered ophthalmic products is available from various reference sources (e.g., those listed in Table 3, chap. 8, "Product Optimization"). Another advantage of using established excipients in a topically applied formulation is to improve the chance of patient tolerability and patient compliance. An essential product design requirement is to minimize ocular side effects such as irritation, burning, stinging, and blurring of vision, any of which may provide a reason for patients to stop their medication.

Typical finished product specification and control tests for an ophthalmic multidose (preserved) solution product, required to demonstrate that the product is of a quality suitable for the intended use, may include the following:

- Appearance: description, for example, clear, colored, absence of foreign particles
- Identification test(s) for drug
- Quantitative drug assay/impurities and degradation products: limits based on analytical capability and stability data
- Quantitative preservative assay: limits based on analytical capability and levels required for antimicrobial preservative efficacy
- pH: limits based on stability, solubility, and physiological acceptability
- Osmolality: limits based on physiological acceptability
- Volume/weight of contents: to ensure that label claim number of doses can be dispensed, but not more than 10 µL, unless otherwise justified
- Sterility

Additional tests would be required for an ophthalmic suspension or other type of dosage form. Such tests might be one for particle size and one to show whether the suspension sediments can be readily dispersed on shaking to enable the correct dose to be delivered.

Finally, as for any pharmaceutical product, ophthalmic products have to be designed to be stable. Ideally, the product should be stable at room temperature over a shelf life of two to three years. Multidose products must also be stable, after opening the pack, over the period of use. If antimicrobial preservatives are included to maintain sterility over this period, the effectiveness of the chosen preservative has to be demonstrated. There must be a discard statement on the label of multidose products, indicating that the contents must not be used after a stated period. Normally, this does not exceed 28 days after opening the pack, unless there is a good justification.

PRODUCT OPTIMIZATION CONSIDERATIONS

The exact product optimization studies to be conducted will depend on the type of ophthalmic dosage form to be developed (liquid drops, semisolid gel/ointment, or solid device). However,

Table 3 Formulation Components Used in Common Ophthalmic Dosage Forms

Component	Solution	Suspension	Gel	Ointment	Insert
Drug	Y	Y	Y	Y	Y
Drug carrier	O	O	O	O	O
Water	Y	Y	Y		O
Buffering agent	Y	Y	Y		
Tonicity agent	O	O	O		
Antimicrobial preservative	Y	Y	Y	Y	
Viscosity modifier	O	O			
Solubilizer	O		O		
Salts	O	O	O		O
Bioadhesive agent	O	O	O		O
Suspending agent		Y			
Phase modifier				Y	
Permeation enhancer	O	O	O		O
Cross-linked polymer					Y
Wax/oil/petrolatum				Y	

(Y) Component is included, (O) Component optional.
Source: From Lang (1995).

the dosage form type should be clearly defined from the product design evaluation and supporting preformulation studies, to enable the formulator to focus on the most relevant product optimization studies.

The physicochemical properties of the drug gained from preformulation studies are often the most significant determinant of the dosage form type to be developed. Preformulation data on drug solubility, lipophilicity, charge, degree of ionization, compatibility with other excipients and packaging components will all be relevant.

Depending on the basic physicochemical properties of the drug, a variety of different components may have to be included in the formulation to achieve the target pharmaceutical product profile required. An important recommendation for any formulation developed is to keep it as simple as possible, adding only components that are required to serve a clear function in the product. This is also true for ophthalmic products, but because of the wide-ranging design requirements, it can be difficult to achieve in practice. The complexity of ophthalmic formulation development is illustrated in Table 3, which shows typical components included in different types of conventional ophthalmic dosage forms, taken from a review by Lang (1995). Some components will always be included in the formulation, indicated by a Y in Table 5. Other components are optional, indicated by an O.

Further discussion about the considerations for formulation development of conventional ophthalmic dosage is given below.

Ocular Solutions
Solubility
The advantages of solution ophthalmic products over multiphase systems have been emphasized in section "Product Design Considerations". If the tear film concentration of the drug is too low because of poor drug solubility, the rate of absorption may not be sufficient to achieve adequate tissue levels of drug in the eye.

For compounds possessing a low aqueous solubility, there are several approaches that can be used to enhance the concentration of the drug in solution. Many drugs are weak bases or acids and can be formulated as water-soluble, pharmaceutically acceptable salts. Ideally, salt selection should be fixed during preclinical candidate selection. It is not a good idea to change the salt form during clinical development because it could result in significant changes to the drug absorption and bioavailibility profiles and may result in the need to do additional human bioavailability studies (for more information about salt selection, refer to chap. 3 on preformulation).

Manipulation of formulation pH Generally, the eye can tolerate eye preparations formulated over a range of pH values as low as 3.5 and as high as pH 9. However, it is preferable to formulate as close to physiological pH values as possible (pH 7.4), or at slightly alkaline pH values, to minimize the potential for pH-induced lacrimation, eye irritation, and discomfort (Meyer and McCulley, 1992). If it is necessary to formulate at the extremes of the above pH range, for example, to maintain stability of the drug or to achieve optimum antimicrobial preservative efficacy, the buffer strength should be kept to a minimum to reduce buffer irritation effects (Allergan Pharmaceuticals, 1969). The majority of drugs exhibit a pH–solubility profile, and the pH of optimum solubility is determined from preformulation studies. However, a greater degree of corneal permeation is observed when drugs are formulated at a pH providing a higher concentration of unionized drug, which may be away from the pH–solubility optimum.

Another important consideration when selecting the optimum formulation pH is the drug stability for pH-sensitive drugs, such as peptides and proteins. Also, pH might affect the function of other components in the formulation. For example, the antimicrobial preservative, parabens (parahydroxybenzoic acid derivatives), is inactive at alkaline pH and more active as the pH becomes more acid. Another example is the viscosity of aqueous ophthalmic gels formulated with acrylic acid polymers (carbomer), Carbopol™ resins (BFGoodrich), which are particularly sensitive to pH changes. To maintain a low viscosity in the dosing solutions, the pH is typically in the 4 to 5 range. When placed in the eye, the immediate increase in pH causes a rapid gellation, which results in an increase in the residence time and bioavailability.

A variety of regulatory approved buffers are available covering the useful pH range. For acidic pH adjustment, acetic acid/sodium acetate or citric acid/sodium citrate are often employed. For alkaline-buffered solutions, phosphate or borate buffers are frequently used.

If pH manipulation fails to increase the drug solubility sufficiently, the next logical step is to try adding solubility-enhancing materials to the formulation. The choice of approved materials for use in ophthalmic products is somewhat limited because of the irritation potential of many adjuvants. Cosolvents, for example, are not generally acceptable. Materials approved and typically used include polyethylene glycols, propylene glycol, polyvinyl alcohol, poloxamers, glycerin, cellulose derivatives, and surfactants. For a complete list of adjuvants approved for use in ophthalmic products, the formulator should refer to one of the inactive ingredient guides listed in Table 3, chapter 8, "Product Optimization".

Cyclodextrins and their derivatives, which can form inclusion complexes with some drugs, have shown promising results in rabbit studies. Both drug solubility and/or ocular bioavailability are increased, and sometimes tolerability is improved. However, the properties of cyclodextrins in ophthalmic drug delivery are poorly understood, and their benefits are still to be proven in the clinic (Jarvinen et al., 1995; Shimpi et al., 2005).

If the desired aqueous solubility is not achievable by any means, then alternatively, an oily solution or emulsion formulation could be considered. These systems rely on the drug partitioning out of the oily phase available in the eye, and are generally not as well tolerated as aqueous-based delivery systems. For these reasons, aqueous suspension formulations are probably preferred to oily vehicles, employing very small drug particles to encourage dissolution and drug availability in the eye.

Osmolarity

Ophthalmic products instilled into the eye may be tolerated over a fairly wide range of tonicity (0.5–1.5% NaCl equivalents; Hind and Goyan, 1950). However, to minimize irritation and discomfort, ophthalmic solutions should ideally be isotonic with the tears, equivalent to 0.9% w/v solution of sodium chloride.

Hypotonic ophthalmic solutions or suspensions can be rendered isotonic by the addition of tonicity agents such as sodium chloride, potassium chloride, dextrose, glycerol, and buffering salts. As with other adjuvants, the formulator should give due consideration to possible interactions between the tonicity agent and other components of the formulation, including the active ingredient itself.

Table 4 FDA-Approved Ophthalmic Viscosity-Enhancing Agents

Viscosity enhancer	Typical concentration range (%)
Methylcellulose	0.2–2.5
Hydroxypropyl cellulose	0.2–2.5
Hydroxypropyl methylcellulose	0.2–2.5
Hydroxyethylcellulose	0.2–2.5
Carboxymethylcellulose sodium	0.2–2.5
Polyvinyl alcohol	0.1–5.0
Povidone	0.1–2.0
Polyethylene glycol 400	0.2–1.0
Carbomer 940/934P	0.05–2.5[a]
Poloxamer 407	0.2–5.0

[a]Capable of forming a very stiff gel depending on the concentration of the polymer and the pH.

Vehicle Viscosity

It is generally agreed that an increase in vehicle viscosity increases the residence time in the eye, although there are conflicting reports in the literature to support the optimal viscosity for ocular bioavailability (Seattone et al., 1991). Products formulated with a high viscosity are not well tolerated in the eye, causing lacrimation and blinking until the original viscosity of the tears is regained. Drug diffusion out of the formulation into the eye may also be inhibited because of high product viscosity. Finally, administration of high-viscosity liquid products tends to be more difficult. Therefore, most commercial liquid eye drop products are adjusted to within the range of 10 to 25 cP, using an appropriate viscosity-enhancing agent.

Ophthalmic ointments are designed to be of very high viscosity to prolong the residence time in the eye, compared to solutions and suspensions. However, ointments are the least tolerated and so tend to be restricted to application at night when the patient is asleep.

A list of regulatory approved synthetic viscosity-enhancing agents, with typical concentrations used in aqueous ophthalmic formulations, is given in Table 4. There are also a variety of naturally occurring viscosity enhancers such as xanthan gum, alginates, and gelatin, but these are not as popular as the synthetic alternatives because they are good mediums for microbial growth. Some viscosity-enhancing agents, such as carbomer 940 and hydroxyethylcellulose, also possess mucoadhesive properties, which will contribute to increasing the residence time in the eye. Cellulose derivatives may also provide the product with lubrication properties by reducing the friction between the cornea and the eyelids. The reversible thermosetting properties of poloxamers (particularly poloxamer 407) can be exploited to provide a low-viscosity free-flowing liquid at room temperature suitable for easier administration to the eye. On contact with the eye, a viscous gel is produced which prolongs the residence time of the drug in the eye.

Stabilizers

For drugs that are susceptible to oxidative degradation, stabilizers such as antioxidants and/or chelating agents can be included in the formulation to improve the product shelf life. The use of plastic bottles, which allow gases to permeate through the container, will be particularly susceptible to oxidative degradation. Oxidation reactions are often catalyzed in the presence of heavy metal ions, and so chelating agents such as disodium edetate (EDTA) are often included to complex with any metal ions.

There are a variety of regulatory approved antioxidants commonly used in liquid ophthalmic products, such as sodium metabisulfite, sodium sulfite, ascorbic acid, acetylcysteine, 8-hydroxyquinoline, and antipyrine.

Antimicrobial Preservatives

Ophthalmic products have to be manufactured sterile and be free from microorganisms. Once opened, the sterility of a multidose product must be maintained during its period of use. This is usually required for at least four weeks, after which the product is discarded. If the drug itself does not possess antimicrobial properties, then an antimicrobial preservative must be included in the formulation to ensure that any microorganisms accidentally introduced during use are destroyed.

There are a limited number of regulatory approved antimicrobial preservatives that can be used in ophthalmic products, and some of these are becoming less favored because of increasing awareness of ocular toxicity concerns following the repeated administration of a multidose product (Vanrell, 2007). Therefore, it can be a challenging exercise for the formulator to find a preservative to use with the following attributes:

- Effective at the optimal formulation pH
- Stable to processing, possibly heat sterilization
- Stable over the product shelf life
- Does not physically interact with other components in the formulation
- Does not interact with the pack components

A list of commonly used antimicrobial preservatives suitable for ophthalmic formulations with recommended concentration ranges is shown in Table 5. The use of methyl- and propylparabens, thimerosal, and other mercurial preservatives has decreased in recent years because of adverse reactions associated with their use (Wade and Weller, 1994).

By far, the most widely used antimicrobial preservative in ophthalmics is BKC. It is often used in combination with EDTA because of the synergistic effects, allowing lower concentrations of BKC to be used. Even the use of BKC has been questioned because of some evidence of eye toxicity in rabbits (Dormans and van Logten, 1982), and some people have developed hypersensitivity to this preservative. However, BKC does possess good pharmaceutical properties, being stable in solution, stable to autoclaving, and at the usual concentration of 0.01%, is an effective preservative over the range of pH values typically used in ophthalmic formulations.

BKC is a mixture of alkylbenzyl dimethylammonium chlorides of different alkyl chain lengths, containing even carbon numbers from C8 to C18, mostly C12 and C14. Being cationic in nature, it is not compatible with anionic drugs, and its activity is reduced in the presence of some materials, such as multivalent metal ions and anionic and nonionic surfactants. It may still be possible to use a preservative even if there is a known drug interaction. The best-known examples of commercial ophthalmic formulations are sodium cromoglycate and nedocromil sodium interacting with BKC. Both of these drugs will form an insoluble emulsion complex with BKC because of ion pair formation between the drug anions and the benzalkonium cation. This is acceptable, because the insoluble complex can be removed by filtration during

Table 5 Regulatory Approved Ophthalmic Antimicrobial Preservatives

Antimicrobial preservative	Typical concentration range (%)
Benzalkonium chloride	0.01–0.02
Benzethonium chloride	0.01–0.02
Chlorhexidine	0.002–0.01
Chlorobutanol	Up to 0.5
Methylparaben	0.015–0.05
Phenylethyl alcohol	Up to 0.5
Phenylmercuric acetate	0.001–0.002
Phenylmercuric borate	0.002–0.004
Phenylmercuric nitrate	0.002–0.004
Propylparaben	0.005–0.01
Thimerosal	0.001–0.15

processing in a controlled and reproducible fashion. An excess of preservative is added during manufacture, leaving 0.01% BKC in the final solution, which effectively preserves the product.

Chlorhexidine is also cationic like BKC and exhibits similar incompatibilities. It is not as stable as BKC to autoclaving and may irritate the eyes. It tends to be more favored in Europe than in the United States, and is particularly used in contact lens products. Chlorobutanol and phenylethyl aclohol are also widely used in ophthalmic products. However, chlorobutanol will hydrolyze in solution, and autoclaving is not usually possible without loss of preservative activity. It is also volatile and may be lost through the walls of plastic containers.

There has been an emergence of new preservatives that do not seem to cause ocular damage or irritation, based on stabilized chloride and oxygen compounds (Purite®), as well as sodium perborate (Bartlett, 2006).

The effectiveness of any antimicrobial preservative in a formulation must be demonstrated by using specified test procedures described in relevant pharmacopoeias. In spite of ICH and attempts to harmonize, the preservative challenge test procedures and acceptance criteria are different in the major pharmacopoeias of Europe, United States, and Japan. All the tests involve mixing the preserved formulation with standard cultures of gram-positive and gram-negative bacteria, yeasts and moulds, and counting the number of viable microorganisms remaining at different time points after inoculation. The preservative is effective in the formulation if the concentration of each test microorganism remains at or below stipulated levels during the test period.

To effectively preserve a formulation, the preservative system must have a broad spectrum of activity against a range of microorganisms. Each type of microorganism used in the preservative challenge test presents a particular challenge. Pharmacopoeial challenge tests have been designed to do this, and to demonstrate that any test microorganisms inoculated are totally cleared from the formulation over the period of the test. In this respect, the USP limits must be considered to be inadequate for ophthalmic products, allowing two weeks to reduce a bacterial count by 99.9%. This is recognized in the EP test that is far more stringent, stipulating that bacteria should be reduced by 99.9% within 6 hours and cleared within 24 hours, and fungi should be reduced by 99% in 7 days with no subsequent growth thereafter.

Therefore, if the product will pass the EP test, it should pass any other pharmacopoeial challenge tests.

Standard pharmacopoeial tests are time consuming, taking up to 28 days to conduct the test and a further few days to analyze the data. During formulation optimization, when several trial formulations may have to be evaluated, D-value testing is a faster way of generating data quickly to select the preservative and optimize the concentration. The D-value (the decimal reduction time) is the time required for a reduction of one logarithm in the concentration of a test microorganism. Typically, the time taken for the concentration of bacteria to fall to one-tenth of its starting concentration can be achieved over a few hours or so if the preservative is effective. The rate of kill (D-values) for different preservative systems can be determined to provide a rank order and to aid final selection. However, it will then be necessary to demonstrate that the final formulation is effectively preserved, using the standard type pharmacopoeial challenge tests. Testing should be performed after processing, and over time, at different storage conditions. It is also good practice to test the product at and below the lower limit of the proposed specification range for preservative label claim to demonstrate that the product will retain its preservative efficacy over its shelf life. This is particularly important if there is likely to be any loss of preservative into the pack, or through the pack, over time.

It is also useful to conduct a simulated use test in which the product is opened each day and drops administered according to the dosing instructions for 28 days. The remaining formulation should pass the preservative efficacy test at the end of this period.

Ophthalmic Suspensions

For ophthalmic suspension products, the drug particle size must be reduced to less than 10 μm to prevent irritation of the eye. The product should comply with pharmacopoeial limits for the number of particles greater than the stated size permitted in ophthalmic products. The EP includes a microscopic test with the following limits: not more than 20 particles per 10 μg of the solid phase have a maximum dimension greater than 25 μm, not more than two of these particles have a maximum dimension greater than 50 μm, and no particles are greater than 90 μm. During formulation optimization, the potential for any changes in particle size due to Ostwald ripening or particle agglomeration need to be evaluated through stability testing. Excipients such as povidone can be included in the formulation to inhibit crystal growth.

Surfactants may be included in an ophthalmic suspension to disperse the drug effectively during manufacture and in the product during use. Nonionic surfactants are generally preferred because they tend to be less toxic. The level of surfactant included in the formulation should be carefully evaluated, as excessive amounts can lead to irritation in the eye, foaming during manufacture and upon shaking the product, or interactions with other excipients. The most likely interaction is with the preservative. For example, polysorbate 80 interacts with chlorobutanol, benzyl alcohol, parabens, and phenyl ethanol and may result in a reduced preservative effectiveness in the product.

Consideration must be given to establishing good physical stability of a suspension. If the particles settle and eventually produce a cake at the bottom of the container, they must re-disperse readily to achieve dosage uniformity. Viscosity-enhancing agents can be used to keep the particles suspended. Preparation of flocculated suspensions is not recommended because the larger flocs may irritate the eye.

Drug and Excipient Interactions

The consequences of having several components in an ophthalmic formulation are the increased possibility of physical or chemical incompatibilities occurring, resulting in an unstable product, or one component not functioning in the presence of another. Several examples of potential interactions have been mentioned throughout this chapter. The presence of an interaction between the drug, excipients, or pack does not necessarily mean that they cannot be used together. However, the formulator will be required to determine the extent and nature of such an interaction, and conduct sufficient testing to develop an effective formulation.

A systematic approach to formulation development of an ophthalmic product is therefore recommended, which should also meet Quality-by-Design (QbD) requirements. The product design requirements should be evaluated systematically to try and achieve the targets and limits for specification tests, such as appearance, drug solubility, pH, viscosity, osmolarity, and preservative effectiveness. By experimentation and iteration, the selection and quantity of each type of component can be established, until the acceptance criteria are met for each product design requirement. For example, in the first stage of experimentation, the requirement might be to achieve the target drug solubility. If solubility in an aqueous vehicle is insufficient, pH manipulation or the addition of various solubility enhancers can be evaluated over a range of concentrations, to establish the optimum combination that meets the design criteria. In the next stages of experimentation, viscosity enhancers and tonicity agents can be evaluated to meet the specification test limits for viscosity and osmolality. Finally, a variety of antimicrobial preservatives are evaluated, but at the same time, the formulator checks to ensure that drug solubility, viscosity, and osmolality are not significantly affected. Further experimentation and testing is continued until all of the various components have been added in this iterative manner, and the product design requirements have been met.

An experimental design approach (DoE) should be attempted to reduce the number of experiments, but this can be very complex if a large number of components are involved.

Accelerated stress stability testing of the final product, with all the components added, should establish whether there are any compatibility problems between the drug, excipients, and packaging. Stability data from accelerated studies can be used to predict shelf lives at ambient conditions (see sect. "Stability Testing," chap. 8, "Product Optimization," for more details). It is worthwhile including temperature cycling from low (4°C) to high (40°C) temperatures in the stability program, particularly if solubility enhancers have been used. For example, an experimental formulation of the anti-glaucoma drug, acetazolamide, was formulated with povidone to enhance its solubility. The product was perfectly stable when stored at constant temperatures of 4°C, 25°C, and 45°C. However, when the product was stored in a warehouse with no control of temperature, the drug precipitated out of solution because of the repeated wide fluctuations in temperature.

Administration and Use

As part of the optimization program, it is important to evaluate the ocular irritation potential of formulation prototypes. The Draize test, established in the 1940s, is the most widely used method for the identification of primary irritants. There have been modifications to the original test, but they all involve instilling a drop of the formulation into the conjunctival sac of one eye of an albino rabbit, the other eye acting as a control. The condition of both eyes is then evaluated after stipulated time periods and scored relative to the control eye. A high score indicates that the formulation is likely to be an irritant and would not be recommended for progression.

More recently, there has been much effort to replace animal tests with in vitro test models, such as isolated tissues and cell cultures (Hutak and Jacaruso, 1996). These have some advantages in that they are less costly than in vivo tests, use relatively simple methodology, and can be used to identify primary changes at the cellular level. The disadvantages are that they do not mimic the eye response, cannot be used to evaluate insoluble materials (e.g., suspensions), and the various methods differ widely in their ability to predict irritancy potential. It is conceivable that in vitro methods could be used for primary screening tests, while more standard in vivo methods are used to verify the result.

Compatibility tests with contact lenses can also be carried out in vitro. Contact lenses are manufactured from a range of materials and may be broadly classified as rigid, soft, and scleral lenses, based on differences in the purpose and material used. The potential for interaction between the drug or excipients and a contact lens depends largely on the material of the lens. It is most likely that highly water-soluble and charged materials will interact with a soft, hydrophilic contact lens. There are several consequences of this happening, including a reduction in available drug, potential alterations to aesthetics of the contact lens (especially if the drug is colored), and possible deformation of the lens polymer affecting patient vision.

The uptake and release of ophthalmic drugs into contact lenses can be evaluated with in vitro models designed to simulate the human eye. This involves soaking the contact lens in buffered saline containing drug product and continuously diluting the system with buffered saline to simulate tear turnover in the eye. Fresh drug product is instilled at the times of dosing during the day. The lens is removed for cleaning at the end of a day according to routine wear, and left to soak overnight. This can be continued over several days and the soaking solutions analyzed for drug at intervals to determine the buildup of drug in the lens.

Alternatively, a simpler in vitro study can be conducted to determine the uptake/release profile of drug, based on the FDA procedure for the assessment of uptake/release of antimicrobial preservatives that might be included in soft contact lens solutions (FDA, 1989). This test involves subjecting a range of contact lenses to incubation in a series of dilutions of drug product. The potential for buildup of drug on the lens over time is determined by analytical techniques such as high-performance liquid chromatography (HPLC), atomic absorption spectroscopy, laser fluorescence spectroscopy, or ^{14}C-labeled drug. If the uptake of drug into the lens appears to be problematic, the use of the drug product with contact lens wearers may be contraindicated, or, alternatively, a specific cleaning/soaking program may be recommended.

It should be noted that any eye product containing BKC preservative is contraindicated in patients wearing soft contact lenses. Wherever possible, wearers of such lenses should remove them before administration and allow time for the medication to be removed by the tears. Otherwise, the use of a unit-dose preparation is another option.

Finally, compatibility tests can be carried out to demonstrate that the drug product is compatible with other commercially available eye products, which may be coadministered. Each mixture is examined for signs of chemical and physical compatibility over a short period of time. These in vitro results should be validated by the successful use of the drug product with concomitant therapy in clinical studies.

PROCESSING CONSIDERATIONS

The objectives of the process design and optimization stages of product development have been discussed in chapter 8, "Product Optimization." For ophthalmic products, like parenterals, process development can be quite challenging because the formulation must be manufactured sterile. Quite often, it is discovered that some formulations cannot withstand a stressful sterile process such as autoclaving. Chemical degradation or changes to the formulation properties of multiphase systems, such as suspensions and gels, can occur. In all cases, the compendial sterility test requirements described in the various pharmacopoeias must be complied with.

There are certain expectations and requirements for "acceptable" sterile products from the regulatory agencies, particularly in Europe (Matthews, 1999) and also the United States. The Committee for Proprietary Medicinal Products (CPMP) published a Note for Guidance on Development Pharmaceutics (January 1998), and its Annex, Decision Trees for the Selection of Sterilisation Methods (February 1999), advising that, for products intended to be sterile (including ophthalmic products), an appropriate method of sterilization should be chosen and the choice justified. Whenever possible, all such products should be terminally sterilized in their final container, using a fully validated terminal sterilization method using steam, dry heat, or ionizing radiation, as described in the EP. The guidance emphasizes that heat lability of a packaging material should not itself be considered adequate justification for not utilizing terminal sterilization, for otherwise heat-stable products. Alternative packaging material should be thoroughly investigated before making any decision to use a nonterminal sterilization process. However, it could be that the drug candidate, or one or more of the formulation excipients, is not stable to heat.

For ophthalmic products, there is a dilemma because recent market trends show that flexible LDPE plastic dropper bottles are popular with users, as they offer several advantages, including ease of administration, better control of drop delivery, and lower risk of contamination during patient use; plastic dropper bottles are lightweight, yet more robust than glass. However, one disadvantage of LDPE containers is that they cannot withstand terminal heat sterilization using pharmacopoeial recommended heat cycles.

According to the decision trees, where it is not possible to carry out terminal sterilization by heating because of formulation instability, a decision should be made to utilize an alternative method of terminal sterilization, filtration, and/or aseptic processing. If this alternative route is taken, then a clear scientific justification for not using terminal heat sterilization will be required in the regulatory submission. Commercial reasons will not be acceptable because terminal sterilization offers the highest possible level of sterility assurance.

If using nonterminal sterilization methods, it is important to ensure that a low level of presterilization bioburden is achieved prior to and during manufacture. For example, the raw materials used for aseptic manufacture by sterile filtration should be sterile if possible, or should meet a low specified bioburden control limit, for example, <100 CFU/mL. Also, there should be a presterilization bioburden limit for the bulk product that is within the validated capacity of the filters used to remove microorganisms. The FDA guidance on Sterile Drug Products Produced by Aseptic Processing and Annex 1 of the EC GMP Guide Manufacture of Sterile Medicinal Products should both be referred to for further guidance (European Commission, 1998).

It will be necessary to conduct preliminary feasibility studies to establish an acceptable and effective method for sterilization of the product. There is a clear responsibility with the manufacturer to provide evidence to the regulatory agencies that the product can or cannot be terminally sterilized. Preformulation studies will indicate whether the candidate drug and proposed formulation can withstand the sterilization process using small samples of product.

There are several comprehensive texts on the sterile processing of pharmaceutical products. A book edited by Groves and Murty (1995) is particularly recommended.

Process design and optimization for ophthalmic products is discussed further below with the aid of three examples of manufacturing processes for different types of ophthalmic products, based on the author's experience.

Ophthalmic Solution Eye Drops

The first example is a multidose eye drop pack containing an aqueous solution of a drug used for the treatment of allergic conjunctivitis. The drug is a polar, ionic compound, available as a sodium salt, which is highly water soluble and has a low lipophilicity. Formulation details are as follows:

Formulation	Rationale
Drug (2.0%)	Active
Disodium edetate	Ion sequester
Sodium chloride	Tonicity adjustment
Benzalkonium chloride	Preservative
Purified water	Vehicle

Solubility of the drug in the aqueous vehicle, even at 2%, was not an issue. EDTA was included to prevent the drug from forming insoluble salts with metal ions such as calcium, zinc, and magnesium. The tonicity of the solution was adjusted to within acceptable physiological limits by the addition of sodium chloride.

Microbiological preservation was achieved by the inclusion of BKC, the only preservative found to be safe and effective. It was selected in spite of a known interaction between the drug anion and the benzalkonium cation, producing an insoluble emulsion complex of a yellow-brown color, removed by filtration during manufacture. However, to compensate for the loss of BKC resulting from the filtration process, an excess was added during manufacture, so that 0.01% w/v remains in solution after removal of the complex.

The critical process parameters potentially affecting the quality or performance of the proposed process were evaluated to ensure the consistency of the interaction between the drug and BKC and assurance of product sterility.

It was demonstrated that the drug in the formulation could not withstand terminal heat sterilization. Furthermore, the product was poured into LDPE bottles fitted with an LDPE dropper plug and polypropylene cap, which could not withstand heat sterilization either. It was therefore necessary to develop a process to sterilize the solution by aseptic filtration followed by aseptic filling into presterilized packaging components. This process was accomplished by exposure of the drug, the LDPE bottles, the dropper plug, and the polypropylene cap to ethylene oxide.

The optimized process entailed the addition of a solution of BKC to a solution containing the remainder of the ingredients. The solution temperature was maintained between 15°C and 25°C, and the mixture stirred for at least 30 minutes, to ensure that the ion pair reaction between the drug and BKC consistently goes to completion before clarification by filtration. Mixing speed was evaluated and determined not to be a critical parameter over a wide range of speeds tested. During the clarification filtration evaluation, it was found that a reduced flow rate of solution passing through the filters was important for retaining the drug–benzalkonium emulsion complex, and for avoiding excessive foaming on the surface of the filtered solution.

The clarified bulk solution was sterilized by passing through a 0.22 μm sterilizing grade cartridge filter fitted in-line and after the clarification filter. Samples taken from the sterile filtered solution showed that the BKC levels were low in the first few liters collected. This was due to physical adsorption of BKC onto the sterilizing grade filter surface. Once the filter surface was saturated, the preservative level rose to the target level. To ensure that the final level of BKC was within the specification limits, the initial quantity of filtered solution had to be discarded prior to filling the dropper bottles.

In-process controls included tests on the integrity of the sterilizing filter before and after filtration, a microbial count before filtration, and monitoring of fill volume and cap torque during the filling operation. These controls helped to ensure that the product met the required standard for sterility, that an adequate volume was dispensed into each container, and that leakage of product from the container was prevented.

Viscous Ophthalmic Solutions

A second example of a manufacturing process for ophthalmic topical drug delivery involves the cromone drug, sodium cromoglycate, used for the treatment of allergic conjunctivitis. This particular aqueous formulation was made viscous by the addition of carbomer, to increase the residence time in the eye and to reduce the dose regimen from four applications daily to once or twice daily. It was filled into an LDPE unit-dose pack using a form-filled seal process. The formula and rationale are given below:

Formulation	Rationale
Sodium cromoglycate	Active
Glycerol	Tonicity adjuster
Carbomer 940 (0.5%)	Viscosity modifier
Sodium hydroxide (to pH 6.0)	pH adjustment
Water for Injection (WFI)	Vehicle

Glycerol was used to adjust the tonicity of solution to physiological limits, in preference to sodium chloride, because the latter was shown to reduce the viscosity of carbomer solution to unacceptable levels. The formulation did not include a preservative because it was intended for single-dose application once the pack was opened.

Unlike the previous example, sodium cromoglycate was able to withstand terminal heat sterilization. However, the final product was too viscous to be autoclaved, not allowing effective heat transfer, and so a combination of heat sterilization and aseptic manufacture was developed. The drug and carbomer were dispersed by homogenization in the majority of the Water for Injection (WFI) contained in a large stainless steel mixing vessel. A thin watery dispersion that resulted was sealed in the vessel and autoclaved at 121°C for 15 minutes. The bulk dispersion was then cooled to ambient temperature (18–22°C). Filter-sterilized sodium hydroxide was added aseptically to pH 6.0 to increase the viscosity by neutralizing the carbomer. After making up to weight with the remaining WFI and thoroughly mixing, the liquid formulation was aseptically filled into sterile LDPE unit-dose dropper packs using a form-filled seal process.

A number of process parameters were found to critically affect the quality or performance of the final product. Obviously, the order of addition of the materials was important for successful manufacture. It was necessary to autoclave the carbomer dispersion before pH adjustment; otherwise the product would have been too viscous to allow effective heat transfer.

Even prior to pH adjustment, it was important to stir the watery dispersion continuously during the heating cycle to ensure that even temperatures were obtained throughout the bulk, thus avoiding cold and hot spots. It was also necessary to stir the bulk product during the cooling phase, and to use a vessel with a cooling jacket, to reduce the cooling time to an acceptable limit. Finally, the pH target of 6 was critical; below pH 6 the drug was unstable and above pH 6 produced a too viscous product for drug delivery to the eye. However, it could be demonstrated that this narrow pH window could be achieved during repeated manufacture.

Semisolid Gel Suspension

The final example of a novel process development formulation involves a semisolid ophthalmic gel containing a carbonic anhydrase inhibitor drug for the treatment of glaucoma. It is administered to the patient by extruding the gel from an ophthalmic tube into the conjunctival sac of the eye. The drug had a very low aqueous solubility. It was necessary to reduce the particle size of the drug to less than 10 µm and suspend it in a very thick carbomer gel vehicle, to increase the residence time of the gel and maximize corneal permeation. The formulation details are given below:

Formula	Rationale
Anti-glaucoma drug	Active
Carbomer 934P (2.5%)	Viscosity enhancer
Chlorbutol (0.5%)	Preservative
Sodium hydroxide (to pH 4.5)	pH adjustment
Water for Injection	Vehicle

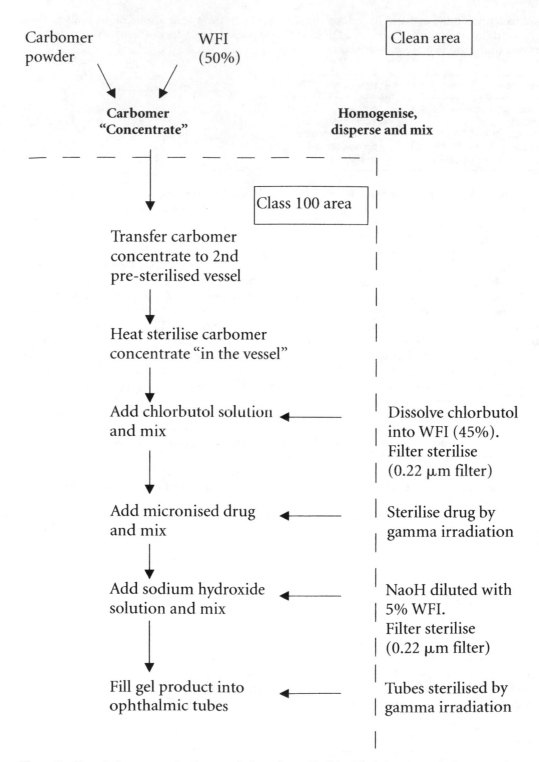

Figure 2   Steps in the process for the manufacture of a semisolid ophthalmic gel suspension.

The pH was adjusted to 4.5 with sodium hydroxide solution to ensure drug stability and an acceptable product shelf life, in addition to neutralizing the carbomer and producing a thick gel. Chlorbutol was included as an antimicrobial preservative because of its activity in this pH range.

Process development studies showed that terminal sterilization of the gel was not possible. Heat sterilization and gamma irradiation methods both caused unacceptable physical degradation of the gel and also caused chlorbutol hydrolysis. Aseptic filtration was not possible because the drug was suspended in the gel vehicle and viscosity would also have been a problem. The process described below was therefore developed with consideration of the sterilization of the product components and the maintenance of asepsis throughout manufacture.

The drug was sterilized by gamma irradiation prior to aseptic dispersion in the gel. The chlorbutol was dissolved in a portion of the WFI and sterile filtered through a 0.2 μm cartridge filter. Attempts to use heat sterilization methods caused an unacceptable loss of chlorbutol potency and also caused volatilization. The carbomer was sterilized by autoclaving a "concentrate" of carbomer in water, contained in the manufacturing vessel, whereas an aqueous sodium hydroxide solution was sterilized by autoclaving, but then added to the other components in the manufacturing vessel by aseptic filtration. The ophthalmic tubes were sterilized by gamma irradiation.

Careful selection of the processing equipment and design features was important for successful manufacture. Stainless steel mixing vessels fitted with a paddle stirrer for general mixing, and a homogenizer head for high-speed mixing of the drug and carbomer, were required, respectively. One vessel was jacketed for heating and cooling, pressure-rated to allow in situ sterilization of the contents, and fitted with ports to allow the aseptic addition of liquid and powders.

The process was constrained by the limited aqueous solubility of chlorbutol such that half of the available water was required to produce a chlorbutol solution. Also, a higher temperature of the chlorbutol solution had to be maintained. The remainder of the available water was used for the preparation of an intermediate carbomer gel concentrate ($\sim 6\%$ carbomer concentration) and the sodium hydroxide solution. Initially, the carbomer concentrate was prepared clean, but not sterile, by the slow addition of carbomer to the water in the stainless steel vessel fitted with a homogenizer head. A heavy-duty diaphragm pump was then used to transfer the carbomer concentrate (by weight) to the second steam-sterilized jacketed stainless steel mixing vessel fitted with a paddle stirrer, situated in the Class 100 (EU Grade A) sterile area. The filter-sterilized aqueous chlorbutol solution was aseptically transferred and mixed with the carbomer dispersion, followed by the drug powder and then the filter-sterilized sodium hydroxide solution. Finally, the total contents were mixed continuously using the paddle stirrer while filling the product into sterilized ophthalmic tubes. A schematic diagram showing the process steps is given in Figure 2.

CONCLUDING REMARKS

In the introduction to this chapter, the current status of ophthalmic drug delivery was discussed. The abundance of compounds in clinical development, and the recent introduction of new ophthalmic products to the market, indicates the importance of this area. The next section discussed the challenges and issues associated with ophthalmic topical drug delivery, which need to be understood if a new drug delivery system is to be successfully developed. Some novel formulation and packaging design approaches were discussed to show the progress being made to overcome these challenges.

Because of the wide variety of ophthalmic formulation types available, it was not possible to cover all aspects of every formulation type in detail. However, there should be sufficient guidance and practical examples in this chapter to give the preformulation or formulation scientist a good understanding of the subject, and to provide some direction in their endeavors to develop a new ophthalmic product. It is hoped that some of the possible pitfalls mentioned will be avoided along the way.

REFERENCES

AlGhaneem AM, Crooks PA. Phase I and phase II ocular metabolic activities and the role of metabolism in ophthalmic prodrug and codrug design and delivery. Molecules 2007; 12(3):373–388.

Allergan Pharmaceuticals. The effects of pH on contact lens wearing. J Am Optom Assoc 1969; 40(7): 719–722.

AlvarezLorenzo C, Hiratani H, Concheiro A. Contact lenses for drug delivery: achieving sustained release with novel systems. Am J Drug Deliv 2006; 4(3):131–151.

Amrite A, Kompella U. Nanoparticles for ocular drug delivery. In: Gupta R, Kompella U, eds. Nanoparticle Technology for Drug Delivery. New York: Taylor & Francis, 2006:319–360.

Bartlett JD. Ophthalmic Drug Facts. St. Louis, MO: Wolters Kluwer Health Inc., 2006.

Birch DG, Liang FQ. Age-related macular degeneration: a target for nanotechnology derived medicines. Int J Nanomedicine 2007; 2(1):65–77.

Booth BA, Vidal DL, Bouhanik S. Sustained-release ophthalmic drug delivery systems for treatment of macular disorders: present and future applications. Drugs Aging 2007; 24(7):581–602.

Borchardt RT. Assessment of transport barriers using cell and tissue culture systems. Drug Dev Ind Pharm 1990; 16(8):2595–2612.

Bundgaard H, Falch E, Larsen C, et al. Pilocarpic acid esters as novel sequentially labile pilocarpine prodrugs for improved ocular delivery. J Med Chem 1985; 28(8):979–981.

Burnstein NL, Anderson JA. Review: corneal penetration and ocular availability of drugs. J Ocul Pharmacol 1985; 1:309–326.

Chrai SS, Robinson JR. Ocular evaluation of methylcellulose vehicle in albino rabbits. J Pharm Sci 1974; 63:1218–1223.

Conway BR. Recent patents on ocular drug delivery systems. Recent Pat Drug Deliv Formul 2008; 2(1):1–8.

CPMP. Note for guidance on development pharmaceutics and annex (1999) decision trees for the selection of sterilisation methods. Brussels, Belgium: Committee for Proprietary Medicinal Products, 1998.

Del Amo EM, Urtti A. Current and future ophthalmic drug delivery systems. A shift to the posterior segment. Drug Discov Today 2008; 13(3–4):135–143.

Dormans JA, van Logten MJ. The effects of ophthalmic preservatives on corneal epithelium of the rabbit: a scanning electron microscopical study. Toxicol Appl Pharmacol 1982; 62:251–261.

European Commission. EC GMP guide to good manufacturing practice. Revised Annex 1: Manufacture of sterile medicinal products. The Rules Governing Medicinal Products in the EU. Vol 4: Good Manufacturing Practices. Luxembourg: European Commission, 1998.

FDA. Guidelines to contact lens manufacturers: preservative uptake/release procedures. Chem. Appendix B. Rockville, MD: Food and Drug Administration, 1989.

Fialho SL, Cunha AS Jr. Drug delivery systems for the posterior segment of the eye: fundamental basis and applications. Arq Bras Oftalmol 2007; 70(1):173–179.

Fraunfelder FT, Meyer SM. Drug-Induced Ocular Side Effects and Drug Interactions. 3rd ed. Portland, OR: Oregon Health Sciences University, 1989:476–480.

Glasspool M, ed. Eyes: Their Problems and Treatments. London: Martin Dunitz, 1984:11.

Groves MJ, Murty R, eds. Aseptic Pharmaceutical Manufacturing II: Applications for the 1990s. Vol 2. Buffalo Grove, IL: Interpharm Press, Inc., 1995.

Hind H, Goyan F. Contact lens solutions. J Am Pharm Assoc 1950; 11:732.

Hornof M, Weyenberg W, Lugwig A, et al. Mucoadhesive ocular insert based on thiolated poly(acrylic acid): development and *in vivo* evaluation in humans. J Control Release 2003; 89:419–428.

Hsu J. Drug delivery methods for posterior segment disease. Curr Opin Ophthalmol 2007; 18(3):235–239.

Hutak CM, Jacaruso RB. Evaluation of primary ocular irritation: alternatives to the Draize test. In: Reddy IK, ed. Ocular Therapeutics and Drug Delivery. Lancaster, PA: Technomic Publishing Company, 1996:489–525.

Jarvinen K, Jarvinen T, Urtti A. Ocular absorption following topical delivery. Adv Drug Deliv Rev 1995; 16:3–19.

Khromow GL, Davydov AB, Maychuk YF, et al. Base for ophthalmological medicinal preparations and an ophthalmological medicinal film. U.S. Patent No. 3,935,303, 1976.

Lang JC. Ocular drug delivery conventional ocular formulations. Adv Drug Deliv Rev 1995; 16:39–43.

Lee VHL, Li VHK. Prodrugs for improved ocular drug delivery. Adv Drug Deliv Rev 1989; 3:1–38.

Li VHK, Robinson JR. Solution viscosity effects on the ocular disposition of cromolyn sodium in the albino rabbit. Int J Pharm 1989; 53(3):219–225.

Liaw J, Rojanasakul Y, Robinson JR. The effect of drug charge type and charge density on corneal transport. Int J Pharm 1992; 88:111–124.

Loftsson T, Sigurdsson HH, Konradsdottir F. Topical drug delivery to the posterior segment of the eye: anatomical and physiological considerations. Pharmazie 2008; 63(3):171–179.

Matthews BR. Recent developments in the European regulation of ophthalmic, parenteral and other sterile products. Eur J Parenter Sci 1999; 4(3):103–109.

Maurice DM, Mishima S. Ocular pharmacokinetics. In: Sears ML, ed. Pharmacology of the Eye, Handbook of Experimental Pharmacology. Vol 69. Berlin-Heidelberg: Springer-Verlag, 1984:19–116.

Meisner D, Mezei M. Liposomal ocular delivery systems. Adv Drug Deliv Rev 1995; 16:75–93.

Merkli A, Tabatabay C, Gurny R. Use of insoluble biodegradable polymers in ophthalmic systems for the sustained release of drugs. Eur J Pharm Biopharm 1995; 41(5):271–283.

Meyer DR, McCulley JP. pH tolerance of rabbit corneal epithelium in tissue culture. J Toxicol Cutan Ocul Toxicol 1992; 11(1):15–30.

Patton TF. Ophthalmic Drug Delivery Systems. Washington, DC: American Pharmaceutical Association, 1980.

Robinson JR, Mylnek CM. Bioadhesive and phase change polymers for ocular drug delivery. Adv Drug Deliv Rev 1995; 16:45–50.

Rojanasakul Y, Wang L-Y, Bhat M, et al. The transport barrier of epimelia: a comparative study on membrane permeability and charge selectivity in the rabbit. Pharm Res 1992; 9:1029–1034.

Rozier A, Mazuel C, Grove J, et al. Gelrite: a novel, ion-activated, in-situ gelling polymer for opthalmic vehicles. Effect on bioavailability of timolol. Int J Pharm 1989; 57:163–168.

Saettone MF, Salminen L. Ocular inserts for topical delivery. Adv Drug Deliv Rev 1995; 16:95–106.

Schell JW. Relationship between steroid permeability across excised rabbit cornea. Surv Ophthalmol 1982; 27:217–218.

Schoenwald RD, Ward R. Relationship between steroid permeability across excised rabbit cornea and octanol–water partition coefficients. J Pharm Sci 1978; 67:786–788.

Seattone MF, Giannaccini P, Chetoni P, et al. Evaluation of high- and low-molecular-weight fractions of sodium hyaluronate and an ionic complex as adjuvants for topical ophthalmic vehicles containing pilocarpine. Int J Pharm 1991; 72:131–139.

Shimpi S, Chauhan B, Shimpi P. Cyclodextrins: applications in different routes of drug administration. Acta Pharm 2005; 55:139–156.

Sieg JW, Robinson JR. Vehicle effects on ocular drug bioavailability. 1. Evaluation of fluorometholone. J Pharm Sci 1975; 64:931–936.

Suhonen P, Jarvinen T, Lehmussaari K, et al. Ocular absorption and irritation of pilocarpine prodrug is modified with buffer, polymer, and cyclodextrin in the eyedrop. Pharm Res 1995; 12(4):529–530.

Tammara VK, Crider MA. Prodrugs: a chemical approach to ocular drug delivery. In: Reddy IK, ed. Ocular Therapeutics and Drug Delivery. Lancaster, PA: Technomic Publishing Company, 1996: 285–334.

Vanrell R. Preservatives in ophthalmic formulations: an overview. Arch Soc Esp Oftalmol 2007; 82:531–532.

Van Santvilet L, Ludwig A. Determinants of eye-drop size. Surv Ophthalmol 2004; 49(2):197–213.

Vulovic N, Primorac M, Stupar M, et al. Some studies into the properties of indomethacin suspensions intended for ophthalmic use. Int J Pharm 1989; 55:123–128.

Wade A, Weller PJ, eds. Handbook of Pharmaceutical Excipients. 2nd ed. Washington, DC: American Pharmaceutical Association, and London: The Pharmaceutical Press, 1994.

Wagh DV, Inamdar B, Samanta MK. Polymers used in ocular dosage forms and drug delivery systems. Asian J Pharm 2008; 2(1):12–17.

Zimmer A, Kreuter J. Microspheres and nanoparticles used in ocular delivery systems. Adv Drug Deliv Rev 1995; 16:61–73.

13 | Aqueous Nasal Dosage Forms

Nigel Day
AstraZeneca R&D Charnwood, Loughborough, Leicestershire, U.K.

Nasal spray products contain therapeutically active ingredients (drug substances) dissolved or suspended in solutions or mixtures of excipients (e.g., preservatives, viscosity modifiers, emulsifiers, and buffering agents) in nonpressurized dispensers that use metering spray pumps. (FDA, 1999.)

The nasal route of drug delivery is convenient for administering active pharmaceutical agents. These agents can be for *local* therapy (e.g., established treatments such as corticosteroids for rhinitis) or for *systemic* therapy [e.g., migraine therapies such as Imigran® (U.K.)/Imitrex® (U.S.)]. Table 1 summarizes a range of aqueous nasal products marketed in the United States and the United Kingdom. The numbers of active ingredients are relatively small, and comprise both simple low molecular mass molecules and newer peptide molecules.

For local therapy, the advantages of nasal delivery are clear. For systemic therapy, the advantages can only be realized for certain categories of drug. Typically, those agents metabolized in the gastrointestinal (GI) tract, or by first-pass metabolism, are candidates for evaluation in nasal delivery systems. The opportunity for delivering peptide drugs by this route has stimulated much research interest in recent years. There are many factors to consider, such as the physicochemical properties of the drug and the dose required for clinical effect. The rate of absorption from the nasal cavity can be quite rapid. While still slower and less dose-efficient than for intravenous (IV) delivery, it is likely to be more rapid than oral dosing in most cases. A good example is the migraine therapy Imitran® (sumatriptan). The oral dose is 25 mg, 50 mg, or 100 mg. By contrast, the nasal dose is 5 mg or 20 mg (GlaxoSmithKline, 2008). The subcutaneous dose is 4 mg or 6 mg; in this example, nasal delivery offers an improved bioavailability over oral delivery without the trauma of a subcutaneous injection.

Absorption of drugs from the nasal mucosa is also influenced by the contact time between drug and epithelial tissue. This contact time is dependent on the clearance of the drug formulation from the nasal cavity. The mean $t_{1/2}$(clearance) is about 25 minutes (90% within the range 5 to 40 minutes). The short half-life is caused by rapid clearance from the nose to the throat by ciliary movement. A typical dose volume for a nasal spray is up to about 200 μL. Larger volumes are lost from the absorptive region; they are either swallowed or run out of the nose. It is preferable to test formulation prototypes in man, rather than using in vitro or animal models, because the latter do not mimic the human nasal mucociliary clearance system and may give misleading absorption data. Additionally, only a human study will confirm whether drug metabolism is a critical factor in the nose. The physiological condition of the nose vascularity, the speed of mucus flow, and the presence of infection and atmospheric conditions [e.g., relative humidity (RH)] will affect the efficacy of nasal absorption. In the formulation, the concentration, viscosity, surface tension, tonicity, Ph, and excipients will have an effect. Finally, the delivery device volume, droplet size, spray characteristics, and site of deposition will be relevant.

In summary, nasal drug delivery has the following advantages:

- Avoids parenteral administration/noninvasive
- Rapid absorption, peaking generally within 15–30 minutes
- Avoidance of first-pass effect
- Apparent permeability to some peptides
- Ease of self-administration/good patient compliance

Table 1 Marketed Aqueous Nasal Products in the United States and United Kingdom

Product/manufacturer	Active ingredient	Excipients listed	Pack/pump information
4-Way™ Fast Acting Nasal Spray Novartis Consumer	Phenylephrine HCl 1% nasal decongestant	BKC, boric acid, sodium borate	Plastic squeeze-bottle atomizer
4-Way Menthol™ Nasal Decongestant Novartis Consumer	Phenylephrine HCl 1% nasal decongestant	BKC, boric acid, camphor, eucalyptol, menthol, Tw80, sodium borate	Plastic squeeze-bottle atomizer
4-Way saline moisturizing relief™ Nasal Decongestant Novartis Consumer	Xylometazoline HCl 0.1%	BKC, NaP, Na$_2$edta, hypromellose, NaCl, sorbitol	Plastic squeeze-bottle atomizer
4-Way Saline™ Moisturizing Mist Novartis Consumer		Boric acid, glycerin, NaCl, sodium borate, eucalyptol, menthol, Tw80, BKC	Plastic squeeze-bottle atomizer
Atrovent™ Nasal Spray 0.03/0.06% Boehringer Ingelheim	Ipratropium bromide 0.03%/0.06% anticholinergic, $M_r = 430$	BKC, Na$_2$edta, NaCl, NaOH, HCl, (pH 4.7) isotonic	Metered spray HDPE bottle 70 μL dose each
Beconase Aq™ Nasal Spray GlaxoSmithKline, U.S.	Beclomethasone dipropionate 0.042% (micronized) SAI, $M_r = 521$	MCC, NaCMC, dex, BKC, Tw80, PE-OH (0.25% w/v), (pH 5–6.8)	Amber neutral glass bottle with metering atomising pump and nasal adapter *Nasal* bioavailability ~1%; *swallowed* portion ~43%
Flonase™ Nasal Spray GlaxoSmithKline, U.S.	Fluticasone propionate 0.05% w/w, SAI, $M_r = 501$	MCC, NaCMC, dex, BKC (0.02% w/w), Tw80, PE-OH (0.25% w/w), pH 5–7	Atomizing spray pump, actuations of 100 mg suspension nasal bioavailability <2%
Flumist™ Nasal Spray MedImmune, U.S.	Influenza Virus Vaccine Live	$10^{6.5-7.5}$ FFU live attenuated influenza virus reassortants of strains selected according to the dosing season	Prefilled, single-use sprayers 200 μL: Dose 100 μL per nostril
Imitrex™ Nasal Spray GlaxoSmithKline, U.S.	Sumitriptan 5 mg/20 mg 5HT$_1$ receptor antagonist $M_r = 295$	KP, NaP, H$_2$SO$_4$, NaOH (pH 5.5) 372 mOsmol/kg–5 mg 742 mOsmol/kg–20 mg	100 μL unit dose nasal spray device Nasal bioavailability ~17%
Miacalcin™ Nasal Spray Novartis, U.S.	Calcitonin-salmon 32 amino acids, 2200 IU/mL $M_r = 3527$	NaCl 8.5 mg/mL, BKC 0.1 mg/mL, HCl *qs.*, N$_2$	Glass bottles, screw-on pump 90 μL per actuation Nasal bioavailability ~3% (range 0.3% - 30.6%)
Migranal™ Nasal Spray Valeant, U.S.	Dihydroergotamine mesylate, 4 mg/mL $M_r = 680$	Caffeine 1%, dex 5%, CO$_2$ *qs.*	Unit dose nasal spray pump and amber glass vial Mean bioavailability 32% relative to *sc* formulation
Nasacort Aq™ Nasal Spray Sanofi-Aventis, U.S.	Triamcinolone acetonide Corticosteroid, micronized, $M_r = 435$	MCC, NaCMC, Tw80, dex, BKC, Na$_2$edta, HCl, NaOH *qs.* (pH 4.5–6.0)	HDPE bottle with metered-dose pump spray
Nasonex™ Nasal Spray Schering US	Mometasone furoate 50 μg, $M_r = 539$ Glucocorticosteroid	glycerin, MCC, NaCMC, NaCit, cit, BKC, Tw80, pH 4.3–4.9	White HDPE bottle and metered-dose pump
Omnaris™ Nasal Spray Sepracor, U.S.	Ciclesonide Glucocorticoid, $M_r = 541$	MCC, NaCMC, hypromellose, potassium sorbate, Na$_2$edta, HCl *qs.* to pH 4.5	Amber glass bottle and nasal spray pump delivering 70 μL

(Continued)

Table 1 Marketed Aqueous Nasal Products in the United States and United Kingdom (*Continued*)

Product/manufacturer	Active ingredient	Excipients listed	Pack/pump information
Rhinocort Aqua™ Nasal Spray AstraZeneca, U.S.	Budesonide, micronized SAI, $M_r = 430$	MCC, NaCMC, dex, Tw80, Na₂edta, potassium sorbate, HCl *qs.* (pH 4.5)	Glass bottle, nasal spray 100 μg actuations
Stimate™ Nasal Spray CSL Behring US	Desmopressin acetate 0.15% Antidiuretic hormone, $M_r = 1183$	Chlorobutanol (0.5%) NaCl (0.9%), HCl *qs.* to pH 4	Spray pump bottle delivering 100 μL Bioavailability 3.3–4.1% by intranasal route Maximum plasma levels 40–45 minutes post-dosing
Veramyst™ Nasal Spray GlaxoSmithKline, U.S.	Fluticasone foroate Micronised $M_r = 539$	BKC (0.015% w/w), dex, Na₂edta, MCC, NaCMC, Tw80, pH ~ 6	Atomizing nasal spray pump 50 μL Nasal bioavailability <1%
Vicks Sinex™ 12-Hour Nasal Spray for Sinus Relief Proctor & Gamble, U.S.	Oxymetazoline HCl 0.05% Nasal decongestant	BKC, camphor, chlorhexidine gluconate, Na₂edta, eucalyptol, menthol, KP, NaCl, NaP, tyloxapol	Plastic squeeze bottle *or* measured-dose Ultra Fine mist pump
Vicks Sinex™ Nasal Spray for Sinus Relief Proctor & Gamble, U.S.	Phenylephrine HCl 0.5% Nasal decongestant	BKC, camphor, chlorhexidine gluconate, citric acid, Na₂edta, eucalyptol, menthol, tyloxapol	Plastic squeeze bottle *or* measured-dose Ultra Fine mist pump
Zicam Extreme Congestion Relief™ Matrixx, U.S.	Oxymetazoline HCl 0.05%	Alkoxylated diester, aloe barbadensis gel, BKC, BzOH, Na₂edta, NaP, glycerin, HEC, HLe	Nasal pump bottle Delivers a "no-drip liquid nasal gel"
Zican Intense Sinus Relief™ Matrixx US	Oxymetazoline HCl 0.05%	Alkoxylated diester, aloe barbadensis gel, BKC, BzOH, Na₂edta, NaP, di-alpha tocopherol, eucalyptol, glycerin, HEC, HLe, menthol, Tw80	Nasal pump bottle Delivers a "no-drip liquid nasal gel"
Zomig™ Nasal Spray AstraZeneca, U.S.	Zolmitriptan, $M_r = 287$	Cit, NaP, pH 5.0 420–470 mOsmol/L	Unit dose nasal spray pump, blue plastic with gray cap, 100 μL Mean relative bioavailability 102% comparing oral tablet
Beconase Aqueous™ Nasal Spray GlaxoSmithKline, U.K.	Beclometasone dipropionate 50μg (as monohydrate, micronized)	MCC, NaCMC, dex, BKC, PE-OH, Tw80	25 mL amber neutral glass bottle, or 30 mL PP bottle fitted with a metering atomising pump (Valois)
Boots™ Nasal Spray Boots, U.K.	Oxymetazoline HCl 0.05%	NaP, MePB, cetrimide, levomenthol, camphor, eucalyptol, ethanol	22-mL PP bottle, plug, and cap
Desmospray™, Desmopressin Nasal Spray. Ferring, U.K.	Demopressin acetate 10 μg per actuation 0.1 mg/mL	NaCl, cit, NaP, BKC	10-mL amber glass injection vial, pre-compression pump with 20mm nasal adaptor. Fill volume 7.1 mL (60 × 100 μL)
Flixonase Aqueous™ Nasal Spray GlaxoSmithKline, U.K.	Fluticasone propionate, micronized, 0.05%	Dex, MCC, NaCMC, PE-OH, BKC, Tw80	Amber glass bottle fitted with a metering, atomizing pump.

(Continued)

Table 1 Marketed Aqueous Nasal Products in the United States and United Kingdom (*Continued*)

Product/manufacturer	Active ingredient	Excipients listed	Pack/pump information
Imigran™ 10 mg/20 mg Nasal Spray GlaxoSmithKline, U.K.	Sumatriptan 10mg (20 mg)	KP, NaP, H_2SO_4, NaOH	Type I Ph.Eur. glass vial, rubber stopper and applicator. Unit dose 100 µL solution.
Miacalcic 200 IU™ Nasal Spray, solution. Novartis, U.K.	Salmon calcitonin 200 IU (1 IU = 0.167-µg drug substance)	BKC, NaCl, HCl	Type I clear glass bottle and spray, and automatic dose-counting mechanism
Nasacort™ 55 µg/ dose, nasal spray, suspension Sanofi-Aventis, U.K.	Triamcinolone acetonide suspension, 55 µg/ dose	MCC, CCS, Tw80, dex, BKC, Na_2edta, HCl, NaOH.	20 mL HDPE bottle fitted with a metered-dose spray pump unit
Nicorette™ Nasal Spray McNeil, U.K.	Nicotine 10 mg/mL Each spray of 50 µL delivers 0.5-mg nicotine	NaP, cit, NaCl, Tw80, NNS aroma DZ-03226 (B-ionone), MePB, PrPB, Na_2edta	Glass container with pump
Non-Drowsy Sudafed Decongestant™ Nasal Spray McNeil, U.K.	Xylometazoline hydrochloride 0.1%	BKC, Na_2edta, NaP, NaCl, sorbitol	Amber glass bottle, 140 µL, PE, PP, and polyoxymethylene pump
Octim™ Nasal Spray Ferring, U.K.	Desmopressin acetate 150-µg per actuation	NaCl, cit, NaP, BKC	Type I glass vial with a precompression pump and nasal applicator
Otrivine Adult Measured Dose Sinusitis Spray™ Novartis, U.K.	Xylometazoline hydrochloride 0.1%	BKC, NaP, Na_2edta, NaCl, sorbitol, hypromellose	High density PE bottle with a PP/PE metered dose pump
Otrivine Adult Menthol™ Nasal Spray Novartis, U.K.	Xylometazoline hydrochloride 0.1%	BKC, NaP, Na_2edta, NaCl, menthol, eucalyptol, sorbitol, macrogol glycerol hydroxystearate	Squeeze bottle of HDPE and PP, with a PE nosepiece.
Rhinocort Aqua™ Nasal Spray AstraZeneca, U.K.	Budesonide 64 µg (1.28 mg/mL)	Na_2edta, potassium sorbate, dex, MCC, NaCMC, Tw80, HCl	Type II amber/brown glass bottle with spray pump
Rhinolast™ Nasal Spray Meda, U.K.	Azelastine HCl 0.1%	hypromellose, Na_2edta, cit, NaP, NaCl	PE bottle with PP cap and PE seal containing either 10 mL or 20 mL
Rinatec™ Nasal Spray Boehringer Ingelheim, U.K.	Ipratropium Br 0.03%	NaCl, BKC, Na_2edta, HCl, NaOH *qs.* to 4.0–5.0	Type I amber glass bottle, 70 µL manually activated nasal pump/closure
Rynacrom™ 4% Nasal Spray Sanofi-Aventis, U.K.	Sodium cromoglycate 4%	Na_2edta, BKC	22-mL HDPE bottle, metered-dose pump, PP cover
Suprecur™ Nasal Spray Sanofi-Aventis, U.K.	Buserelin 150 µg as acetate (157.5 µg).	NaCl, cit, BKC	Bottle with metered-dose pump
Synarel™ Pharmacia, U.K.	Nafarelin 2 mg/mL (as acetate)	Sorbitol, BKC, acetic acid, NaOH, HCl	White, HDPE bottle with a 100 µL metered spray pump *or* PVC-coated glass bottle with internal conical reservoir and Valois pump. Al crimp-on PP snap-on cap
Vicks Sinex Decongestant™ Nasal Spray Procter & Gamble, U.K.	Oxymetazoline HCl 0.05%	Menthol, eucalyptol, NaCit, Tyloxapol, chlorhexidine digluconate, BKC, camphor, Na_2edta, NaOH	15 mL or 20 mL PE/PP copolymer bottle, LDPE dip tube. Green PP screw cap

(*Continued*)

Table 1 Marketed Aqueous Nasal Products in the United States and United Kingdom (*Continued*)

Product/manufacturer	Active ingredient	Excipients listed	Pack/pump information
Vicks Sinex Micromist™ Procter & Gamble, U.K.	Oxymetazoline HCl 0.05%	Menthol (levo), NaCit, Tyloxapol, chlorhexidine gluconate, BKC, camphor, Na₂edta, eucalyptol, NaOH	Type III amber glass bottle, atomiser/metering unit 0.015 g mean spray weight. PP body, HDPE piston, PE terephthalate dip tube
Vicks Sinex Soother™ Procter & Gamble, U.K.	Oxymetazoline HCl 0.05%	Tyloxapol, cit, chlorhexidine digluconate solution Menthol. BKC, camphor, Na₂edta, cineole, NaOH	Type III brown glass bottle 10 mL/15 mL with a PP pump
Vividrin™ Nasal Spray Iris Healthcare, U.K.	Sodium cromoglycate 2%	BKC, Na₂edta, Tw80, sorbitol, NaOH	15-mL PE bottle fitted with integral nasal spray pump and cap
Zomig™ 5 mg Nasal Spray AstraZeneca, U.K.	Zolmitriptan 50 mg/mL	Cit, NaP (pH 5.0)	Type I glass vials, chlorobutyl rubber stoppers (unit dose) nasal spray device, vial holder, actuation device and protection cover

Abbreviations: BA, benzyl alcohol; BHT, butylated hydroxytoluene; BKC, benzalkonium chloride; BzCl, benethonium chloride; BzOH, benzyl alcohol; CCS, croscarmellose sodium; cit, citric acid; dex, dextrose; IPM, isopropyl myristate; HDPE, high-density polyethylene; HEC, hydroxyethylcellulose; HLe, hydroxylated lecithin; KP, potassium phosphates; MCC, microcrystalline cellulose; MeC, methyl cellulose; MePB, methyl parabens; M_r, relative molecular mass; NaCit, Na citrate; NaCMC, sodium carboxymethyl-cellulose; Na₂edta, disodium edentate; NaP, sodium phosphate, PEG, polyethylene glycol, PE-OH, phenylethyl alcohol; PE, polyethylene, PG, propylene glycol; PP, polypropylene; pov, povidone; PrPB, propyl parabens; SAI, steroidal anti-inflammatory; Tw, Tween (polysorbate).
Source: From Refs. PDR (2008) and ABPI (2008).

If the route is technically feasible, the disadvantages are few.

- Environmental conditions, infection, and inter-subject variability can lead to inconsistent absorption.
- Short time span is available for absorption due to rapid clearance.
- Local metabolism in the nose and instability of compound (especially for peptide drugs) occur.

NASAL ANATOMY AND PHYSIOLOGY

The respiratory tract is divided into regions: the nasopharyngeal airway (upper respiratory tract) and the tracheobronchial and pulmonary airways (lower respiratory tract). The anterior one-third of the nasal cavity viewed in cross-section reveals a central septum dividing the two cavities. This region, including the proximal portion of the inferior and middle turbinates, is nonciliated (Fig. 1). The meatuses are spaces formed by the folds of the two inferior and middle turbinates. In the posterior two-thirds of the nasal cavity, clearance of deposited particles occurs by slow spreading of the mucus layer into the ciliated regions along the inferior and middle meatuses, followed by a more rapid mucociliary clearance into the nasopharynx from where they are swallowed (Mygind, 1979).

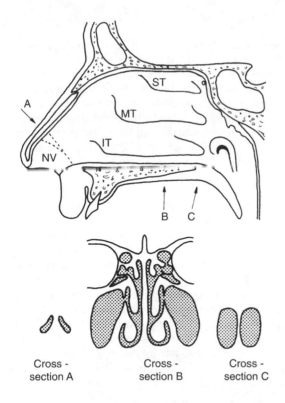

Cross-section A

Cross-section B

Cross-section C

Figure 1 The upper airways seen from the midline with cross-sections at three points (**A, B, C**). *Abbreviations*: NV, Nasal valve; IT, Inferior turbinate; MT, Middle turbinate; ST, Superior turbinate. *Source*: From Mygind, 1979.

The nose functions both as a passageway for the movement of air into the respiratory tract and also as an "air conditioner" by filtering environmental pollutants, warming and humidifying the air. Large particles trapped in the nasal filter undergo a relatively rapid clearance (i.e., minutes compared to hours or weeks for the bronchi and alveoli, respectively). In the anterior region of the nose (about 1.5 cm in from the nares), the airways are constricted on each side to a cross-sectional area of only about 30 to 40 mm^2 at the location of the nasal valve (Proctor, 1982). Subsequently, the airstream undergoes a sharp turbulent change in direction of nearly 90° upon entry to the turbinates. In vitro studies using molds of the human nose and in vivo studies in humans using gamma scintigraphy under conditions of natural breathing have shown that particles delivered by intranasal spray devices are deposited in the anterior regions of the nasal cavity primarily between the nasal valve and the ciliated epithelium (frontal turbinates) (Kim et al., 1985; Hallworth and Padfield, 1986; Newman et al., 1987, 1988). Particles impact onto a layer of mucus covering the surface, underlying which there is a layer of ciliated epithelial cells beating toward the pharynx. The site of particle deposition and the rate of clearance are of primary importance for nasally administered drugs that act locally. Particles >5–10 μm in diameter (typical of intranasal sprays) do not penetrate the pulmonary airways, but tend to deposit at their impaction sites within the upper respiratory tract. Particles <5 μm thus are regarded as respirable and are deposited within the lung. Particles <1 μm are inhaled deeply into the pulmonary airways, but undergo little gravitational settling and are likely to be exhaled without deposition during normal tidal breathing (Bates et al., 1966; Brain and Valberg, 1979). For good nasal absorption of drug to occur, dosing must be achieved in the region above the level of the nasal palate. The region below this (effectively the "anterior" visible area of the outer nasal cavity) shows poor absorption. This knowledge of nasal anatomy and the importance of particle size on deposition have enabled nasal device manufacturers to design their delivery systems accordingly. It is discussed further in the section "Device Selection Considerations."

FORMULATION SELECTION CONSIDERATIONS

There are many factors to be considered in the successful "product design" and development of an aqueous nasal formulation. A typical development program should consider the technical challenges of the molecule and balance these against the clinical and marketing requirements for the product. Several issues need to be addressed. For example, is the drug to be administered to one or two nostrils, is the drug sufficiently soluble to permit administration as a solution, and is the dose feasible (e.g., are there existing formulations for similar molecules)? If the dose levels are limited, solubility enhancement may be possible with permitted excipients, or permeability enhancers may be required. If solubility is limited, a suspension product is the only alternative, but there are more technical challenges than are present for solution products.

Preformulation and Bulk Drug Properties

A preformulation package provides essential information on the physicochemical properties of the drug, such as pKa, aqueous solubility, aqueous stability, light stability, and lipophilicity (this may predict potential for binding to plastic/rubber pump components). The pKas of any ionizable group are particularly important as they affect stability, solubility, and lipophilicity and should indicate the optimum pH for the nasal solution. For physiological reasons, formulated products are usually in the range of pH 4.0 to 7.4.

If the drug is insufficiently soluble to allow delivery of the required dose as a solution (the maximum delivered dose for each nostril is 200 μL), then a suspension formulation will be required. There are additional issues for suspension products, for example, crystal growth, physical stability, resuspension, homogeneity, and dose uniformity. Suspension products will also require information on density, particle size distribution, particle morphology, solvates and hydrates, polymorphs, amorphous forms, moisture and/or residual solvent content, and microbial quality (sterile filtration of the bulk liquid during manufacture is not feasible).

Selection of Excipients

Aqueous nasal products are listed as marketed in the United States and the United Kingdom (Table 1) (PDR, 2008; ABPI, 2008). This table shows there is a relatively limited range of excipients used and accepted by the regulatory authorities. Excipients featured in marketed nasal products in the United States are listed in Table 2 (Weiner and Bernstein, 1989; FDA, 1996). Since the first edition of this chapter in 2000, there has been a reduction in the number of marketed nasal products and range of therapeutic agents (PDR, 2008). Products containing the mercury-based preservatives thimerosal and phenylmercuric acetate have been discontinued. Some manufacturers are no longer marketing nasal products because of inevitable changes in the commercial environment. Some therapeutic agents are no longer available in a nasal presentation in the United States and the United Kingdom any more. These include butorphanol tartrate, cyanocobalamin, flunisolide, fusafungine, levocabastine hydrochloride, naphazoline, and tramazoline hydrochloride. According to the pH chosen and the ionization properties of the drug, an appropriate buffer system is usually incorporated, often a mixed phosphate buffer system. However, if it is appropriate to choose the pKa of the drug itself, then this becomes a self-buffered system. If it is feasible, there are advantages in choosing a pH equal to the pKa; during manufacturing it is easier to titrate to the target pH in the region of maximum buffer capacity (pKa). Aqueous nasal preparations are usually isotonic to ensure physiological acceptability. A choice needs to be made between ionic tonicity (e.g., saline) or nonionic (e.g., dextrose). Counter-ion effects may influence the decision on pH adjustment and buffers. Flavors or sweetening agents are sometimes added to a formulation to mask the taste of the formulation, a small proportion of which may be swallowed following nasal delivery (Batts et al., 1991). Perceptions of taste do vary with age, therefore, pediatric formulations may have to be slightly different from adult formulations. Sometimes a metal-chelating agent (e.g., disodium edetate) is included. This may also enhance preservative efficacy. Oxygen is sometimes excluded by means of a nitrogen purge, and antioxidants may also be included to improve stability. Suspension systems usually require an appropriate surfactant and viscosity adjuster.

Table 2 Excipients Used in Aqueous Nasal Products

Excipient	Function	Typical concentration
Acetic and citric acids	pH adjustment/buffer	0.12%/0.10%
Sodium hydroxide/hydrochloric acid	pH adjustment	No range
Sodium borate/boric acid		
Sodium acetate, citrate, and phosphates (mixed), potassium phosphate (mixed)	Buffer	No range
Edetate disodium	Metal chelator/preservative enhancer	0.01%
BKC	Preservative (known effect on cilia)	0.01–0.02% w/v
Benzethonium chloride	Preservative	No range
Benzyl alcohol	Preservative	No range
Chlorhexidine (di)gluconate	Preservative	No range
Chlorobutanol	Preservative (known effect on cilia)	0.05–0.1%
Methylparaben	Preservative (known effect on cilia)	0.033%
Phenylethyl alcohol	Preservative	0.25%
Propylparaben	Preservative (known effect on cilia)	0.017%
Potassium chloride	Tonicity adjustment	No range
Sodium chloride	Tonicity adjustment	0.5–0.9%
Me-OH-Pr cellulose	Viscosity adjustment	<1%
Na CMC	Viscosity adjustment	<1%
Microcrystalline cellulose	Viscosity adjustment	<1%
Ethanol	Solvent	No range
Glycerin/glycerol	Solvent/tonicity adjustment	1.0–1.8–2.5%
Glycine	Solvent/tonicity adjustment	No range
PEG (mixed)	Solvent	<5%
PG	Solvent	<10%
Glyceryl dioleate	Solvent	<10%
Glyceryl monoleate	Surfactant	<7%
Lecithin	Surfactant	<5%
Polysorbate 20 & 80	Surfactant	<2%
Tyloxapol	Surfactant	No range
Triglycerides		<2%
Menthol	Flavoring agent	No range
Saccharin sodium	Flavoring agent (sweetener)	No range
Sorbitol	Flavoring agent (sweetener)	<10% (2.5%)

Abbreviation: BKC, benzalkonium chloride.

Penetration Enhancers

For many years, penetration (or permeation) enhancers have been used in experimental studies to overcome the resistance to nasal absorption of peptide and protein drugs (refer to section "Special Considerations for Peptide Nasal Delivery"). There is a vast research literature on this subject alone, but despite this, aqueous nasal products using permeation enhancers are not currently available in the United States or the United Kingdom. Examples of enhancers used in animal studies are chitosan (Aspden et al., 1997a, b; Dyer et al., 2002), cyclodextrins (Marttin et al., 1998; Merkus et al., 1999; Werner et al., 2004), bile salts (sodium cholate, deoxycholate, and taurodihydrofusidate) (Illum and Fisher, 1997), bioadhesive degradable starch microspheres, glycyrrhizin, and liposomes. Their modes of action vary between those of bioadhesion (therefore retaining the drug at the absorption site for longer) to interference with the "tight" epithelial cell junctions. The slow introduction of enhancers into clinical products may be largely attributed to concerns over histological damage, which has been observed under certain circumstances in experimental systems (Chandler et al., 1991). Since the first edition of this chapter in 2000, there have still been no nasal products on the U.S. market, which contain a penetration enhancer (PDR, 2008). This highlights the difficulties in their introduction.

Preservatives

If a traditional multi-dose nasal spray is used, then a preservative will have to be included in the formulation and preservative challenge testing will be required [e.g., in accordance with

U.S. Pharmacopeia (USP) chapter <51> Antimicrobial Effectiveness Testing]. The test is usually performed over four weeks using 50 mL of formulation, covering five organisms. Testing is required at zero time (initial), and at the 1-, 2-, and 3-year time point of the stability program. This work must also cover concentration ranges of preservative at the limits of specification. It is important to consider the effect of pH on preservative efficacy. The most common preservatives in aqueous nasal formulations are benzalkonium chloride (BKC) and phenylethyl alcohol. BKC is often chosen because it is a good preservative, but it does have two known complications. The benzalkonium cation can react with anionic actives and can lead to a reduction in either active potency or preservative efficacy. In addition to this, it is reported that BKC can have a long-term adverse effect on nasal mucosa (Hallén and Graf, 1995). Clinically this was exhibited by increased nasal stuffiness from symptom scores and swelling of the nasal mucosa. This may be related to the observed experimental effect of BKC on nasal cilia (Batts et al., 1989, 1990; Deitmer and Scheffler, 1993; Bernstein, 2000). Preservative efficacy testing can produce variable results, and it is important to evaluate several alternatives during formulation development (Hodges et al., 1996). Some traditional preservatives are now discontinued in nasal products (e.g., the mercury-based preservatives thiomersal/thimerosal and phenylmercuric salts) because of toxicological concern with chronic use. It is vital the international acceptability of preservative is checked.

Stability and Compatibility
Both the formulation and the delivery device together need to be considered in the stability-testing program. The active must be compatible with the excipients, but in addition, *both* must be compatible with the delivery device. Stability testing must be conducted according to International Conference on Harmonization (ICH) guidelines depending on the intended territories. Specific considerations relevant to the pack are the type of bottle, plastic [e.g., HDPE (high density polyethylene)] or glass (e.g., amber), binding of active to the bottle or pump components, and the appearance of leachables and extractables from the plastics and elastomers used in the delivery device.

Processing Issues
It is essential to look forward to the manufacturing and processing issues that will be encountered during development of a nasal product, particularly the effect of scaling-up from the laboratory (e.g., 5 L scale) to stability and small-scale clinical trial (e.g., 50 L) through to production scale (e.g., 500 L). For solution products, it is important to consider the rate of dissolution and mixing time required. Filter (membrane) compatibility data should be generated, if possible using a filtration system that can be appropriately scaled-up from laboratory to production. A membrane system on the basis of polyvinylidene fluoride (PVDF), polysulfone, or polycarbonate is often chosen. The availability of this information is especially important for peptide drugs, where issues of stability and drug adsorption are often present.

For suspension products, there are particular issues already mentioned in the section "Preformulation and Bulk Drug Properties." In general, there are more issues in scaling-up suspension products than there are for solution products. Such issues are the need to "wet" larger quantities of drug, the possibility of foaming, and homogeneity during the extended time of filling.

DEVICE SELECTION CONSIDERATIONS

Following the discussion in the section on "Nasal Anatomy and Physiology," it is apparent that droplet size and spray angle from a nasal device are important data for the regulatory authorities. This section reviews the types of nasal devices available, discusses clinical studies on spray angle and droplet size, and finally reviews device testing.

Types of Nasal Device
The three key requirements of the nasal delivery device are

1. stability with the formulated product,

2. user-friendly design for patient compliance, and
3. reliability in use.

The longest-established systems typically dispense nasal drops or a crude spray via a flexible plastic "squeeze bottle." These systems are often described as "open" since they readily allow contaminated air back into the bottle after discharge. Bacteria can thus enter the system and, while the use of preservatives can minimize the risk of growth, these systems are now regarded as the least satisfactory design. In addition, the instillation of drops per se into the nasal cavity is inefficient since the drug solution is inevitably cleared along the floor of the nasal cavity, with a correspondingly short residence time. Squeeze-bottle systems that dispense a spray (as opposed to drops) have better distribution within the nasal cavity, but these suffer from imprecise dosing. Key dosing parameters such as spray angle, droplet size, and delivered dose (volume or weight) are all subject to variability because of (*i*) the squeeze pressure applied to the bottle and (*ii*) the ratio of liquid to air in the squeeze bottle (which changes significantly during the life of the bottle).

The more sophisticated devices are capable of overcoming all the typical problems associated with squeeze-bottle systems. These devices are multiple or unit-dose systems based upon a mechanical pump dispenser mounted on a glass or rigid plastic bottle. There are several manufacturers of specialist nasal pumps, most notably Becton Dickinson, Pfeiffer, Rexam, and Valois. Many of these companies have manufacturing facilities physically separated (often on different sites) from their other pump business interests (e.g., cosmetic applications). It is particularly important to ensure the highest standards are per Current Good Manufacturing Practice (cGMP) regulations as expected by the pharmaceutical regulatory authorities. A summary of some of the devices available from the major manufacturers is in Table 3. There are examples of unit-dose and multiple-dose devices. All the manufacturers offer a range of designs to cover both the adult and pediatric market. Dose counting systems are now available to allow the patient to monitor the actuation life of the product.

There are two key elements in the design of nasal spray pumps. First, it is essential the suppliers fully understand the complex nature of the plastic, elastomer, and metallic components that comprise the pump mechanism. Injection molding and the tooling dimensions must be tightly controlled to ensure consistency of component product from plastic and elastomer components. These components will often require the addition of additives such as plasticizers and lubricants during manufacture, either to ensure a smooth manufacturing process or to optimize the properties of the component in the fully assembled pump unit. Ideally, the number of different polymers will be minimized; this reduces the number of potential interactions with other components and (more importantly) the formulation. It also reduces the problems of supply-chain management. The pump manufacturers usually source all their raw materials from third parties. Once a design is established and committed to commercial production, it is essential for the pump manufacturer to have an assured level of stockpile of all the components for several years' production. It is advisable for the pump manufacturer to dual-source all raw material supplies. This is because the pump customer, the pharmaceutical industry, will have invested considerable time and money in extensive stability tests of its formulations with the specific pump and bottle system. To repeat these studies may take two to three years to generate sufficient data to satisfy a pack-change to a regulatory authority. Second, in addition to the complexities of pump and bottle manufacture and supply, there is the additional requirement to test the pack system for interactions with the formulation. This is not restricted to the relatively simple issue of adsorption of active to the container, but also the adsorption of excipients, particularly preservatives such as BKC, which are notorious for binding to elastomeric and polymeric surfaces. The other area where the regulatory authorities (particularly FDA) have shown great interest is leachables and extractables from elastomeric and polymeric components into the formulation itself. Sophisticated modern analytical techniques will not always detect these, so perhaps the best remedy is to provide data showing the levels are low and consistent from batch to batch. Precise identification of the leachables and extractables may not always be possible, but certain classes of compounds are now almost always to be avoided,

Table 3 Examples of Commercially Available Nasal Delivery Systems

Company	Device	Features
Becton Dickinson www.bdpharma.com	AccuSpray®	Based on BD Hypak® syringe system Single-use mono- or bi-dose system. Adaptable to aseptic use 50–250 µL dose per nostril. Dose divider available to deliver one dose per nostril Type I borosilicate glass/elastomeric stopper contact Spray angle: $60° \pm 10°$ Droplet size: 4% < 10 µm; 85% = 10–150 µm; 11% > 150 µm
Pfeiffer (AptarGroup Inc.) www.pfeiffer.de	Nasal pumps, screw top, crimp or snap-on	Range of standard dose volumes: 45, 50, 70, 90, 100, 120, 130, 140 µL Multidose preserved system
	AmPump®	45, 50, 70, 90 µL Suitable for highly sensitive products. Special closure fits on ampoule Preservative-free system
	Counting Pump	90 µL dose with a range from 1–16 actuations Preservative-free system
	Advanced Preservative-Free System	Range of standard dose volumes: 45, 50, 70, 90, 100, 120, 130, 140 µL Suitable for use with glass or plastic bottles Preservative-free system
	Unit dose	100 µL standard dose Preservative-free system.
	Bidose	2 × 100 µL. Other volumes can be customized. Powder system also available. Preservative-free system
Rexam www.rexam.com	SP270 Pump	45, 50, 55, 80, 90, 100, 130 and 140 µL With M17 ring, avoids use of aluminum ferrules and elastomer gaskets by plastic/plastic design Components polyethylene, polypropylene, stainless steel Integrated dip tube
	Squeeze bottles	Various simple design LDPE bottles: Kervap, Ovale, Tablet, Tentation, Delphex
Valois (AptarGroup Inc.) www.valois.com	Combidose	Can reconstitute a powder and liquid, or two liquids prior to dosing (volume 100 µL)
	Dolphin	Unit-dose device, range 50–100 µL
	Equadel	Dose range 50–120 µL. No elastomeric gaskets Screw-on, crimp-on or snap-on design.
	Freepod	Sealed system, built-in top seal Snap-on closure Dose range 50, 70, 140 µL
	VP3 Pump	Classic multiple dose range 50–140 µL Screw-on or crimp-on design Spray angle typically $43.2° \pm 1.8°$ Droplet size typically 56.8 ± 1.8 µm
	VP6 Pump	Dose range 50–200 µL No elastomeric gaskets Screw-on, crimp-on or snap-on design
	VP7 Pump	Airless multiple dose 25–130 µL Screw-on, crimp-on or snap-on design

Source: Data from manufacturers' literature.

e.g., polynuclear aromatic hydrocarbons found in the carbon black used in black rubber gaskets; these are now not acceptable for any new product applications because they are proven carcinogens.

In the basic mechanical pump, the dispensed volume (or weight) is controlled by the volume of the metering chamber. The spray angle and droplet size are controlled by the dimensions and geometry of the orifice and also by the pressure build-up in the metering chamber prior to dispensing (influenced by the spring characteristics). It is usually more convenient to document the effect of varying these (dimension/geometry/spring) on the subsequent spray angle and droplet size, and then to place relevant specification controls on the component, rather than to routinely test the product for spray angle and droplet size for the purpose of release.

Recent innovations in pump design have allowed preservative-free formulations to be developed. These have obvious advantages in the avoidance of the use of preservatives, some of which can affect mucociliary clearance and some of which can interact with active ingredients. Another benefit is that a new formulation with the advantage of no preservative will usually achieve a patent extension over the existing product. These systems can only exist if the contents of the nasal spray bottle are sealed to ingress from the environment. Two examples of the preservative-free systems are from Pfeiffer and Valois. Some systems use a sealing mechanism in the nasal actuator to prevent air from entering the container upon actuation; air is allowed to enter the container and equalize with atmospheric pressure through a microbiological filter. Another approach is to use a collapsible bag (containing the formulation) inside the rigid bottle. The bag remains sealed and clean, and displaced solution is compensated for by ingress of air into the space between the bag and the bottle. Finally, a sliding piston system can be used (analogous to the displacement of a syringe); this also has the advantage of allowing the device to be used at any angle (Bommer, 1999). Typical multidose and unit-dose nasal devices are illustrated in Figures 2 and 3.

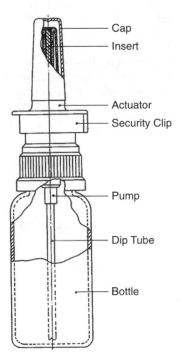

Figure 2   Cross-section of a traditional multidose nasal device.

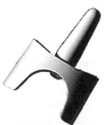

Figure 3   A typical unit-dose nasal device.

Spray Angle/Droplet Size Studies in Man

Various studies (Bond et al., 1984; Newman et al., 1987, 1988) have all found droplet size distributions of aqueous nasal spray products to have mass mean (median) diameter values between 44 μm and 62 μm. These studies showed that the majority of the dose was deposited locally in the anterior one-third of the nose. The relationship between retention time and viscosity has shown the addition of various concentrations of methylcellulose (MC) to a metered spray pump containing desmopressin resulted in a dose-related increase in mean particle size from 51 μm (0% MC) to 81 μm (0.25% MC) to 200 μm (0.5% MC), without a change in mean spray weight. The longest retention time was observed for the 0.25% MC solution, which was attributed to its particle size (81 μm) and not to an increase in viscosity, since a decrease in retention time was observed for the highest viscosity (0.5% MC) solution (Harris et al., 1988). Bond has shown that there is a curvilinear relationship between the percentages remaining in the nasal cavity versus time, with no significant dependence on the spray angle delivered to the patient over the range 30° to 60° (Bond et al., 1984). This is not surprising, since any effect of spray angle on dispersion within the nasal cavity is mitigated by the short distance (a few millimeters) between the nasal actuator tip and the site of impaction. Newman and coworkers simulated the suspension of budesonide crystals found in Rhinocort® Nasal Spray with radiolabeled Teflon particles (mean diameter 2 μm). The droplet mass median diameter was 62 μm for this aqueous nasal pump with a spray cone of 60°. Particle deposition was chiefly confined to the anterior region of the nose, with 44% clearance after 30 minutes via the nasopharynx (Newman et al., 1987, 1988). Aoki compared nasal drops (administered in the supine position) with a nasal pump spray (administered in the seated position), and found a more uniform deposition pattern for the nasal drops. However, retention time in the nasal cavity was not affected by differences in initial deposition pattern, volume administered (100 μL for spray–750 μL for drops), mode of administration (spray vs. drops), or concentration (3–30% radiolabeled human serum albumin) (Aoki and Crawley, 1976). Clearance of nasally administered drug has been shown to be biphasic, with an initial rapid phase representing removal of product from the ciliated regions, followed by a slower phase representing removal of product retained in the non-ciliated anterior region of the nose (Lee et al., 1984).

Testing of Nasal Devices
Spray Weight, Droplet Size, and Spray Angle
It is important for data on nasal sprays to include the following: (*i*) *Spray weight* variation (important to measure the amount of drug reaching the patient), (*ii*) *Droplet size* distribution, and (*iii*) *Spray angle*. Spray weight is volume dependent and is effectively a measure of the amount of drug reaching the patient for a solution formulation. The spray pump controls spray weight, and any variation should be limited by the dimensional tolerances of the pump chamber (expected to be very small). The dimensions of the orifice in the nasal actuator are considered critical to produce the droplet size distribution and spray angle. Control of these parameters is therefore best achieved by controlling the dimensions during manufacture. Once the specifications for the actuator orifice dimensions (diameter, length) are established, samples at each extreme can be manufactured (i.e., four populations at minimum/maximum orifice diameter/length). It is then feasible to test these to record the effect on spray angle and droplet size. Spray angle is usually measured by a high-speed video camera, and droplet size can be measured by laser light scattering (e.g., Malvern). Testing should be done at the beginning, middle, and end of the pack life, ideally using an automated actuating machine to eliminate operator variability. Of the three parameters measured, spray weight is the most clinically relevant, since it determines the nominal dose to patient. Methods normally used for evaluating aerosols designed for pulmonary use, such as assessments of spray plume patterns and droplet size distribution, are not generally considered useful for evaluating the clinical performance of intranasal products, because they do not take into account the unique morphology of the nasal passages. Nonetheless, for regulatory purposes, the provision of these data is *essential*.

In addition to the fundamental testing of spray weight, droplet size, and spray angle, there are a variety of additional tests to be performed as part of the development process.

Dose Accuracy

Dose accuracy over time should be recorded; this is done at the beginning, middle, and end of *delivery* life for the product. This test is usually performed during the stability test program to check dose accuracy at the end of *shelf* life.

Pump Priming

This is tested by reference to the number of shots required to initially prime the pump, and the loss of prime during a typical user test (i.e., the pump should not require repriming during normal daily use). If the product is only used intermittently, then repriming may be required.

Weight Loss

Weight loss from the bottle is important in two respects. First, loss of water vapor will affect the concentration of all the formulation ingredients, and second, the fill volume will need adjustment to ensure there are sufficient initial contents to guarantee delivery of the stated number of shots during the whole of the shelf life of the product.

Fill Volume

This is calculated taking account of the label claim (number of doses), the upper limit of dose delivered for each actuation, the number of shots required to prime the pump, the moisture loss through the pack life, and the residual volume (ullage) remaining in the bottle at the end of life (affected, e.g., by the positioning of the dip tube relative to the bottom of the bottle).

Cap Removal Torque

This test is designed to measure the potential for leakage during product life. Cap *on* and *off* torques are measured at zero time, and also during the period of the stability-testing program.

Supplier Issues

It should be assumed that the regulatory authorities will question as much, if not more, the nasal delivery device, rather than the formulation per se. They will critically examine for equivalence between the nasal device used in clinical trials and that proposed for the market. As the nasal device is usually more complicated in design than the formulation and is manufactured by a third party, it is absolutely essential to work closely with the device provider. Some of the key questions to ask of the supplier are the following:

- What is the composition of *every* component of the device (formulation contact and noncontact)?
- Is there dual sourcing in place for all the components?
- What is the component stockpile?
- What are the dimensional tolerances of all the components?
- Is microscopic surface analysis (i.e., low-power electron microscopy) performed routinely?
- Is a legally binding supply contract in place to control *all* of the above?
- Does the supplier have a Drug Master File (DMF)?
- Is this a new device, never before released on the market (i.e., are you developing both a new pharmaceutical formulation and a new delivery device simultaneously)?

REGULATORY ASPECTS

Many of the points raised in this section have been mentioned in the earlier sections on formulation and device. The FDA issued the document "Guidance for Industry" during 2002: "Nasal Spray and Inhalation Solution, Suspension, and Spray Drug Products—Chemistry, Manufacturing and Controls Documentation" (FDA, 2002). This document provides a plethora of information on issues FDA will consider in documentation submitted supporting the approval of nasal products, and is essential reading.

It is stated that nasal sprays have unique characteristics with respect to formulation, container-closure system, manufacturing, in-process and final controls, and stability. The product must deliver reproducible doses during its whole life. Excipient controls are discussed in the FDA draft guidance; in many respects, the CMC (Chemistry, Manufacturing and Controls) standards expected of excipients are starting to approach those required of the active pharmaceutical ingredient (API).

Test parameters are discussed in the FDA draft guidance. These include appearance, color, clarity, identification, drug content (assay), impurities and degradation products, and preservatives and stabilizing excipients assay. For the device, the parameters include pump delivery, spray content uniformity through container life, spray pattern and plume geometry, droplet size distribution, particle size distribution (suspensions), microscopic evaluation (suspensions), foreign particles, microbial limits, preservative effectiveness, net content and weight loss (stability), leachables (stability), pH, and osmolality.

The Container Closure System is an important area for FDA. The FDA comments, "The clinical efficacy of nasal and inhalation spray drug products is directly dependent on the design, reproducibility, and performance characteristics of the container closure system." Also mentioned is the selection of a pump suitable for the formulation, and "compatibility of the pump, container, and closure with formulation components, should be thoroughly investigated and established before initiating critical clinical, bioequivalence, and primary stability studies." Thus, it is no longer acceptable for the formulator to delay this compatibility testing until later in the development program. The key message is for the formulator to test early and ensure equivalence of the whole product throughout the development cycle. Leachables are specifically mentioned; data on their identity and concentration in the product and placebo are required through the shelf life and also under accelerated stability test conditions. Information should be submitted on source, chemical composition, and physical dimensions of the container closure system, together with control and routine extraction tests. Acceptance criteria are also required.

The section on Drug Product Stability provides clear guidance for the formulator. The content of the stability protocol, test parameters, acceptance criteria and procedures, test intervals (long-term, accelerated, intermediate), container storage (upright, inverted, horizontal), and test storage conditions (40°C/75%RH, 30°C/60%RH, 25°C/60%RH). For products packaged in semipermeable containers, the three humidity levels are 40°C/15%, 30°C/40%, and 25°C/40%, respectively; the reason for this is to provide a challenging environment to test the moisture permeability of the container. Moisture vapor loss will change the concentrations of all formulation ingredients (and hence the delivered dose), and may even result in precipitation of the active ingredient. The FDA requires stability data from three batches as the minimum to evaluate batch-to-batch variability and also the expiry date to be based on data from full shelf-life stability studies of at least three batches of drug product.

Another section states that drug product characterization studies are required to "characterise the optimum performance properties of the drug product and to support appropriate labelling statements." These include studies on priming and repriming of the pump in various orientations and after different periods of nonuse. Also, the number of sprays required to prime the device should be determined. Resting time and temperature cycling are also discussed.

Table 4 summarizes the major testing requirements of the European Pharmacopoeia and the FDA guidelines/USP. The manufacturers of nasal sprays try to design their products to perform within the requirements of the PharmEur/FDA/USP; for example, Valois aim to produce pumps, which deliver a mean delivered dose ± 10% of target, with all doses ± 15% of target.

In summary, it is apparent there are no shortcuts to attaining regulatory approval. A formulator who dismisses the requirements of the *draft* guidelines without a strong scientific justification will give FDA an unequivocal opportunity to delay the approval while the outstanding questions are answered.

Table 4 Regulatory Requirements for Nasal Devices

	PharmEur	FDA guidelines/USP
Materials, safety	Chapters 3.1, 3.2	21CFR: Food additive regulations USP tests: Physicochemical <661> Biological reactivity <87>, <88>
Uniformity of delivered dose	$^8/_{10} \pm 25\%$ $^{10}/_{10} \pm 35\%$	
Weight loss, container closure	No requirements	Characterize weight loss Check bacterial resistance Measure light or gas contamination
Priming	<5 strokes	Measure priming
Droplet (particle) size	Suitable for nasal deposition	Measure droplet size distribution
Spray characteristics	No requirements	Measure spray pattern and plume geometry
Extractables	No requirements	Measure extractables from polymeric and elastomeric systems
Actuators	No requirements	Dimensional controls

Source: Williams, 1998.

SPECIAL CONSIDERATIONS FOR PEPTIDE NASAL DELIVERY

Peptide and protein nasal drug delivery have challenges related to their unique physical and chemical properties and comprise issues of chemical stability, loss due to physical adsorption (especially for low-dose/ high-potency molecules), and self-aggregation. The two key factors for nasal delivery of peptides are molecular mass and lipophilicity. The transitional area between a predicted "good absorption" and a predicted "increasing difficulty" of absorption is a molecular mass of about 1000 (McMartin et al., 1987). Complete absorption of a peptide, by any nonparenteral route, is unlikely. The maximum absorption expected is usually about 30%. However, there are isolated examples of more complete peptide absorption, often with the assistance of chemical enhancement. The use of chemical enhancers can have a pathophysiological effect on the nasal mucosa. As this "effect" on the mucosa is fundamental in their mode of action, the key to success will be to seek the optimum balance in the "enhancement" versus "pathology" equation.

A further difficulty with peptide delivery is the risk of metabolism during the absorption phase. This can only be assessed in a complete system; metabolic studies using homogenised cell fractions are not representative of the intact membrane(s).

Penetration enhancers are often used to improve peptide bioavailability in nasal formulations. A variety of different enhancers have been tried and they work by one or several combined mechanisms. Some act by increasing the membrane fluidity and reducing the viscosity of the mucus layer, thereby increasing membrane permeability. Others act by transient loosening of the tight junctions between epithelial cells. The types of penetration enhancers used in the research literature include the following:

- Bile salts (sodium glycocholate, deoxycholate, cholate)
- Surfactants [polyoxyethylene lauryl ether (laureth-9)]
- Chelating agents (EDTA, salicylates)
- Fatty acids (sodium caprylate, laurate, caprate, oleic acid, monoolein)
- Glycosides (saponin)
- Glycyrrhetinic acid derivatives (sodium and dipotassium glycyrrhetinates)
- Fusidic acid derivatives (sodium taurodihydrofusidate, sodium dihydrofusidate)
- Phospholipids (lysophosphatidylcholine and palmitoyl and stearoyl derivatives)

See, for example, Donovan et al. (1990a, b) and Yamamoto et al. (1993). Of these, the steroidal surfactants have been the subject of most studies, and have been examined in clinical trials. However, in most cases there are adverse reactions of a stinging or burning sensation,

Table 5 Peptides Studied in the Nose

Peptide/protein	M_r (approx.)	Species	Bioavailability
Protirelin (TRH: thyrotropin-releasing hormone)	362	Human	20–30%
Metkephamid	600	Rat/Human	70–90%
Vasopressin analogues	1000	Human	10%
Nafarelin[a]	1113	Monkey/Human	5–10% 20–30% with 2% sodium glycocholate
GRF 1-29-NH$_2$	3600	Human	<2%
Human pancreatic GHRH	5000	Human	<2%
Ovine corticotrophin-releasing hormone	5000	Human	<1%
Insulin	5700	Dog/Human	10–30% with bile salts
B-Interferon	20,000	Rabbit	<2% with 3% sodium glycochlolate
Buserelin[a]	1300	Human	Not stated
Gonadorelin	1182	Human	Not stated
Calcitonin[a]	3527	Human	Not stated
Desmopressin[a]	1069	Human	Not stated

[a]Currently marketed products in United States/United Kingdom.

discomfort, or a certain degree of pain, indicative of irritation potential. In experimental studies, the use of penetration enhancers is often accompanied by pathohistological changes to the nasal mucosa (Chandler et al., 1991). The use of cyclodextrins to improve the nasal absorption of insulin has been demonstrated in rats (Merkus et al., 1991).

One reason for poor absorption by the nasal route may be the rapid removal of the drug from the site of absorption by mucociliary clearance (Dondeti et al., 1996; Quraishi et al., 1997). Bioadhesive gels adhere to the mucus and can reduce clearance and improve bioavailability. Microcrystalline cellulose, hydroxypropyl cellulose, and neutralized Carbopol 934 have all shown different degrees of enhancement of nasal absorption of insulin in the dog. Bioadhesive starch microspheres have also shown enhanced absorption of desmopressin in sheep (Critchley et al., 1994). Gamma scintigraphy has been used to study microsphere clearance in man, and great differences have been observed. Starch microspheres have been used for nasal delivery of insulin in the rat with a bioavailability of about 30% (Björk et al., 1988). Combinations of an absorption enhancer and a bioadhesive agent have been shown to provide a synergistic improvement in bioavailability (Dondeti et al., 1996).

Freeze-dried preparations are generating a lot of interest for peptides because of potentially improved stability, the avoidance of preservatives that can have a damaging effect on nasal mucosa during chronic treatment, and improved bioavailability. There are devices to deliver the powder but this concept is still at the research stage and is likely to be expensive to market.

Successful nasal delivery of peptide compounds has led to a number of peptide drugs marked for systematic absorption, for example, buserelin (Suprefact®, Hoechst), calcitonin (Miacalcic®, Sandoz), nafarelin (Synarel®, Syntex), and desmopressin acetete (Minirin®, Ferring). Vaccines can also be delivered by the intranasal route, an example being live attenuated influenza virus (FluMist®, Medimmune). Table 5 summarizes the characteristics of some peptides studied in the nose.

REFERENCES

ABPI. Data Sheet Compendium. London: Association of the British Pharmaceutical Industry, 2008.

Aoki FY, Crawley JCW. Distribution and removal of human serum albumin-technetium 99m instilled intranasally. Br J Clin Pharmacol 1976; 3:869–878.

Aspden T, Illum L, Skaugrud O. The effect of chronic nasal application of chitosan solutions on cilia beat frequency in guinea pigs. Int J Pharm 1997a; 153:137–146.

Aspden T, Mason JTD, Jones NS, et al. Chitosan as a nasal delivery system: the effect of chitosan solutions on *in vitro* and *in vivo* mucociliary transport rates in human turbinates and volunteers. J Pharm Sci 1997b; 86:509–513.

Bates DV, Fish BR, Hatch TF, et al. Deposition and retention models for internal dosimetry of the human respiratory tract. Task group on lung dynamics. Health Phys 1966; 12:173–207.

Batts AH, Marriott C, Martin GP, et al. The effect of some preservatives used in nasal preparations on mucociliary clearance. J Pharm Pharmacol 1989; 41:156–159.

Batts AH, Marriott C, Martin GP, et al. The effect of some preservatives used in nasal preparations on the mucus and ciliary components of mucociliary clearance. J Pharm Pharmacol 1990; 42:145–151.

Batts AH, Marriott C, Martin GP, et al. The use of radiolabelled saccharin to monitor the effect of the preservatives thiomersal, benzalkonium chloride and EDTA on human nasal clearance. J Pharm Pharmacol 1991; 43:180–185.

Bernstein IL. Is the use of benzalkonium chloride as a preservative for nasal formulations a safety concern? A cautionary note based on compromised mucociliary transport. J Allergy Clin Immunol 2000; 105:39–44.

Björk E, Edman P. Degradable starch microspheres as a nasal delivery system for insulin. Int J Pharm 1988; 47:233–236.

Bommer R. Advances in nasal drug delivery technology. Pharm Tech Eur 1999; 11:26–33.

Bond SW, Hardy JG, Wilson CG. Deposition and clearance of nasal sprays. In: Aiache JM, Hirtz J, eds. Proceedings of the Second European Congress of Biopharmaceutics and Pharmacokinetics, Salamanca, April 1984, 93–98.

Brain JD, Valberg PA. Deposition of aerosol in the respiratory tract. Am Rev Respir Dis 1979; 120:1325–1373.

Chandler SG, Illum L, Thomas NW. Nasal absorption in the rat. I: A method to demonstrate the histological effects of nasal formulations. Int J Pharm 1991; 70:19–27.

Critchley H, Davies SS, Farraj N, et al. Nasal absorption of desmopressin in rats and sheep. Effect of a bioadhesive microsphere delivery system. J Pharm Pharmacol 1994; 46:651–656.

Deitmer T, Scheffler R. The effect of different preparations of nasal decongestants on ciliary beat frequency *in vitro*. Rhinology 1993; 31:151–153.

Dondeti P, Zia H, Needham TE. Bioadhesive and formulation parameters affecting nasal absorption. Int J Pharm 1996; 127:115–133.

Donovan MD, Flynn G, Amidon G. The molecular weight dependence of nasal absorption: the effect of absorption enhancers. Pharm Res 1990a; 7:808–814.

Donovan MD, Flynn G, Amidon G. Absorption of polyethylene glycols 600 through 2000: the molecular weight dependence of gastrointestinal and nasal absorption. Pharm Res 1990b; 7:863–868.

Dyer AM, Hinchcliffe M, Watts P, et al. Nasal delivery of insulin using novel chitosan-based formulations: A comparative study in two animal models between simple chitosan formulations and chitosan nanoparticles. Pharm Res 2002; 19:998–1008.

FDA. Inactive Ingredient Guide, 1996.

FDA. Nasal Spray and Inhalation Solution, Suspension and Spray Drug Products—Chemistry Manufacturing and Controls Documentation. Guidance for Industry, July 2002.

GlaxoSmithKline. Patient Information Leaflet for Imigran®, 2008.

Hallén H, Graf P. Benzalkonium chloride in nasal decongestive sprays has a long-lasting adverse effect on the nasal mucosa of healthy volunteers. Clin Exp Allergy 1995; 25:401–405.

Hallworth GW, Padfield JM. A comparison of the regional deposition in a model nose of a drug discharged from metered aerosol and metered-pump nasal delivery systems. J Allergy Clin Immunol 1986; 77:348–353.

Harris AS, Svensson E, Wagner ZG, et al. Effect of viscosity on particle size, deposition, and clearance of nasal delivery systems containing desmopressin. J Pharm Sci 1988; 77:405–408.

Hodges NA, Denyer SP, Hanlon GW, et al. Preservative efficacy tests in formulated nasal products: reproducibility and factors affecting preservative efficacy. J Pharm Pharmacol 1996; 48:1237–1242.

Illum L, Fisher AN. Intranasal delivery of peptides and proteins. In: Adjei AL, Gupta PK, eds. Inhalation Delivery of Therapeutic Peptides and Proteins. New York: Marcel Dekker, 1997:135–184.

Kim CS, Eldridge MA, Sackner MA, et al. Deposition of aerosol particles in the human nose. Am Rev Respir Dis 1985; 131:A370.

Lee SW, Hardy JG, Wilson CG, et al. Nasal sprays and polyps. Nucl Med Commun 1984; 5:697–703.

McMartin C, Hutchinson LEF, Hyde R, et al. Analysis of structural requirements for the absorption of drugs and macromolecules from the nasal cavity. J Pharm Sci 1987; 76:535–540.

Marttin E, Verhoef JC, Merkus FWHM. Efficacy, safety and mechanism of cyclodextrins as absorption enhancers in nasal delivery of peptide protein drugs. J Drug Target 1998; 6:17–36.

Merkus FWHM, Verhoef JC, Marttin E, et al. Cyclodextrins in nasal drug delivery. Adv Drug Deliv Rev 1999; 36:41–57.

Merkus FWHM, Verhoef JC, Romeijn SG, et al. Absorption enhancing effect of cyclodextrins on intranasally administered insulin in rats. Pharm Res 1991; 8:588–592.

Mygind N. Nasal Allergy. Oxford: Blackwell Scientific, 1979.

Newman SP, Morén F, Clarke SW. Deposition pattern from a nasal pump spray. Rhinology 1987; 25: 77–82.

Newman SP, Morén F, Clarke SW. Deposition pattern of nasal sprays in man. Rhinology 1988; 26: 111–120.

PDR. Physician's Desk Reference. New Jersey: Medical Economics Company, 1999.

Proctor DF. The upper airway. In: Proctor DF, Andersen IB, eds. The Nose: Upper Airway Physiology and the Atmospheric Environment. Amsterdam: Elsevier Biomedical Press, 1982:23–43.

Quraishi MS, Jones NS, Mason JDT. The nasal delivery of drugs. Clin Otolaryngol 1997; 22:289–301.

Weiner M, Bernstein IL. Adverse Reactions to Drug Formulation Agents. New York: Marcel Dekker, 1989.

Werner U, Damge C, Maincent P, et al. Properties of *in situ* gelling nasal inserts containing estradiol/methyl betacyclodextrin. J Drug Deliv Sci Technol 2004; 14:275–284.

Williams G. Nasal drug delivery devices, performance and regulatory requirements – the manufacturer's view. London: Management Forum, 1998.

Yamamoto A, Morita T, Hashida M, et al. Effect of absorption promoters on the nasal absorption of drugs with various molecular weights. Int J Pharm 1993; 93:91–99.

OTHER REFERENCE SOURCES

Various papers related to nasal drug delivery. Adv Drug Deliv Rev 1998; 29:1–194.

Chien YW, ed. Transnasal Systemic Medications. Amsterdam: Elsevier, 1985.

Chien YW, Su KSE, Chang SF. Nasal Systemic Drug Delivery. New York: Marcel Dekker, 1989.

Costantino HR, Illum L, Brandt G, et al. Intranasal delivery: physicochemical and therapeutic aspects. Int J Pharm 2007; 337:1–24.

Davis SS, Illum L. Absorption enhancers for nasal drug delivery. Clin Pharmacokinet 2003; 42:1107–1128.

Newman SP, Pitcairn GR, Dalby RN. Drug delivery to the nasal cavity: *in vitro* and *in vivo* assessment. Crit Rev Ther Drug Carrier Syst 2004; 21:21–66.

Edman P, Björk E. Nasal delivery of peptide drugs. Adv Drug Deliv Rev 1992; 8:165–177.

14 | Topical and Transdermal Delivery

Kenneth A. Walters
An-eX Analytical Services Ltd., Cardiff, U.K.

Keith R. Brain
Cardiff University, Cardiff, U.K.

> Our primitive forebears had little difficulty in recognizing a disorder of the skin . . . [but] . . . when a single remedy . . . [was] . . . of no avail, it . . . [was] . . . easy and tempting to add others ad infinitum. There can be no other ready explanation for the complexities of dermatological therapy of the past and, indeed, of the present day.

These words, written by Frazier and Blank in 1954, suggested that the external treatment of skin disorders in the mid-20th century was probably as haphazard as it was in ancient times. Now, more than 50 years later, we have to ask ourselves, "Have things changed that much?" In the first edition of this book we pointed out that the advances in our understanding of the physicochemical properties of formulation systems and their ingredients had resulted in the development of physically, chemically, and biologically stable products that, after two or three years on the shelf, were as potent as they were when they were first manufactured. There were also considerable advances in our knowledge of the skin and the processes that control percutaneous absorption. The ground rules were laid down by Scheuplein and Blank in the late 1960s and early 1970s (Scheuplein and Blank, 1971), and these are updated on a reasonably regular basis (Barry, 1983; Schaefer and Redelmeier, 1996; Roberts et al., 2002; Roberts and Walters, 2008).

Thus we know, for example, that permeation of compounds across the skin is, in most cases, controlled by the stratum corneum and that it is the chemical composition and morphology of this layer that usually determines the rate and extent of absorption (Elias, 1981; Raykar et al., 1988; Elias and Feingold, 2006). We also know how to modify this barrier, by chemical or physical means, to alter the rate of diffusion of many permeating molecules (Walters and Hadgraft, 1993; Smith and Maibach, 2006; Williams and Walters, 2008).

A basic flaw, however, in the application of our understanding of the barrier properties of the skin to dermatological and transdermal therapy is that this knowledge has largely been generated by investigations on normal rather than pathological skin. It is known that the intercellular lipid profile of diseased stratum corneum is considerably different from normal stratum corneum (Bouwstra and Ponec, 2006) and the permeation through synthetic stratum corneum with modified lipid has been investigated (de Jager et al., 2006). The relevance of such information to diseased skin, where permeation characteristics are likely to be significantly altered, has yet to be fully established. Limited information available on permeation through diseased skin has been obtained in the clinic (van der Valk et al., 1985; Turpeinen et al., 1986; Turpeinen, 1991; Fartasch and Diepgen, 1992) but, for obvious reasons, this has not been systematically evaluated.

This chapter concentrates on the specific considerations that are fundamental to the development of pharmaceutical dosage forms designed for application to the skin. Many of the early pharmaceutical development stages for these dosage forms, such as preformulation and drug substance stability, are common to dosage forms designed for other routes of delivery. These have been fully discussed elsewhere in this volume and will not be discussed in depth here. In modern-day pharmaceutical practice, therapeutic compounds are applied to the skin for dermatological (within the skin) or local (regional) action, or for transdermal (systemic) delivery. Whatever the target site or organ, it is usually obligatory that the drug compound crosses the outermost layer of the skin, the stratum corneum. It is a major function of the stratum corneum to provide a protective barrier to the ingress of xenobiotics and to control the rate of water loss from the body. Evolution has generated a robust and durable membrane, which fulfills its biological function throughout the life span. A basic, yet thorough, understanding of the structure and transport properties of this membrane is essential to the rational development of topical dosage forms.

THE SKIN AND PERCUTANEOUS ABSORPTION

Skin Structure
The skin is the largest organ in the body, accounting for more than 10% of body mass, and it enables the body to interact most intimately with its environment. The skin consists of four layers: the stratum corneum (nonviable epidermis), the remaining layers of the epidermis (viable epidermis), dermis, and subcutaneous tissues. There are also a number of associated appendages: hair follicles, sweat ducts, apocrine glands, and nails. Many of the functions of the skin are essential to survival of humans in a terrestrial environment. These functions, which are both integrated and overlapping, are usually classified as protective, homeostatic, or sensing.

The stratum corneum is a 10- to 20-μm thick nonviable epidermis, consisting of 15 to 25 flattened and stacked cornified cells. Each stratum corneum cell is composed mainly of insoluble bundled keratins (~70%) and lipids (~20%) encased in a cell envelope. The intercellular region consists mainly of lipids together with the desmosomes, which provide corneocyte cohesion, as described later. There is continuous desquamation (shedding) of the outermost layer of the stratum corneum, with total turnover occurring once every two to three weeks. The most important function of the viable epidermis is the generation of the stratum corneum, which is described in detail below. Other functions include metabolism and the synthesis of melanin from melanocytes for skin pigmentation and sun protection.

The dermis provides support to the epidermis and also plays a role in regulating temperature, pressure, and pain. The dermis consists mainly of collagen fibers, which provide support, and elastic connective tissues, which provide elasticity, in a semi-gel matrix of mucopolysaccharides. The dermis contains an extensive vascular network with many arteriovenous anastomoses, which are critical to the functions of heat regulation and blood vessel control.

Epidermal Cell Composition
It is the stratum corneum, the outermost skin layer, which is responsible for the ability of terrestrial animals to exist in a nonaquatic environment without desiccation. The ability to control both loss of water and the influx of potentially harmful chemicals and microorganisms is the result of the evolution of a unique mixture of protein and lipid materials, which collectively form this coherent membrane composed of distinct domains. These domains are principally protein, associated with the keratinocytes, and lipid, largely contained within the intercellular spaces.

The cells of the stratum corneum originate in the viable epidermis and undergo many changes before desquamation. Thus, the epidermis consists of several cell strata at varying levels of differentiation. The germinative cells of the epidermis lie in the basal lamina between the dermis and viable epidermis. In this layer, there are other specialized cells such as melanocytes, Langerhans cells, and Merkel cells. The cells of the basal lamina are attached to the basement membrane by hemidesmosomes. The cohesiveness of, and communication between, the viable epidermal cells is maintained in a fashion similar to the cell-matrix connection, except that desmosomes replace hemidesmosomes. In the epidermis, the desmosomes are responsible for interconnecting individual cell keratin cytoskeletal structures, thereby creating a tissue very resistant to shearing forces.

The Langerhans cells are the prominent antigen-presenting cells of the skin's immune system, and their main function appears to be to pick up contact allergens in the skin and present these agents to T lymphocytes in the skin-draining lymph nodes. They therefore play an important role in contact sensitization. Melanocytes are a further functional cell type of the epidermal basal layer whose main activity is to produce melanin, which results in pigmentation of the skin. The final type of cell found in the basal layer of the stratum corneum is the Merkel cell. Merkel cells are closely associated with nerve endings, which suggests that they function as sensory receptors of the nervous system. Indeed, all epidermal cells (i.e., keratinocytes, melanocytes, Langerhans cells, and Merkel cells) express sensor proteins, indicating that they are all involved with the epidermal sensory system (Boulais and Misery, 2008).

Differentiation in the Epidermis

Development of the stratum corneum from the keratinocytes of the basal layer involves several steps of cell differentiation, which has resulted in a structure-based classification of the layers above the basal layer (the stratum basale). Thus the cells progress through the stratum spinosum, the stratum granulosum, and the stratum lucidum to the stratum corneum. The stratum spinosum (prickle-cell layer), which lies immediately above the basal layer, consists of several layers of cells, which are connected by desmosomes and contain prominent keratin tonofilaments. In the outer cell layers of the stratum spinosum, membrane-coating granules appear, and this reflects the border between this layer and the overlying stratum granulosum. The most characteristic feature of the stratum granulosum is the presence of many intracellular membrane-coating granules. Within these granules, lamellar subunits arranged in parallel stacks are observed. These are believed to be the precursors of the intercellular lipid lamellae of the stratum corneum (Wertz and Downing, 1982). In the outermost layers of the stratum granulosum, the lamellar granules migrate to the cell surface where they fuse and eventually extrude their contents into the intercellular space. At this stage in the differentiation process, the keratinocytes lose their nuclei and other cytoplasmic organelles and become flattened and compacted to form the stratum lucidum, which eventually becomes the stratum corneum. The extrusion of the contents of lamellar granules is a fundamental requirement for the formation of the epidermal permeability barrier. For comprehensive recent reviews of the intercellular lipid of the stratum corneum and its role in the maintenance of the skin barrier function, the reader is referred to Bouwstra and Ponec (2006) and Norlen (2008).

The majority of the protein in the stratum corneum is composed of intracellular keratin filaments, which are cross-linked by intermolecular disulfide bridges (Baden, 1979; Alibardi, 2006). In the terminal stages of differentiation, the keratinocytes contain keratin intermediate filaments together with two other proteins, loricrin and profilaggrin. Loricrin is a major component of the cornified cell envelope, whereas profilaggrin is implicated in both the alignment of the keratin filaments and epidermal flexibility. The cornified cell envelope of the stratum corneum is composed of a cross-linked protein complex, which includes periplakin and plectins, which lies adjacent to the interior surface of the plasma membrane (Boczonadi et al., 2007). The cross-linked protein complex of the corneocyte envelope is very insoluble and chemically resistant. The corneocyte protein envelope appears to play an important role in the structural assembly of the intercellular lipid lamellae of the stratum corneum. The work of Downing, Wertz and colleagues (Lazo et al., 1995; Hill et al., 2006) has demonstrated that each corneocyte possesses a chemically bound lipid envelope comprised of N-(ω-hydroxyacyl) sphingosines, which are covalently linked to glutamate side chains of the envelope protein. This lipid envelope may provide the scaffold for the generation of the intercellular lipid lamellae, the composition of which is unique in biological systems (Table 1). A remarkable feature is the lack of phospholipids and preponderance of ceramides and cholesterol. Overall, the intercellular lipid lamellae appear to be highly structured and very stable and constitute a highly effective barrier to chemical penetration and permeation.

Skin Permeability

The Relationship Between Stratum Corneum Microstructure and Barrier Function–Absorption Pathways

It has been known for some time that the intercellular lipids of the stratum corneum play a very important role in skin barrier function. This knowledge has been accumulated and confirmed in systematic studies on skin permeability of compounds of varying lipophilicity (Scheuplein, 1965; Roberts et al., 1977; Surber et al., 1993; Akomeah et al., 2007) and

Table 1   Composition of Human Stratum Corneum Lipids

Lipid
Cholesterol esters
Cholesterol
Cholesterol sulfate
Ceramide 1
Ceramide 2
Ceramide 3
Ceramide 4
Ceramide 5
Ceramide 6
Ceramide 7
Ceramide 8
Ceramide 9
Fatty acids

Source: From Gooris and Bouwstra (2007), Caussin et al. (2008), and Norlen (2008).

investigations of alterations in transepidermal water loss (Elias and Feingold, 1992; Aszterbaum et al., 1992). Because the major route of permeation across the stratum corneum is via the intercellular lipid, the rate at which permeation occurs is largely dependent on the physicochemical characteristics of the penetrant, the most important of which is most commonly the relative ability to partition into the intercellular lamellae.

Three major variables account for differences in the rate at which different compounds permeate the skin: the concentration of permeant applied, the partition coefficient of the permeant between the stratum corneum lipids and the vehicle, and the diffusivity of the compound within the stratum corneum. For a homologous series of chemicals, such as the alkanols, in which lipid/water partition coefficients increase exponentially with increasing alkyl chain length (Flynn and Yalkowski, 1972) and for permeation through a lipid membrane of fixed or normalized thickness, the permeability coefficients will directly reflect partitioning tendencies and increase exponentially. This relationship holds as long as the rate-determining step in crossing the membrane is passage through a lipid region. For a pure lipid membrane, a plot of the logarithm of the permeability coefficient versus the alkyl chain length of the permeant is therefore a straight line. However, as the stratum corneum is not a pure lipid membrane, a plot of the log of the permeability rate versus permeant lipophilicity is actually sigmoidal (Fig. 1), which reflects the coexistence of barriers of a more hydrophilic nature.

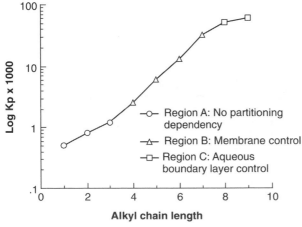

Note: The y-axis is a log scale.

Figure 1   Effect of permeant lipophilicity on the rate of skin permeation. Average permeability coefficient data for aqueous alcohol solutions through human stratum corneum as a function of alcohol chain length. *Source*: From Scheuplein and Blank (1973).

Relatively polar permeants preferentially partition into, and diffuse through, these hydrophilic regions, and there is, therefore, no lipid partitioning dependency in the initial part of the curve. There is a further loss of direct lipid partitioning sensitivity in the mass transfer process at high permeant lipophilicity (Fig. 1, region C). This is often attributed to a barrier of hydrophilic nature, known as the aqueous boundary layer, but may also represent a reduction in mobility due to an increase in molecular size. In skin, the most obvious hydrophilic boundary layer is the viable epidermis (the layer between the stratum granulosum and stratum basale). Overall, compounds with partition coefficients, which indicate an ability to dissolve in both oil and water (i.e., log P of 1–3), permeate the skin relatively rapidly.

Physicochemistry of Skin Permeation

There are three basic steps in the process of percutaneous absorption, and the first two of these are governed by the physicochemical properties of the permeating molecule. Initially the permeant has to escape from the vehicle and penetrate into the stratum corneum (step 1). This is largely a function of partition and solubility characteristics. Diffusion across the stratum corneum (step 2) is related to binding characteristics and, to a lesser extent, molecular size of the diffusing molecule. On the other hand, clearance from the epidermis/dermis (step 3) is governed mainly by physiological factors, such as blood flow.

The most important factor in step 1 is the ability to partition from the application vehicle into the intercellular lipid lamellae of the stratum corneum. The partition coefficient (K) of a drug between the skin and vehicle can be written as C_{sc}/C_v, where C_v is the concentration of drug in the vehicle. Thus, the steady-state flux (J_s) across the skin can be expressed as:

$$J_s = \frac{ADKC_v}{h} \tag{1}$$

In this equation, A is the area of application, D is the apparent diffusion coefficient, and h is the diffusional path length (often taken as the thickness of the membrane). The permeability coefficient (k_p) is the steady-state flux per unit area divided by the concentration of drug applied in solution and may be calculated from:

$$k_p = \frac{J_s}{AC_v} = \left(\frac{D}{h}\right) \tag{2}$$

In considerations of therapeutic activity following dermal application, emphasis is placed either on quantifying the extent of absorption of a drug through the skin or on some relevant pharmacodynamic response. The amount absorbed (Q) may be expressed in terms of the area of application and the exposure time (T). The amount absorbed will be determined by the permeability coefficient of the drug, the diffusional lag time across the barrier (lag), and the concentration of the drug in the vehicle:

$$Q = k_p AC_v(T - \text{lag}) \tag{3}$$

In reality, the overall amount absorbed should simply be $k_p AC_v T$. Equation 3 is based on steady-state conditions and assumes that there is no appreciable accumulation of the drug on the distal side of the barrier, or depletion of the drug on the application side.

It is evident, therefore, that a number of principles apply in dermal absorption. These include the fact that the amount of a drug absorbed will depend on the area of application, the concentration applied, the duration of application, and the permeability coefficient, which, as shown above, is defined by the physicochemical properties of the solute and the vehicle.

Permeability Coefficients and Diffusivity

To understand more fully the role of the structure of the drug and the nature of the applied vehicle on the amount of drug absorbed through the skin, the steady-state flux J_s of the drug across the stratum corneum barrier may be deconvoluted into its fundamental components of drug diffusivity (D), the path length for diffusion (h), and the concentrations of drug immediately below the outside $C_{sc(o)}$ and the inside $C_{sc(i)}$ of the stratum corneum.

$$J_s = \frac{Q}{(T - \text{lag})} = \frac{DA}{h}(C_{sc(o)} - C_{sc(i)}) \tag{4}$$

If the drug stratum corneum/product partition coefficient K is defined as $C_{sc(o)}/C_v$, $C_{sc(i)}$ is assumed to be much less than $C_{sc(o)}$ and the permeability coefficient (k_p) is KD/h; equation 4 is equivalent to equation 3. The lag time is normally defined by Fick's law as $h^2/6D$. The importance of equation 4 is well illustrated by the work of Rougier and Lotte (1993) in which it was shown that the in vivo percutaneous absorption ($=J_s$) of a series of compounds was directly related to their concentration in stripped stratum corneum, irrespective of their structure, concentration, or site of application. In theory, drug transport could go via a polar pathway, with a permeability coefficient $k_{p,polar'}$ as well as through the intercellular lipid pathway, with a permeability coefficient $k_{p,lipid'}$, although the existence and possible magnitude of a polar pathway remains controversial. As indicated previously, for lipophilic drugs, an aqueous boundary layer is likely to be present at the stratum corneum–viable epidermis interface with $k_{p,aqueous}$. Thus

$$k_p = \left(\frac{1}{k_{p,lipid'} + k_{p,polar'}} + \frac{1}{k_{p,aqueous}}\right)^{-1} \tag{5}$$

For most drugs, $k_{p,lipid} \gg k_{p,polar}$ and $k_{p,lipid} \ll k_{p,aqueous}$ so that $k_p \sim k_{p,lipid}$ and hence drug lipophilicity favors skin permeability. The model proposed by Kasting and his colleagues (Kasting et al., 1992) advocated two main determinants for $k_{p,lipid}$: lipophilicity, as defined by the logarithm of the octanol-water partition coefficient $\log k_{oct}$ and molecular size, as defined by molecular weight MW:

$$\log k_{p,lipid} = \log K_{oct} - \left(\frac{0.018}{2.303}\right)MW - 2.87 \tag{6}$$

Substitution of equation (6) into equation 5, together with the expressions for $k_{p,polar}$ and $k_{p,aqueous}$ as a function of MW, provides a simple model for predictions of k_p in terms of octanol-water partition coefficients and MW. An expression similar to equation 6 was also developed by Potts and Guy (1992):

$$\log k_p = 0.711 \log K_{oct} - 0.0061MW - 2.72 \tag{7}$$

Of particular interest in pharmaceutical delivery is the maximum flux J_{max} attainable for a selected drug. Assuming that the maximal concentration of drug possible in the stratum corneum is defined by the solubility of the drug in the stratum corneum lipid S_{sc} and that sink conditions apply, equation 4 can be reexpressed in the form:

$$J_{max} = \frac{DA}{h}S_{sc} \tag{8}$$

Thus, when the lipid pathway predominates, as defined by equation 6, J_{max} is defined by the maximum solubility of the drug in octanol S_{oct} and the MW. Therefore, applying the Kasting et al. (1992) equation:

$$\log J_{max} = \log S_{oct} - \left(\frac{0.018}{2.303}\right)MW - 2.87 \tag{9}$$

or applying the Potts and Guy (1992) equation:

$$\log J_{max} = 0.71 \log S_{oct} - 0.0061MW - 2.72 \tag{10}$$

Interrelating equations 9 and 10 with equation 8 suggests that the highest maximal flux in any series of drugs will correlate with the highest possible S_{sc}, as characterized by S_{oct} and the most rapid D, corresponding to the smallest drug (lowest MW). The observation that the maximum flux is related to S_{sc} suggests that a drug substantially more polar or lipophilic than stratum corneum will have a lower maximal flux than a drug with a polarity in the vicinity of octanol. Since octanol has a log K_{oct} of 3.15 (Leo et al., 1971), equations 9 and 10 predict maximum flux for any series of drugs at log K_{oct} 3.15 and 2.23, respectively (Fig. 2, where the data are consistent with a parabolic dependency on lipophilicity with a peak in the vicinity of K_{oct} 2.23–3.15). However, it should be noted that the above analysis is confined to data generated for a limited number of compounds, which had similar hydrogen-bonding (H-bonding) capacity and molecular size.

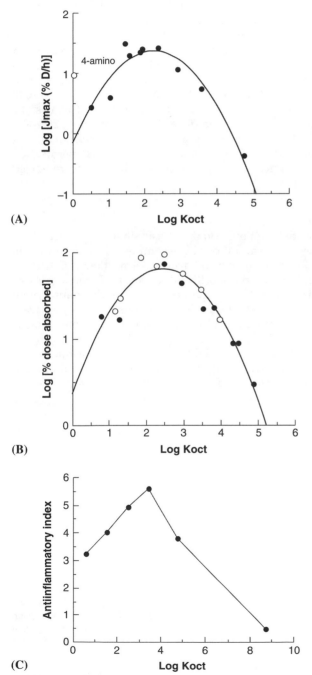

(A)

(B)

(C)

Figure 2 Skin flux, absorption or pharmacodynamic activity as a function of permeant lipophilicity. (**A**): Phenols (Hinz et al., 1991); (**B**): Salicylates (O) and other NSAIDs (•) (Yano et al., 1986); (**C**): Hydrocortisone-21-esters (Flynn, 1996).

Epidermal Reservoir, Binding, and Molecular Size
Equation 4 also suggests that a significant accumulation of drug at the inner surface of the stratum corneum will reduce flux. It is likely that, for most lipophilic drugs, an epidermal reservoir will exist after application because there is a substantial lag time as the drug diffuses through the skin (equation 1) and/or the epidermis and dermis do not act as efficient sinks. Historical evidence of reservoir formation is illustrated by the work of Vickers (1963) in which steroid-induced vasoconstriction was observed on occlusion of a previously treated area of skin two weeks following a single topical application of the drug. Furthermore, the permeability coefficients for a series of phenols, alcohols, and steroids were found to be inversely related to the number of H-bonding groups present (Roberts, 1976). It has been shown that, after allowing for molecular size and partitioning into the stratum corneum, the permeability coefficient is related to the number of H-bonding groups in the permeant. Further information on H-binding effects is discussed in Pugh et al. (1998).

   Another factor potentially limiting diffusion across the stratum corneum is the molecular size of the permeant, although, as indicated in equations 6 and 7, molecular size, expressed as *MW*, appears to have little effect on the diffusion process. It should be noted, however, that these equations were derived from limited data sets (in which MW varied only from 18 to 700). It is probable that the diffusion of larger molecules (e.g., polymeric materials) across the stratum corneum will be severely limited by their molecular size (Magnusson et al., 2004).

   The complexity and selectivity of the processes, which may be determinants of permeation, is well illustrated by the demonstration of significantly differential permeation of isomeric drugs. The mechanisms and significance of this selectivity have been reviewed (Heard and Brain, 1995).

Vehicle (Formulation) Thermodynamic Effects
The flux of a drug through the skin is dependent not only on the physicochemical nature of the permeant but also on the nature of the formulation and the vehicle composition. A formulation may alter the properties of the skin, and hence enhance or retard the permeation of a drug by increasing or decreasing its diffusivity and/or solubility within the stratum corneum. In the theoretical analysis above, most emphasis was placed on the description of drug absorption from dilute aqueous solution. The historical data, shown in Figure 3, illustrate that, whereas the permeability coefficient of alcohols increased with chain length from an aqueous vehicle, the permeability coefficient decreased with chain length when applied in lipophilic vehicles (olive oil and isopropyl palmitate). Similarly, the permeability coefficients for a number of phenolic compounds were reported to increase with lipophilicity for aqueous solutions but decrease with increasing lipophilicity for ethanol and arachis (peanut) oil formulations (Roberts, 1991).

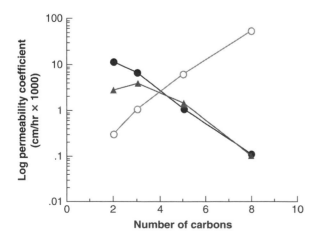

Figure 3 Effect of application vehicle on alcohol [expressed in terms of number of carbons present] permeability coefficients through human skin. The vehicles used were saline (O), isopropyl palmitate (●) and olive oil (▲). *Source*: Adapted from Blank (1964).

Maximal flux was traditionally derived from saturated solutions. However, it is now known that an even higher flux can be achieved using supersaturated solutions (Davis and Hadgraft, 1993). Equation 1 is a simplification of the exact physicochemical parameters, which control flux. More precisely, the driving force for diffusion is not the concentration but the chemical potential gradient. Higuchi was the first to apply this more rigorous solution (equation 11) to the process of percutaneous penetration (Higuchi, 1960).

$$J = \frac{Da}{h(\gamma_{sc})} \tag{11}$$

where a is the thermodynamic activity of the permeant in the vehicle (and, assuming equilibrium, also in the outer layer of the stratum corneum), and γ_{sc} is the permeant activity coefficient in the stratum corneum (a/γ_{sc} is equivalent to $C_{sc(o)}$). From this, Higuchi predicted that supersaturation of a drug in a vehicle would increase its percutaneous absorption. The effect may be described as an increase in "push" of the permeant into the stratum corneum. Supersaturation causes an increase in permeant solubility in the stratum corneum beyond and independent of saturated solubility. From this, vehicle systems affecting $C_{sc(o)}$ and/or D and supersaturated vehicle systems affecting $C_{sc(o)}$ should work independently (and possibly in synergy) and may be capable of multiplicative increases in penetration (Megrab et al., 1995; Pellett et al., 1997).

Inoue et al. (2005) used an amorphous form of ketotifen to generate a supersaturated system and enhanced drug delivery in a drug-in-adhesive transdermal delivery system. A practical issue concerning the commercial development of supersaturated systems is the difficulty that may be encountered in maintenance of long-term physical stability of such products. Addition of anti-nucleants such as hydroxypropyl methyl cellulose and polyvinylpyrrolidone may reduce the tendency of supersaturated systems to crystallize, but this is unlikely to generate systems with pharmaceutically acceptable shelf lives. For example, the addition of hydroxypropyl methyl cellulose to supersaturated solutions of salicylic acid delayed crystallization by at least eight weeks when compared with systems not containing the cellulose, which were stable for up to 46 hours depending on the degree of supersaturation (Leveque et al., 2006). Furthermore, Leichtnam et al. (2007), in their attempts to reduce crystallization in a supersaturated testosterone spray formulation, found that a cyclodextrin derivative (RAMEB, Wacker Burghausen, Germany) and a polyvinylpyrrolidone/vinyl acetate copolymer (Kollidon VA64, BASF AG, Ludwigshafen, Germany) were not able to maintain testosterone in a supersaturated solution.

Removal from the Epidermis
The clearance of a drug from the epidermis is an important determinant of dermal absorption and can influence therapeutic activity in both dermatological and transdermal therapy (Dancik et al., 2008). The steady-state ratio of the concentrations of drug in the epidermis ($C_{epidermis}$) and in the applied vehicle (C_v) may be related (Roberts, 1991) as:

$$\frac{C_{epidermis}}{C_v} = \frac{k_p}{k_p + CL_{dermis^*}} \tag{12}$$

where k_p is the permeability coefficient of the drug and CL_{dermis^*} is the clearance into the dermis per unit area of application. Equation 12 shows that the epidermal concentration $C_{epidermis}$ depends on the relative magnitude of dermal clearance, which is determined mainly by blood flow, and the permeability coefficient k_p. Situations in which k_p is of a similar order of magnitude to clearance, such as disruption of the barrier or vasoconstriction, enable blood flow to play a greater role in determining topical absorption. When blood flow is much higher than k_p, epidermal clearance will be the determinant of epidermal concentration. In this situation, equation 12 reduces to:

$$\frac{C_{epidermis}}{C_v} = \frac{k_p}{CL_{dermis^*}} \tag{13}$$

There is evidence of altered topical absorption due to changing blood flow as a consequence of elevated temperature or exercise or coadministration of vasoactive drugs (Rogers and Riviere, 1994; Singh and Roberts, 1994).

Prediction of Skin Permeation
In an ideal world, the availability of a large body of historical absorption data would allow a reasonably accurate prediction of the behavior of a new drug based on previous experimental observations for other compounds. However, even after several decades of research and data accumulation, the available data set is still very limited so that it is still only possible to make a rather limited approximation of the magnitude of the percutaneous absorption of a new drug from the permeability coefficient predicted using physicochemical properties (as described above). From this approximation, it is further necessary to approximate the potential total absorption for a given application regimen (Nitsche and Kasting, 2008).

Many of the mathematical models are based on experiments in which permeants were applied in aqueous solution and, therefore, their value in prediction of permeation from actual formulations applied under in-use conditions is severely compromised. For example, while the predicted K_p for nitrosodiethanolamine was $\sim 1.5 \times 10^{-4}$ cm/hr, the experimentally determined value from isopropyl myristate (IPM) was 3.5×10^{-3} cm/hr (Franz et al., 1993). The predicted value for octyl salicylate was $\sim 1.35 \times 10^{-7}$ cm/hr, while the experimental values from a hydroalcoholic lotion were 4.7×10^{-6} cm/hr (infinite dose) and 6.6×10^{-7} cm/hr (finite dose) and from an oil-in-water (O/W) emulsion 1.7×10^{-5} cm/hr (infinite dose) and 6.6×10^{-7} cm/hr (finite dose) (Walters et al., 1997a). The discrepancies between predicted and experimental skin permeation values for methyldodecyl nitrosamine were highly relevant to toxicological considerations of inadvertent exposure, as the predicted value of $\sim 12.6 \times 10^{-2}$ cm/hr was four orders of magnitude greater than experimentally determined values of 9.0×10^{-6} cm/hr (IPM solution) and 4.2×10^{-6} cm/hr (O/W emulsion vehicle) (Walters et al., 1997b).

Despite all their limitations, predictions of skin permeability may still be valuable and have several important potential uses. Ranking of drugs in order of potential dermal penetration is probably the most valuable use in the pharmaceutical field. For example, in situations where it is necessary to predict the dermal penetration potential for a series of homologous or closely related drugs, it is possible to rank the compounds using theoretical calculations. However, to validate the calculated values, it is essential to experimentally determine the skin permeation properties of several representative compounds of the group in a relevant vehicle.

It is important to appreciate that predictive estimates are of limited quantitative value even when the estimates and assumptions within the model are rigorous. Many variables associated with actual product use will significantly alter the extent of skin penetration. For example, reapplication of a formulation, drug release from a formulation, and the presence of nominally "inactive" excipients may all affect skin permeability. Unless these complicating parameters can be factored into the overall calculations, the predictive values cannot provide a closer approximation to the actual skin permeability under "in-use" conditions.

Biological Factors Affecting Percutaneous Absorption
Anatomical Site Variations
Perhaps the clearest data available on variation in skin permeability deal with anatomical site-to-site variation. Feldman and Maibach (1967) found that the skin permeation of hydrocortisone decreased in the following order: scrotum > jaw > forehead > scalp > back > forearm > palm (Fig. 4), and Roberts et al. (1982) found that the abdomen was more permeable to methyl salicylate than the arms or the feet. Site-to-site variation of skin permeability was examined using the tape-stripping method (Rougier, 1987b) and correlated with corneocyte diameter (Rougier, 1991) and hence diffusional path length. Although skin permeation of compounds may follow a different pattern in different skin regions, it is generally agreed that some body sites (the head and genital region) are uniformly more permeable than others (extremities).

Intrasubject and Intersubject Variability
The degree and nature of the distribution patterns of skin permeabilities was addressed to some extent by Southwell et al. (1984) who investigated both in vitro and in vivo variation in the permeability of human skin between different individuals (interspecimen) and the same

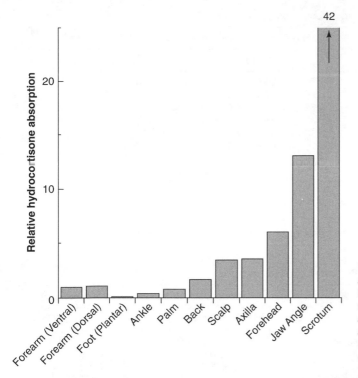

Figure 4 Regional variation in the absorption of hydrocortisone through human skin in vivo. Absorption was normalized to that through ventral forearm. Hydrocortisone was applied in acetone to a marked site. *Source*: Redrawn from Feldman and Maibach (1967).

individuals (intraspecimen). On the basis of permeation characteristics for a series of compounds, they concluded that in vitro interspecimen variation was 66% $\pm$ 25% and intraspecimen variation 43% $\pm$ 25%. The pattern in vivo was similar, although the overall level of variation was somewhat smaller. This analysis has been extended by assessing the statistical distribution of human skin permeabilities. Williams et al. (1992) examined the permeation of 5-fluorouracil and estradiol through human abdominal skin. Here, where the possibility of site variability was excluded, the data were log-normally distributed. A log-normal distribution implies that the use of normal Gaussian statistics is inappropriate and that use of geometric (rather than arithmetic) means should be considered. On the other hand, Frum et al. (2007) found no correlations between the molecular physicochemical properties of selected permeants and the extent of statistical fit to either a normal or log-normal distribution. However, Meidan and Roper (2008) used data from a very large population sample to confirm that, at least for water, human skin permeation did exhibit positively skewed non-normal distribution behavior.

Sex and Age Variability
The questions of how age and sex affect the permeability of human skin have been rather poorly addressed to date. Some studies have concluded that in vitro in humans there was no discernible dependence of skin permeability on age, sex, or storage conditions (Harrison et al., 1984; Marzulli and Maibach, 1984; Bronaugh et al., 1986). The effect of age on percutaneous absorption has been examined in vivo in humans with variable results. It was postulated (Roskos et al., 1989) that reduced hydration levels and lipid content of older skin may be responsible for a demonstrated reduction in skin permeability where the permeants were hydrophilic in nature (no reduction was seen for model hydrophobic compounds) (Table 2). The reduced absorption of benzoic acid demonstrated in the elderly (Rougier, 1991) was in line with this suggestion, but not the reduction in absorption of testosterone (lipophilic) (Roskos et al., 1986), or lack of change in the absorption of methyl nicotinate (more hydrophilic) with age (Guy et al., 1983). There are a number of potential physiological changes, which may be responsible for age-related alterations, including an increase in the size of individual stratum

Table 2 Age-Related Differences in Percutaneous Absorption

Permeant	log K[a]	Percentage of applied dose permeated over 7 day[b]		
		22–40 yr		>65 yr
Testosterone	3.32	19.0 ± 4.4		16.6 ± 2.5
Estradiol	2.49	7.1 ± 1.1		5.4 ± 0.4
Hydrocortisone	1.61	1.5 ± 0.6		0.54 ± 0.15
Benzoic acid	1.83	36.2 ± 4.6		19.5 ± 1.6
Acetylsalicylic acid	1.26	31.2 ± 7.3		13.6 ± 1.9
Caffeine	0.01	48.2 ± 4.1		25.2 ± 4.8
Age range	-	20–29 yr	30–39 yr	60–70 yr
Water	-	7.2 ± 2.5[c]	7.9 ± 2.8	6.9 ± 2.1

[a]octanol-water partition coefficient.
[b]compounds (4 μg/cm^2) were applied in 20 μL acetone to ventral forearm (n = 3–8). From Roskos et al. (1989).
[c]Transepidermal water loss (g/m^2/hr) in Chinese women. From Hillebrand and Wickett (2008).

Table 3 Race-Related Differences in Percutaneous Absorption

Permeant	Race	Amount of permeant recovered (nmol/cm^2)	
		Urine at 24 hr	Stratum corneum at 30 min[a]
Benzoic acid	Caucasian	9.0 ± 1.5	6.8 ± 1.0
	Black	6.4 ± 0.9	6.1 ± 1.0
	Asian	9.7 ± 1.2	8.1 ± 1.5
Caffeine	Caucasian	5.9 ± 0.6	5.5 ± 0.6
	Black	4.5 ± 1.0	5.8 ± 1.0
	Asian	5.2 ± 0.8	6.1 ± 0.9
Acetylsalicylic acid	Caucasian	6.2 ± 1.9	11.9 ± 1.9
	Black	4.7 ± 0.9	9.0 ± 1.7
	Asian	5.4 ± 1.7	10.1 ± 1.7

[a]Amount in stratum corneum determined by tape stripping (n = 6–9).
Source: From Lotte et al. (1993).

corneum corneocytes, increased dehydration of the outer layers of the stratum corneum with age, decreased epidermal turnover, and decreased microvascular clearance (reviewed in Roskos and Maibach, 1992). The issue of age-related variability, however, is far from resolved.

Racial Differences

Caucasian skin has been reported to be slightly more permeable than black skin (Corcuff et al., 1991; Kompaore and Tsuruta, 1993; Leopold and Maibach, 1996), which correlates with observations that black skin has both more cell layers within the stratum corneum (Weigand et al., 1974) and a higher lipid content (Rienertson and Wheatley, 1959). Lotte et al. (1993) determined the penetration and permeation of benzoic acid, caffeine, and acetylsalicylic acid into and through Asian, black, and Caucasian skin and found no statistical differences between the races (Table 3). The equivocal findings in this area are discussed in more detail by Wesley and Maibach (2003), and the implications of skin color in skin disease profiles are outlined in a study by Taylor (2002).

Skin Metabolism

It is widely established that there is potential for biotransformation of molecules within the skin (Bronaugh et al., 1989; Noonan and Wester, 1989; Sharma, 1996; Hotchkiss, 1998; Wilkinson and Williams, 2008), but the nature of skin enzymes differs quantitatively and qualitatively from those in the liver. In general, the activities of many metabolic processes are

Table 4 Comparison Between Specific Activities of Cutaneous Enzymes Compared with Hepatic Enzymes

Enzyme system	Substrate	Cutaneous-specific Activity (percent hepatic)
Cytochrome P-450s	Aldrin	0.4–2.0
	Aminopyrine	1
	Diphenyloxazole	2–3
	Ethylmorphine	0.5
	7-Pentoxyresorufin	20–27
Epoxide hydrolases	*cis*-Stilbene oxide	9–11
	trans-Stilbene oxide	24–25
	Styrene oxide	6
Glutathione transferases	*cis*-Stilbene oxide	49
	Styrene oxide	14
Glucuronosyl transferases	Bilirubin	3
	1-Naphthol	2–50
Sulfotransferases	1-Naphthol	10
Acetyltransferases	*p*-Aminobenzoic acid	18
	2-Aminofluorene	15

Source: From Hotchkiss (1998).

much lower in skin than in liver, although certain enzymes, such as *N*-acetyltransferases and those involved in reductive processes, have demonstrated fairly high activity (Table 4).

The majority of metabolic work on skin has employed epidermal homogenates or cell cultures, which are useful for the study of enzyme activity per se, but have little predictive value for the in vivo situation where drugs may not be in contact with particular cellular systems during permeation. A more useful in vitro model uses metabolically active fresh skin mounted in a diffusion cell under conditions, which maintain viability. For example, this technique has been used to investigate in vitro permeation and metabolism of several compounds including estradiol and testosterone (Collier et al., 1989).

Enhancement and Retardation of Skin Absorption

Because of the very extensive barrier properties of the stratum corneum, it is often necessary to increase the intrinsic rate of dermal or transdermal drug delivery to achieve the required therapeutic drug levels. In these instances, skin penetration and permeation enhancement strategies must be evaluated. The therapeutic target may be the skin, the local subcutaneous tissues or the microvasculature, depending on the requirement for local, regional, or systemic therapy. In some cases, for example, the use of sunscreen agents, insect repellents, and drugs whose therapeutic target is the epidermis, skin permeation retardation would be an attractive option from a toxicological standpoint. Both enhancement and retardation of skin permeation can be achieved using either particular formulation strategies or the co-application of specific chemicals designed to modify stratum corneum barrier function (Williams and Walters, 2008). In addition, recent enhancement tools include the use of synergistic combinations (Karande et al., 2008) and microneedles (Birchall and Brain, 2008). Other chemical and physical mechanisms for enhancement, including prodrugs with more suitable physicochemical properties, liposomes, iontophoresis, electroporation, ultrasound, and particle-mediated pressure-driven systems have been fully reviewed and discussed elsewhere (Walters and Hadgraft, 1993; Korting, 1996; Prausnitz, 1996; Smith and Maibach, 2006; Menon et al., 2007; Sloan and Wasdo, 2008) and will not be discussed here.

Formulation Strategies

As discussed earlier, it is well established that a principal driving force for diffusion across the skin is the thermodynamic activity of the permeant in the donor vehicle. This activity is reflected by the concentration of the permeant in the donor vehicle as a function of its saturation solubility within that medium. The closer to saturation concentration, the higher the thermodynamic activity and greater the escaping tendency of the permeant from the vehicle.

This principle has been extensively and successfully used in pharmaceutical formulations in attempts to enhance percutaneous absorption of drugs (Davis and Hadgraft, 1993; Pellett et al., 1997). Supersaturated systems can be created using binary mixtures in which one component is a good solvent for the solute and the other component is a non-solvent. Slow addition of the non-solvent to the solvent (both pre-saturated with solute) creates a supersaturated solution. Because of the high potential for crystal growth in these systems, it is necessary to add an appropriate antinucleant polymer, such as hydroxypropyl methyl cellulose.

Supersaturated transdermal delivery devices have also been described, although, in these cases, stability considerations limit the degree to which the systems can be supersaturated. Supersaturated systems containing nitroglycerine or isosorbide dinitrate have been formed in polymer films. Jenkins (1992) described the development of saturated and supersaturated transdermal drug-in-adhesive systems and demonstrated their use with norethisterone and estradiol. In the preparation of these systems, the active agent was dissolved in a mixture of solvents, at least one of which had a boiling point above that of the solvent used as a vehicle for the adhesive. The degree of saturation or supersaturation was dictated by the selected solvent mix and, because there are a large number of suitable solvents, the system was suitable for a wide range of drugs. Also embodied in this patent application was the suggestion that at least one of the remaining solvents may act as a skin permeation enhancer, and in this respect propylene glycol-diethyltoluamide and *n*-methyl-pyrrolidone-diethyltoluamide were included in the preferred solvent systems.

The potential for development of systems in which both the drug and the permeation enhancer were in the supersaturated state was mentioned in the first edition of this book. Since then we have seen the development of the Acrux system in which drug and enhancer are delivered by a metered-dose transdermal spray system (www.acrux.com.au) that can produce "on skin" supersaturated systems. To date, Acrux has successfully marketed an estradiol product in the United States and Australia/New Zealand and is currently developing several transdermal products, including systems for hypogonadism, chronic pain, contraception, and smoking cessation (Nicolazzo et al., 2005).

Penetration Enhancers

Chemical penetration and permeation enhancers comprise a diverse group of compounds including water, organic solvents, phospholipids, simple alkyl esters, long-chain alkyl esters, fatty acids, urea and its derivatives, and pyrrolidones (for reviews, see Walters and Hadgraft, 1993; Smith and Maibach, 2006). In some cases, molecules with specific potential as skin penetration enhancers have been designed and synthesized. Of the latter, 2-*n*-nonyl-1,3-dioxolane (SEPA®, Gyurik et al., 1996; Gauthier et al., 1998), 1-dodecylazacycloheptan-2-one (Azone®, Hadgraft et al., 1993), l-[2-(decylthio)ethyl]azacyclopentan-2-one (HPE-101, Bugaj et al., 2006; Utsuki et al., 2007), 4-decyloxazolidin-2-one (Dermac™ SR-38, Rajadhyaksha, 1990), and dodecyl-*N*,*N*-dimethylamino isopropionate (NexACT 88, Büyüktimkin et al., 1993) have all been shown to possess enhancing properties on the skin penetration and permeation of a variety of permeants, although few have made it to the product stage to date.

An exception to this generalization is provided by Bentley Pharmaceuticals CPE-215 permeation enhancement technology, which uses enhancers based on the structure shown in Figure 5 and is incorporated into Auxillium Pharmaceutical's Testim Gel (see www.bentleypharm.com). Testim Gel is a testosterone-containing product indicated for the topical

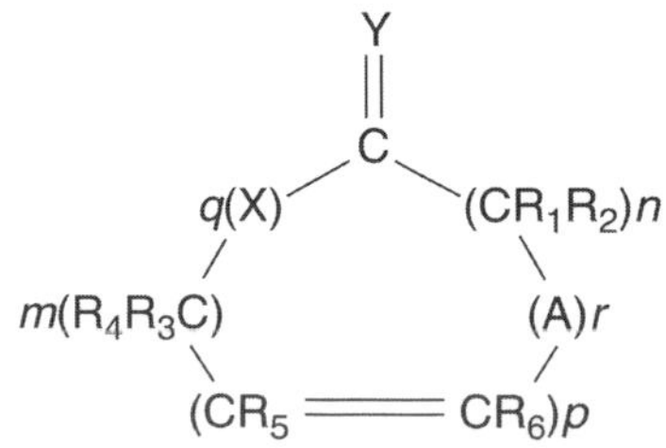

Figure 5 Basic structure of the CPE-215 series of chemical penetration enhancers (Bently Pharmaceuticals).

treatment of hypogonadal men. In trials comparing effectiveness of Testim gel with competitive gels or patches, Testim proved superior providing higher serum levels and greater bioavailability, with fewer local adverse events (Marbury et al., 2003; Grober et al., 2008).

DRUG CANDIDATE SELECTION AND PREFORMULATION

Drug Candidate Selection

While it may appear to be a simple task to select lead compounds for pharmaceutical product development, based on therapeutic rationale and compound safety/efficacy, the practicality of this procedure is somewhat more complex. For the most part, therapeutic efficacy is dependent on the ability of the compound to cross biological barriers to reach the target site. However, as pointed out and excellently reviewed by Flynn (1996), in topical therapy it is more appropriate, in many instances, to select compounds on the basis of their inability to cross relevant biological barriers. Since the site of action may be the skin surface, the stratum corneum, the viable epidermis, the appendages, the dermis, or the local subcutaneous tissues that may require systemic distribution, the rules of candidate selection will vary. For the purposes of this discussion, it will be assumed that the therapeutic rationale for dermal or transdermal drug delivery has been established and that a series of compounds with appropriate pharmacological activity has been identified. It will also be assumed that each compound within the series possesses equivalent chemical and physical stability. In other words, drug candidate selection need only be made on the basis of the ability to deliver the compound to its site of action.

In the section "Skin Permeability," the physicochemical determinants of the ability of a compound to permeate the skin were addressed. It was shown that the primary requirement for a compound to penetrate into the skin was the ability to leave the delivery vehicle and partition into the stratum corneum. This characteristic has been shown to be dependent on the compound's stratum corneum vehicle partition coefficient, for which the octanol-water partition coefficient is often used as a surrogate. It is immediately apparent that a high value for this parameter will favor uptake of the drug into the stratum corneum, although it will not favor diffusion to the more hydrophilic regions of the viable epidermis. Furthermore, the rate of diffusion though the stratum corneum and lower layers of the skin is linked to the molecular volume of the permeant. From this, it is evident that a compound with a high octanol-water partition coefficient and a relatively high molecular volume will possess a high affinity for the stratum corneum (i.e., be substantive to the stratum corneum). This principle is used extensively in the design of sunscreen agents, where it is not uncommon to add a medium length or branched alkyl chain to the ultraviolet (UV) reflective molecule to maximize residence time in the skin.

At the other end of the spectrum, however, in transdermal systemic delivery, the molecular attributes required are rather different. In this case, compounds are required to partition into the relatively lipophilic stratum corneum, diffuse rapidly across the stratum corneum, and partition easily into the more hydrophilic viable epidermis and dermis prior to vascular removal. The intrinsic requirements of compounds for transdermal delivery are, therefore, a medium polarity (a log octanol-water partition coefficient of 1–3), a low molecular volume, and a lack of potential to bind to skin components (e.g., via hydrogen bonding).

Strategies to obtain ideal physicochemical properties of drugs for dermatological or transdermal delivery have included the use of prodrugs, binary drugs, and codrugs. In the former the active moiety is reversibly chemically linked to an inactive component in an attempt to optimize physicochemical properties and increase penetration into the stratum corneum (Sloan and Wasdo, 2008). Once this combination has entered the stratum corneum, it can readily diffuse toward the viable epidermis where a variety of enzyme systems await to initiate liberation of the active drug, which is then free to diffuse into the deeper layers of the skin. The rationale behind codrugs is similar to that of prodrugs, except that the added moiety is another active drug that has an added or synergistic effect with the original parent drug. Where the additional moiety is the same drug, a binary or "Gemini" codrug is formed.

Hammell and colleagues (2004) evaluated the transdermal delivery of a dimer of naltrexone using human skin in vitro. Skin permeation rates of naltrexone, as a single entity, and the dimer were determined, and drug concentrations in the skin were measured at the termination of the experiment. During the permeation process the prodrug was hydrolyzed, and it appeared mainly as naltrexone in the receptor solution. The dimer provided a significantly higher naltrexone-equivalent flux across human skin than naltrexone alone. Although naltrexone permeability from the dimer exceeded the permeability of naltrexone base by twofold, there was no significant increase in drug concentration in the skin after dimer treatment compared with application of naltrexone alone. The same group evaluated the enhancement of transdermal delivery of the naltrexone active metabolite 6-β-naltrexol when carbonate linked to hydroxybupropion (Kiptoo et al., 2006). This was an interesting dual therapy concept allowing the treatment of alcohol abuse to be combined with an aid to smoking cessation. The codrug was partially hydrolyzed on passing through skin, and a combination of intact codrug and parent drugs was found in the receptor medium. Flux of 6-β-naltrexol was significantly higher than the parent drug when applied as the codrug.

There is also tremendous potential for codrug therapy in dermatological diseases. There are several conditions that would benefit from dual therapy including the most prevalent, such as oxidative stress, acne and psoriasis, and the less common, such as actinic keratosis. However, a review of the available literature indicates that investigation of the codrug concept is limited and evaluation in the clinic rare. Many cosmetic formulations contain retinoid-based compounds, such as retinyl palmitate, either to protect the skin or to stimulate skin responses that will correct skin damaged by sunlight. Another long-chain ester compound, ascorbyl palmitate, is also used in cosmetic products as an effective antioxidant that protects tissue integrity. Abdulmajed and Heard (2004) synthesized the ester-linked codrug retinyl ascorbate from all-trans-retinyl chloride and L-ascorbic acid (Fig. 6). The flux across human epidermal membranes was measured, and skin penetration was determined by stratum corneum tape stripping of full thickness human skin. Similar determinations were made for retinyl palmitate and ascorbyl palmitate. Retinyl ascorbate demonstrated higher skin retention than the other two esters and delivered more retinoic acid and ascorbic acid to the viable epidermis than retinol from retinyl palmitate and ascorbic acid from ascorbyl palmitate. Clearly, prolonged efficacy of agents designed to act in the epidermis is influenced by retention time in the target tissue and this can be increased by interaction with skin components. Abdulmajed et al. (2004) continued their studies on retinyl ascorbate to determine the skin binding properties of the codrug. They determined the binding of the codrug and its parent compounds, retinoic acid and ascorbic acid, together with retinol, ascorbyl palmitate, and retinyl palmitate to keratinous tissues. Binding to keratin was assessed using both native tissue and delipidized tissue. Not surprisingly, in delipidized tissue, binding was higher for the polar compounds, and dipolar/H-bonding to keratin was proposed. The binding characteristic of native tissues was complicated by lipid, creating a dual effect comprising keratin binding and partitioning. Therefore, for highly polar compounds, such as ascorbic acid, lipid content decreased binding, whereas for the more lipophilic retinyl ascorbate binding increased with lipid content, suggesting that a substantial amount is dissolved in the lipid matrix. The authors concluded that this ability to bind with skin components enhanced the suitability of the codrug for topical application.

A codrug of triamcinolone acetonide and 5-fluorouracil (CDS-TC-32), a combination that may be a potential therapy for proliferative skin diseases with inflammatory components, was synthesized and evaluated using skin blanching (Cynkowski et al., 2008). The vasoconstriction (skin-blanching assay) and skin surface biopsy (SSB) study was run in healthy volunteers, and results were compared following application of a cream containing 0.75% CDS-TC-32 (equivalent to 0.5% triamcinolone acetonide) and a marketed 0.5% triamcinolone acetonide

All *trans*- retinyl ascorbate (RA-AsA)

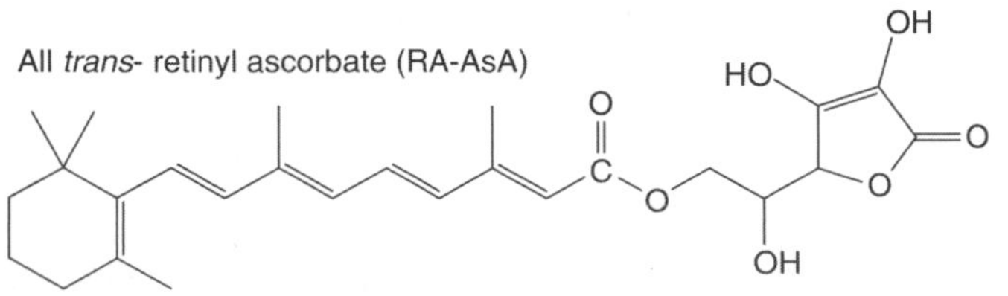

Figure 6 The ester-linked codrug retinyl ascorbate synthesized from all-trans-retinyl chloride and l-ascorbic acid. *Source*: Abdulmajed and Heard (2004).

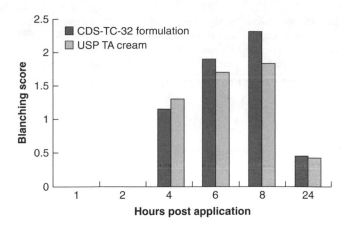

Figure 7 In vivo vasoconstriction scores in human volunteers following application of triamcinolone acetonide cream [0.5% (w/w)] and CDS-TC-32 cream containing the equivalent of 0.5% (w/w) triamcinolone acetonide. Skin blanching was assessed by trained personnel on a scale of 0–3 where 0 = no blanching and 3 = profound blanching. Scores were verified using a chromameter. Note that for the 24-hour blanching score the residual formulation had been removed at 8 hours. *Source*: Data from Cynkowski et al. (2008).

cream. Steroids cause local vasoconstriction when applied, and the degree of skin blanching is a function of steroid potency and concentration at the active site. The SSB technique removes surface layers of the stratum corneum using cyanoacrylate adhesive and glass slides. Formulations were applied to randomized sites on the backs of volunteers and skin blanching assessed at intervals up to 24 hours. Each volunteer was dosed with three formulations, on separate sites for each formulation and time point. Formulation A was a placebo cream, B a 0.75% CDS-TC-32 cream, and C a marketed 0.5% triamcinolone acetonide cream. SSBs were taken from six volunteers over the 24-hour period. Five SSBs were taken from each site, following assay for skin blanching and removal of remaining surface formulation, at 1, 2, 4, 6, and 8 hours. At 8 hours the formulation was removed from remaining sites, and further SSBs were taken at 24 hours. The SSBs were extracted and analyzed for CDS-TC-32 and triamcinolone acetonide.

No skin blanching was observed at the placebo-treated site. Sites treated with 0.75% CDS-TC-32 cream and the marketed 0.5% triamcinolone acetonide cream showed equivalent blanching (Fig. 7), suggesting that similar amounts of triamcinolone acetonide had reached the dermis from the two formulations. From the SSB data it was concluded that some conversion of CDS-TC-32 to triamcinolone acetonide and 5-fluorouracil occurred, with conversion increasing with skin depth. Overall skin delivery of triamcinolone acetonide was not altered by application as a codrug, except that there appeared to be a greater substantivity of the codrug, which indicated the possibility of a cutaneous reservoir of the codrug. The cutaneous reservoir would provide a more sustained release of both triamcinolone acetonide and 5-fluorouracil, a factor that may be important in the therapy of actinic keratosis.

Preformulation

Preformulation encompasses those studies that must be carried out before the commencement of formulation development. The major goal of the preformulation process is to permit the rational development of stable, safe, and efficacious dosage forms, and it is mainly concerned with the characterization of the physicochemical properties of the drug substance. At the preformulation stage, the final route of drug administration is usually undecided, and, as such, any protocol must be able to cover all required aspects. As with any development programme, progression can be limited by several factors, including

- project objectives,
- priority rating,
- compound availability, and
- availability of analytical procedures.

For the purposes of this discussion, we will assume that the project objectives are known, priority has been established, there are sufficient amounts of raw materials to carry out the investigations, and initial analytical procedures have been developed. A fundamental point that must be kept in mind throughout the early stages is that for new chemical entities (NCEs) the toxicological profile will not normally have been established at the preformulation stage. It is of paramount importance, therefore, to take all due precautions throughout the study. The preformulation study has several distinct phases (in approximate chronological order):

- General description of the compound
- Calorimetry
- Polymorphism
- Hygroscopicity
- Analytical development
- Intrinsic stability
- Solubility and partitioning characteristics
- Drug delivery characteristics

A detailed description of most of the studies that form part of the preformulation stage is given elsewhere in this volume and will not be considered here. In addition, the importance of preformulation studies in the overall development of transdermal drug delivery systems has been excellently reviewed and discussed by Roy (1997). The only aspect of preformulation, which is specific to and important for dermatological and transdermal formulations that will be discussed in depth in this chapter, concerns drug delivery characteristics.

Measurement of Skin Penetration, Distribution, and Permeation In Vitro
In dermatological and transdermal drug delivery, there is a need to optimize the delivery of the drug into and through various skin strata to provide maximum therapeutic effect. The requirement for such data, produced under reproducible and reliable conditions, using relevant membranes, has led to an increase in the development and the standardization of in vitro and in vivo test procedures. There have been numerous recommendations on in vitro and in vivo methodologies, and many of these have been collated as guidelines. Perhaps the most widely known of the early guidelines was produced following an Food and Drug Administration (FDA)/American Association of Pharmaceutical Scientists (AAPS) workshop on the performance of in vitro skin penetration studies (Skelly et al., 1987). However, following many iterations and numerous workshops and conferences, the guidelines produced by the Organization for Economic Co-operation and Development (OECD, 2004) have now been generally adopted as the current standard. It should be pointed out that these documents are *guidelines* and still leave much to the discretion of the individual experimenter. A definitive *protocol* that could be used in interlaboratory studies to validate the in vitro technique as a means of determining bioequivalence of dermatological dosage forms has yet to be agreed.

In many respects, in vitro techniques have advantages over in vivo testing. For example, permeation through the skin is measured directly in vitro where sampling is carried out immediately below the skin surface. This contrasts with most in vivo methods, which rely on the measurement of systemic (or at least nonlocal) levels of permeant. Some form of in vitro diffusion cell experiment is, therefore, the most appropriate method for assessment of skin penetration, distribution, and permeation in a transdermal or topical drug developmental programme.

A major advantage of in vitro investigation is that the experimental conditions can be controlled precisely, such that the only major variables are the skin and the test material. Although a potential disadvantage is that little information on the metabolism, distribution, and effects of blood flow on permeation may be obtained, it has been reported that such procedures were more effective than several other methods for the assessment of differential delivery of hydrocortisone and other steroids from commercial formulations (Lehman et al., 1996; Franz et al., 2008). In vitro systems range in complexity from a simple two-compartment "static" diffusion cell (Franz, 1975) to multi-jacketed "flow-through" cells (Bronaugh and Stewart, 1985) (Fig. 8). Construction materials must be inert; glass is most common, although other materials (Walters et al., 1981) are also used. In all cases, excised skin, preferably human,

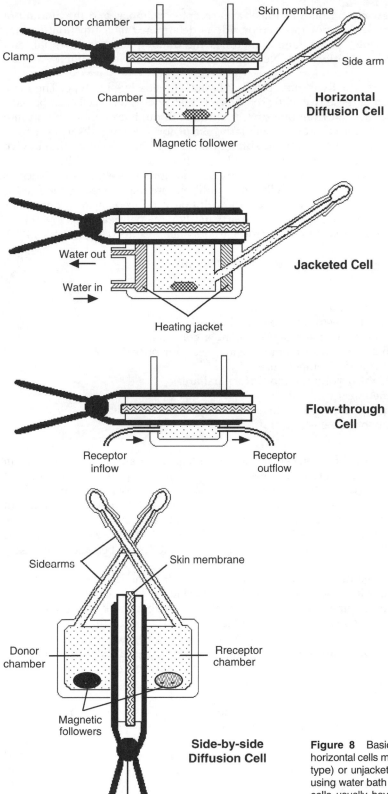

Donor chamber — Skin membrane

Clamp —

— Side arm

Chamber —

Horizontal Diffusion Cell

Magnetic follower

Water out

Jacketed Cell

Water in

Heating jacket

Flow-through Cell

Receptor inflow

Receptor outflow

Sidearms

Skin membrane

Donor chamber

Rreceptor chamber

Magnetic followers

Side-by-side Diffusion Cell

Clamp

Figure 8 Basic diffusion cell designs. Static horizontal cells may be jacketed (as in the Franz-type) or unjacketed (and temperature controlled using water bath or heating block). Flow-through cells usually have a small receptor chamber to maximize mixing. Side-by-side cells are used mainly for solution vehicles.

is mounted as a barrier between a donor chamber and receptor chamber, and the amount of compound permeating from the donor to receptor side is determined as a function of time. Efficient mixing of the receptor phase (and sometimes the donor phase) is essential, and sample removal should be straightforward. Neither of these processes should interfere with diffusion of the permeant.

Static diffusion cells are usually of the upright ("Franz") or side-by-side type. The main difference in the application of these two static cell types is that side-by-side cells can be used for the measurement of permeation from one stirred solution, through a membrane and into another stirred solution. Upright cells are particularly useful for studying absorption from semisolid formulations spread on the membrane surface and are optimal for simulating in vivo performance. The donor compartments can be capped, to provide occlusive conditions, or left open, according to the objectives of the particular study. In addition, use-related steps such as washing can be simulated. In flow-through cells sink conditions are maximized as the fluid is continually replaced (Bronaugh, 1996). However, the dilution produced by the continuous flow can raise problems with analytical sensitivity, particularly if the permeation is low. Flow-through and static systems have been shown to produce equivalent results (Hughes et al., 1993; Clowes et al., 1994).

To summarize, a well-designed skin diffusion cell should

- be inert,
- be robust and easy to handle,
- allow the use of membranes of different thicknesses,
- provide thorough mixing of the receptor chamber contents,
- ensure intimate contact between membrane and receptor phase,
- be maintainable at constant temperature,
- have precisely calibrated volumes and diffusional areas,
- maintain membrane integrity,
- provide easy sampling and replenishment of receptor phase, and
- be available at a reasonable cost.

The receptor phase of any diffusion cell should provide an accurate simulation of the in vivo permeation conditions. The permeant concentration in the receptor fluid should not exceed ∼10% of saturation solubility (Skelly et al., 1987), as excessive receptor phase concentration can lead to a decrease in absorption rate and result in an underestimate of bioavailability. The most common receptor fluid is pH 7.4 phosphate-buffered saline (PBS), although, if a compound has water solubility below ∼10 μg/mL, then a wholly aqueous receptor phase is probably unsuitable, and addition of solubilizers becomes necessary (Bronaugh, 2008).

Receptor fluids described in the literature range from water alone to isotonic phosphate buffers containing albumin, which increases solubility (Dick et al., 1996). Microbial growth can produce problems due to partitioning of the permeant into, or metabolism of the permeant by, the microbes, and preservatives may be required. One particularly useful fluid is 25% (v/v) aqueous ethanol, which provides a reasonable "sink" for many permeants, whilst removing the need for other antimicrobial constituents. It is important to appreciate that the pH of an aqueous receptor solution may affect the apparent "flux" of a weakly ionizable compound. The pH of the hydrophilic viable epidermal layers may be "altered," and this can result in modulation of the partitioning tendencies of ionizable species (Kou et al., 1993).

It is also important to select an appropriate membrane for use during in vitro skin permeation studies. Attempts have been made to model human skin permeation characteristics using artificial membranes, laboratory animal skin, and skin equivalents. These investigations have been fully discussed elsewhere (Brain et al., 1998; Schaefer-Korting and Schreiber, 2008). The consensus of opinion is that, whereas animal models may be useful alternatives in the early stages of development, there is no substitute for human skin when definitive values are required. Although the most appropriate scenario would involve experimentation directly on freshly excised surgical skin samples, this is not always practically feasible. In reality, most in vitro human skin permeation investigations are carried out on cadaver or surgical specimens that have been frozen prior to experimental use. Although some authors have concluded that freezing had no measurable effect on permeability (Harrison et al., 1984; Kasting and Bowman, 1990), Wester et al. (1998) have cautioned against the use of frozen stored human skin for studies in which cutaneous metabolism may be a contributing factor.

Several different methods can be used to prepare human skin. The most commonly used membranes are as follows:

- Full-thickness skin, incorporating the stratum corneum, viable epidermis and dermis
- Dermatomed skin, in which the lower dermis has been removed to a definite depth
- Epidermal membranes, comprising the viable epidermis and the stratum corneum (prepared by heat separation)
- Stratum corneum alone (prepared from epidermal membranes by enzyme treatment)

The most suitable type of membrane is dependent on the nature of the permeant. For example, the relatively aqueous environment of the dermis will inhibit the penetration of lipophilic compounds in vitro, whereas in vivo this barrier is largely circumvented by the capillary bed. Thus the use of dermatomed epidermal or stratum corneum membranes is most appropriate for particularly lipophilic permeants. Other considerations may justify the use of epidermal membranes even where the dermis does not present an artificial barrier to a permeant. For example, if a study involves an assessment of the skin content of permeant, it is much easier to extract or solubilize epidermal membranes than full-thickness skin. The disadvantages inherent to the use of epidermal membranes are that preparation is time consuming and that the necessary processing increases the possibility of damage to skin integrity.

For human skin, the separation of the dermis from the epidermis (stratum corneum and viable epidermis) is a relatively simple technique (Scheuplein, 1965; Bronaugh et al., 1986). Following removal of the subcutaneous fat, the skin is totally immersed in water at 60°C for ~45 seconds. The tissue is then removed from the water, pinned (dermal side down) to a dissecting board, and the epidermis gently peeled back using forceps. The epidermal membrane is floated onto warm water, taken onto a support membrane (paper filter or aluminum foil), and air-dried before storage in a freezer. To mount previously frozen skin membranes in a diffusion cell, they are thawed and then floated from the support membrane.

There are two basic approaches to applying substances to the skin: infinite dose (which involves application of sufficient permeant to make any changes in donor concentration during the experiment negligible) and finite dose (which involves application of a dose that may show marked depletion during an experiment). The infinite dose technique may be useful if the experimental objectives include calculation of diffusional parameters, such as permeability coefficients, or investigation of mechanisms of penetration enhancement. The finite dose technique is normally used for the evaluation of materials in prototype formulations and should be used with a regime that mimics as closely as possible the proposed "in-use" situation (Walters et al., 1997a). With finite dosing, the permeation profile usually exhibits a characteristic plateauing effect that is the result of donor depletion (Fig. 9). There are several published recommendations regarding the amount of formulation, which should be applied to correspond with an "in-use" dose level. OECD recommends 1 to 5 mg/cm^2 for a solid/semisolid and up to 10 μL/cm^2 for a liquid. Given the high intrasubject and intersubject variability in human skin permeability, a large number of replicates for each dosage regimen are recommended. The most widely quoted recommendation for numbers of replicates in in vitro studies on human skin is 12 (Skelly et al., 1987), although OECD suggests a minimum of four replicates per test group. Donor samples should be distributed throughout the test groups so that comparisons are matched. Care should be taken to ensure accurate distribution of the test dose over the entire skin area.

In vitro finite dose skin permeation experiments are usually conducted with a constant skin temperature of 32°C. Prior to carrying out in vitro experiments, the integrity of each skin sample should be evaluated. Quantitative integrity tests include measurement of trans-epidermal water loss, the flux of marker compounds such as tritiated water or sucrose

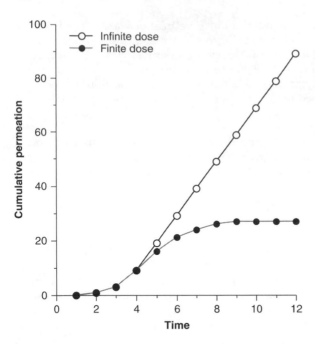

Figure 9 Sample cumulative skin permeation patterns following finite and infinite closing regimes. With infinite dose, permeation normally reaches a steady-state flux region, from which it is possible to calculate permeability coefficients and diffusional lag times. In finite dosing the permeation profile normally exhibits a plateauing effect as a result of donor depletion.

(Pendlington et al., 1998; Green, 2005) or electrical measurement of skin conductivity (Fasano et al., 2002; Davies et al., 2004).

The ideal sampling and analytical procedures provide accurate assessment of both the quantity and nature of the material present at a given time point, and the sensitivity of the method must be capable of producing data of practical significance. Preliminary prediction from existing data or physicochemical modelling can give "ballpark" estimates of the likely amount of permeant. As replication and multiple time point sampling are common, analysis should not be unnecessarily complex. High-performance liquid chromatography (HPLC) is particularly useful, as relatively large (~200 μL) aqueous samples can often be handled without preliminary processing or concentration. Determination of permeants in tissue samples necessitates some form of extraction or solubilization process. When radiolabelled permeants are used, tissue samples are routinely taken up in commercially available solubilizers. Such aggressive products are often not applicable in other cases where more traditional extraction methods are required. Recovery of permeant from stratum corneum tape strips may be less demanding and can often be accomplished by vortexing, roller mixing, and sonicating with relatively small volumes of appropriate solvent.

A typical in vitro permeation experiment will involve analysis of receptor samples at intervals up to 24 to 72 hours. At the termination of the exposure period, the remaining formulation on the skin surface is often removed using a suitable rinsing procedure (which will depend on the nature of the applied formulation). This removed material is analyzed to determine the amount of permeant remaining on the skin. The epidermal membranes or skin samples are removed from the diffusion cells, and the stratum corneum may be tape-stripped 10 to 15 times, and the tape strips extracted and analyzed for permeant content. Tape stripping is under evaluation by the U.S. Food and Drug Administration (FDA) and others as a potential method for determining relative bioavailability/bioequivalence of dermatological products (Bunge and Guy, 2007; N'Dri-Stempfer et al., 2008; Herkenne et al., 2008). Following the tape stripping, the remaining epidermal membranes or skin samples may be homogenized, extracted, and analyzed for permeant content. The results of these studies demonstrate how the developed prototype formulations compare in terms of in vitro skin penetration, distribution, and permeation. The criteria for determining the preferred formulation using an in vitro skin model will depend on the particular circumstances. For example, preferred formulations for dermatological activity may demonstrate rapid uptake of drug into the epidermal layers together with limited transfer of the drug through the skin. On the other hand, preferred vehicles for transdermal systemic delivery will be those demonstrating both rapid penetration into and rapid permeation across the skin.

FORMULATION

In the previous sections, the theoretical aspects of dermatological and transdermal drug delivery, together with some aspects of product preformulation, have been discussed. This section concentrates on the formulation development of dermatological and transdermal products and will take into account several important factors in the development process. In many companies, the first stage of product development is the formation of a project team. At the inaugural meeting of this team, it is essential that all members be aware of what is required from both a medical and a marketing point of view. Realistic time schedules should be drawn up with well-defined decision points, and due allowance should be made for the inevitable slippage time.

In the early stages of product development, there is usually a bottleneck in the analytical department. Most companies work on the basis of allowing two analysts per formulator, but this ratio is often inadequate. It is of paramount importance that the analytical department be involved in the early stages of the formulation process. These are the people who will have to analyze the prototype formulations and look for evidence of stability problems as soon as possible. They are, of course, capable and equipped to do this, but time will be saved if they know precisely what materials the formulator is planning to include in the prototypes. There is no substitute for a fully validated stability indicating assay, but initial "rough" analytical methods can be extremely useful for determining what excipients to avoid and what conditions, such as pH, are critical to the formulation.

Although the medical and marketing departments will have defined targets in terms of disease to be treated, and territories in which the product is to be launched, it is up to the formulator to specify and identify the optimum formulation. Often, however, the formulator is hindered by the fact that, for an NCE, the dose level is unknown and will remain so until a dose-ranging study has been carried out. This leads to the unsatisfactory, but unavoidable, situation of the formulator trying to obtain a formulation containing a "hypothetical" maximum dose.

Throughout the development process, it is important to maintain a high level of quality. The application of systematic quality assurance (QA) in the research and development (R&D) portion of topical product development is necessary to facilitate registration and also acts as a safeguard should any problems arise during scale-up and manufacture. The QA/quality control (QC) systems for topical product development are exactly the same as for any new drug development and can be achieved only by the systematic applications of Good Laboratory Practice (GLP), Good Clinical Practice (GCP), and Good Manufacturing Practice (GMP).

Formulation Type

The selection of formulation type for systemic transdermal products, which are designed for application to intact non-diseased skin, is guided by the requirement of the system, be it a semisolid, spray, or patch preparation, to deliver therapeutic amounts of drug into the systemic circulation. On the other hand, the selection of formulation type for dermatological products is influenced more by the nature of the skin lesion. As pointed out by Kitson and Maddin (1998): "It is idle to pretend that the therapy for skin diseases, as currently practiced, has its origins in science." To this day a practicing dermatologist would prefer to apply a "wet" formulation (ranging from simple tap water to complex emulsion formulations—with or without drug) to a wet lesion and a "dry" formulation (e.g., petrolatum) to a dry lesion (Kitson, 2008). For these reasons, the dermatological and transdermal formulator must be skilled in the art and knowledgeable in the science of a variety of formulation types.

In general, the preparation of such formulations as poultices and pastes is extemporaneous, and it is unlikely that the industrial pharmaceutical formulator will be required to develop stable, safe, and efficacious products of this type. Solutions and powders lack staying power (retention time) on the skin and can only afford transient relief. In modern-day pharmaceutical practice, semisolid formulations are preferred vehicles for dermatological therapy because they remain in situ and deliver their drug payload over extended periods. In the majority of cases, therefore, the developed formulation will be an ointment, emulsion, or gel. Typical constituents for these types of formulations are shown in Table 5, and it is important to appreciate that the judicious selection of the appropriate

Table 5 Constituents of Semisolid Formulations

Function	Sample ingredients	
Polymeric Thickeners	**Gums**	**Acrylic acids**
	Acacia	Carbomers
	Alginates	Polycarbophil
	Carageenan	**Colloidal solids**
	Chitosan	Silica
	Collagen	Clays
	Tragacanth	Microcrystalline cellulose
	Xanthan	**Hydrogels**
	Celluloses	Polyvinyl alcohol
	Sodium carboxymethyl	Polyvinylpyrrolidone
	Hydroxyethyl	Thermoreversible polymers
	Hydroxypropyl	Poloxamers
	Hydroxypropylmethyl	
Oil phase	Mineral oil	IPM
	White soft paraffin	Isopropyl palmitate
	Yellow soft paraffin	Castor oil
	Beeswax	Canola oil
	Stearyl alcohol	Cottonseed oil
	Cetyl alcohol	Jojoba oil
	Cetostearyl alcohol	Arachis (Peanut) oil
	Stearic acid	Lanolin (and derivatives)
	Oleic acid	Silicone oils
Surfactants	**Nonionic**	**Anionic**
	Sorbitan esters	Sodium dodecyl sulfate
	Polysorbates	**Cationic**
	Polyoxyethylene alkyl ethers	Cetrimide
	Polyoxyethylene alkyl esters	Benzalkonium chloride
	Polyoxyethylene aryl ethers	
	Glycerol esters	
	Cholesterol	
Solvents	**Polar**	Polyethylene glycols
	Water	Propylene carbonate
	Propylene glycol	Triacetin
	Glycerol	**Nonpolar**
	Sorbitol	Isopropyl alcohol
	Ethanol	Medium chain triglycerides
	Industrial methylated spirit	
Preservatives	**Antimicrobial**	**Antioxidants**
	Benzalkonium chloride	α-tocopherol
	Benzoic acid	Ascorbic acid
	Benzyl alcohol	Ascorbyl palmitate
	Bronopol	Butylated hydroxyanisole
	Chlorhexidine	Butylated hydroxytoluene
	Chlorocresol	Sodium ascorbate
	Imidazolidinyl urea	Sodium metabisulfite
	Paraben esters	**Chelating agents**
	Phenol	Citric acid
	Phenoxyethanol	Edetic acid
	Potassium sorbate	
	Sorbic acid	
pH adjusters	Diethanolamine	Sodium hydroxide
	Lactic acid	Sodium phosphate
	Monoethanolamine	Triethanolamine

Abbreviation: IPM, isopropyl myristate.

inactive ingredients in semisolid preparations can be a significant factor in formulation efficacy (Wiechers et al., 2004).

Ointments

In its strictest definitive form, an ointment is classified as any semisolid containing fatty material and intended for external application [U.S. Pharmacopeia, (USP)]. In practice, ointments are considered to be semisolid anhydrous external preparations. In the 19th century, ointments were based on lard, a compounding material, the usefulness of which was severely limited by its tendency to turn rancid. Early in the 20th century, lard was replaced by petrolatum (white or yellow soft paraffin or petroleum jelly). In present practice, non-medicated ointments (ointment bases) are used alone, for emollient or lubricating purposes, or in combination with a drug for therapeutic purposes.

There are four types of ointment base (classified in the USP as hydrocarbon bases, absorption bases, water-removable bases, and water-soluble bases), but only the hydrocarbon bases are completely anhydrous. The anhydrous hydrocarbon bases contain straight or branched hydrocarbon chain lengths ranging from C_{16} to C_{30} and may also contain cyclic alkanes. They are used principally in non-medicated form as described above. A typical formulation contains fluid hydrocarbons (mineral oils, liquid paraffins) mixed with longer alkyl chain, higher melting point hydrocarbons (white and yellow soft paraffin, petroleum jelly). The difference between white and yellow soft paraffin is simply that the white version has been bleached. Hard paraffin and microcrystalline waxes are similar to the soft paraffins except that they contain no liquid components. These anhydrous mixtures tend to produce formulations, which are greasy and unpleasant to use. The addition of solid components, such as microcrystalline cellulose, can reduce the greasiness. Improved skin feel can also be attained by the incorporation of silicone materials, such as polydimethylsiloxane oil or dimethicones. Silicones are often used in barrier formulations, which are designed to protect the skin against water-soluble irritants.

Although the non-medicated anhydrous ointments are extremely useful for emolliency, their value as topical drug delivery platforms is limited by the relative insolubility of many drugs in hydrocarbons and silicone oils. However, it is possible to increase drug solubility within the formulation by incorporating hydrocarbon-miscible solvents, such as isopropylmyristate or propylene glycol, into the ointment. Although increasing the solubility of a drug within a formulation may often decrease the release rate, it does not necessarily decrease the therapeutic effect. It is well accepted that simple determination of release rates from formulations may not be predictive of drug bioavailability. For example, when formulated in a simple white petrolatum/mineral oil ointment, the release rate of betamethasone dipropionate was shown to be considerably higher than when the drug was formulated at the same concentration (0.05%) in an augmented, and more clinically effective, ointment containing propylene glycol (Fig. 10) (Zatz et al., 1996). It is also important to appreciate that various grades of petrolatum are commercially available and that the physical properties of these materials will vary depending on the source and refining process. Slight variations in physical properties of the constituents of an ointment may have significant effects on drug release behavior (Kneczke et al., 1986; Piechota-Urbanska et al., 2007).

The preparation of ointment formulations may, at first sight, appear a simple matter of heating all of the constituents to a temperature higher than the melting point of all of the excipients and cooling with constant mixing. The reality, however, is that the process is somewhat more complex and requires careful control over various parameters, especially the cooling rate. Rapid cooling, for example, creates stiffer formulations in which there are numerous small crystallites. On the other hand, a slow cooling rate results in the formation of fewer, but larger, crystallites and a more fluid product. Further information regarding temperature effects and ointment phase behavior can be found in Osborne (1992, 1993) and Pena et al. (1994).

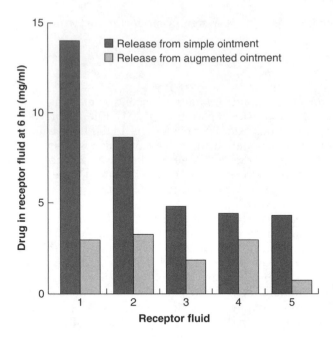

Figure 10   Release rates of betamethasone dipropionate from ointments into various receptor fluids. (*i*), 50% hexane in acetonitrile; (*ii*), octanol; (*iii*), acetonitrile; (*iv*), 60% aceto-nitrile in water; (*v*), 95% ethanol. *Source*: Data from Zatz et al. (1996).

Gels

The common characteristic of all gels is that they contain continuous structures, which provide solid-like properties (Barry, 1983). Depending on their constituents, gels may be clear or opaque and be polar, hydroalcoholic, or nonpolar. The simplest gels contain water thickened with natural gums (e.g., tragacanth, guar, xanthan), semisynthetic materials [e.g., methyl-cellulose (MC), carboxymethylcellulose (CMC), hydroxyethylcellulose (HEC)], synthetic materials (e.g., carbomer-carboxyvinyl polymer), or clays (e.g., silicates, hectorite). Gel viscosity is generally a function of the amount and molecular weight of the added thickener.

There are a variety of semisynthetic celluloses in use as thickeners in gel formulations. These include MC, CMC, HEC, hydroxypropyl cellulose (HPC), and hydroxypropyl methyl cellulose (HPMC). These celluloses are obtainable in diverse molecular weight grades, and the higher-molecular-weight moieties are used at 1% to 5% (w/w) for gelation. In the preparation of aqueous gels, the cellulose is dissolved in a preheated portion of the required water. On dispersion of the cellulose in the hot water, the remainder of the water is added, cold, and stirred to form the gel. When polar organic solvents (e.g., ethanol, propylene glycol) form part of the formulation, the cellulose should be dispersed or dissolved in the organic phase, and the aqueous phase subsequently added. It is useful, when developing prototype gel formulations, to evaluate a variety of different types of cellulose. If a major requirement is for clarity of the gel, for example, HPMC is preferable to MC. It is also important to appreciate that some celluloses may exhibit specific incompatibilities with other potential formulation ingredients. For example, HEC is incompatible with several salts, and MC and HPC are incompatible with parabens. This latter incompatibility will limit the choice of preservative for gel formulations based on MC and HPC. Finally, the presence of oxidative materials (e.g., peroxides or other ingredients containing peroxide residues) in formulations gelled with celluloses should be avoided, because oxidative degradation of the polymer chains may cause a rapid decrease in formulation viscosity (Dahl et al., 1998).

Because they are of naturally occurring plant origin, the branched chain polysaccharide gums, such as tragacanth, pectin, carrageenan, and guar, will have widely varying physical properties depending on their source. They are incorporated into formulations at concentrations of between 0.5% and 10.0% contingent upon the required viscosity. Viscosity may be enhanced synergistically by the addition of inorganic suspending agents such as magnesium aluminum silicate. Tragacanth, a mixture of water-insoluble and water-soluble polysaccharides, is negatively charged in aqueous solution and therefore incompatible with many preservatives when formulated at a pH of 7 and above. Similarly, xanthan gum, which is produced by bacterial fermentation, is incompatible with some preservatives but, unlike other gums, it is very stable over a wide range of temperatures and pH. The viscosity of xanthan gum solutions decreases with higher shear rates, but when the shear forces are removed, the product will thicken. Xanthan gum is used to prepare aqueous gels usually in conjunction with bentonite clays, and it is also used in O/W emulsions to help stabilize oil droplets against coalesence. Alginic acid is a hydrophilic colloidal carbohydrate obtained from seaweed. The sodium salt, sodium alginate, is used at 5% to 10% as a gelling agent, and firm gels may be obtained by incorporating small amounts of soluble calcium salts (e.g., tartrate, citrate). Many gums are ineffective in hydroalcoholic gels containing greater than 5% alcohol. Nonetheless, ethanol or glycerin is often used as wetting agents to ease aqueous dispersion of the gums.

The natural clay thickeners (e.g., bentonite and magnesium aluminum silicate) are useful for thickening aqueous gels containing co-solvents, such as ethanol, isopropanol, glycerin, and propylene glycol. These materials possess a lamellar structure that can be extensively hydrated. The flat surfaces of bentonite are negatively charged, whereas the edges are positively charged. The clays swell in the presence of water because of hydration of the cations and electrostatic repulsion between the negatively charged faces. Thixotropic gels form at high concentrations because the clay particles combine in a flocculated structure in which the edge of one particle is attracted to the face of another. The rheological properties of these clay dispersions are, therefore, particularly sensitive to the presence of salts. Bentonite, a native colloidal hydrated aluminum silicate (mainly montmorillonite), can precipitate under acidic conditions, and formulations must be at pH 6 or above. A synthetic clay (colloidal silicon dioxide) is also useful for thickening both aqueous and nonpolar gels. The usual concentrations of clay required to thicken formulations is from 2% to 10%. Polymeric materials used in gels and other dermatological formulations are reviewed in Valenta and Auner (2004).

By far the most extensively employed gelling agents in the pharmaceutical and cosmetic industries are the synthetic carboxyvinyl polymers known as carbomers. These are high-molecular-weight polymers of acrylic acid cross-linked with either allylsucrose or allyl ethers of pentaerythritol. Pharmaceutical grades of carbomers are available (e.g., Carbopol 934P NF and Carbopol 981NF, Lubrizol, www.pharma.lubrizol.com). At a concentration of 0.5% (w/w) and at pH 7.5, the carbomers can generate aqueous gel viscosities from 4000 to 65,000 cP. In the dry state, a carbomer molecule is tightly coiled. When dispersed in water, the molecule begins to hydrate and partially uncoil. This uncoiling exposes free acidic moieties. To attain maximum thickening, the carbomer molecule must be fully uncoiled, and this can be achieved by one of two mechanisms (Fig. 11). The most common way is to convert the acidic molecule to a salt by the addition of an appropriate neutralizing agent. For aqueous or polar solvent containing formulations, carbomer gelation can be induced by the addition of simple inorganic bases, such as sodium or potassium hydroxide. Less polar or nonpolar solvent systems may be neutralized with amines, such as triethanolamine or diethanolamine. A number of alternative amine bases (e.g., diisopropanolamine, aminomethyl propanol, tetrahydroxypropyl ethyl-enediamine, and tromethamine) may be employed. For example, clear and stable hydro-alcoholic gels containing 40% ethanol can be thickened with triethanolamine or tromethamine. Neutralization ionizes the carbomer molecule, generating negative charges along the polymer backbone, and the resultant electrostatic repulsion creates an extended three-dimensional structure. Care must be taken not to under- or overneutralize the formulation as this will result in viscosity or thixotropy changes (Planas et al., 1992). Overneutralization will reduce viscosity because the excess base cations screen the carboxy groups and reduce electrostatic repulsion. Hydrated molecules of carbomer may also be uncoiled in aqueous systems by the addition of 10% to 20% of a hydroxyl donor, such as a nonionic surfactant or a polyol (Fig. 12), which is able to hydrogen bond with the polymer. Using this mechanism, maximum thickening will not be instantaneous, as it is with base neutralization, and may take several hours. Heating will accelerate the process, but the system should not be heated above 70°C.

A typical carbomer gel can be prepared as follows. The carbomer resin (0.5–1.0%) is dispersed in water to form a lump-free mixture, which is allowed to stand to free entrapped

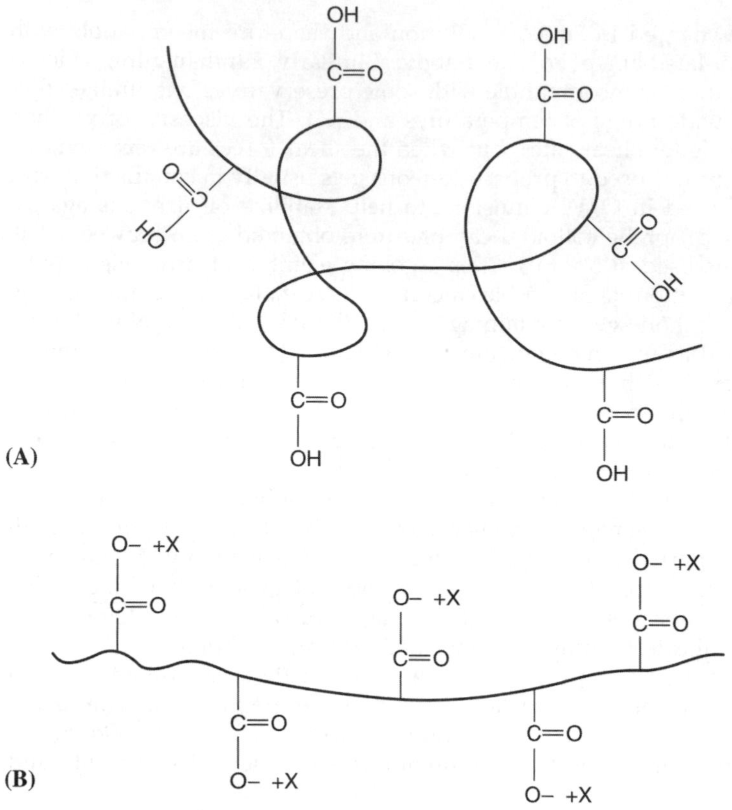

Figure 11 (**A**) A tightly coiled carbomer molecule will hydrate and swell when dispersed in water. (**B**) The molecule will completely uncoil to achieve maximum thickening when it is converted from the acid form to the salt form upon neutralization.

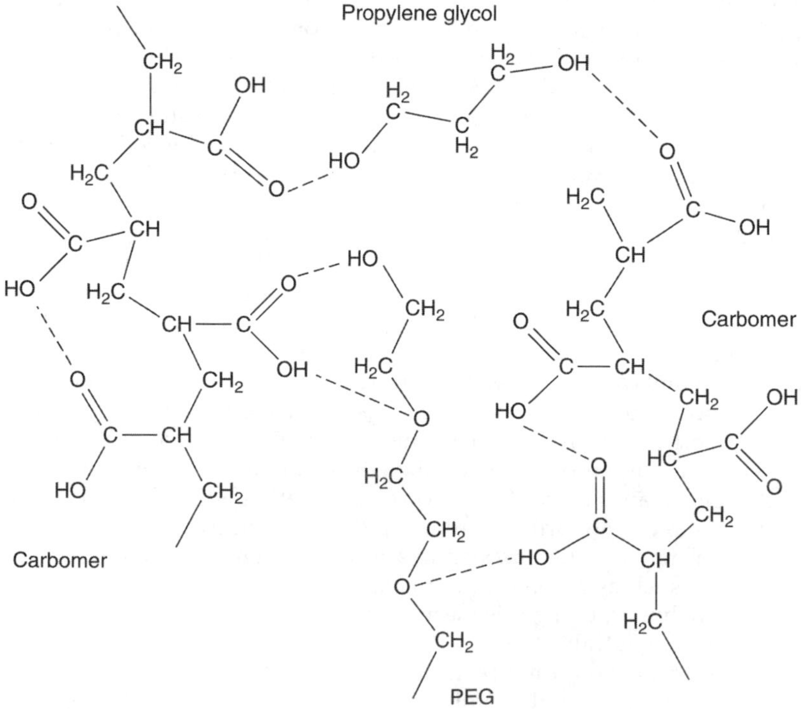

Figure 12 Hydrated carbomer molecules may be uncoiled in water by adding hydroxyl donors such as propylene or PEGs. *Abbreviation*: PEG, polyethylene glycols.

air. A small proportion (~2%) of 10% aqueous NaOH is added using moderate agitation to form the gel. The dispersion process may take some time, and many formulators prepare a concentrated stock dispersion of carbomer for dilution. The exact quantity of neutralizing agent to be added depends on the type and equivalent weight (carbomer resins have an approximate equivalent weight of 76). Because they are synthetic, carbomer bases vary little from lot to lot. However, differences in batch-to-batch mean molecular weight may result in variations in the rheological characteristics of aqueous dispersions (Pérez-Marcos et al., 1993). Despite this, carbomer gel rheology remains remarkably stable within the pH range of 5 to 8 (Islam et al., 2004) even when formulated with cosolvents such as propylene glycol and glycerine. It is possible to modulate the flow behavior and elastic properties of carbomer gels using surfactants (Barreiro-Iglesias et al., 2001), and such alterations may be used to alter the diffusion rates within and release of drugs from formulated gels (A-sasutjarit et al., 2005).

The carbomers have an excellent safety profile, are generally regarded as essentially nontoxic and nonirritant materials, and have been extensively used by the pharmaceutical and cosmetic industries. In addition, there is no evidence of hypersensitivity or allergic reactions in humans as a result of topical application.

Although aqueous-based formulations remain the most popular form of gel preparation, there has been some interest in the development of nonaqueous gel systems, particularly for water-sensitive drugs (Chow et al., 2008). These systems are made up of polymers, such as the copolymers *N*-vinylacetamide/sodium acrylate and methylvinyl ether/maleic anhydride (Gantrez S-97, ISP Technologies, Wayne, New Jersey, U.S.), which are dissolved in nonaqueous vehicles such as binary mixtures of propylene glycol and glycerol. Dependent on the polymer, concentrations of 1% (w/w) to 20% (w/w) are used to provide gelation, and viscosity can also be varied by adjusting the ratio of the hydrophilic solvents.

Emulsions

The most common emulsions used in dermatological therapy are creams. These are two-phase preparations in which one phase (the dispersed or internal phase) is finely dispersed in the other (the continuous or external phase). The dispersed phase can be either hydrophobic based (O/W creams) or aqueous based [water-in-oil (W/O) creams]. Whether a cream is O/W or W/O is dependent on the properties of the system used to stabilize the interface between the phases. Given the fact that there are two incompatible phases in close conjunction, the physical stability of creams is always tenuous, but may be maximized by the judicious selection of an appropriate emulsion-stabilizing system. In most pharmaceutical emulsions, stabilizing systems comprise surfactants (ionic and/or nonionic), polymers (nonionic polymers, polyelectrolytes, or biopolymers), or mixtures of these. The most commonly used surfactant systems are sodium alkyl sulfates (anionic), alkylammonium halides (cationic), and polyoxyethylene alkyl ethers or polysorbates (nonionic). These are often used alone or in conjunction with nonionic polymerics, such as polyvinyl alcohol or poloxamer block copolymers, or polyelectrolytes, such as polyacrylic/polymethacrylic acids.

The physicochemical principles underlying emulsion formulation and stabilization are extremely complex and will not be covered in depth here. The interested reader is referred to the volume edited by Sjöblom (1996). Briefly, an emulsion is formed when two immiscible liquids (in most cases oil and water) are mechanically agitated. When this occurs in the absence of any form of interfacial stabilization during agitation, both liquids will form droplets that rapidly flocculate and coalesce into two phases on standing. "Flocculation" is the term used to describe the close accumulation of two or more droplets of dispersed phase without loss of the interfacial film and is largely the result of Van der Waals forces. The flocculated droplets may then coalesce into one large droplet with the loss of the interfacial film. In reality, there is a brief period where one of the phases becomes the continuous phase because the droplets of this liquid coalesce more rapidly than the droplets of the other. Physical stability of an emulsion is determined by the ability of an additive to counteract the Van der Waals attractions, thereby reducing flocculation and coalescence of the dispersed phase. This may be achieved in two ways: an increase in the viscosity of the continuous phase, which will reduce the rate of droplet movement, and/or the establishment of an energy barrier between the droplets. While it is true that increasing the viscosity of the continuous phase will reduce the rate at which droplets flocculate, in pharmaceutical shelf-life terms, a stable system will be generated in this way only when the continuous phase is gelled and the droplet diameter is <0.1 μm.

In pharmaceutical emulsions, it is more common to develop stability using the energy barrier technique and to complement this stabilization, if necessary, by increasing the viscosity of the continuous phase. The basis of the energy barrier is that droplets experience repulsion when they approach each other. Repulsion can be generated either electrostatically, by the establishment of an electric double layer on the droplet surface, or sterically, by adsorbed nonionic surfactant or polymeric material. Electrostatic repulsion is provided by ionic surfactants that, when adsorbed at the oil-water interface, will orient such that the polar ionic group faces the water. Some of the surfactant counterion (e.g., the sodium ion of sodium dodecyl sulfate) will separate from the surface and form a diffuse cloud surrounding the droplet. This diffuse cloud, together with the surface charge from the surfactant, forms the electric double layer. Electrostatic repulsion will occur when two similarly charged droplets approach each other. For obvious reasons, this method of emulsion stabilization is only appropriate for O/W formulations. In addition, it is important to appreciate that emulsions stabilized by electrostatic repulsion are extremely sensitive to additional electrolytes, which will disrupt the electrical double layer.

Steric repulsion may be produced using nonionic surfactants or polymers, such as polyvinyl alcohol or poloxamers. The specific distribution of the polyethoxylated nonionic surfactants and block copolymers (Fig. 13A,B) results in the formation of a thick hydrophilic shell of polyoxyethylene chains around the droplet. Repulsion is then afforded both by mixing interaction (osmotic repulsion) and entropic interaction (volume restriction), the latter as a result of a loss of configurational entropy of the polyoxyethylene chains when there is a significant overlap. For polymeric materials without definitive hydrophobic and hydrophilic regions, the adsorption energy is critical to generation of steric repulsion. The adsorption energy should neither be so low as to result in no polymer adsorption nor so high as to result in complete polymer adsorption to the droplet. In either case, there will be none of the loops or tails (Fig. 13C) that are essential to steric repulsion. For this reason, polymeric steric repulsion is usually achieved using block copolymers such as poloxamers, which consist of linked polyoxyethylene and polyoxypropylene chains. More recently, polyacrylic acid polymers linked to hydrophobic chains [(Pemulen™, Lubrizol Corporation (www.pharma.lubrizol.com)] have been used as primary emulsification systems in O/W formulations and are listed in the USP as carbomer 1342. These materials form very stable emulsions because the polyacrylic acid chain, anchored to the oil droplet by the alkyl methacrylate moieties, considerably increases the surface charge on the oil droplet, forming a strong electrical barrier at the interface. Furthermore, emulsion stability is enhanced by an increase in the viscosity of the continuous phase (Friedrich et al., 2004; Ribeiro et al., 2004). The development of methods to rapidly and reliably predict the long-term physical stability of emulsions is a continuing task in the pharmaceutical and personal care industry. Recently, Muehlbach et al. (2006) concluded that the time–temperature superposition principle, often used to predict polymeric system stability, was not a technique that could be applied to predict the long-term stability of a W/O emulsion.

In most cases for O/W emulsions, and all cases for W/O emulsions, it is necessary to select an emulsification system based on surfactants. While we have already seen that ionic surfactants can only be used for O/W emulsions, nonionic surfactants may be used for both O/W and W/O formulations. Although, at first glance, the choice of surfactant system appears limitless (there are hundreds to choose from), there are some basic guidelines to aid the formulator. In the first instance, use of pharmaceutically approved surfactants (or those having a drug master file in place with the regulatory authority) will save a considerable amount of regulatory justification time. Very often, guidelines are provided by the raw material supplier, although these will obviously be biased toward the use of their products. Nonetheless, it should be appreciated that the suppliers have considerable experience in the applications and uses of their products, and they provide a very useful resource. In addition, a rough and ready

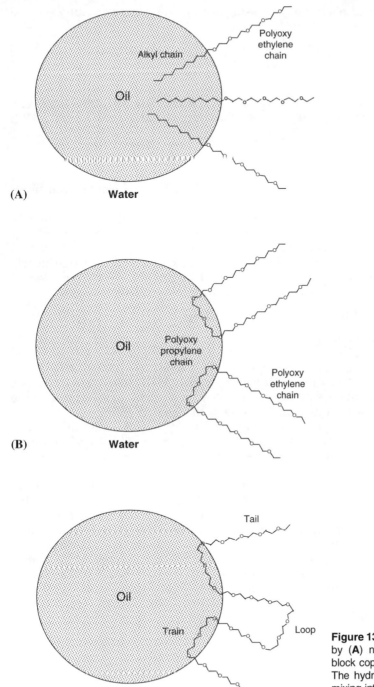

Figure 13 O/W emulsions may be stabilized by (**A**) nonionic surfactants, (**B**) poloxamer block copolymers, or (**C**) polymeric materials. The hydrophilic chains produce repulsion by mixing interaction (osmotic) or volume restriction (entropic). *Abbreviation*: O/W, oil-in-water.

guide is provided by the hydrophilic–lipophilic balance (HLB) system, which generates an arbitrary number (usually between 0 and 20) that is assigned to a particular surfactant. The HLB value of a polyoxyethylene-based nonionic surfactant may be derived from

$$HLB = \frac{mol\% \text{ hydrophobic group}}{5} \qquad (14)$$

and the HLB of a polyhydric alcohol fatty acid ester (e.g., glyceryl monostearate) may be derived from

$$HLB = 20\left(1 - \frac{S}{A}\right)$$

(15)

where S is the saponification number of the ester and A the acid number of the fatty acid. When it is not possible to obtain a saponification number (e.g., lanolin derivatives), the HLB can be calculated from:

$$HLB = \frac{E + P}{5}$$

(16)

where E is the weight percentage of the polyoxyethylene chain and P the weight percentage of the polyhydric alcohol group in the molecule.

It is immediately obvious from the above equations that hydrophilic surfactants will have high HLB values and lipophilic surfactants low values. It is generally recognized that surfactants with HLB values between 4 and 6 are W/O emulsifiers, and those with HLB values between 8 and 18 are O/W emulsifiers. It is also generally recognized, although poorly understood, that mixtures of surfactants create more stable emulsions than individual surfactants. The overall HLB of a surfactant mixture (HLB$_M$) can be calculated from

$$HLB_M = fHLB_A + (1 - f)HLB_B$$

(17)

where f is the weight fraction of surfactant A. The required emulsifier HLB values for several oils and waxes are given in Table 6. It is important to appreciate, however, that the HLB system can only be used as an approximation in emulsion design and that stability of an emulsion cannot be guaranteed by the use of an emulsifier mix with the appropriate HLB value. As an example, creaming of an emulsion, a typical physical stability problem, is much more dependent on the viscosity of the continuous phase than the characteristics of the interfacial film.

As mentioned above, it is recognized that mixtures of surfactants create more stable emulsions that the individual surfactants. A reasonable and coherent explanation for this is given by the gel network theory (Eccleston, 1990, 1997). Briefly, the theory relates the consistencies and stabilities of O/W creams to the presence or absence of viscoelastic gel networks in the continuous phase. These networks form when there is an amount of mixed emulsifier, in excess of that required to stabilize the interfacial film, which can interact with the aqueous continuous phase. In its simplest form, a cream consists of oil, water, and mixed emulsifier. Official emulsifying waxes may be cationic (cationic emulsifying wax BPC; a mixture of cetostearyl alcohol and cetyltrimethylammonium bromide, 9:1), anionic (emulsifying wax BP; a mixture of cetostearyl alcohol and sodium dodecyl sulfate, 9:1) or nonionic (nonionic emulsifying wax BPC; a mixture of cetostearyl alcohol and cetomacrogol, 4:1). The theory dictates that when the cream is formulated, it is composed of at least four phases (Fig. 14):

1. Bulk water
2. A dispersed oil phase

Table 6 HLB Values for Several Oils and Waxes

	Emulsion type	
Constituent	O/W	W/O
Liquid paraffin	12	4
Hard paraffin	10	4
Stearic acid	16	-
Beeswax	12	5
Castor oil	14	-
Cottonseed oil	9	-

Abbreviation: HLB, hydrophilic-lipophilic balance.

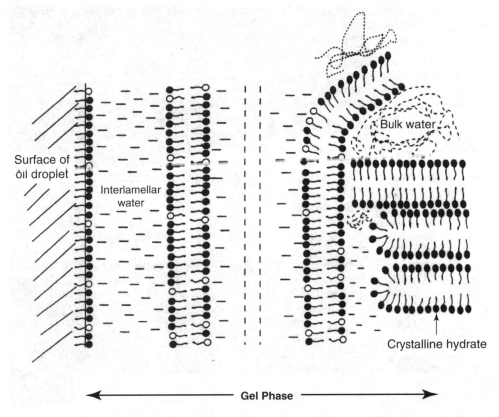

Surface of oil droplet

Interlamellar water

Bulk water

Crystalline hydrate

← **Gel Phase** →

Figure 14 The gel network theory suggests that when a cream is formulated, it is composed of four phases: bulk water, a dispersed oil phase, a crystalline hydrate, and a crystalline gel composed of bilayers of surfactant and fatty alcohol separated by layers of interlamellar fixed water (courtesy of Dr. G. M. Eccleston).

3. A crystalline hydrate
4. A crystalline gel phase composed of bilayers of surfactant and fatty alcohol separated by layers of interlamellar fixed water

Examination of ternary systems (containing the emulsifying wax and water but no oil phase) by X-ray diffraction indicates that, for all emulsifying systems, addition of water causes swelling of the interlamellar spaces. Ionic emulsifying systems possess a greater capacity to swell than nonionic systems. Swelling in ionic systems is an electrostatic phenomenon, whereas that in nonionic systems is due to hydration of the polyoxyethylene chains and is limited by the length of this chain. The gel network theory also offers an explanation for the observation that nonionic O/W creams thicken on storage. This change is related to the formation of additional gelation in the continuous phase as a result of slow hydration of the polyoxyethylene chains of the surfactant. This process reduces the amount of free water in the formulation.

A great deal of information on emulsion stability, measurement, and strategies for improving shelf life can be gleaned from the food and cosmetic industries (McClements, 2007). A relatively stable emulsion formulation may be prepared from a simple four-component mixture: oil, water, surfactant, and fatty amphiphile. In practice, however, formulation is never this straightforward (Ribeiro et al., 2004; Moulai Mostefa et al., 2006). In addition to the four principal components, a pharmaceutical emulsion formulation will also contain the drug and is likely to contain a co-solvent for the drug, a viscosity enhancer, a microbiological preservative system, a pH adjusting/stabilizing buffer, and an antioxidant system (Korhonen et al., 2004.). All of the additional components are related to the requirement that the formulation must be capable of delivering the correct amount of drug to the therapeutic application site in a formulation that is free from microbial contamination and is essentially physically unchanged from the day of manufacture.

Other Semisolid Formulations

In addition to the traditional dermal delivery formulations discussed above, several other pharmaceutical semisolid and liquid formulation types have been the subject of a considerable amount of research and are at various stages of development. Several of these formulations may be considered to be simple modifications of the formulator's standard armamentarium but, more often than not, simple changes can lead to significant benefits in parameters such as physical, chemical, and microbiological stability. Furthermore, these newer formulations often demonstrate improved performance in drug release and delivery.

Multiple emulsions or double emulsions are complex systems that can be either water-in-oil-in-water (W/O/W) or oil-in-water-in-oil (O/W/O). Although these systems are relatively difficult to formulate and have somewhat variable stability issues (Jiao and Burgess, 2003), they can have advantages over conventional emulsions in areas such as the control of drug release and the kinetics of skin distribution (Laugel et al., 2000; Pays et al., 2002).

There have been considerable advances in the field of microemulsion delivery systems in topical drug therapy. These clear, relatively stable, isotropic mixtures comprise oil, water, and surfactant. When combined in the appropriate proportions, these mixtures spontaneously form colloidal drug carrier systems that have been shown to be very effective in drug delivery (Kogan and Garti, 2006; Date and Patravale, 2007; Heuschkel et al., 2008).

Other systems include foams, pluronic lecithin organogels (Kumar and Katare, 2005), cyclodextrin beads (Trichard et al., 2008), vesicular formulations, such as transfersomes (Cevc, 2008), pickering emulsions (Melle et al., 2005), nano-suspensions (Piao et al., 2008), lipid nanoparticles (Souto et al., 2008), and nano-injectors (Lotan, 2008). One awaits with interest the next generation of pico- and femto-delivery devices. Or, perhaps, they are already here....

Drug Release from Semisolid Formulations and SUPAC-SS

Determination of the ability of a semisolid formulation to release a drug, the pattern of release, and the rate at which this release occurs are important aspects of formulation development and optimization. However, it is also important to appreciate that the data obtained should not be overinterpreted. Release studies normally involve the measurement of drug diffusion of a mass of formulation into a receiving medium, which is separated from the formulation by a synthetic membrane (Shah et al., 1991; Chattaraj and Kanfer, 1995). Detailed study of the data obtained using this type of system will generate invaluable data concerning the physical state of the drug in the formulation. For example, an examination of the early models, and their refined updates, derived to describe drug release from semisolids reveals that release patterns are different depending on whether the drug is present as a solution or suspension within the formulation (Higuchi, 1960, 1961; Bunge, 1998). These subtle differences, together with differences in the rate of release, may be used to determine such parameters as drug diffusivity within the matrix of a formulation, the particle size of suspended drug, and the absolute solubility of a drug within a complex formulation (Caetano et al., 1999). It is generally agreed that drug release rate data cannot be used to predict skin permeation or bioavailability. When a formulation is applied to the skin, the situation is ephemeral. The formulation will undergo considerable shearing forces, and solvents will evaporate. There may be excipients in the formulation that will interact with the skin and potentially modulate bioavailability. Nonetheless, release rate determinations are important for purposes other than formulation development and characterization.

The FDA has issued a guidance document (FDA, 1997), which recommends the use of in vitro drug release testing in the scale-up and post-approval changes for semisolids (SUPAC-SS). The FDA intends to promote the use of this test as a QA tool to monitor minor differences in formulation composition or changes in manufacturing sites, but not at present as a routine batch-to-batch QC test. Thus, the FDA is suggesting in vitro release rate data for levels 2 and 3 changes in formulation components and composition, but such data are not required for a level 1 change. In the former, the in vitro release rate of the new or modified formulation should be compared with a recent batch of the original formulation, and the 90% confidence limit should fall within the limits of 75% to 133%. Similarly, in vitro release testing is suggested for level 2 changes in manufacturing equipment, processes and scale-up, and level 3 changes in manufacturing site. The use of in vitro testing as a QA tool has been questioned, especially in the case of a hydrophilic formulation containing the highly water-soluble drug, ammonium lactate (Kril et al., 1999). The method was found not to be specific enough to differentiate between small differences in drug loading or minor compositional and processing changes.

Bioequivalence of Dermatological Formulations

Bioequivalence of dermatological dosage forms presents particular difficulties, mainly because it may be difficult to determine the very low blood levels of a specific drug following dermal application. The FDA has, therefore, suggested the use of alternative methods such as determining dermatopharmacokinetics by the tape-stripping method. The use of in vivo skin stripping in dermatopharmacokinetic evaluation was discussed at an AAPS/FDA workshop on bioequivalence of topical dermatological dosage forms (Bethesda, Maryland, U.S.A., September 1996). Although opinions were divided, it was concluded that stratum corneum skin stripping "may provide meaningful information for comparative evaluation of topical dosage forms" (Shah et al., 1998). Furthermore, it was established that a combination of dermatopharmacokinetic and pharmacodynamic data may provide sufficient proof of bioequivalence "in lieu of clinical trials." However, much remains to be validated in skin-stripping protocols. The in vivo tape-stripping technique is based on the dermal reservoir principle (Rougier, 1987a; Tojo and Lee, 1989). It is hypothesized that if a compound is applied to the skin for a limited time (e.g., 0.5 hours) and then removed, the amount of drug in the upper layers of the stratum corneum will be predictive of the overall bioavailability of the compound. It follows that determination of the stratum corneum content of a permeating material following a short-term application will predict in vivo bioavailability from a corresponding administration protocol. Data obtained in studies of this type have shown reasonable predictability for several compounds.

An outline protocol for skin-stripping bioequivalence studies was suggested (Shah et al., 1998). The basic protocol has two phases: uptake and elimination.

1. Uptake:
   i. Test and reference drug products are applied concurrently at multiple sites.
   ii. After exposure for a suitable time (determined by a pilot study), excess drug is removed by wiping three times with tissue or cotton swab.
   iii. The adhesive tape is applied with uniform pressure. The first strip is discarded (skin surface material). Repeat if necessary to remove excess surface material.
   iv. Collect nine successive tape strips from the same site. If necessary collect more than nine strips.
   v. Repeat the procedure for each site at designated time intervals.
   vi. Extract the drug from the combined tape strips for each time point and site and determine the content of drug using an appropriate validated analytical method.
   vii. Express the data as amount of drug per square centimeter of tape.

2. Elimination:
   i. As for steps i, ii, and iii bove.
   ii. After a predetermined time interval (e.g., 1, 3, 5, and 21 hours post-drug removal) perform steps iv through vii as above.

The results are then expressed as the amount of drug recovered from the tape strips against time. Uptake and elimination phases are observed, and "bioavailability" may be predicted from the area under the curve (AUC). There are several sources of variability in such studies, all of which must be considered in standard operating procedures. The major causes of concern are variability in

- drug application procedure,
- type of tape,
- size of tape,
- pressure applied by investigator,
- duration of application of pressure,
- drug removal procedure,
- drug extraction procedure,
- analytical methodology,
- temperature and relative humidity, and
- skin type and skin surface uniformity.

Nonetheless, following further validation, the technique is seen to have several advantages. For example, basic pharmacokinetic parameters such as AUC, C_{max}, T_{max}, and half-life may be approximated from the data obtained. In addition, the approach could be applicable to all types of topical preparation.

Pershing and colleagues (1992) validated an in vivo skin-stripping protocol by correlating the stratum corneum strip data obtained for betamethasone dipropionate with a skin bioassay blanching experiment. Skin blanching was assessed at 1, 24, and 48 hours following removal of formulations applied under occlusion for 24 hours. The correlation between the amount of betamethasone dipropionate in skin and skin blanching score was good ($r = 0.994$), although the skin blanching scores were not entirely objective because they were assessed visually rather than using a chromameter. Nonetheless, differences in responses between formulations (cream and ointment) and manufacturers could be discerned with both the pharmacokinetic and the pharmacodynamic techniques. Further details of the dermatological drug product bioequivalence, including the proposed protocol, may be obtained from the FDA draft guidance document (FDA, 1998).

Tape stripping is a common method for investigating the distribution of applied materials within stratum corneum and may be very useful in the determination of the bioavailability of topical drugs. However, as pointed out by Loffler et al. (2004), who investigated the influence of procedures (anatomical site, pressure, pressure duration, and tape removal rate) inherent in the tape-stripping protocol, the results are influenced dramatically by all of the investigated parameters. This was confirmed by Bunge and Guy (2007) who, following a very thorough series of experiments, concluded that "the variability in experimental parameters that exist at present preclude the acceptance of the tape-stripping method as a means to evaluate the bioequivalence of topically applied drugs, except for those compounds such as antifungal agents whose main site of activity is the stratum corneum itself. "

Preservation of Semisolid Formulations

All pharmaceutical semisolid formulations, which are not sterilized unit dose products, can support the growth of microorganisms. Preservatives are ingredients, which prevent or retard microbial growth and thus protect formulations from spoilage. The use of preservatives is required to prevent damage of products caused by microorganisms during manufacture, storage, and inadvertent contamination by the patient during use. Similarly, preservatives serve to protect consumers from possible infection from contaminated products. The characteristics of an ideal preservative system are shown in Table 7. Unfortunately, no single preservative meets all of these characteristics for all formulations (Orth, 1993), and it is often necessary to use a preservative system containing a combination of individual preservatives. It is also important to appreciate that preservatives are intrinsically toxic materials, and a balance must be found between antimicrobial efficacy and dermal toxicity.

Table 7 Characteristics for an Ideal Preservative

The ideal preservative
1 Effective at low concentrations against a wide spectrum of microbes
2 Soluble in the formulation at the required concentration
3 Nontoxic and non-sensitizing to the consumer at in-use concentrations
4 Compatible with other formulation components
5 No physical effect on formulation characteristics
6 Stable over a wide range of pH and temperature
7 Inexpensive

Source: From Takruri and Anger (1989).

The most commonly used preservatives in pharmaceutical products are the parabens (alkyl esters of *p*-hydroxybenzoic acid, such as methyl- and propylparaben). These compounds are highly effective against both gram-positive bacteria and fungi at low concentrations (e.g., at concentrations of 0.1–0.3%, paraben combinations provide effective preservation of most emulsions). Because of their widespread use, the toxicological profile of the parabens has been extensively researched, and the safety in use of the lower esters (methyl, ethyl, propyl, and butyl) has been established (Soni et al., 2005). Other preservatives that have been used widely in topical pharmaceutical formulations include benzoic acid, sorbic acid, benzyl alcohol, phenoxyethanol, chlorocresol, benzalkonium chloride, and cetrimide. All have particular advantages and disadvantages, which makes combination preservatives particularly effective. For example, although methylparaben is highly active against gram-positive bacteria and moderately active against yeasts and molds, it is only weakly active against gram-negative bacteria. A combination of methylparaben with phenoxyethanol generates a preservative system that is also highly active against gram-negative species. The acid preservatives, benzoic and sorbic, are only active as free acids, and it is therefore necessary to ensure that formulations containing these preservatives are buffered to acid pH values (pH < 5). A list of pharmaceutical preservatives useful in topical formulations is given in Table 8, together with their microbiological and physicochemical properties. More information on preservatives and preservative systems may be found in the British Pharmaceutical Codex (The Pharmaceutical Press) and in the excellent text by Orth (1993).

It is interesting to note that, despite their widespread use and excellent safety profile, there is an increasing interest in the potential systemic exposure to preservatives following application in pharmaceutical and cosmetic products. In many cases, however, skin penetration data for preservatives are not available in the literature. In addition, much of the data that are publicly available have been obtained under conditions inappropriate to risk assessment. By far the most available data concerns the parabens, and this was reviewed by the

Table 8 Microbiological and Physicochemical Properties of Selected Preservatives

Preservative	Antimicrobial activity[a]				In-use conc. (%)	pH range[b]	O/W[c]
	Gram +	Gram −	Molds	Yeasts			
Benzoic acid	1	2	3	3	0.1	2–5	3–6
Sorbic acid	2	2	2	1	0.2	<6.5	3.5
Phenoxyethanol	2	1	3	3	1.0	wide	-
Methyl paraben	1	3	2	2	0.4–0.8	3.0–9.5	7.5
Propyl paraben	1	3	2	2	0.4–0.8	3.0–9.5	80
Butyl paraben	1	3	2	2	0.4–0.8	3.0–9.5	280
Chlorocresol	1	2	3	3	0.1	<8.5	117–190
Benzalkonium Cl	1	2	3	2	0.01–0.25	4–10	<1
Cetrimide	1	2	3	2	0.01–0.1	4–10	<1

[a]1, highly active; 2, moderately active; 3, weakly active.
[b]Optimal pH range for activity.
[c]Oil-water partition coefficient.

authors in the previous edition of this book (Walters and Brain, 2001). However, one of the most important recent issues regarding the safety of the parabens is the suggestion that some of them may possess estrogenic activity (Pugazhendhi et al., 2005). Although there have been questions raised regarding the rationale, experimental design, and interpretation of these studies (Godfrey, 2006), it is clear that any potential risk associated with parabens use will ultimately be related to exposure, which is dependent on usage patterns of the product and the rate and extent of their percutaneous absorption (Golden et al., 2005).

The early literature on the skin permeation of parabens leads to the conclusion that, although these compounds can permeate the skin, the rate and extent of absorption is markedly dependent on the vehicle of application. Further studies have confirmed the effect of vehicles (Cross and Roberts, 2000), evaluated the effect of skin permeation enhancers on parabens absorption (Nanayakkara et al., 2005), and reported attempts to reduce the penetration of the preservatives (Hasegawa et al., 2005). However, although there is considerable evidence that parabens can penetrate the skin, permeation and systemic availability of intact compounds are likely to be considerably reduced by transcutaneous and systemic metabolism. Furthermore, since these preservatives are present at concentrations of 0.1% to 0.2% (w/w) in topical pharmaceutical formulations, in-use dermal exposure to these compounds will be relatively low.

In the cosmetic industry, there is a trend toward preservative-free and self-preserving formulations (Kabara and Orth, 1997). However, before starting down this road, the pharmaceutical formulator must consider the potential implications on the efficacy and safety of the product.

Transdermal Drug Delivery Systems

The skin was not commercially or scientifically exploited as a route of delivery into the systemic circulation until the 1950s. Development of therapeutically effective ointments containing agents such as nitroglycerin and salicylates dispelled the notion that the skin was essentially impermeable. It was shown that angina, for example, could be controlled for several hours by applying an ointment containing 2% nitroglycerin (Reichek et al., 1974). Similarly, topical salicylates could be absorbed through the skin into arthritic joints, and following this, nonsteroidal anti-inflammatory agents (such as ibuprofen, ketoprofen, and diclofenac) and steroids, including estradiol and testosterone, were developed and marketed in semisolid preparations. A major problem with semisolid preparations, however, is that of control of drug delivery. Drug concentrations in plasma and duration of action are not reliably predictable for several reasons, many of which are patient dependent. Quantity and area of application and dosage frequency obviously affect therapeutic efficacy, but the most significant factors are inter- and intraindividual variations in skin permeability. The seminal work of Scheuplein and Blank (1971) opened a floodgate of research into skin permeation, which has ultimately resulted in the development of modern controlled transdermal drug delivery.

The particular advantages of transdermal therapy are well understood and have been fully discussed elsewhere (Cleary, 1993a). Briefly, transdermal devices are easy to apply, can remain in place for up to seven days (depending on the system), and are easily removed following or during therapy. Reduced dosing frequency and production of controllable and sustained plasma levels tend to minimize risks of undesirable side effects that may be observed after oral dosage. Although viable epidermis contains enzyme systems that may be capable of catabolizing drugs (Wilkinson and Williams, 2008), the avoidance of hepatic first-pass metabolism is an obvious advantage. The intrinsic barrier property of the skin is the major limitation to transdermal drug delivery, a problem discussed later. Marketed patch type transdermal delivery systems are currently available for several drugs (including scopolamine, nitroglycerin, clonidine, estradiol, fentanyl, testosterone, nicotine, oxybutynin, lidocaine, selegiline, methylphenidate, rotigotine, buprenorphine, and tulobuterol), although several other candidates are at various stages of development (Thomas and Finnin, 2004; Stinchcomb et al., 2004; Nalluri et al., 2005; Furuishi et al., 2008; Hai et al., 2008; Park et al., 2008). Many drugs under investigation do not intrinsically possess a great ability to cross the skin, and ways must be found, therefore, to enhance their transdermal delivery. For example, prodrugs can be designed with properties that result in more rapid absorption than the parent compound but

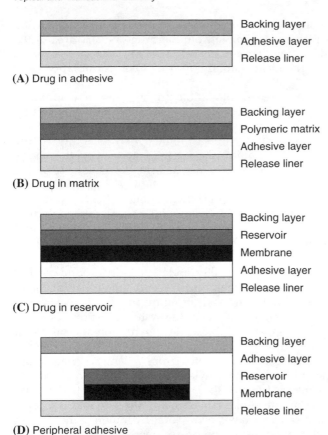

(A) Drug in adhesive

Backing layer
Adhesive layer
Release liner

(B) Drug in matrix

Backing layer
Polymeric matrix
Adhesive layer
Release liner

(C) Drug in reservoir

Backing layer
Reservoir
Membrane
Adhesive layer
Release liner

(D) Peripheral adhesive

Backing layer
Adhesive layer
Reservoir
Membrane
Release liner

Figure 15 Typical transdermal drug delivery system designs.

are subsequently metabolized to the active species before reaching the receptor site (Sloan and Wasdo, 2008). Permeation enhancement strategies have increased the number of candidate drugs for transdermal delivery. An important factor that must be taken into account during transdermal product development is the potential for allergic or irritant responses to the drug and/or other formulation constituents (Chan et al., 2008).

Although there have been several variations, current patch-type transdermal delivery systems continue to utilize one of three basic design principles: drug in adhesive, drug in matrix (usually polymeric), or drug in reservoir (Fig. 15). Other systems include those that utilize small electrical currents to increase drug delivery (e.g., Alza's E-TRANS; Padmanabhan et al., 2008), sound or pressure waves (Mitragotri and Kost, 2008; Doukas et al., 2008) or completely bypass the stratum corneum by the use of microneedles (Birchall and Brain, 2008; Prausnitz et al., 2008) or ballistic delivery (Kendall, 2008). These physical methods have been fully discussed elsewhere and will not be covered in this chapter.

Several features are common to all traditional systems, including the release liner, pressure-sensitive adhesive, and backing layer, all of which must be compatible (Cleary, 1993b; Valenta and Auner, 2004). In the more established transdermal drug delivery systems, the reservoir of a form-fill-seal-type device is separated from the skin by a rate-controlling membrane. In a system where the drug is intimately mixed with adhesive, or diffuses from a reservoir through adhesive, the potential for interaction between drug and adhesive, which can lead to either reduction of adhesive effectiveness or formation of a new chemical species, must be fully assessed. Similarly, residual monomers, catalysts, plasticizers, and resins may react to give new chemical species, and it is possible that excipients (including enhancers) and/or their reaction products may interfere with adhesive systems (Li et al., 2002a, b; Tokumura et al., 2007).

Incompatibilities between the adhesive system and other formulation excipients may be circumvented by designs in which the adhesive is remote from the drug delivery area of the system (Fig. 15d). Three critical considerations in system selection are adhesion to skin, compatibility with skin, and physical/chemical stability of the total formulation and components.

Devices are secured to the skin by use of a skin-compatible pressure-sensitive adhesive, usually based on silicones, acrylates, or polyisobutylenes. These adhesives are evaluated by shear testing and assessment of rheological parameters (Venkatraman and Gale, 1998). Standard rheological tests include creep compliance (measurement of the ability of the adhesive to flow into surface irregularities), elastic index (the extent of stretch or deformation as a function of load and time), and recovery following deformation. Skin adhesion performance is described by properties such as initial and long-term adhesion, lift, and residue. The adhesive must be soft enough to ensure initial adhesion, yet have sufficient cohesive strength to remove cleanly, leaving no residue. Premature lift will interfere with drug delivery, and therefore, the cohesive and adhesive properties must be carefully balanced and maintained over the intended period of application. This must be evaluated by wear testing, using placebo patches applied to the skin (Ho and Dodou, 2007).

Adhesion to the skin is affected by shape, conformability, and occlusivity. Round patches tend to be more secure than those of more sharply angled geometry. A patch that is able to conform to the contours of the skin will resist buckling and lifting during movement. Water may affect adhesive properties, and therefore, the occlusivity of the system must be taken into consideration. Occlusion for prolonged periods can lead to excessive hydration and microbial growth, which may increase the possibilities of irritation or sensitization.

The backing material and release liner can be fabricated from a variety of materials including polyvinylchloride, polyethylene, polypropylene, ethylene-vinyl acetate, and aluminum foil. The most important property of these materials is that they are impervious to both drug and formulation excipients. The most useful backing materials conform with the skin and provide a balanced resistance to transepidermal water loss, which will allow some hydration of the stratum corneum, yet maintain a healthy subpatch environment. The release liners are usually films or coated papers and must separate easily from the adhesive layer without lifting off any of the pressure-sensitive adhesive. Silicone release coatings are used with acrylate and rubber-based adhesive systems, and fluorocarbon coatings are suitable for most types of adhesive.

The three principal methods of incorporation of active species into a transdermal system have led to the loose classification of patches as membrane, matrix, or drug-in-adhesive types. Combinations of the main types of patch can also be fabricated, for example, by placing a membrane over a matrix or using a drug-in-adhesive with a membrane/matrix device to deliver an initial bolus dose. Membrane patches contain delivery rate–controlling membranes between the drug reservoir and the skin (Yuk et al., 1991a). These may be microporous membranes, which control drug flux due to the size and tortuosity of pores in the membrane, or dense polymeric membranes, through which the drug permeates by dissolution and diffusion. Examples of rate-controlling membranes are ethylene-vinyl acetate copolymers, silicones, high-density polyethylene, polyester elastomers and polyacrylonitrile. Ideally, the membrane should be permeable only to the drug and enhancer (if present) and retain other formulation excipients. Membranes have been designed, which allow differential permeation of enhancer and drug (Yuk et al., 1991b; Okabe et al., 1994), and this type (sometimes designated as a one-way membrane) is useful when the drug is located in the adhesive, while the enhancer is formulated into a reservoir.

A variety of materials are used in the drug reservoir, ranging from mineral oil to complex formulations, such as aqueous/alcoholic gels. A reservoir system should provide zero-order release of the drug over the entire delivery period, which requires that the reservoir material remains saturated with the drug over the period of product application. This can usually be achieved by formulating the drug as a suspension.

The second type is the matrix transdermal system where the drug is uniformly dispersed in a polymeric matrix through which it diffuses to the skin surface (Leuenberger et al., 1995). The polymeric matrix (which may be composed of silicone elastomers, polyurethanes, polyvinyl alcohol, polyvinylpyrrolidones, etc.) may be considered as the drug reservoir. A series of steps are involved in the drug delivery process: dissociation of drug molecules from the crystal lattice, solubilization of the drug in the polymer matrix, and diffusion of drug molecules through the matrix to the skin surface. Many factors can affect dissolution and diffusion rates, making it particularly difficult to predict release rates from experimental or prototype formulations. It is fundamental, however, that for a drug to be released from the matrix under zero-order kinetics, it must ideally be maintained at saturation in the fluid phase of the matrix, and the diffusion rate of the drug within the matrix must be much greater than the diffusion rate of the drug in the skin.

The release rate of a drug or an enhancer from a polymeric matrix can be modified in several ways (Pfister et al., 1987; Ulman et al., 1989a,b; Ulman and Lee, 1989; Gelotte and Lostrito, 1990), some of which are illustrated by a study of release of several drugs from silicone matrices (Pfister et al., 1987). Silicone medical-grade elastomers (polydimethylsiloxanes) are flexible, lipophilic polymers with excellent compatibility with biological tissues. They can be co-formulated with hydrophilic excipients, such as glycerol, and inert fillers, such as titanium dioxide, to alter release kinetics. Increasing the level of glycerol in the matrix increases the release rates of indomethacin, propranolol, testosterone, and progesterone, while the presence of the inert fillers, titanium dioxide or barium sulfate, tends to reduce release rates. Release rates for hydrophilic drug from polydimethylsiloxane matrices can be increased by up to three orders of magnitude using polydimethyl siloxane/polyethylene oxide graft copolymers (Ulman et al., 1989b). These examples demonstrate the relative ease with which release rates of drugs can be tailored to produce a desired profile.

The microsealed delivery device is a variation of the matrix-type transdermal system in which the drug is dispersed in a reservoir phase that is then immobilized as discrete droplets in a cross-linked polymeric matrix. Release can be further controlled by inclusion of a polymeric microporous membrane. This system therefore combines the principles of both the liquid reservoir and matrix-type devices. Rate of release of a drug from a microsealed delivery system is dependent on the partition coefficient between the reservoir droplets and the polymeric matrix; the diffusivity of the drug in the reservoir, the matrix, and the controlling membrane; and on the solubility of the drug in the various phases. There are, obviously, many ways to achieve the desired zero-order release rate, but only nitroglycerin has been commercially formulated into this type of delivery device (Karim, 1983).

The simplest form of transdermal drug delivery device, most commonly employed at present, is the drug-in-adhesive system where the drug (and enhancer if present) is formulated in an adhesive mixture that is coated onto a backing membrane to produce an adhesive tape. The apparent simplicity is, however, deceptive, and a number of factors, which arise from potential interactions between drug or enhancer and adhesive, must be considered (Kokubo et al., 1991, 1994; Li et al., 2002a,b; Cheong and Choi, 2003). Chemical interactions may interfere with adhesive performance, cause breakdown of the active species, or formation of NCE (Dimas et al., 2000). The variability in physicochemical characteristics of drugs and adhesive systems will result in different release rates for hydrophilic and hydrophobic drugs: For example, silicone adhesives are typically lipophilic, which markedly limits the solubility of hydrophilic drugs within the adhesive matrix (Roy et al., 1996).

Incorporation of additional excipients, such as skin permeation enhancers, into a drug-in-adhesive system may alter drug release rates and adhesive properties. Reduction of the influence of both drug and enhancer on adhesive properties has been achieved by design of transdermal systems where there is no contact between these constituents and the adhesive (e.g., where the adhesive is present in a boundary laminate surrounding a drug/enhancer-releasing layer). A disadvantage of this type of system is that the drug/enhancer-releasing layer may not remain in intimate contact with the skin. Where high levels of liquid skin penetration enhancers are incorporated into drug-in-adhesive transdermal patches, there is often a loss in cohesiveness, which results in patch slipping and skin residues following patch removal. Cohesive strength can be increased by high levels of cross-linking in acrylate adhesives, but this may alter both long-term bonding and drug release rates. These problems have been overcome by the development of grafted copolymer adhesives such as ARcare® ETA Adhesive Systems where reinforcement is mainly achieved through phase separation of the side chain within the continuous polymer network. A variety of side chains are available, and up to 30% of enhancers have been incorporated without seriously affecting the adhesive properties. This work involved fatty acid ester type enhancers, and utility with other enhancer types remains to be established. Adhesive properties may also be maintained in the presence of skin penetration enhancers by using blends of acrylic copolymers with different molecular weights (Ko et al., 1995). Present adhesive technology provides a variety of acrylic-, silicone-, and rubber-based adhesives that can be mixed and combined to provide different characteristics in terms of adhesive/cohesive properties and drug release patterns (see, e.g., the National Starch range of acrylate pressure sensitive adhesives at www.nationaladh.com/Adhesives/USA/Your+Business/Transdermal/Products/Products.htm; Dow Corning's range of silicone pressure-sensitive adhesives at www.dowcorning.com/content/pressure/pressureadhesive. It is important to appreciate that it is a fundamental requirement that the enhancer, as well as the drug, be released by the adhesive. It is also probable that an enhancer will increase skin permeation of other formulation excipients, which may have an impact on local toxicity (Chan et al., 2008).

A major concern with drug-in-adhesive systems is that of physical stability within the adhesive matrix. A common problem is for the drug to crystallize on storage leading to changes in adhesion and drug delivery. Several strategies have been developed to reduce this problem, including the addition of additives (Kotiyan and Vavia, 2001; Cilurzo et al., 2005), but perhaps the most effective option is to ensure that the drug is not too close to saturation within the adhesive matrix.

Manufacturing processes for reservoir, matrix, and drug-in-adhesive transdermal systems are largely similar and involve the following stages:

- Preparing drug;
- Mixing drug (and any other excipients) with reservoir, matrix, or adhesive;
- Casting into films and drying (or molding and curing);
- Laminating with other structural components (e.g., backing layer, rate-controlling membrane, and release liner);
- Die cutting
- Final packaging.

The most critical steps in the manufacturing process are casting and lamination, and tensions and pressures must be carefully controlled to produce a wrinkle-free laminate with uniform drug content and reproducible adhesive-coating thickness.

In common with other controlled-release delivery systems, final product checks include content uniformity, release rate determination, and physical testing. Content-uniformity evaluation involves taking a random sample of patches from a batch and assaying for drug content. Several methods are available for determining drug release rates from controlled release formulations, but the U.S. PMA Committee (PMA Committee Report, 1986) has recommended three: the "Paddle over Disk" (identical to the USP paddle dissolution apparatus, except that the transdermal system is attached to a disk or cell resting at the bottom of the vessel that contains medium at 32°C), the "Cylinder-Modified USP Basket" (similar to the USP basket method, except that the system is attached to the surface of a hollow cylinder immersed in medium at 32°C), and the "Reciprocating Disk" (where patches attached to holders are oscillated in small volumes of medium, allowing the apparatus to be useful for systems delivering low concentrations of drug). In a comparative study using a scopolamine patch, a diffusion cell method was evaluated against the "Paddle over Disk" and "Reciprocating Disk" methods (Mazzo et al., 1986). Although the latter two methods gave equivalent results, these were ∼25% greater than the steady-state flux determined using the diffusion cell. The "Paddle over Disk" method was preferred on the basis of ease of use and ready availability of equipment. The FDA has developed a modified paddle procedure (essentially the "Paddle over Disk" method) for determining drug release from transdermal systems (Shah et al., 1986). One problem with the original method was the mode of keeping the patch in position in the dissolution beaker, and a device to improve and maintain placement of the patch has been subsequently suggested (Man et al., 1993).

CONCLUDING REMARKS

In this chapter, we have described some of the considerations that we believe to be important in the design and development of pharmaceutical products intended for application to the skin. Space limitations dictated that we could not provide an exhaustive review of all the factors that are essential in pharmaceutical product development. The reader who has read this far will appreciate that preformulation, formulation recipes, scale-up, safety, and clinical aspects are not covered. These aspects are fully covered either elsewhere in this volume or in some of the excellent and fully recommended texts listed in the bibliography. What we have attempted to achieve herein is to share our knowledge of the structure of skin and the biological and physicochemical determinants of skin penetration and permeation. We have then described the methodologies employed and the usefulness of skin permeation measurement in the development of formulations. Finally, we have described some of the formulation types that are applied to the skin together with their properties. We hope that our comments will provide the novice formulator with some insights borne of experience and the experienced formulator with some novel insights in the field of dermatological and transdermal product development.

REFERENCES

Abdulmajed K, Heard CM. Topical delivery of retinyl ascorbate co-drug 1. Synthesis, penetration into and permeation across human skin. Int J Pharm 2004; 280:113–124.

Abdulmajed K, Heard CM, McGuigan C, et al. Topical delivery of retinyl ascorbate co-drug 2. Comparative skin tissue and keratin binding studies. Skin Pharmacol Physiol 2004; 17:274–282.

Akomeah FK, Martin GP, Brown MB. Variability in human skin permeability in vitro: comparing penetrants with different physicochemical properties. J Pharm Sci 2007; 96:824–834.

Alibardi L. Structural and immunocytochemical characterization of keratinization in vertebrate epidermis and epidermal derivatives. Int Rev Cytol 2006; 253:177–259.

A-sasutjarit R, Sirivat A, Vayumhasuwan P. Viscoelastic properties of Carbopol 940 gels and their relationships to piroxicam diffusion coefficients in gel bases. Pharm Res 2005; 22:2134–2140.

Aszterbaum M, Menon GK, Feingold KR, et al. Ontogeny of the epidermal barrier to water loss in the rat: correlation of function with stratum corneum structure and lipid content. Pediatr Res 1992; 31:308–317.

Baden HP. Keratinization in the epidermis. Pharm Ther 1979; 7:393–411.

Barreiro-Iglesias R, Alvarez-Lorenzo C, Concheiro A. Incorporation of small quantities of surfactants as a way to improve the rheological and diffusional behavior of carbopol gels. J Contr Rel 2001; 77:59–75.

Barry BW, Dermatological Formulations, Percutaneous Absorption. New York: Marcel Dekker, 1983.

Birchall J, Brain KR. Microneedle arrays as transcutaneous delivery devices. In: Walters KA, Roberts MS, eds. Dermatologic, Cosmeceutic, and Cosmetic Development: Therapeutic and Novel Approaches. New York: Informa Healthcare, 2008:577–589.

Blank IH. Penetration of low-molecular weight alcohols into the skin. I. The effect of concentration of alcohol and type of vehicle. J Invest Dermatol 1964; 43:415–420.

Boczonadi V, McInroy L, Maatta A. Cytolinker cross-talk: periplakin N-terminus interacts with plectin to regulate keratin organization and epithelial migration. Exp Cell Res 2007; 313:3579–3591.

Boulais N, Misery L. The epidermis: a sensory tissue. Eur J Dermatol 2008; 18:119–127.

Bouwstra JA, Ponec M. The skin barrier in healthy and diseased state. Biochim Biophys Acta 2006; 1758:2080–2095. [Epub 2006, Jul 11]

Brain KR, Walters KA, Watkinson AC. Investigation of skin permeation in vitro. In: Roberts MS, Walters KA, eds. Dermal Absorption and Toxicity Assessment. New York: Marcel Dekker, 1998:161–187.

Bronaugh RL. Methods for *in vitro* percutaneous absorption. In: Marzulli FN, Maibach HI, eds. Dermatotoxicology. 5th ed. Washington, DC: Taylor and Francis, 1996:317–324.

Bronaugh RL. Interpretation of in vitro skin absorption studies of lipophilic chemicals. In: Roberts MS, Walters KA, eds. Dermal Absorption and Toxicity Assessment, 2nd ed. New York: Informa Healthcare, 2008:135–140.

Bronaugh RL, Stewart RF. Methods for *in vitro* percutaneous absorption studies. IV: The flow through diffusion cell. J Pharm Sci 1985; 74:64–67.

Bronaugh RL, Stewart RF, Simon M. Methods for *in vitro* percutaneous absorption studies. VII: use of excised human skin. J Pharm Sci 1986; 75:1094–1097.

Bronaugh RL, Stewart RF, Storm JE. Extent of cutaneous metabolism during percutaneous absorption of xenobiotics. Toxicol Appl Pharmacol 1989; 99:534–543.

Bugaj A, Juzeniene A, Juzenas P, et al. The effect of skin permeation enhancers on the formation of porphyrins in mouse skin during topical application of the methyl ester of 5-aminolevulinic acid. J Photochem Photobiol B 2006; 83:94–97.

Bunge AL. Release rates from topical formulations containing drugs in suspension. J Contr Rel 1998; 52:141–148.

Bunge AL, Guy RH. Therapeutic equivalence of topical products. Final Report 223-04-3004. Food and Drug Administration, 2007.

Büyüktimkin S, Büyüktimkin N, Rytting JH. Synthesis and enhancing effect of dodecyl 2-(N,N-dimethylamino)-propionate (DDAIP) on the transepidermal delivery of indomethacin, clonidine, and hydrocortisone. Pharm Res 1993; 10:1632–1637.

Caetano PA, Flynn GL, Farinha AR, et al. The in vitro release test as a means to obtain the solubility and diffusivity of drugs in semisolids. Proc Intl Symp Contr Rel Bioact Mater 1999; 26:375–376.

Caussin J, Gooris GS, Janssens M, et al. Lipid organization in human and porcine stratum corneum differs widely, while lipid mixtures with porcine ceramides model human stratum corneum lipid organization very closely. Biochim Biophys Acta 2008; 1778:1472–1482.

Cevc G. Transfersome: self-optimizing and self-driven drug-carrier, for localized and transdermal delivery. In: Rathbone MJ, Hadgraft J, Roberts MS, et al.eds. Modified-Release Drug Delivery Technology. 2nd ed. Volume 2. New York: Informa Healthcare, 2008:311–324.

Chan HP, Levin CY, Maibach HI. Irritancy of topical chemicals in transdermal drug delivery systems. In: Roberts MS and Walters KA, eds. Dermal Absorption and Toxicity Assessment. 2nd ed. New York: Informa Healthcare, 2008:371–390.

Chattaraj SC, Kanfer I. Release of acyclovir from semi-solid dosage forms: a semiautomated procedure using a simple plexiglass flow-through cell. Int J Pharm 1995; 125:215–222.

Cheong H-A, Choi H-K. Effect of ethanolamine salts and enhancers on the percutaneous absorption of piroxicam from a pressure sensitive adhesive matrix. Eur J Pharm Sci 2003; 18:149–153.

Chow KT, Chan LW, Heng PWS. Formulation of hydrophilic non-aqueous gel: drug stability in different solvents and rheological behavior of gel matrices. Pharm Res 2008; 25:207–217.

Cilurzo F, Minghetti P, Casiraghi A, et al. Polymethacrylates as crystallization inhibitors in monolayer transdermal patches containing ibuprofen. Eur J Pharm Biopharm 2005; 60:61–66.

Cleary GW. Transdermal delivery systems: a medical rationale. In: Shah VP, Maibach HI,eds. Topical Drug Bioavailability, Bioequivalence, and Penetration. New York: Plenum Press, 1993a: 17–68.

Cleary GW. Transdermal drug delivery. In: Zatz JL, ed. Skin Permeation, Fundamentals and Application. Wheaton, IL: Allured Publishing, 1993b; 207–237.

Clowes HM, Scott RC, Heylings JR. Skin absorption: flow-through or static diffusion cells. Toxicol In Vitro 1994; 8:827–830.

Collier SW, Sheikh NM, Sakr A, et al. Maintenence of skin viability during in vitro percutaneous absorption/metabolism studies. Toxicol Appl Pharmacol 1989; 99:522–533.

Corcuff P, Lotte C, Rougier A, et al. Racial differences in corneocytes. A comparison between black, white and oriental skin. Acta Derm Venereol 1991; 71:146–148.

Cross SE, Roberts MS. The effects of occlusion on epidermal penetration of parabens from a commercial allergy test ointment, acetone and ethanol vehicles. J Invest Dermatol 2000; 115:914–918.

Cynkowski T, Cynkowska G, Walters KA. Codrugs: potential therapies for dermatological diseases. In: Walters KA, Roberts MS, eds. Dermatologic, Cosmeceutic, and Cosmetic Development: Therapeutic and Novel Approaches. New York: Informa Healthcare, 2008:255–266.

Dahl T, He, G-X, Samuels G. Effect of hydrogen peroxide on the viscosity of a hydroxyethylcellulose-based gel. Pharm Res 1998; 15:1137–1140.

Date AA, Patravale VB. Microemulsions: applications in transdermal and dermal delivery. Crit Rev Ther Drug Carrier Syst 2007; 24:547–596.

Dancik Y, Jepps OG, Roberts MS. Beyond stratum corneum. In: Roberts MS, Walters KA. eds. Dermal Absorption and Toxicity Assessment. 2nd ed. New York: Informa Healthcare, 2008:209–250.

Davies DJ, Ward RJ, Heylings JR. Multi-species assessment of electrical resistance as a skin integrity marker for in vitro percutaneous absorption studies. Toxicol In Vitro 2004; 18:351–358.

Davis AF, Hadgraft J. Supersaturated solutions as topical drug delivery sytems. In: Walters KA and Hadgraft J, eds. Pharmaceutical Skin Penetration Enhancement. New York: Marcel Dekker, 1993:243–268.

Dick IP, Blain PG, Williams FM. Improved in vitro skin absorption for lipophilic compounds following the addition of albumin to the receptor fluid in flow-through cells. In: Brain KR, James VJ, Walters KA, eds. Prediction of Percutaneous Penetration, Volume 4b. Cardiff, UK: STS Publishing, 1996:267–270.

Dimas DA, Dallas PP, Rekkas DD, et al. Effect of several factors on the mechanical properties of pressure-sensitive adhesives used in transdermal therapeutic systems. AAPS PharmSciTech 2000; 1(2):E16.

Doukas AG, Paliwal S, Mitragotri S. Pressure waves for transdermal drug delivery. In: Walters KA, Roberts MS, eds. Dermatologic, Cosmeceutic, and Cosmetic Development: Therapeutic and Novel Approaches. New York: Informa Healthcare, 2008:557–576.

Eccleston GM. Multiple phase oil-in-water emulsions. J Soc Cosmet Chem 1990; 41:1–22.

Eccleston GM. Functions of mixed emulsifiers and emulsifying waxes in dermatological lotions and creams. Colloids Surf 1997; 123:169–182.

Elias PM. Lipids and the epidermal permeability barrier. Arch Dermatol Res 1981; 270:95–117.

Elias PM, Feingold KR. Lipids and the epidermal water barrier: metabolism, regulation, and pathophysiology. Sem Dermatol 1992; 11:176–182.

Elias PM, Feingold KR, eds. Skin Barrier. New York: Taylor & Francis, 2006.

Fartasch M, Diepgen TL. The barrier function in atopic dry skin. Acta Derm Venereol 1992; 176(suppl.): 26–31.

Fasano WI, Manning LA, Green JW. Rapid integrity assessment of rat and human epidermal membranes for in vitro dermal regulatory testing: correlation of electrical resistance with tritiated water permeability. Toxicol In Vitro 2002; 16:731–740.

FDA. SUPAC-SS—Nonsterile semisolid dosage forms. Rockville, MD: Food and Drug Adiminstration, U.S. Department of Health and Human Services, 1997.

FDA. Topical dermatological drug product NDAs and ANDAs—In vivo bioavailability, bioequivalence, in vivo release, and associated studies. Rockville, MD: Food and Drug Administration, U.S. Department of Health and Human Services, 1998.

Feldman RJ, Maibach HI. Regional variation in the percutaneous penetration of ^{14}C cortisol in man. J Invest Dermatol 1967; 48:181–183.

Flynn GL. Cutaneous and transdermal delivery: processes and systems of delivery. In: Banker GS and Rhodes CT, eds. Modern Pharmaceutics. 3rd ed. New York: Marcel Dekker, 1996:239–298.

Flynn GL, Yalkowski SH. Correlation and prediction of mass transport across membranes. I: influence of alkyl chain length on flux-determining properties of barrier and diffusant. J Pharm Sci 1972; 61:838–852.

Franz TJ. On the relevance of in vitro data. J Invest Dermatol 1975; 64:190–195.

Franz TJ, Lehman PA, Franz SF, et al. A Formulary For External Therapy of The Skin. Springfield, IL: Charles C. Thomas, 1954.

Franz TJ, Lehman PA, Franz SF, et al. Percutaneous penetration of N-nitroso-diethanolamine through human skin (in vitro): comparison of finite and infinite dose application from cosmetic vehicles. Fundam Appl Toxicol 1993; 21:213–221.

Franz TJ, Lehman PA, Rainey SG. Use of the human cadaver skin model to assess the bioavailability and bioequivalence of topical products. Perspectives in Percutaneous Penetration, 2008; 11: pp6

Friedrich S, Brummer R, Wittern KP, et al. Dielectric spectroscopy of concentrated cosmetic W/O-emulsions: possibilities to distinguish product changes caused by coalescence, sedimentation and variation of ingredients. Int J Cosmet Sci 2004; 26:157–164.

Frum Y, Khan GM, Sefcik J, et al. Towards a correlation between drug properties and in vitro transdermal flux variability. Int J Pharm 2007; 336:140–147.

Furuishi T, Io T, Fukami T, et al. Formulation and in vitro evaluation of pentazocine transdermal delivery system. Biol Pharm Bull 2008; 31:1439–1443.

Gauthier ER, Gyurik RJ, Krauser SF, et al. SEPA® absorption enhancement of polar and non-polar drugs. In: Brain KR, James VJ, Walters KA, eds. Perspectives in Percutaneous Penetration, Volume 5b. Cardiff, UK: STS Publishing, 1998:270–272.

Gelotte KM, Lostritto RT. Solvent interaction with poly-dimethylsiloxane membranes and its effects on benzocaine solubility and diffusion. Pharm Res 1990; 7:523–529.

Godfrey D. Parabens – a safe bet!, 2006. Available at: www.health-report.co.uk/parabens_industry_view.htm.

Golden R, Gandy J, Vollmer G. A review of the endocrine activity of parabens and implications for potential risks to human health. Crit Rev Toxicol 2005; 35:435–458.

Gooris GS, Bouwstra JA. Infrared spectroscopic study of stratum corneum model membranes prepared from human ceramides, cholesterol, and fatty acids. Biophys J 2007; 92:2785–2795.

Green DM. *Investigation of Factors Affecting Skin Penetration In Vitro* [master's thesis]. Cardiff, UK: Cardiff University, 2005:196–210.

Grober ED, Khera M, Soni SD, et al. Efficacy of changing testosterone gel preparations (Androgel or Testim) among suboptimally responsive hypogonadal men. Int J Impot Res 2007; 20:213–217.

Guy RH, Tur E, Bjerke S, et al. Are there age and racial differences to methyl nicotinate-induced vasodilation in human skin? J Am Acad Dermatol 1983; 12:1001–1006.

Gyurik RJ, Krauser SF, Gauthier ER, et al. SEPA® penetration enhancement of econazole in human skin. In: Brain KR, James VJ, Walters KA, eds. Prediction of Percutaneous Penetration. Volume 4b. Cardiff, UK: STS Publishing, 1996:124–126.

Hadgraft J, Williams DG, Allan G. Azone, mechanism, of action and clinical effect. In: Walters KA, Hadgraft J, eds. Pharmaceutical Skin Penetration Enhancement. New York: Marcel Dekker, 1993:175–197.

Hai NT, Kim J, Park ES, et al. Formulation and biopharmaceutical evaluation of transdermal patch containing benztropine. Int J Pharm 2008; 357:55–60.

Hammell DC, Hamad M, Vaddi HK, et al. A duplex "Gemini" prodrug of naltrexone for transdermal delivery. J Contr Rel 2004; 97:283–290.

Harrison SM, Barry BW, Dugard PH. Effects of freezing on human skin permeability. J Pharm Pharmacol 1984; 36:261–262.

Hasegawa T, Kim S, Tsuchida M, et al. Decrease in skin permeation and antibacterial effect of parabens by a polymeric additive, poly(2-methacryloyloxyethyl phosphorylcholine-co-butylmetacrylate). Chem Pharm Bull 2005; 53:271–276.

Heard CM, Brain KR. Does solute stereochemistry influence percutaneous penetration? Chirality 1995; 7:305–309.

Herkenne C, Alberti I, Naik A, et al. In vivo methods for the assessment of topical drug bioavailability. Pharm Res 2008; 25:87–103.

Heuschkel S, Goebel A, Neubert RH. Microemulsions—modern colloidal carrier for dermal and transdermal drug delivery. J Pharm Sci 2008; 97:603–631.

Higuchi T. Physical chemical analysis of percutaneous absorption process from creams and ointments. J Soc Cosmet Chem 1960; 11:85–97.

Higuchi T. Rate of release of medicaments from ointment bases containing drugs in suspension. J Pharm Sci 1961; 50:874–875.

Hill J, Paslin D, Wertz PW. A new covalently bound ceramide from human stratum corneum—ω-hydroxyacylphytosphingosine. Int J Cosm Sci 2006; 28:225–230.

Hillebrand GG, Wickett RR. Epidemiology of skin barrier function: host and environment factors. In: Walters KA, Roberts MS, eds. Dermatologic, Cosmeceutic, and Cosmetic Development: Therapeutic and Novel Approaches. New York: Informa Healthcare, 2008:129–156.

Hinz RS, Lorence CR, Hodson CD, et al. Percutaneous penetration of para-substituted phenols in vitro. Fundam Appl Toxicol 1991; 47:869–892.

Ho KY, Dodou K. Rheological studies on pressure-sensitive silicone adhesives and drug-in-adhesive layers as a means to characterise adhesive performance. Int J Pharm 2007; 333:24–33.

Hotchkiss SAM. Dermal metabolism. In: Roberts MS, Walters KA, eds. Dermal Absorption and Toxicity Assessment. New York: Marcel Dekker, 1998:43–101.

Hughes MF, Shrivasta SP, Fisher HL, et al. Comparative in vitro percutaneous absorption of p-substituted phenols through rat skin using static and flow-through diffusion systems. Toxicol In Vitro 1993; 7: 221–227.

Inoue K, Ogawa K, Okada J, et al. Enhancement of skin permeation of ketotifen by supersaturation generated by amorphous form of the drug. J Contr Rel 2005; 108:306–318.

Islam MT, Rodriquez-Hornedo N, Ciotti S, et al. Rheological characterization of topical carbomer gels neutralized to different pH. Pharm Res 2004; 21:1192–1199.

de Jager M, Groenink W, Bielsa i Guivernau R, et al. A novel in vitro percutaneous penetration model: evaluation of barrier properties with p-aminobenzoic acid and two of its derivatives. Pharm Res 2006; 23:951–960.

Jenkins AW, inventor; Ethical Pharmaceuticals. Transdermal device. UK patent GB 2 249 956A. 1992.

Jiao J, Burgess DJ. Rheology and stability of water-in-oil-in-water multiple emulsions containing Span 83 and Tween 20. AAPS PharmSci 2003; 5(1):Article 7.

Kabara JJ, Orth DS, eds. Preservative-Free and Self-Preserving Cosmetics and Drugs—Principles and Practice. New York: Marcel Dekker.

Karande P, Jain A, Mitragotri S. Multicomponent formulations of chemical penetration enhancers. In: Walters KA, Roberts MS, eds. Dermatologic, Cosmeceutic, and Cosmetic Development: Therapeutic and Novel Approaches. New York: Informa Healthcare, 2008:505–516.

Karim A. Transdermal absorption of nitroglycerin from microseal drug delivery (MDD) system. Angiology 1983; 34:11–22.

Kasting GB, Smith RL, Anderson BD. Prodrugs for dermal delivery: solubility, molecular size, and functional group effects. In: Sloan KB, ed. Prodrugs. New York: Marcel Dekker, 1992:117–161.

Kasting GB, Bowman LA. Electrical analysis of fresh excised human skin: a comparison with frozen skin. Pharm Res 1990; 7:1141–1146.

Kendall MAF. Needle-free ballistic delivery of powdered immunotherapeutics to the skin using supersonic gas flow. In: Walters KA, Roberts MS, eds. Dermatologic, Cosmeceutic, and Cosmetic Development: Therapeutic and Novel Approaches. New York: Informa Healthcare, 2008:591–611.

Kiptoo PK, Hamad MO, Crooks PA, et al. Enhancement of transdermal delivery of 6-β-naltrexol via a codrug linked to hydroxybupropion. J Contr Rel 113:137–145.

Kitson N. Drugs used for skin diseases. In: Walters KA, Roberts MS, eds. Dermatologic, Cosmeceutic, and Cosmetic Development: Therapeutic and Novel Approaches. New York: Informa Healthcare, 2008: 11–20.

Kitson N, Maddin S. Drugs used for skin diseases. In: Roberts MS, Walters KA, eds. Dermal Absorption and Toxicity Assessment. New York: Marcel Dekker, 1998:313–326.

Kneczke M, Landersjö L, Lundgren P, et al. In vitro release of salicylic acid from two different qualities of white petrolatum. Acta Pharm Suec 1986; 23:193–204.

Ko CU, Wilking SL, Birdsall J. Pressure sensitive adhesive property optimizations for the transdermal drug delivery systems. Pharm Res 1995; 12:S–143.

Kogan A, Garti N. Microemulsions as transdermal drug delivery vehicles. Adv Colloid Interface Sci 2006; 123/6:369–385.

Kokubo T, Sugibayashi K, Morimoto Y. Diffusion of drug in acrylic-type pressure-sensitive adhesive matrices. I. Influence of physical property of the matrices on the drug diffusion. J Contr Rel 1991; 17: 69–78.

Kokubo T, Sugibayashi K, Morimoto Y. Interaction between drugs and pressure-sensitive adhesives in transdermal therapeutic systems. Pharm Res 1994; 11:104–107.

Kompaore F, Tsuruta H. In vivo differences between Asian, Black and White in the stratum corneum barrier function. Int Arch Occup Environ Health 1993; 65:S223–S225.

Korhonen M, Hirvonen J, Peltonen L, et al. Formation and characterization of three-component-sorbitan monoester surfactant, oil and water-creams. Int J Pharm 2004; 269:227–239.

Korting HC. ed. The skin as a site for drug delivery: the liposome approach and its alternatives. Adv Drug Del Rev 1996; 18(3):271–425.

Kotiyan PN, Vavia PR. Eudragits: role as crystallization inhibitors in drug-in-adhesive transdermal systems of estradiol. Eur J Pharm Biopharm 2001; 52:173–180.

Kou JH, Roy SD, Du J, et al. Effect of receiver fluid pH on in vitro skin flux of weakly ionizable drugs. Pharm Res 1993; 10:986–990.

Kril MB, Parab PV, Genier SE, et al. Potential problems encountered with SUPAC-SS and the in vitro release testing of ammonium lactate cream. Pharm Tech 1999; (March):164–174.

Kumar R, Katare OP. Lecithin organogels as a potential phospholipids-structured system for topical drug delivery: a review. AAPS PharmSciTech. 2005; 6(2):Article 40.

Laugel C, Rafidison P, Potard G, et al. Modulated release of triterpenic compounds from a O/W/O multiple emulsion formulated with dimethicones: infrared spectrophotometric and differential calorimetric approaches. J Contr Rel 2000; 63:7–17.

Lazo ND, Maine JG, Downing DT. Lipids are covalently attached to rigid corneocyte protein envelopes existing predominantly as β-sheets: a solid-state nuclear magnetic resonance study. J Invest Dermatol 1995; 105:296–300.

Lehman PA, Agrawa IN, Franz TJ, et al. Comparison of topical hydrocortisone products: percutaneous absorption vs. tape stripping vs. vasoconstriction vs. membrane rate of release. Pharm Res 1996; 13:S310.

Leichtnam M-L, Rolland H, Wuthrich P, et al. Impact of antinucleants on transdermal delivery of testosterone from a spray. J Pharm Sci 2007; 96:84–92.

Leo A, Hansch C, Elkins D. Partition coefficients and their uses. Chem Rev 1971; 71:525–616.

Leopold CS, Maibach HI. Effect of lipophilic vehicles on in vivo skin penetration of methyl nicotinate in different races. Int J Pharmaceut 1996; 139:161–167.

Leuenberger H, Bonny JD, Kolb M. Percolation effects in matrix-type controlled drug release systems. Int J Pharm 1995; 115:217–224.

Leveque N, Raghavan SL, Lane ME, et al. Use of a molecular form technique for the penetration of supersaturated solutions of salicylic acid across silicone membranes and human skin in vitro. Int J Pharm 2006; 318:49–54.

Li J, Masso JJ, Guertin JA. Prediction of drug solubility in an acrylate adhesive based on the drug-polymer interaction parameter and drug solubility in acetonitrile. J Contr Rel 2002a; 83:211–221.

Li J, Masso JJ, Rendon S. Quantitative evaluation of adhesive properties and drug-adhesive interactions for transdermal drug delivery formulations using linear solvation energy relationships. J Contr Rel 2002b; 82:1–16.

Loffler H, Dreher F, Maibach HI. Stratum corneum adhesive tape stripping: influence of anatomical site, application pressure, duration and removal. Br J Dermatol 2004; 151:746–752.

Lotan T. Immediate topical drug delivery using natural nano-injectors. In: Rathbone MJ, Hadgraft J, Roberts MS, et al. eds. Modified-Release Drug Delivery Technology. 2nd ed. Volume 2. New York: Informa Healthcare, 2008:395–404.

Lotte C, Wester RC, Rougier A, et al. Racial differences in the in vivo percutaneous absorption of some organic compounds: a comparison between black, Caucasian and Asian subjects. Arch Dermatol Res 1993; 284:456–459.

Magnusson BM, Anissimov YG, Cross SE, et al. Molecular size as the main determinant of solute maximum flux across the skin. J Invest Dermatol 2004; 122:993–999.

Man M, Chang C, Lee PH, et al. New improved paddle method for determining the in vitro drug release profiles of transdermal delivery systems. J Contr Rel 1993; 27:59–68.

Marbury T, Hamill E, Bachand R, et al. Evaluation of the pharmacokinetic profiles of the new testosterone topical gel formulation, Testim, compared to AndroGel. Biopharm Drug Dispos 2003; 24:115–120.

Marzulli FN, Maibach HI. Permeability and reactivity of skin as related to age. J Soc Cosmet Chem 1984; 35: 95–102.

Mazzo DJ, Fong EKF, Biffar SE. A comparison of test methods for determining in vitro drug release from transdermal delivery dosage forms. J Pharm Biomed Anal 1986; 4:601–607.

McClements DJ. Critical review of techniques and methodologies for characterization of emulsion stability. Crit Rev Food Sci Nutr 2007; 47:611–649.

Megrab NA, Williams AC, Barry BW. Oestradiol permeation through human skin and silastic membrane: effects of propylene glycol and supersaturation. J Contr Rel 1995; 36:277–294.

Meidan VM, Roper CS. Inter- and intra-individual variability in human skin barrier function: a large scale retrospective study. Toxicol In Vitro 2008; 22:1062–1069.

Menon GK, Brandsma JL, Schwartz PM. Particle-mediated gene delivery and human skin: ultrastructural observations on stratum corneum barrier structures. Skin Pharmacol Physiol 2007; 20:141–147.

Melle S, Lask M, Fuller GG. Pickering emulsions with controllable stability. Langmuir 2005; 21:2158–2162.

Mitragotri S, Kost J. Ultrasound-mediated transdermal drug delivery. In: Rathbone MJ, Hadgraft J, Roberts MS, et al., eds. Modified-Release Drug Delivery Technology. 2nd ed. Volume 2. New York: Informa Healthcare, 2008:339–347.

Moulai Mostefa N, Hadj Sadok A, Sabri N, et al. Determination of optimal cream formulation from long-term stability investigation using a surface response modeling. Int J Cosmet Sci 2006; 28:211–218.

Muehlbach M, Brummer R, Eggers R. Study on the transferability of the time temperature superposition principle to emulsions. Int J Cosmet Sci 2006; 28:109–116.

Nalluri BN, Milligan C, Chen J, et al. In vitro release studies on matrix type transdermal drug delivery systems of naltrexone and its acetyl prodrug. Drug Dev Ind Pharm 2005; 31:871–877.

Nanayakkara GR, Bartlett A, Forbes B, et al. The effect of unsaturated fatty acids in benzyl alcohol on the percutaneous permeation of three model permeants. Int J Pharm 2005; 301:129–139.

N'Dri-Stempfer B, Navidi WC, Guy RH, et al. Optimizing metrics for the assessment of bioequivalence between topical drug products. Pharm Res 2008; 25:1621–1630.

Nicolazzo JA, Morgan TM, Reed BL, et al. Synergistic enhancement of testosterone transdermal delivery. J Contr Rel 2005; 103:577–585.

Nitsche JM, Kasting GB. Biophysical models for skin transport and absorption. In: Dermal Absorption and Toxicity Assessment. 2nd ed. Roberts MS, Walters KA. New York: Informa Healthcare, 2008:251–269.

Noonan PK, Wester RC. Cutaneous metabolism of xenobiotics. In: Bronaugh RL, Maibach HI, eds. Percutaneous Absorption: Mechanisms, Methodology, Drug Delivery. 2nd ed. New York: Marcel Dekker, 1989:53–75.

Norlen L. The physical structure of the skin barrier. In: Roberts MS, Walters KA, eds. Dermal Absorption and Toxicity Assessment. 2nd ed. New York: Informa Healthcare, 2008:37–68.

OECD. Test Guideline 427: Skin absorption: In vivo method. Adopted: 13th April, 2004, Paris, France: OECD Publishing.

OECD. Test Guideline 428: Skin absorption: In vitro method. Adopted: 13th April, 2004, Paris, France: OECD Publishing.

OECD. Guidance Document 28: Conduct of skin absorption studies, 2004.

Okabe H, Suzuki E, Saitoh T, et al. Development of novel transdermal system containing d-limonene and ethanol as absorption enhancers. J Contr Rel 1994; 32:243–247.

Orth DS. Handbook of Cosmetic Microbiology. New York: Marcel Dekker, 1993.

Osborne DW. Phase behavior characterization of propylene glycol, white petrolatum, surfactant ointments. Drug Dev Ind Pharm 1992; 18:1883–1894.

Osborne DW. Phase behavior characterization of ointments containing lanolin or a lanolin substitute. Drug Dev Ind Pharm 1993; 19:1283–1302.

Padmanabhan R, Phipps JB, Cormier M, et al. Alza transdermal drug delivery technologies. In: Rathbone MJ, Hadgraft J, Roberts MS, eds. Modified-Release Drug Delivery Technology. 2nd ed. Volume 2. New York: Informa Healthcare, 2008:273–293.

Park I, Kim D, Song J, et al. Buprederm, a new transdermal delivery system on buprenorphine: pharmacokinetic, efficacy and skin irritancy studies. Pharm Res 2008; 25:1052–1062.

Pays K, Giermanska-Kahn J, Pouligny B, et al. Double emulsions: how does release occur? J Contr Rel 2002; 79:193–205.

Pellett MA, Roberts MS, Hadgraft J. Supersaturated solutions evaluated with an in vitro stratum corneum tape stripping technique. Int J Pharm 1997; 151:91–98.

Pena LE, Lee BL, Stearns JF. Structural rheology of a model ointment. Pharm Res 1994; 11:875–881.

Pendlington RU, Sanders DJ, Cooper KJ, et al. The use of sucrose as a standard penetrant in in vitro percutaneous penetration experiments. In: Brain KR, James VJ, Walters KA, eds. Perspectives in Percutaneous Penetration, vol. 5b. Cardiff, UK: STS Publishing, 1998:123–124.

Pérez-Marcos B, Martinez-Pacheco R, Gómez-Amoza JL, et al. Interlot variability of carbomer 934. Int J Pharm 1993; 100:207–212.

Pershing LK, Silver BS, Krueger GG, et al. Feasibility of measuring the bioavailability of topical betamethasone dipropionate in commercial formulations using drug content in skin and a skin blanching bioassay. Pharm Res 1992; 9:45–51.

Pfister WR, Sheeran MA, Watters DE, et al. Methods for altering release of progesterone, testosterone, propranolol, and indomethacin from silicone matrices: effects of co-solvents and inert fillers. Proc Int Symp Contr Rel Bioact Mat 1987; 14:223–224.

Piao H, Kamiya N, Hirata A, et al. A novel solid-in-oil nanosuspension for transdermal delivery of diclofenac sodium. Pharm Res 2008; 25:896–901.

Piechota-Urbanska M, Kotodziejska J, Zgoda MM. Viscosity of pharmacopeial multimolecular ointment vehicles and pharmaceutical availability of a model therapeutic agent. Polim Med 2007; 37:3–19.

Planas MD, Rodriguez FG, Dominguez MH. The influence of neutralizer concentration on the rheological behaviour of a 0.1% Carbopol® hydrogel. Pharmazie 1992; 47:351–355.

PMA Committee Report. Transdermal drug delivery systems. Pharmacop Forum 1986; 12:1798–1807.

Potts RO, Guy RH. Predicting skin permeability. Pharm Res 1992; 9:663–669.

Prausnitz MR. The effects of electric current applied to skin: a review for transdermal drug delivery. Adv Drug Del Rev 1996; 18:395–425.

Prausnitz MR, Gill HS, Park J-H. Microneedles for drug delivery. In: Rathbone MJ, Hadgraft J, Roberts MS, et al. eds. Modified-Release Drug Delivery Technology. 2nd ed. Volume 2. New York: Informa Healthcare, 2008:295–309.

Pugazhendhi D, Pope GS, Darbre PD. Oestrogenic activity of p-hydroxybenzoic acid (common metabolite of paraben esters) and methylparaben in human breast cancer cell lines. J Appl Toxicol 2005; 25: 301–309.

Pugh WJ, Hadgraft J, Roberts MS. Physicochemical determinants of stratum corneum permeation. In: Roberts MS, Walters KA, eds . Dermal Absorption and Toxicity Assessment, New York: Marcel Dekker, 1998:245–268.

Rajadhyaksha VJ, inventor; Oxalodinone penetration enhancing compounds. US patent 4 960 771. 1990.

Raykar PV, Fung MC, Anderson BD. The role of protein and lipid domains in the uptake of solutes by human stratum corneum. Pharm Res 1988; 5:140–150.

Reichek N, Goldstein RE, Redwood DR. Sustained effects of nitroglycerin ointment in patients with angina pectoris. Circulation 1974; 50:348–352.

Ribeiro HM, Morais JA, Eccleston GM. Structure and rheology of semisolid o/w creams containing cetyl alcohol/non-ionic surfactant mixed emulsifier and different polymers. Int J Cosmet Sci 2004; 26:47–59.

Rienertson RP, Wheatley VR. Studies on the chemical composition of human epidermal lipids. J Invest Dermatol 1959; 32:49–59.

Roberts MS. Percutaneous Absorption of Phenolic Compounds [master's thesis]. Sydney: University of Sydney, 1976.

Roberts MS. Structure-permeability considerations in percutaneous absorption. In: Scott RC, Guy RH, Hadgraft J, et al. eds. Volume 2. London: IBC Technical Services, 1991:210–228.

Roberts MS, Anderson RA, Swarbrick J. Permeability of human epidermis to phenolic compounds. J Pharm Pharmacal 1977; 29:677–683.

Roberts MS, Cross SE, Pellett MA. Skin transport. In: Walters KA, ed. Dermatological and Transdermal Formulations. New York: Marcel Dekker, 2002:89–195.

Roberts MS, Favretto WA, Meyer A, et al. Topical bioavailability of methyl salicylate. Aust NZ J Med 1982; 12: 303–305.

Roberts MS, Walters KA, eds. Dermal Absorption and Toxicity Assessment. 2nd ed. New York: Informa Healthcare.

Rogers RA, Riviere JE. Pharmacological modulation of the cutaneous vasculature in the isolated perfused porcine skin flap. J Pharm Sci 1994; 83:1682–1689.

Roskos KV, Guy RH, Maibach HI. Percutaneous absorption in the aged. Dermatol Clin 1986; 4:455–465.

Roskos KV, Maibach HI. Percutaneous absorption and age: implications for therapy. Drugs and Aging 1992; 2:432–449.

Roskos KV, Maibach HI, Guy RH. The effect of aging on percutaneous absorption in man. J Pharm Biopharm 1989; 17:617–630.

Rougier A. 1987a. An original predictive method for in vivo percutaneous absorption studies. J Soc Cosmet Chem 1989; 38:397–417.

Rougier A. In vivo percutaneous penetration of some organic compounds related to anatomic site in humans: stripping method. J Pharm Sci 1987b; 76:451–454.

Rougier A. Percutaneous absorption-transepidermal water loss relationship in man in vivo. In: Scott RC, Guy RH, Hadgraft J, eds. Prediction of Percutaneous Penetration. Volume 2. London: IBC Technical Services, 1991:60–72.

Rougier A, Lotte C. Predictive approaches. I. The stripping technique. In: Shah VP, Maibach HI, eds. Topical Drug Bioavailability, Bioequivalence and Penetration. New York: Plenum Press, 1993:163–182.

Roy SD. Preformulation aspects of transdermal drug delivery systems. In: Ghosh TK, Pfister WR, Sum SI, eds. eds. Transdermal and Topical Drug Delivery Systems. Buffalo Grove, IL: Interpharm Press, 1997:139–166.

Roy SD, Gutierrez M, Flynn GL, et al. Controlled transdermal delivery of fentanyl: characterizations of pressure-sensitive adhesives for matrix patch design. J Pharm Sci 1996; 85:491–495.

Schaefer H, Redelmeir TE. Skin Barrier, Principles of Percutaneous Absorption. Basel: Karger, 1996.

Schaefer-Korting M, Schreiber S. Use of skin equivalents for dermal absorption and toxicity. In: Roberts MS, Walters KA, eds. Dermal Absorption and Toxicity Assessment. 2nd ed. New York: Informa Healthcare, 2008:141–159.

Scheuplein RJ. Mechanism of percutaneous absorption. I. Routes of penetration and the influence of solubility. J Invest Dermatol 1965; 45:334–346.

Scheuplein RJ, Blank IH. Permeability of the skin. Physiol Rev 1971; 51:702–747.

Scheuplein RJ, Blank IH. Mechanism of percutaneous absorption. IV. Penetration of non-electrolytes (alcohols) from aqueous solutions and from pure liquids. J Invest Dermatol 1973; 60:286–296.

Shah VP, Elkins J, Hanus J, et al. In vitro release of hydrocortisone from topical preparations and automated procedure. Pharm Res 1991; 8:55–59.

Shah VP, Flynn GL, Yacobi A, et al. AAPS/FDA workshop report: Bioequivalence of topical dermatological dosage forms—methods of evaluation of bioequivalence. Pharm Res 1998; 15:167–171.

Shah VP, Tymes NW, Yamamoto LA, et al. In vitro dissolution profile of transdermal nitroglycerin patches using paddle method. Int J Pharm 1986; 32:243–250.

Sharma R. Xenobiotic metabolizing enzymes in skin. In: Brain KR, James VJ, Walters KA, eds. Prediction of Percutaneous Penetration, Vol 4b. Cardiff, UK: STS Publishing, 1996:14–18.

Singh P, Roberts MS. Effects of vasoconstriction on dermal pharmacokinetics and local tissue distribution of compounds. J Pharm Sci 1994; 83:783–791.

Sjöblom J, ed. Emulsions and Emulsion Stability. New York: Marcel Dekker, 1996.

Skelly JP, Shah VP, Maibach HI, et al. FDA and AAPS report of the workshop on principles and practices of in vitro percutaneous penetration studies: relevance to bioavailability and bioequivalence. Pharm Res 1987; 4:265–267.

Sloan KB, Wasdo SC. Percutaneous absorption of prodrugs and soft drugs. In: Roberts MS, Walters KA, eds. Dermal Absorption and Toxicity Assessment. 2nd ed. New York: Informa Healthcare, 2008:605–622.

Smith EW, Maibach HI, eds. Percutaneous Penetration Enhancers. 2nd ed. Boca Raton: Taylor & Francis, 2006.

Soni MG, Carabin IG, Burdock GA. Safety assessment of esters of p-hydroxybenzoic acid (parabens). Food Chem Toxicol 2005; 43:985–1015.

Southwell JD, Barry BW, Woodford R. Variations in permeability of human skin within and between specimens. Int J Pharm 1984; 18:299–309.

Souto EB, Petersen RD, Muller RH. Lipid nanoparticles with solid matrix for dermal delivery: solid lipid nanoparticles and nanostructured lipid carriers. In: Rathbone MJ, Hadgraft J, Roberts MS, eds. Modified-Release Drug Delivery Technology. 2nd ed. Volume 2. New York: Informa Healthcare, 2008:349–372.

Stinchcomb AL, Valiveti S, Hammell DC, et al. Human skin permeation of $\triangle^8$-tetrahydrocannabinol, cannabidiol and cannabinol. J Pharm Pharmacol 2004; 56:291–297.

Surber C, Wilhelm K-P, Maibach HI. In vitro and in vivo percutaneous absorption of structurally related phenol and steroid analogs. Eur J Pharm Biopharm 1993; 39:244–248.

Takruri H, Anger CB. Preservation of dispersed systems. In: Lieberman HA, Rieger MM, Banker GS, eds. Pharmaceutical Dosage Forms: Disperse Systems. Volume 2. New York: Marcel Dekker, 1989:73–114.

Taylor SC. Skin of color: biology, structure, function, and implications for dermatologic disease. J Am Acad Dermatol 2002; 46(suppl 2):S41–S62.

Thomas BJ, Finnin BC. The transdermal revolution. Drug Discov Today 2004; 9:697–703.

Tojo K, Lee AC. A method for predicting steady-state rate of skin penetration in vivo. J Invest Dermatol 1989; 92:105–110.

Tokumura F, Homma T, Tomiya T, et al. Properties of pressure-sensitive adhesive tapes with soft adhesives to human skin and their mechanism. Skin Res Technol 2007; 13:211–216.

Trichard L, Delgado-Charro MB, Guy RH, et al. Novel beads made of alpha-cyclodextrin and oil for topical delivery of a lipophilic drug. Pharm Res 2008; 25:435–440.

Turpcinen M. Absorption of hydrocortisone from the skin reservoir in atopic dermatitis. Br J Dermatol 1991; 124:358–360.

Turpeinen M, Salo OP, Leisti S. Effect of percutaneous absorption of hydrocortisone on adrenocortical responsiveness in infants with severe skin disease. Br J Dermatol 1986; 115:475–484.

Ulman KL, Gornowicz GA, Larson KR, et al. Drug permeability of modified silicone polymers. I. Silicone-organic block copolymers. J Contr Rel 1989a; 10:251–260.

Ulman KL, Larson KR, Lee C-L, et al. Drug permeability of modified silicone polymers. II. Silicone-organic graft copolymers. J Contr Rel 1989b; 10:261–272.

Ulman KL, Lee C-L. Drug permeability of modified silicone polymers. III. Hydrophilic pressure-sensitive adhesives for transdermal controlled drug release applications. J Contr Rel 1989; 10:273–281.

Utsuki T, Uchimura N, Irikura M, et al. Preclinical investigation of the topical administration of phenserine: transdermal flux, cholinesterase inhibition, and cognitive efficacy. J Pharmacol Exp Ther 2007; 321:353–361.

Valenta C, Auner BG. The use of polymers for dermal and transdermal delivery. Eur J Pharm Biopharm 2004; 58:279–289.

van der Valk PGM, Nater JP, Bleumink E. Vulnerability of the skin to surfactants in different groups of eczema patients and controls as measured by water vapour loss. Clin Exp Dermatol 1985; 10:98–103.

Venkatraman S, Gale R. Skin adhesives and skin adhesion 1. Transdermal drug delivery systems. Biomaterials 1998; 19:1119–1136.

Vickers CFH. Existence of reservoir in stratum corneum. Experimental proof. Arch Dermatol 1963; 88:21–23.

Walters KA, Brain KR. Topical and transdermal delivery. In Gibson ME, ed. Pharmaceutical Preformulation and Formulation. IHS Health Group, 2001:515–579.

Walters KA, Hadgraft J, eds. Pharmaceutical Skin Penetration Enhancement. New York: Marcel Dekker, 1993.

Walters KA, Brain KR, Howes D, et al. Percutaneous penetration of octyl salicylate from representative sunscreen formulations through human skin in vitro. Food Chem Toxicol 1997a; 35:1219–1225.

Walters KA, Brain KR, Dressier WE, et al. Percutaneous penetration of N-nitroso-N-methyldodecylamine through human skin in vitro: application from cosmetic vehicles. Food Chem Toxicol 1997b; 35:705–712.

Walters KA, Flynn GL, Marvel JR. Physicochemical characterization of the human nail. I. Pressure sealed apparatus for measuring nail plate permeabilities. J Invest Dermatol 1981; 76:76–79.

Weigand DA, Haygood C, Gaylor JR. Cell layers and density of Negro and Caucasian SC. J Invest Dermatol 1974; 62:563–568.

Wertz PW, Downing DT. Glycolipids in mammalian epidermis: structure and function in the water barrier. Science 1982; 217:1261–1262.

Wesley NO, Maibach HI. Racial (ethnic) differences in skin properties: the objective data. Am J Clin Dermatol 2003; 4:843–860.

Wester RC, Christoffel J, Hartway T, et al. Human cadaver skin viability for *in vitro* percutaneous absorption: storage and detrimental effects of heat-separation and freezing. Pharm Res 1998; 15:82–84.

Wiechers JW, Kelly CL, Blease TG, et al. Formulating for efficacy. Int J Cosmet Sci 2004; 26:173–182.

Wilkinson SC, Williams FM. Cutaneous metabolism. In: Roberts MS, Walters KA, eds. Dermal Absorption and Toxicity Assessment. 2nd ed. New York: Informa Healthcare, 2008:89–115.

Williams AC, Cornwell PA, Barry BW. On the non-Gaussian distribution of human skin permeabilities. Int J Pharmaceut 1992; 86:69–77.

Williams AC, Walters KA. Chemical penetration enhancement: possibilities and problems. In: Walters KA, Roberts MS, eds. Dermatologic, Cosmeceutic, and Cosmetic Development: Therapeutic and Novel Approaches. New York: Informa Healthcare, 2008:497–504.

Yano T, Nakagawa A, Masayoshi T, et al. Skin permeability of non-steroidal antiinflammatory drugs in man. Life Sci 1986; 39:1043–1050.

Yuk SH, Lee SJ, Okano T, et al. One-way membrane for transdermal drug delivery systems. I. Membrane preparation and characterization. Int J Pharmaceut 1991a; 77:221–229.

Yuk SH, Lee SJ, Okano T, et al. One-way membrane for transdermal drug delivery systems. II. System optimization. Int J Pharmaceut 1991b; 77:231–237.

Zatz JL, Varsano J, Shah VP. In vitro release of betamethasone dipropionate from petrolatum-based ointments. Pharm Dev Technol 1996; 1:293–298.

Index

ABAK system, 439
Absorption
  cell culture method for, 152
  determinant of, 147
  enhancer system for, 162–163
  from GI tract
    across intestinal epithelia, 144–145
    dissolution of compound, 129–130
    factors influencing, 143–145
    low permeability values during, 130
    simulations of, 136
    transcellular route, 144
  HT-29 cell lines, 152
  lipid membrane extraction method for, 150
  mechanisms of, 143–144, 146
  models for studying, 145
    cell culture model, 151–152
    chromatographic systems, 148–149
    computer-based prediction models, 147–148
    excised intestinal segments, 152–153
    extraction into lipid phase, 148
    functional use of, 163–164
    intestinal perfusion technique, 155–156
    intestinal rings, 150–151
    membrane vesicles, 150
    nonbiological models, 146–147
    QSAR models, 148
    Ussing chamber technique, 153–154
    in vitro biological methods, 149
    in vivo biological methods, 156–157
  parameter for predicting, 146
  perfusion methods to study, 155
  predictive models for, 148
  studies in human, in vivo techniques for
    intestinal permeability measurements, 158–159
    regional bioavailability assessment, 159–162
  Ussing chamber technique to study, 153–154
Acetylcysteine, 444
Acidic buffers, 327
Active pharmaceutical ingredient (API)
  compatibility and degradation of, 231–232
Active-to-hit (AtH) phase, 17
Actuator, 358–359
Acyclovir, 432
Additive, impact on solubility, 30
AeroFlow, 205
AFM. See Atomic force microscopy (AFM)
Age-related macular degeneration (AMD), 431
Agglomeration, 189–190

Agitation intensity selection, for in vitro
    dissolution testing, 253
AI. See Artificial intelligence (AI) technologies
Amine hydrochloride, primary
  vs. concentration of surface tension, 219
Amorphous indomethacin salts, influence of alkali
    metal counterion on T_g of, 60
Amorphous state
  glass transition temperature, 60–61
  methods for production of, 62
  polyamorphism of, 62
  stability of, 61–62, 63
Amorphous substance, heat of solution for, 108
Angle of response, 373
Animal models
  advantages of, 276
  selection of, 276–278
  study design aspects in bioavailability studies, 278
Antacid formulation, 285
Antioxidants, water- and oil-soluble, 217
Antipyrine, 444
API. See Active pharmaceutical ingredient (API)
Apparatus, for in vitro dissolution testing, 249–253
Aquasol A (vitamin A palmitate as retinol), 331
Aqueous suspensions, 336, 436
AR-C69457AA
  DSC thermograms of hydrochloride salt of, 101
  IR spectra of, 77
  particle size and heating rate effects on, 100
  SSNMR spectra of phases of, 79, 80
Artificial intelligence (AI) technologies, 303–307
Ascorbic acid, 334, 444
Asthma, 348
AstraZeneca tablet formulation expert system, 306
Atomic force microscopy (AFM), 90–91
  for solid dosage forms, 198
Attenuated total reflectance (ATR) technique, 76
Autoclaving, stability to, 216
Automated Forced Degradation System, 214
Avalanching behavior, 373

BAI. See Breath-activated inhalers (BAI)
Ball milling, 192–193
Basic drugs
  protocol for, 47
  salt selection for, 44
  solubility of, 49
BBMV. See Brush-border membrane vesicles (BBMV)

BCS. *See* Biopharmaceutics classification system (BCS)
Bentley Pharmaceuticals CPE-215 permeation enhancement technology, 488
Benzalkonium cation, 464
Benzalkonium chloride (BKC), 440, 445–446, 448, 450, 457, 464
BET adsorption method. *See* Bruner, Emmet, and Teller (BET) adsorption method
β–lactam antibiotics
    heats of solution of, 83–84
    solid-state reactivity of hydrates of, 81
    water-soluble salts of, 51
BFI. *See* Brittle fracture index (BFI)
BHN. *See* Brinell Hardness Number (BHN)
Bile acids, 137–139, 463
    composition and concentration of, 141
    in dog, 255
Bile salts. *See* Bile acids
Bioadhesive gels, 472
Bioavailability studies
    animal models design aspects in, 278
    assumptions in, 264
    during formulation development, 261–262
    in vivo dissolution/release rate
        AUC, 265–266
        C_{max} and t_{max}, 264–265
        fractional amount of drug absorption, 270–271
        model-dependent analysis, 266–267
        moment analysis, 267
        and in vitro dissolution, correlation between, 271–273
        in vivo dissolution/absorption-time profiles, 267–270
    study design
        crossover designs, 262
        food, 263
        plasma-sampling schedule, 263
        sample size, 263
        single-dose studies, 262
        washout period, 262
Biologically active compound, components of, 12
Biopharmaceuticals
    advances to create, 12
    components of, 6
    optimal absorption criteria, 130
Biopharmaceutics classification system (BCS)
    classes of drugs, 135
    importance of solubility in, 25
    solubility classification, 85
Biopharmaceutics studies
    barrier to, 14
    at candidate drug selection stage, 13
BKC. *See* Benzalkonium chloride (BKC)
Blinking, 433
Blow-fill-seal technology, 339
Boundary lubricants, 392
Breath-activated inhalers (BAI), 360
Bricanyl Tubohaler, 200
Brinell Hardness Number (BHN), 379
British Standard 2955 (1958), 369

Brittle fracture index (BFI), 384
Bronchitis, 348
Brønstead and Lowry theory of acids and bases, 20
Bruner, Emmet, and Teller (BET) adsorption method, 202
Brush-border membrane vesicles (BBMV), 150
Buffers, 327
Bulk density, 369
    of powder, 373

Caco-2 cell monolayers
    components of, 151
    drug absorption determination by, 151–152
    epithelium membrane barrier function, 151
    permeability models, 143
Caffeine
    conversion to caffeine hydrate, 59
    QI-MTDSC analysis of polymorphs of, 104
Caking, solid dosage forms, 208
Cambridge Crystallographic Data Centre (CCDC), 205
Candidate drug (CD)
    chemical and physical stability of, 31–32
    development, long-term planning of, 7–8
    early development
        "the 100 mg approach" for, 18
    phase I clinical studies of, 14–15
    prenomination studies of, 19
    selection phase
        biopharmaceutical information, 130–131
        chemical/biological lead, 12–13
        dissolution rate, 131–132
        drug solubility, 131–133
        pharmaceutical involvement to, 13–14
        preclinical research during, 7
        preformulation and biopharmaceutics, 13
    solid-state stability of
        moisture effect on, 91
        photostability, 82–83
        solid-state degradation, 81
    solubility of, 24
Capping, 381–384
Capsugel, 423
Capsule-filling mechanisms. *See* Gelatin capsules
Capsule shells, 418
Captisol, 332
Carbamazepine, 60
Cationic buffers, 327
CCDC. *See* Cambridge Crystallographic Data Centre (CCDC)
CD. *See* Candidate drug (CD)
CDS-TC-32, 490–491
Cefotaxime sodium, solubility of, 31
CEI. *See* Commission Internationale d'Eclairage (CEI)
Cell culture model, for drug absorption, 151–152
CFC. *See* Chlorofluorocarbons (CFC)
Chelating agents
    function in stability, 217–218
Child-resistant packaging, 300

Chloramphenicol, 432
Chlorobutanol, 446
Chlorofluorocarbons (CFC), 7, 297, 348
    formulation, 227–228
    surfactants, 357
Chromatographic systems
    drug absorption studies using, 148–149
Chronic obstructive pulmonary diseases
        (COPD), 348
CMT. *See* Critical micelle temperature (CMT)
Coating methods, 409–416, 418
Cocrystals, 53
    formation of
        goal of, 54
        methods for, 54
CoG. *See* Cost of goods (CoG)
Collapse temperature, 333
Colon residence time
    for nondisintegrating tablet and pellet
        formulation, 284
Color, of drug substance, 206–207
Colorants, 297, 394–396
Coloring agents. *See* Colorants
Commercial considerations, in product design
        report. *See* Economic considerations, in
        product design report
Commercial process, validation of, 320
Commercial viability, of new product, 183
Commission Internationale d'Eclairage (CEI), 207
Committee for Proprietary Medicinal Products
        (CPMP), 319, 449
Compaction simulators, 377, 388
Compatibility study, 231–234
    DSC for, 233–234
    between remacemide HCl and spray-dried
        lactose, 233
    steps for, 232
    storage conditions used to examine, 233
Complexing agents, 331–332
Compressibility (Carr index), 373
Compression coating, 415–416, 418
Compression protocol, 206
Computer-based prediction models, oral drug
        absorption, 146–147
Conformational polymorphism, 36–37
Container Closure System, 470
Contract research organizations (CRO), 181–182
Coprophagy, 278
Cordarone IV, 331
Core flow hoppers, 371
Cosolvents, 211–213, 330
Cost of goods (CoG), 7, 172, 183
CPP. *See* Critical process parameters (CPP)
CQA. *See* Critical quality attributes (CQA)
Cremophor EL, 328
Critical micelle temperature (CMT), 139
Critical process parameters (CPP), 316–317
Critical quality attributes (CQA)
    and product optimization, 289
Critical quality parameters, in product design
        report, 180–181

CRO. *See* Contract research organizations (CRO)
Crossover studies, 15, 262
Crystalline states, 34
Crystalline substance, heat of solution for, 108
Crystallization peak energy
    vs. amorphous content, 196
    vs. time, 196
Crystal morphology assessment
    of α– and γ–indomethacin, 86–87
    crystallization from IMS-water and heptane, 87
    of trimethoprim, 86
Cumulative drug absorption
    for hydrophilic matrix ER tablet, 285
Customer requirements, TPP, 175–179
    QFD and, 176–180
Cyclodextrins, 331–332, 443, 463
    for solubility enhancement of poorly soluble
        drugs, 220

DECCAS. *See* Drug-excipient compatibility
        automated system (DECCAS)
Deconvolution algorithms, 268–269
4-Decyloxazolidin-2-one, 488
Design aspects, of in vitro dissolution testing,
        257–258
Design specifications, in product design report,
        180–181
Development compound
    bioavailability of, 54
    effect of salt formation on solubility of, 50
    E/T diagram of, 43
    heat of solution of amorphous and crystalline
        form of, 108
    morphologies of polymorphs of, 87
Development costs, 181–182
Dexamethasone, 432
    acetate ester, 435
Dextran, 436
Dextrose, 328
Diazepam, 332
Diclofenac, basic salts of, 51
Die-wall lubricants, 394
Differential scanning calorimetry (DSC)
    calibration of, 102
    of carbamazepine, 105
    for compatibility studies, 233–234
    experimental design for, 99–100
    modulated, 102
    particle size and heating rate effects on
        AR-C69457AA, 100–101
    for solubility determination, 101
    thermogram
        of frozen 9% w/v saline solution, 222
        showing glass transition of heated frozen drug
            solution, 221
    types of, 99
    variables influencing, 99
Diflupredate, FTIR thermo-microscopy of, 76
Dihydrochloride salt, DSC and TGA profile of, 52
Dilantin injection (phenytoin sodium), 327

Dipivalyl epinephrine, 434
Direct compression, 400–401
Disintegrants, 398
Disodium edetate, 334, 444
Dissolution profiles assessment, 258–261
Distribution coefficient (log D)
  technique for determining, 24
  for weak acid, 23
DLVO theory, 357
DMF. *See* Drug master file (DMF)
1-Dodecylazacycloheptan-2-one, 488
Dodecyl-*N,N*-dimethylamino isopropionate, 488
Doehlert experimental design, 309
DPI. *See* Dry-powder inhalers (DPI)
Drug delivery systems, development of, 6
Drug discovery and development. *See also*
      Pharmaceutical research and
      development (R&D)
  costs of, 3, 5
  HTS for, 11
  lean concepts in, utilizing, 17
  risk associated with doing minimum, 5
  selection of suitable drug candidate for, 130
  stages of
    candidate drug selection, 12–14
    exploratory development, 14–15
    exploratory research, 11–12
    LG and LO, 17
    post-marketing surveillance trials, 15
    strategic research, 11
Drug-excipient compatibility automated system
    (DECCAS), 234
Drug master file (DMF), 184, 296
Drugs
  absorption of. *See* Absorption
  bioavailability, 144
  cash flow profile for, 4–5
  complexation of, 140–141
  degradation in solution. *See* Drug degradation
    in solution; Solution, degradation in
  dissolution of, 129
    absorption problems, 134–135
    absorption rate dependence on, 261
    bile acids and, 137–138
    biopharmaceutical interpretation of, 134–135
    determinations of, 133–134
    luminal conditions influence on, 136, 140
    for oral absorption, 131, 134
    physiological aspects of, 136–139
    substance properties affecting, 139
    in vitro/in vivo correlations of. *See* In vitro/
      in vivo correlations (IVVC)
  effective patent life for, 5
  life cycle, 3
  risk associated with minimum development
    program of, 5
  solid-state stability of
    photostability, 82–83
    solid-state degradation, 81
  solubility of, 132–133
  stability, 140

[Drugs]
  substance
    cost of, 189
    for inhalation therapy, 228
    production of, 189
    QbD, 190
    surface-active properties, 139
    targets and genomics, 12
Drying, of drug substances after crystallization, 190
Dry powder inhalers (DPI), 229–231, 348. *See also*
    Inhalation products
DSC. *See* Differential scanning calorimetry (DSC)

Economic considerations, in product design report,
    181–183
Edex (alprostadil), 332
EDTA. *See* Ethylenediaminetetraacetic acid (EDTA)
Elastic recovery, percentage, 379
Electrostatic forces, 369
Electrostatic repulsion, 504
Electrostaticity, in solid dosage forms, 207–208
EMEA. *See* European Agency for the Evaluation of
    Medicinal Products (EMEA)
Emphysema, 348
Emulsion formulations, 213–214
Emulsions, 332–333, 336–337
Environmental consideration, in product design
    report, 185
EPAG. *See* European Pharmaceutical Aerosol
    Group (EPAG)
Equilibrium relative humidity (ERH), 92
ERH. *See* Equilibrium relative humidity (ERH)
Essential Requirements of European legislation
    applied to medical devices, 301
Estrone, polymorphs of, 35
E/T diagrams
  for monotropic and enantiotropic dimorphic
    systems, 42
Ethylenediaminetetraacetic acid (EDTA), 297
  function in stability, 217–218
Ethylene vinyl acetate (EVA), 437
Etoposide IV, 331
European Agency for the Evaluation of Medicinal
    Products (EMEA), 319, 343
European Pharmaceutical Aerosol Group (EPAG), 363
Eutectic melting temperature, 333
EVA. *See* Ethylene vinyl acetate (EVA)
Everted sac (everted intestine) method, 152–153
Excipients
  adsorption or absorption of, 300
  basic selection and acceptance criteria for, 296–297
  defined, 295
  microcalorimetry in compatibility studies of, 234
  monographs of key, 296
  safety testing, 185
  selection in nasal products, 462–463
  sources of information, 302
  sourcing of, 297
  true density as function of sample mass for, 204
  well-established, 296

Exploratory development. *See* Phase I
    clinical studies
Exploratory research
  approaches to lead generation during, 12
  high-throughput screening, 11–12

FDA Guideline for Drug Master Files, 296
Felodipine
  response surface of, dissolved in vitro, 260
  in vitro dissolution-time profiles of, 256
Fickian diffusion, 357
Film coating, 411–415, 418
*FIP Guidelines for Dissolution Testing of Solid Oral
    Products,* 249
First-order decomposition, of compound, 215
First-time-in-human (FTIH) studies, 20
Flow, of powders. *See* Powders, in solid
    dosage forms
Flow-through cell (USP IV) dissolution apparatus,
    249, 251
Fluid lubricants, 392
Fluorescein sodium, 432
Flurotec, 339
Formulation "expert systems," 304
Formulator, 370
Freeze-dried formulations, 220–223
FTIH. *See* First-time-in-human (FTIH) studies
FTIR-imaging system, 76
Fumed silicon dioxides, 390
Functional groups, reactivity of, 232
Fungizone, 214

γ–camera investigation, 283
γ–scintigraphy, principles of, 279–281
Gas pycnometry
  to measure true density, 204–205
Gastric emptying time, 284
Gastrointestinal (GI) tract
  drug absorption from, 129
    across intestinal epithelia, 144–145
    dissolution of compound, 129–130
    factors influencing, 143–144
    low permeability values during, 130
    simulations of, 136
  drug dissolution in
    physicochemical and physiological aspects of,
      136–137
  enzymes in, 141–142
  pH and concentration of ions in, 137
Gelatin capsules, 426–427
  alternatives to, 425
  hard
    auger/screw method of filling, 421
    capsule, 419–420
    dependent capsule filling, 420
    dosator method of filling, 421–423
    filling up with pellets, 423
    liquids and semisolids, 423–424
    manufacture of empty capsule shells, 416–419

[Gelatin capsules
  hard]
    piston-tamp method of filling, 421
    powder and granulate filling, 420
    sealing, 425
  soft
    benefits, 426–427
    manufacturing, 425–426
Gelrite, 436
"Gemini" codrug, 489
Geodon, 332
GI tract. *See* Gastrointestinal (GI) tract
Glass transition temperature (T_g), 60–61
Glaucoma, 441
Granulation
  binders, 405–406
  dry, 408–409
  wet, 402–407
GRAS (generally recognized as safe) status, 297
Gravimetric vapor sorption (GVS) analyzer, 93
*Guidance for Industry: Nonclinical Studies for the
    Safety Evaluation of Pharmaceutical
    Excipients,* 184
GVS. *See* Gravimetric vapor sorption (GVS) analyzer

Hamaker constant, 369
*Handbook of Pharmaceutical Manufacturing
    Formulations: Sterile Products,* 328
Hardness tests, 379
Hausner ratio, 373
Health consideration, in product design
    report, 185
Hemolysis, 338
Henderson–Hasselbach equation, 20, 30
HFA. *See* Hydrofluoroalkanes (HFA)
HFA-227, 357, 359–360
HFA-134a, 357, 359–360
HFA propellants. *See* Hydrofluorocarbon (HFA)
    propellants
HFC. *See* Hydrofluorocarbons (HFC)
High-performance liquid chromatography
    (HPLC), 109, 149, 334
High-solubility drug, 135
High-throughput screening (HTS)
  for pharmaceutical drug discovery, 11
  of solubilities, 27
Hit-to-lead (HtL) phases, 17
Hoppers, flow pattern, 370–371
HOQ. *See* House of Quality (HOQ)
Hot-stage microscopy (HSM)
  of carbamazepine, 106
  operating principle of, 105
  photographs of inhalation drug, 229
House of Quality (HOQ), 176, 177
HPLC. *See* High-performance liquid
    chromatography (HPLC)
HSM. *See* Hot-stage microscopy (HSM)
HTS. *See* High-throughput screening (HTS)
Human immunodeficiency virus (HIV),
    348

Hydrates, 222
  classifications of, 57–58
  formation and occurrence of, 56
  hydration state of, 59
  polymorphism exhibited by, 58
  suspension formulation following rapid
      solution-mediated transformation
      of anhydrate to, 59
Hydrochloride salts, 52–53, 327
Hydrofluoroalkanes (HFA), 348
Hydrofluorocarbons (HFC), 348
  propellants, 184
Hydrophilic–lipophilic balance (HLB) system,
      505–506
Hydrophilic matrix ER tablet
  cumulative drug absorption and tablet erosion
      for, 285
Hydroxyethylcellulose, 436
Hydroxyl-β-cyclodextrin, 332
Hydroxypropyl cellulose (HPC), 437
8-Hydroxyquinoline, 444
Hygroscopicity
  classification of, 93
  definition of, 91
Hyper-DSC, 102
Hypotonic formulations, 327
Hypromellose, 432, 436

Ibuprofen enantiomers, base-catalyzed
      racemization of, 32
ICH guidances, 289
  Q8 guidance on pharmaceutical development,
      290–291
    FDA principles of QbD, 291, 294
    section 2, 291
    section 3.2 P.2, 290
  Q10 guidance on pharmaceutical quality
      systems, 292–295
  Q9 guidance on quality risk mangement, 292
IGC. *See* Inverse gas chromatography (IGC)
Image analysis, particle size distribution, 201
Imaging studies, 278–286
  γ–scintigraphy, principles, 279–281
  labeling of formulations, 281–282
  in vivo studies, 282–286
    data evaluation, 283–286
    practical procedures, 282–283
Immobilized artificial membrane (IAM) columns,
      148–149
Implantable delivery systems, 337
Impurities, solid dosage forms and, 190–191
  effects on polymorph, 191
  ICH classification, 190
Inactive Ingredient Database, 184
IND. *See* Investigational New Drugs (IND)
Inhalation dosage forms, 226–231
  dry-powder inhalers, 229–231
  metered-dose inhalers, 226–229
  nebulizer solutions, 231
Inhalation products
  dry powder inhalers (DPI)

[Inhalation products
  dry powder inhalers (DPI)]
    commonality between devices, 353–354
    formulation challenges, 352–353
    future developments, 355
    operation, 354
    scale-up/technology transfer, 354–355
  future prospects
    delivery systems, 364
    disease types, 364
  importance of particle sizing
    high-speed camera video, 352
    impaction, 350–352
    light-scattering technique, 352
    microscopic analysis, 352
    Phase Doppler anemometry, 352
  lung deposition, 349–350
  metered dose inhalers (MDI)
    add-on devices, 360–361
    devices, 357–359
    formulation, 355–357
    future, 361
    scale-up process, 360
  nebulizers
    devices, 362
    formulation techniques and approaches, 362
    operation, 362–363
    phase I formulation, 362
    standards, 363
Initial physicohemical characterization, 20
In situ salt-screening technique, 47
Interaction effects, 308
Internal hygrostat for microcalorimetry
      experiments, 107
International Pharmaceutical Aerosol
      Consortium for Regulation and Science
      (IPAC-RS), 363
International Pharmaceutical Excipients Council
      (IPEC), 184, 295
Intestinal microflora, metabolic reactions of, 142
Intestinal perfusion method, 154–156
Intralipid, 332
Intravenous solution
  PPP for, 174
Intrinsic solubility
  instrument for determining
    pSOL and GLpKa titrator, 29
    shake-flask methodology, 30
  of weak acids and bases, 29–30
Inverse gas chromatography (IGC)
  particles in solid dosage forms, 197–198
Investigational New Drugs (IND), 290
In vitro biological methods, 149–150
In vitro dissolution testing, of solid dosage forms,
      248–261
  apparatus for, 249–253
    factors for selecting, 251–252
    hydrodynamic artifacts, 252
  assessment of dissolution profiles, 258–261
  batch quality control (QC) for, 248
  choice of agitation intensity, 253
  choice of media for, 254–257

[In vitro dissolution testing, of solid dosage forms]
  design aspects of, 257–258
  purposes of, 248
  validation of, 261
In vitro dissolution-time profiles, of felodipin, 256
In vitro/in vivo correlations (IVVC)
  level A correlation
    development and evaluation, 272
    in vitro and in vivo time curves, 273–274
    in vitro dissolution studies and human
      bioavailability studies, 273
    in vivo predictability of in vitro model, 274–275
  level B correlation, 275
  level C correlation
    disadvantages of, 276
    single-point relationship, in vitro dissolution
      rate, 275
  prerequisites for establishing, 271
  types of, 272
In vivo biological methods, 156–157
In vivo dissolution/release rate
  AUC, 265–266
  C_{max} and t_{max}, 264–265
  deconvolution/convolution, 268–269
  fractional amount of drug absorption (F_a), 270–271
  model-dependent analysis, 266–267
  moment analysis, 267
  and in vitro dissolution, correlation between, 271
    level A correlation, 272–275
    level B correlation, 275
    level C correlation, 275–276
  in vivo dissolution/absorption-time profiles,
    267–270
Ionizable drugs, 435
Ionization constant, 20
  determination of
    methods for, 21–22
    software packages for, 22
  of weak acids used in salt formation, 47
IPA. *See* Isopropyl alcohol (IPA)
IPEC. *See* International Pharmaceutical Excipients
    Council (IPEC)
IR spectroscopy, 76
Isopropyl alcohol (IPA), 189
Isothermal microcalorimetry, 105, 108
Isotonicity, 327
IVVC. *See* In vitro/in vivo correlations (IVVC)

Jenike shear cell, 373
Jet milling, 193–194

Labeling of formulations, 281–282
Labile salt, thermal disproportionation of, 52–53
Lachrymal drainage, 434
Lachrymal glands, 433
Lacrisert insert, 437
Laser diffraction/scattering, 363
  for particle size distribution, 198–201
Lattice channel water, 58
L-[2-(decylthio)ethyl]azacyclopentan-2-one, 488

Lead generation (LG) period
  AtH and HtL phases, 17
  structure-activity relationships (SAR), 17
Leuprolide acetate, 337
Light instability, 82
Lipofundin, 214, 332
Lipophilic drugs, 434
  molecules, wettability, 84
Liposomal delivery systems, 335
Liposyn, 332
Lung cancer, 348
Lupron Depot, 337
Lyophilization, 333–334
Lyophilized polylactic acid microspheres, 337

MAA. *See* Marketing authorization application (MAA)
Madin-Darby canine kidney (MDCK), 151, 152
Magnesium palmitate, 392
Magnesium stearate, 392–393
Maillard reaction, 232
Malvern Mastersizer, 199
Mannitol, 328, 333
Marketed products
  financial success of
    risk of delay to registration and launch impact
      on, 3–4
  withdrawn after launch, 2
Marketing authorization application (MAA), 320
Marketing considerations, in product design
    report. *See* Economic considerations, in
    product design report
Market size, 182–183
Mass charge density
  from various operations, 207
Materials Studio software, 87
MCT-1 compounds
  misture sorption and desorption profiles
    for, 96
  penomination studies of, 58
MDCK. *See* Madin-Darby canine kidney (MDCK)
MDL 201346
  surface-active properties of, 218
MDSC. *See* Modulated DSC (MDSC) experiments
MDT. *See* Mean dissolution time (MDT)
Mean dissolution time (MDT), 260
Media selection, for in vitro dissolution testing,
    254–257
  oxygen concentration in deaerated, 257
  physiological components of, 254
Metal ion–coordinated water, 58
Metal ion–ethylenediaminetetraacetic acid, stability
    constants, 218
Metal ions
  on stability of drug product, 216–217
Metered dose inhalers (MDI), 300–301, 348. *See also*
    Inhalation products; Pressurized
    metered-dose inhaler (pMDI)
Methylvinyl ether/maleic anhydride, 503
Microcalorimetry
  crystallization peak energy *vs.* amorphous
    content using, 196

[Microcalorimetry]
   in excipient compatibility studies, 234
   of moisture sorption using internal hygrostat, 195
Microcrystalline cellulose, 408
Micromeritics Gemini BET analyzer, 203
Micronization (jet milling), of particles, 193–194
   effects of, 194–197
Microspheres, 337
Microthermal analysis (μTA), 103
Mid-IR spectroscopy, 75
Mill selection matrix, 192
Minimum product profile (MPP). *See* Target
     product profile (TPP)
Mixing of powders, 374–375
Mixture designs, 309–310
Modulated DSC (MDSC) experiments
   heating program in, 102
   limitations of, 103
   in preformulation studies, 103
   samples, 103
Molecular crystals
   intermolecular interactions, 34–35
   structures of, 34
Molecular solids
   definition of, 34
Multiple ascending dose (MAD) studies, 15

6-β-Naltrexol, 490
Nanoparticles, solid dosage forms and, 194
Nasal delivery systems, aqueous
   benefits, 456
   cap removal torque, 469
   considerations for peptide nasal delivery, 471–472
   device selection considerations
     spray angle/droplet size studies in man, 468
     testing of devices, 468–469
     types, 464–467
   dose accuracy, 469
   droplet size distribution, 468
   fill volume, 469
   formulation selection considerations
     penetration enhancers, 463
     preformulation and bulk drug properties, 462
     preservatives, 463–464
     processing issues, 464
     selection of excipients, 462–463
     stability and compatibility, 464
   freeze-dried preparations, 472
   importance of contact time, 456
   marketed products in United States and
     United Kingdom, 457–460
   nasal anatomy and physiology, 460–461
   pump priming, 469
   regulatory aspects, 469–471
   spray angle, 468
   spray weight, 468
   supplier issues, 469
   weight loss, 469
Nasal valve, 461
Nasolachrymal duct, 433
Nasopharynx, 460

NCE. *See* New chemical entity (NCE)
Near-IR spectroscopy (NIR), 77
Nebulizers. *See* Inhalation products
Nebulizer solutions, 231
Nedocromil sodium
   crystal structure of, 94
   microcalorimetric output for hydration of, 107
   moisture sorption-desorption profile of, 94
   pH-solubility profile of, 28, 29
Nedocromil sodium trihydrate
   crystal structure of, 95
Needle-free technologies, 340–341
Neutron activation, 282
New chemical entity (NCE), 183
   costs of film-coated tablets for, 183
   effective patent life for, 5
   type safety-testing program, 356
New Drug Applications (NDA), 290
Niclosamide, 58
2-n-nonyl-1,3-dioxolane, 488
Nonaqueous vehicles, 330–331
Nonbiological models, oral drug absorption, 146–147
Norplant contraceptive device, 337
Nose, functions of, 461
N-vinylacetamide/sodium acrylate, 503

Ocular inserts, 437–438
Oil-in-water (o/w) emulsions, 213
Oil-soluble antioxidants, 217
Oily vehicles, 335–336
Oleic acid, 357
Omeprazol stability, 141
Omniflex, 339
Operational qualification (OQ), 320
Ophthalmic dosage forms
   drug candidate selection, 434–435
   ocular topical drug delivery issues and challenges
     patient compliance, 434
     physiological barriers, 432–434
   optimization considerations
     administration and use, 448
     antimicrobial preservatives, 445–446
     drug and excipient interactions, 447
     ocular solutions, 442–446
     ophthalmic suspensions, 446–447
     osmolarity, 443
     pH–solubility optimum, 443
     solubility, 442–443
     stabilizers, 444
     vehicle viscosity, 444
   processing considerations
     ophthalmic solution eye drops, 449–450
     semisolid gel suspension, 451–453
     viscous ophthalmic solutions, 450–451
   product design considerations
     formulation design options, 435–439
     novel ophthalmic drug delivery systems,
       438–439
     ocular inserts, 437–438
     ointments, 437
     packaging options, 439–440

[Ophthalmic dosage forms
 product design considerations]
  selection criteria and critical quality
   parameters, 440–441
  solutions, 436
  suspensions, 436–437
  water-based gels, 436
 target segments, 431
 therapeutic classes of drugs used, 432
Ophthalmic response, to concentrations of sodium
  chloride, 220
Optical microsocopy, 89
Optidyne system, 439
Oral dosage forms
 biopharmaceutical properties of, 248
Oral drug absorption
 nonbiological methods for prediction of, 146–147
Oral solid dosage forms
 compound intended for, 13
 disintegrating dosage forms, 427–428
 powder technology
  compaction properties, 375–384
  density, 368–369
  flow properties, 369–373
  mixing of powders, 374–375
  particle size and shape, 368
 solid dosage form. *See* Tablets, gelatin capsules
Ordered mixing, 375
Organic molecular crystals, hydration of, 57
Orifices, powder flow into, 371
Osmolality, solution formulation, 219–220
Osteoarthritis
 TPP for fictitious product to treat, 174
Ostwald ripening, 223, 228, 352, 437
Outsourcing, pros and cons of, 182
Oxybuprocaine, 432
Oxygen
 in deaerated dissolution test medium, 257
 and stability of drug product, 216–217
Oxytetracycline, 93

Parenteral products
 administration, 343
 choice of excipients, 328–329
 large-volume parenterals (LVP), 326
 liposomal delivery systems, 335
 manufacturing, 341–342
 packaging
  container closure integrity, 341
  pack selection, 338–341
 preservatives used, 329–330
 principles
  intramuscular or subcutaneous injections, 326
  pH and tonicity requirements, 326–328
  selection of injection volume, 326
 and regulatory environment
  EMEA guidelines, 344
  FDA guidelines, 344
  PDA technical reports, 345
 small-volume parenterals (SVP), 326
 sterility considerations, 329–330

[Parenteral products]
 strategies for formulating of macromolecules,
  334–335
 strategies for formulating poorly soluble drugs
  complexing agents, 331–332
  cosolvents, 330
  emulsions, 332–333
  nonaqueous vehicles, 330–331
  pH manipulation, 330
  surfactants, 331
 strategies for formulating unstable molecules
  nonaqueous vehicles and emulsions, 334
  use of excipients, 334
  water removal, 333–334
 sustained release parenteral formulations, 335
  aqueous suspensions, 336
  emulsions, 336–337
  implantable delivery systems, 337
  microspheres, 337
  oily vehicles, 335–336
  pegylation, 337
 U.S. Pharmacopeia (USP) definition, 326
 in vitro and in vivo testing methods
  hemolysis, 338
  pain, 338
  phlebitis, 338
  in vitro precipitation, 338
Particle density, 369
Particle size distribution, solid dosage forms, 198–201
 image analysis, 201
 laser diffraction/scattering for, 198–201
  of micronized powder, 200, 201
  particle size, 200
 PCS/QELS for, 201
 sieve analysis, 198
Particle size reduction, solid dosage forms, 191–198
 ball milling, 192–193
 effect of milling and micronization, 194–197
 inverse gas chromatography of, 197–198
 micronization (jet milling), 193–194
 mill selection matrix, 192
 nanoparticles, 194
Partition coefficient (log P)
 of compounds, 23
 expression for, 22
 and intrinsic lipophilicity of drug, 23
 lipophilic molecules, 22
 technique for determining, 24
Patent system, product design report, 185–186
PCS. *See* Photon correlation spectroscopy (PCS)
PDA Technical Reports, 345
 No. 26, 342
 No. 44, 342
PEG. *See* Polyethylene glycol (PEG) 400
Pegylation, 337
Performance qualification (PQ), 320
Permeation enhancers, of nasal products, 463
Pharmaceutical companies
 product life cycle management approach, 4
 strategic research, 11
Pharmaceutical Dissolution Testing, 249

Pharmaceutical industry
  environmental pressures on, 7
  mergers and acquisitions in, 5
  political/economical pressures on, 7
  regulatory compliance, 6–7
Pharmaceutically acceptable counterions, 44
Pharmaceutical material selection,
    polymorphs in, 36
Pharmaceutical product profile (PPP), 174
Pharmaceutical quality systems (PQS), 289
  and ICH Q10 guidance, 293
Pharmaceutical research and development (R&D)
  candidate drug emerging from, 5–6
  highly soluble drugs in, 135
  hurdles to, 2
  objective of, 2
  risk associated with doing minimum, 5
  risk of failure in, 2
Pharmaceutical solids, characterization of, 63–64
Pharmacopoeial standards, 296
Phase Doppler anemometry, 352
Phase I clinical studies
  definition of, 14
  kinds of, 14–15
Phase II studies, 15
Phase III studies, 15
Phase IV trials, 15
Phase solubility analysis, 26–27
Phase 0 studies
  for exploratory, first-in-human microdosing
    studies, 12–13
  potential advantages of, 13
Phenylethyl aclohol, 446
Phlebitis, 338
Photo-instability. *See* Light instability
Photon correlation spectroscopy (PCS)
  for particle size distribution, 201
pH value function, in solution formulation, 210–211
Physicians' Desk Reference, 328, 394
Pilocarpine, 432, 434
Pk$_a$. *See* Ionization constant
Plasma-sampling schedule, 263
PLGA. *See* Polylactide/polyglycolide (PLGA)
  copolymers
PMDI. *See* Pressurized metered-dose inhaler
  (pMDI)
Pocket hydrates, 57–58
Polyethylene glycol (PEG) 400, 212–213
Polylactide/polyglycolide (PLGA) copolymers, 337
Polymeric microspheres, 337
Polymorph, impurities effects on, 191
Polymorphic hydrates, 59
Polymorphic transitions
  of AR-C69457AA, effect of particle size and
    heating rate on, 100
  induced by heating, 60
  thermodynamic rules for, 41
Polymorphism. *See also* Polymorphs
  definition of, 35
  induced by conformational differences, 36
  of omeprazole, 37

[Polymorphism]
  screens in prenomination phase, 37–38
  thermodynamics related to, 41–44
Polymorphism issues, in solid dosage forms,
    209–210
Polymorphs
  classification of, 41
  of estrone, 35
  FTIR spectra of, 76
  interconversion of
    factors influencing, 38
    organic crystals, 39
    role of impurities in, 38
  nucleation behavior of, 39
  production and characterization, 64
  production methods for, 39–40
  relative stability hierarchy of, 41
  relative stability of, 83
  relative thermodynamic stability of, 40
  solubilities of, 43–44
  solution-mediated transitions in, 36
  solvent-free methods of isolating, 36
  of spiperone, 36–37
  stability hierarchy of
    assigning relative, 41
    sublimation experiments, 42–43
Polysorbate (Tween) 80, 331
Polyvinyl alcohol, 436
Polyvinyl chloride (PVC), 298, 339
Porosity of a powder, 369
Post-marketing surveillance trials. *See* Phase IV trials
Povidone, 436
Powder
  measurement of properties, 376–377
    compaction simulators, 377
    conventional tablet machines, 377
    conventional testing machines, 376–377
  quantitative data
    diametral compression test, 381
    elasticity, 379–380
    Heckel plots, 377–379
    indentation hardness, 380–381
    pressure/strength relationships, 381–382
  in solid dosage forms, 205–206
PPP. *See* Pharmaceutical product profile (PPP)
PQS. *See* Pharmaceutical quality systems (PQS)
Preapproval inspection (PAI), 290
Precorneal area, 433
Preformulation studies
  barrier to, 14
  at candidate drug selection stage, 13
  dissolution rate of drug candidate, 84–85
  pharmacological and safety testing, 14
  progression of compounds through, 18
Prenomination studies
  assessment of compounds for development, 18
  light stability, 82
  of MCT-1 compounds, 58
  physicochemical tests carried out during, 19
    amorphous phases, 60–63
    atomic force microscopy, 90–91

[Prenomination studies
  physicochemical tests carried out during]
    chemical stability, 31–34, 82
    cocrystals, 53–54
    crystalline states and structural assessment, 35–39
    crystal morphology assessment, 86–89
    HPLC, 109–110
    hydrates, 56–60
    hygroscopicity, 91–99
    initial physicohemical characterization, 20
    mid-IR spectroscopy, 75–76
    near-IR spectroscopy, 77
    optical microsocopy, 89
    partition and distribution coefficients, 22–24
    phase solubility analysis, 26–27
    photo-instability, 82–83
    physical stability, 31–34
    pK$_a$ determinations, 20–22
    polymorphism, 39–44
    Raman spectroscopy, 77–78
    salts, 44–53
    scanning electron microscopy, 89–90
    solid-state degradation of drug, 81
    solid-state NMR, 78–80
    solubility analysis, 26, 27–31
    solution calorimetry, 83–85
    solvates, 54–56
    synchrotron radiation, 72–75
    terahertz-pulsed spectroscopy, 77
    thermal analysis, 99–108
    X-ray diffraction, 65–72
  polymorphism screening in, 37–38
  scope of, 18
  solid-state stability, 82
  solubility profile, 28
Pressurized metered-dose inhaler (pMDI), 226–229, 360
  drug substances for inhalation therapy, 228
Price, 183
Primary packaging, selection and optimization criteria for, 298
Process analytical technology (PAT), 289, 291–292, 344
Process capability index (CpK), 317–318
Process optimization, 316–318
  clinical trials process validation, 319
  postapproval changes, 321–323
  preapproval inspection, 320–321
  principles of process validation, 319
  process design, 315–316
  scale-up process, 318
  technology transfer, 318–319
  validation of commercial process, 320
Prodrugs, enzymatic degradation of, 143
Product design
  benefits of, 173
  defined, 173
  importance of, 172–173
  report. *See* Product design report

Product design report, 173–186
  commercial and marketing considerations, 181–183
  design specifications and critical quality parameters, 180–181
  environmental/health/safety considerations, 184
  intellectual property considerations, 185–186
  safety assessment considerations, 184
  technical issues and risk assessment, 183
  TPP/MPP, 173–180
Product development, framework for, 8–9
Product Formulation Expert System (PFES), 304
Production rule, 305
Product life cycle, 3
  management, 4
Product optimization
  and AI technologies, 303–307
  concept of experimental design
    benefits, 308
    DOE techniques, 308
    mixture designs, 309–310
    optimization studies, 309
    screening, 308–309
  and critical quality attributes (CQA), 289
  excipient and pack optimization considerations
    excipient selection, 295–298
    pack considerations, 298–301
    sources of information, 301–303
  and good patient compliance, 301
  ICH guidances, 289–295
  IT sources of information and development guidelines, 303
  objective, 289
  PAT guidance initiative, 291–292
  presentation to the user/administration of, 300–301
  Product Optimization Report, 295
  protection of product, 299–300
  quality-by-design (QbD) regulatory initiatives, 289
  selection of optimal product, 295
  specifications
    product, 314–315
    raw material, 312–314
  stability testing
    accelerated stress, 310–311
    safety and clinical studies, 311
    stability testing of product license application, 311–312
    studies, 289
Product specifications, 314–315
Proton pump inhibitor, ionization and partitioning scheme for, 23–24
P/T diagram, 42
Pulmonary airways, 461
Pulmonary delivery, of aerosol suspensions and dry powders, 294
PVC. *See* Polyvinyl chloride (PVC)

QbD. *See* Quality by design (QbD)
QELS. *See* Quasi-elastic elastic light scattering (QELS)

QFD. *See* Quality function deployment (QFD)
QFD charts, 178
  for metered dose inhaler, 179
QicPic, 201
QSAR models, of oral drug absorption, 148
Quality-by-design (QbD)
  drug substance, 190
  regulatory initiatives, 316, 321–322, 344
    FDA principles, 291, 294
    ophthalmic product, 447
    role in product optimization, 289
    vs traditional product development, 290
Quality function deployment (QFD), 176–180
Quality risk management (QRM), 289
Quasi-elastic elastic light scattering (QELS)
  for particle size distribution, 201

Radiolabeled formulations
  safety aspects in manufacturing and analysis
    of, 282
Radionuclide selection, in labeling, 281–282
Raman spectroscopy
  basic principle of, 77
  low-wavelength, 78
  of organic solid state, 78
Reciprocating cylinder (USP III) dissolution
    apparatus, 249, 251
Reference formulation, 262
Relative density, 369
Remacemide HCl
  crystal structure of, 66
  hygroscopicity of, 91
  and lactose, 92
  scanning electron micrograph of, 205–206
  and spray-dried lactose, 233
Remacemide hydrochloride
  pH-solubility profile of, 28–29
Residual solvents, classification of, 56
Retention valves, 358
Reticuloendothelial system (RES), 335
Retinyl ascorbate, 490
Return on investment (ROI), 172, 173
Rhinocort Nasal Spray, 468
Risk assessment, in product design report, 183
ROI. *See* Return on investment (ROI)
Rotary tablet machines, 386–388
Rotating basket (USP I) dissolution apparatus,
    249, 250
Rotating disk method, 133–134
Rotating paddle (USP II) dissolution apparatus,
    249, 250, 252
R-value, 391

Safety assessment considerations, in product design
    report, 184
Safety consideration, in product design report, 185
Salbutamol salts, 51
Salt formation
  chemical stability and, 49–50
  effect on solubility of development compound, 50

[Salt formation]
  of ephedrine, 48
  pK$_a$s of weak acids used in, 47
  properties altered by, 44
Salts
  formation of. *See* Salt formation
  intrinsic dissolution behavior, 50
  selection
    for new drug candidates, 46–47
    using small-scale throughput well-plate
      methodologies, 47–48
  solubility of
    factors determining, 49
    as function of suspension pH, 51
    modulation of, 50
  stability of, 52
  of weak bases, 49
Saturated salt solutions, relative humidities
    generated by, 98
Scale-up and post-approval changes for semisolids
    (SUPAC-SS), 508
Scale-up and post-approval changes (SUPAC), 322
Scale-up process, 318
Scanning electron microscopy (SEM)
  components of, 89
  of compound undergoes capping and
    lamination, 206
  in ESEM mode, 90
  of micronized powder and particle size, 200
  operating mechanism of, 89–90
  of sibenadit HCl, 90
Sebenadit HCl, solubility of, 231
Sebenidet hydrochloride
  pH-solubility curve of, 211
Secondary packaging, 298
Segregation, 375
SEM. *See* Scanning electron microscopy (SEM)
Semisolid gel-type preparations, 436
Shear cells methods, 370–373
Sieve analysis, particle size distribution, 198
Silastic, 337
Siliconize stoppers, 339
Single ascending dose (SAD) studies, 14
Single-crystal structure determinations, 65–66
Single-crystal XRD (SXRD), 65
Single-dose studies, 262
Single punch presses, 386
Skin-stripping bioequivalence protocol, 509
Slugging, 408
Sodium chloride, ophthalmic response
    to, 220
Sodium dodecyl sulfate–polyacrylamide gel
    electrophoresis (SDS–PAGE), 334
Sodium metabisulfite, 334, 444
Sodium salts
  and free acid, bioavailability of, 44
  solid-state properties of, 48
  solvent composition influence on solubility and
    solid-state properties of, 49
Sodium sulfite, 444
SolEmuls, 214

Solid dosage forms, 188–210
  agglomeration, 189–190
  atomic force microscopy for, 198
  caking, 208
  color, 206–207
  electrostaticity, 207–208
  flow and compaction of powders, 205–206
  impurities, 190–191
  particle size distribution measurements, 198–201
    image analysis, 201
    laser diffraction/scattering for, 198–201
    PCS/QELS for, 201
    sieve analysis, 198
  particle size reduction, 191–198
    ball milling, 192–193
    effect of milling and micronization, 194–197
    inverse gas chromatography of, 197–198
    micronization (jet milling), 193–194
    mill selection matrix, 192
    nanoparticles, 194
  polymorphism issues in, 209–210
  surface area measurements in, 202–203
  Tof SIMS of, 198
  true density, 203–205
  in vitro dissolution testing of, 248–261
    apparatus for, 249–253
    assessment of dissolution profiles, 258–261
    choice of agitation intensity, 253
    choice of media for, 254–257
    design aspects of, 257–258
    validation of, 261
Solid-state NMR
  anisotropic interactions in solution state, 79
  of hydrates of nedocromil sodium, 79
  molecular structure determination using, 78
  of phases of AR-C69457AA, 79–80
Solubility, 210–214
  cosolvents, 211–213
  definitions of, 25
  emulsion formulations, 213–214
  general rules regarding, 25
  high, 25
  impact of additives on, 30
  ionization effect on, 27–30
  kinetic, 27
  molecular size effect on, 27, 28
  pH value function, 29, 210–211
  prediction of, 26–27
  temperature effect on, 30–31
Soluble ophthalmic drug insert (SODI), 438
Solution
  calorimetry systems, 83
  degradation in
    hydrolysis, 32
    kinetics, 33–34
    oxidation, 32–33
  formulation. *See* Solution formulation
Solution formulation, 210–220
  osmolality, 219–220
  solubility considerations, 210–214
    cosolvents, 211–213

[Solution formulation
  solubility considerations]
    emulsion formulations, 213–214
    pH value function, 210–211
  stability considerations, 214–218
    to autoclaving, 216
    EDTA and chelating agents in, 217–218
    effect of metal ions and oxygen on, 216–217
  surface activity, 218–219
Solvates
  definition of, 54
  formation of, 55
  high-throughput crystallization studies, 55
Solvents, classification of, 25–26
Sorbitan trioleate, 357
Spiperone, conformational polymorphism of, 36
Sporonox, 332
Spray-dried lactose, with remacemide HCl, 233
Squeeze-bottle systems, 465
Stability, solution formulations, 214–218
  to autoclaving, 216
  EDTA and chelating agents in, 217–218
  effect of metal ions and oxygen on, 216–217
Stability constants, metal ion–ethylenediamine
    tetraacetic acid, 218
Stability hierarchy, definition of, 41
Stability testing, 310–312
  ophthalmic products, 447
Standard operating procedures (SOP), 305
Starch, 390
Static diffusion cells, 494
Statistics for Experimenters, 258
Steric repulsion, 504
Sterilization, terminal, 216
Strain rate sensitivity (SRS), 379
Structure-activity relationships (SAR), 17
Sublimation experiments, 42–43
Sugar coating, 409–411, 418
Sulfaproxiline, FTIR thermo-microscopy
    of, 76
Sulfathiazole, solvates formation by, 55
SUPAC. *See* Scale-up and post-approval changes
    (SUPAC)
SUPAC-SS. *See* Scale-up and post-approval
    changes for semisolids (SUPAC-SS)
Super disintegrants, 397
Surface-active drugs, 139
Surface activity, solution formulation, 218–219
Surface pH hypothesis for weak acids and bases, 140
Surface tension
  vs. concentration of primary amine hydrochloride,
    219
Surfactants, 331
Suspensions formulations, 223–224
Synchrotron X-ray analysis
  ab initio crystal structure solution from XRPD
    data, 72
    powder diffraction pattern, 73
    problems associated with, 75
    process of solution of, 74
  data collection using, 72

Tablets
  coating
    compression coating, 415–416
    film coating, 411–415
    sugar coating, 409–411
  erosion, 285
  formulation
    appearance, 394–397
    compatibilities, 388, 390–391
    direct compression technique, 400–401
    disintegration, 397–399
    dissolution, 399
    flowability, 388–390
    granulation, 401–409
    lubricity, 391–394
    processing, 399–400
    process of extrusion/spheronization,
      407–408
    selection of appropriate process, 409
  machines for making
    rotary machine, 386–388
    single punch presses, 386
Talc, 389
Tape stripping, 510
Target clinical profile (TCP), 174
Target product profile (TPP), 173–180
  for fictitious product to treat osteoarthritis, 174
  meeting customer needs, 175–179
  QFD, 176–180
Tautomerism-induced polymorphism, 37
TCP. *See* Target clinical profile (TCP)
Technical issues, in product design report, 183
Terahertz-pulsed spectroscopy, 77
Terminal sterilization, 216, 441
Tert-butylhydroxylamine acetate
  moisture sorption and desorption profile
    under normal operating conditions, 97
    under reduced operating conditions, 98
TGA. *See* Thermogravimetric analysis (TGA)
Thermal analytical techniques
  differential scanning calorimetry (DSC). *See*
    Differential scanning calorimetry (DSC)
  hot-stage microscopy, 105
  microthermal analysis (μTA), 103
  TGA. *See* Thermogravimetric analysis (TGA)
Thermogravimetric analysis (TGA)
  calibration of, 105
  effect of heating rate on weight loss during, 104
  of nedocromil sodium trihydrate, 103–104
Time-of-flight secondary ion mass spectroscopy
    (Tof SIMS)
  of solid dosage forms, 198
Timing to market, 182
Timolol, 432
Tof SIMS. *See* Time-of-flight secondary ion mass
    spectroscopy (Tof SIMS)
Tonicity, *vs.* mannitol in water, 220
Topical delivery. *See* Transdermal delivery
TPP. *See* Target product profile (TPP)
Transdermal delivery, 224–226
  drug candidate selection, 489–491

[Transdermal delivery]
  enhancement and retardation of skin absorption
    formulation strategies, 487–488
    penetration enhancers, 488–489
    supersaturated transdermal delivery
      devices, 488
  factors affecting percutaneous absorption
    age and sex variability, 485–486
    intrasubject and intersubject variability, 484–485
    racial differences, 486
    site variations, 484
    skin metabolism, 486–487
  formulation process
    bioequivalence of dermatological dosage
      forms, 509–510
    emulsions, 503–508
    gels, 500–503
    ointments, 499
    semisolid formulations, 508, 510–512
    type, 497–499
  preformulation process, 491–497
  skin permeability
    barrier function–absorption pathways,
      477–479
    coefficients and diffusivity, 479–481
    epidermal reservoir, binding, and molecular
      size, 482
    hydrogen-bonding (H-bonding) capacity and
      molecular size, 481–482
    physicochemical properties, 479
    predictability, 484
    process of percutaneous absorption, 479
    removal from epidermis, 483
    steady-state flux (Js) across the skin, 479
    stratum corneum/product partition
      coefficient K, 480
    vehicle (formulation) thermodynamic effects,
      482–483
  skin structure
    corneocyte protein, 477
    dermis, 476
    differentiation in epidermis, 477
    epidermal cell composition, 476–477
    Langerhans cells, 476
    melanocytes, 476
    stratum corneum, 476–477
  transdermal drug delivery systems, 512–516
Tropicamide, 432

Uniformity of weight, 389
Unit-dose systems, 439
U.S. Pharmacopoeia (USP), 249
USP. *See* U.S. Pharmacopoeia (USP)
USP dissolution apparatus, 249–253
USP I. *See* Rotating basket (USP I) dissolution
    apparatus
USP II. *See* Rotating paddle (USP II) dissolution
    apparatus
USP III. *See* Reciprocating cylinder (USP III)
    dissolution apparatus

USP IV. *See* Flow-through cell (USP IV) dissolution apparatus
Ussing chamber technique, 153–154

van der Waals forces, 369
Vibrational spectroscopy techniques, 75
Vickers hardness test, 379

Wagner–Nelson method, 269
Washout period, 262
Water for Injection (WFI), 451
Water-free oleaginous eye ointment, 437
Water-soluble antioxidants, 217
Weight, uniformity of, 389

X-ray diffraction (XRD)
    single-crystal structure determinations, 65–66

[X-ray diffraction (XRD)]
    standards used in, 70–71
    XRPD analysis
        Bragg–Bentano geometry used in, 67
        of compound undergoing polymorphic change, 71
        crystalline, amorphous, and partially crystalline forms, 68
        data collection, 72
        dehydrates of olanzapine, 72
        powder pattern, 67
        sources of error, 68–70
XRD. *See* X-ray diffraction (XRD)

Zeldox, 332
Zoladex, 337